Dreisbach's
# HANDBOOK
of
# POISONING

PREVENTI
and T

THIRTE

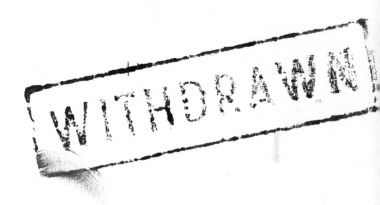

*Dreisbach's*

# HANDBOOK
## *of*
# POISONING

### PREVENTION, DIAGNOSIS *and* TREATMENT

## THIRTEENTH EDITION

**Bev-Lorraine True, PharmD, MD**
Group Health Permanente Medical Group, Seattle
Clinical Instructor, Department of Family Medicine
University of Washington, Seattle, WA, and
Fellow in Medical Toxicology, Washington Poison Center, Seattle, WA

*and*

**Robert H. Dreisbach, PhD, MD**
Clinical Professor
Department of Environmental Health
School of Public Health and Community Medicine
University of Washington, Seattle, WA, and
Emeritus Professor of Pharmacology
Stanford University School of Medicine, Stanford, CA

## The Parthenon Publishing Group
International Publishers in Medicine, Science & Technology

A CRC PRESS COMPANY
BOCA RATON    LONDON    NEW YORK    WASHINGTON, D.C.

Notice: Our knowledge in clinical sciences is constantly changing. As new information becomes available, changes in treatment and in the use of drugs become necessary. The authors and the publisher of this volume have taken care to make certain that the doses of drugs and schedules of treatment are correct and compatible with the standards generally accepted at the time of publication. The reader is advised to consult carefully the instruction and information material included in the package insert of each drug or therapeutic agent before administration. This advice is especially important when using new or infrequently used drugs.

13th edition published by:
The Parthenon Publishing Group
23–25 Blades Court, Deodar Road, London SW15 2NU, UK

Copyright © 2002 The Parthenon Publishing Group

**Library of Congress Cataloging-in-Publication Data**

True, Bev-Lorraine.
Dreisbach's handbook of poisoning : prevention, diagnosis, and treatment / by Bev-Lorraine True and Robert H. Dreisbach. – 13th ed.
p. ; cm.
Includes bibliographical references and index.
ISBN 1-85070-038-9 (alk. paper)
1. Poisoning–Handbooks, manuals, etc. 2. Toxicological emergencies–Handbooks, manuals, etc. I. Dreisbach, Robert H. (Robert Hastings), 1916– II. Title.
[DNLM: 1. Poisoning–diagnosis–Handbooks. 2. Poisoning–therapy–Handbooks. QV 607 T866h 2001]
RA1215.T78 2001
615.9–dc21

2001036722

**British Library Cataloguing in Publication Data**

True, Bev-Lorraine
Dreisbach's handbook of poisoning : prevention, diagnosis and treatment. – 13th ed.
1. Poisoning – Handbooks, manuals etc.
I. Title II. Dreisbach, Robert H. (Robert Hastings), 1916– III. Robertson, William O.
615.9

ISBN 1850700389

Typeset by Martin Lister Publishing Services, Carnforth, Lancashire, UK

Printed and bound by J. W. Arrowsmith Ltd., Bristol, UK

# Contents

Preface      vii

## I.  General considerations

1. Prevention of poisoning      3
2. Emergency management of poisoning      25
3. Diagnosis and evaluation of poisoning      35
4. Management of poisoning      52
5. Legal and medical responsibility in poisoning      102

## II.  Agricultural poisons

6. Halogenated insecticides      109
7. Cholinesterase inhibitor pesticides      123
8. Miscellaneous pesticides      133

## III.  Industrial hazards

9. Nitrogen compounds      163
10. Halogenated hydrocarbons      172
11. Alcohols and glycols      199
12. Esters, aldehydes, ketones, and ethers      216
13. Hydrocarbons      228
14. Corrosives      240
15. Metallic poisons      269
16. Cyanides, sulfides, and carbon monoxide      311
17. Atmospheric particulates      327

## IV.  Household hazards

18. Cosmetics      343
19. Food poisoning      348

20.  Miscellaneous chemicals                                          356

**V.  Medicinal poisons**

21.  Analgesics, antipyretics, and anti-inflammatory agents           367
22.  Anesthetics                                                      379
23.  Depressants                                                      390
24.  Drugs affecting the autonomic nervous system                    422
25.  Antiseptics                                                      442
26.  Cardiovascular drugs                                             459
27.  Anti-infective drugs                                             485
28.  Stimulants, antidepressants, antimanics, anticonvulsants,       508
     and psychotomimetic agents
29.  Irritants and rubefacients                                      532
30.  Cathartics                                                       541
31.  Endocrine drugs                                                  546
32.  Miscellaneous therapeutic and diagnostic agents                 556

**VI.  Animal and plant hazards**

33.  Reptiles                                                         587
34.  Arachnids and insects                                            601
35.  Marine animals                                                   610
36.  Plants                                                           615

Index                                                                 639

# Preface

*Dreisbach's Handbook of Poisoning* provides a concise summary of the diagnosis and treatment of poisoning for medical students, residents, nurses and practicing physicians. This book is intended to be a readily available reference and quick guide to more detailed sources of poisoning information. As speed is critical in the initial management of poison cases, this book is a quick source of practical information. Listings of more detailed references, websites, antidotes, antivenins, etc. are included. Because this book has been in use throughout the world for many decades, chemicals and substances that are now banned in the United States are still included since they may still be available elsewhere. In addition, while the US has mandated that employers adhere to detailed occupational exposure requirements for the use of protection, there are many small businesses that are not aware of such safety requirements. Workers may present with chronic poisonings such as lead in radiator repair, or central nervous system damage from chronic organic solvent exposures.

## Organization of the book

Chapters 1–4 provide general information about prevention, diagnosis, and treatment of poisoning. Chapter 5 considers the important medicolegal aspects of poisoning. Specific poisons are discussed in the remainder of the book and are organized into agricultural, industrial, household, medicinal, and natural hazards. This organizational system facilitates correlation of poisons with types of exposure. Insofar as is possible, chemically- and, in some cases, pharmacologically-related agents have been grouped together.

To enable the physician to identify the toxic principle in a given proprietary preparation, brand-named products likely to be encountered clinically or whose composition is not obvious are listed in the index. This group includes many insecticides and medicinal agents.

## New features

The thirteenth edition of *Dreisbach's Handbook of Poisoning* has been substantially revised and includes the following new features:

- Sections on diagnosis and treatment have been revised and updated to reflect the latest procedures in emergency rooms and poison centers.
- Sections on management of poisoning have been simplified for easier use in emergencies.
- New sections added in the medicinal chapters to include the enormous expansion of drugs since the last edition.
- Reference lists restricted to useful recent articles.

With the thirteenth edition, Dr Bev-Lorraine True joins Dr Robert H. Dreisbach as co-author of the book. Both authors thank Dr William O. Robertson, co-author of the twelfth edition and Medical Director of the Washington Poison Center and all of those who have taken the time to offer helpful criticisms and suggestions for improvement of *Dreisbach's Handbook of Poisoning*.

Bev-Lorraine True
Robert H. Dreisbach

# I. General considerations

# 1 Prevention of poisoning

More than 12 000 deaths due to poisoning occur in the USA each year. Many of these deaths are avoidable regardless of whether the poisoning is purposeful or accidental, occupational or environmental. Prevention of poisoning requires adequate knowledge of the hazardous properties of substances by users.

In the USA over two million exposures to drugs and chemicals occurred in 1997. Over 90% of exposures occurred in the home and 40% of exposures occurred to children. The majority of cases of exposure involved cleaning substances, analgesics, cosmetics and personal care products, plants, and cough and cold substances. However, children comprised less than 4% of fatalities. Thus, rapid and effective treatment of poisonings by lay persons, with the advice by poison control centers and health personnel, reduces fatal outcomes. The majority of fatalities occur in adolescents and adults and are the result of exposures to analgesics, sedatives, antidepressants, anti-psychotics, anticonvulsants, cardiac drugs, theophylline, amphetamines, cocaine, hydrocarbons, cleaning products, and pesticides/rodenticides. Fatalities in children are most often from acetaminophen, aspirin, iron tablets, and cleaning products. Drugs should not be used during pregnancy unless benefit overrides the risk to the fetus. Use available resources for evaluating the safety of drug use in pregnancy (see p. 19).

When prescribing drugs, always be alert to their potential toxicities so that the first signs will be recognized and proper action taken. Be cautious when prescribing drugs with a narrow therapeutic index (the difference between the effective and toxic dose). Many resources alert the prescriber to potential drug interactions that increase likelihood of a toxic reaction.

## HOUSEHOLD POISONING

### Safe storage and use

(1) All containers should have safety closures. Medicines, insecticides, and rodenticides should be stored in locked cabinets. If a locked cabinet is not available, a suitcase with a lock is satisfactory.

(2) Lye, polishes, kerosene, and other household chemicals should never be left on a low shelf or on the floor. Again, locked storage is best. Do not leave these materials exposed in the kitchen or bathroom.

(3) Never leave dangerous solutions in drinking glasses or in beverage bottles. Store them in their original containers.

(4) Combustion devices should be adequately vented.

(5) Inhalation of spray or fumes must be prevented during painting and application of insecticides. Use a respirator with organic filters that seals properly upon the face.

(6) Dispose of unnecessary toxic substances, such as boric acid and unused medicines.

(7) Toxic substances (hydrocarbons, gasoline) should be taken to appropriate toxic waste disposal stations (do not flush them into sewer systems). Any rags that have on them gasoline or other flammable substances must be put in a closed metal container to avoid spontaneous combustion.

(8) Carefully check the label of any medicine before taking or administering to others. Do not put different tablets or capsules in the same bottle, and avoid transferring them to envelopes or purses for convenience.

### Education

Parents should be educated to the dangers present in medicines and household chemicals. All adults should be familiar with the concept of risk versus benefit in using chemicals at home, in the workplace, or in the environment. For those who use toxic substances such as paint thinners, well-fitted respirators with organic filters are mandatory; simple dust masks will not be protective.

All dangerous medicines, including aspirin, soluble iron salts (adult-strength iron tablets), and household chemicals should have a poison label on them. A checklist of dangerous household chemicals and medicines (Table 1.1) and instructions for safe storage and use should be given to parents when their children become mobile.

Education should include instruction in the proper use of syrup of ipecac and a recommendation that it must be available. It should be emphasized that time from ingestion to appropriate treatment is critical in preventing serious injury or death. Therefore, telephone numbers for the local poison control center and emergency room should be posted on the telephone (along with 911 for emergency access in the USA). It should also be emphasized that

**Table 1.1** Checklist of household poisons

## HOUSE

**Insecticides** – ant, roach, moth poisons, animal flea collars.

**Inflammables** – kerosene, gasoline, industrial products in the USA that are flammable are labeled as such.

Fire lighter–methanol, petroleum hydrocarbons, denatured alcohol.

Fire starting tablets – metaldehyde, methenamine.

Fire extinguisher – carbon dioxide.

**Mercury thermometers** – if broken, the mercury is not toxic to the touch; however, it is extremely volatile and the gas phase is toxic. Wipe up with wet rag and dispose. If spilled on carpet, also throw out that section of carpet. Do not flush down toilet.

**Cleaning supplies** – Chlorinated hydrocarbons, solvent distillate, lye (sodium hydroxide), ammonia, bleach (sodium hypochlorite), oxalic acid, drain cleaner (lye, sodium acid sulfate), rug cleaner (chlorinated hydrocarbons), wallpaper cleaner (kerosene), laundry ink (aniline).

## All medicines

**Drugs of abuse** – amphetamines, alcohol, barbiturates, benzodiazepines, cocaine, ethchlorvynol, fentanyl, glutethimide, heroin, meperidine, meprobamate, methadone, LSD (lysergic acid diethylamide), marijuana (*Cannabis sativa*), mescaline (peyote from the plant *Lophophora williamsii*), phencyclidine (PCP), Psilocybin from mushroom *Psilocybe mexicana*; 3,4-methylenedioxymethamphetamine (MDMA or Ecstasy), and numerous inhalants (see solvents, etc.).

**Antiseptics** – boric acid, mercuric chloride, iodine, phenol, cationic detergents.

**Liniments** – methyl salicylate, alcohols, oils, DMSO (dimethyl sulfoxide), capsicum.

**Cosmetics** – alcohol, cuticle removers, artificial tanning agents (dihydroxyacetone), eyelash and hair dyes (naphthylamines, phenylenediamines, toluenediamines, silver salts, anilines), other hair care products (potassium hydroxide, barium sulfide, thioglycolates, alkalis, potassium bromate).

**Hobbies** – toluene (cement), methanol (stencils), photography chemicals, etc.

**Lead** – While lead is no longer used in household paint or in gasoline within the US, lead solder has been used in plumbing. Lead is also present in older sewer pipes, fishing sinkers, bullets and shot, and exercise weights.

## STOREROOM

**Paints and painting supplies**

Paint-thinner, lead, arsenic, chlorinated hydrocarbons.

Paint remover – chlorinated hydrocarbons, acids, alkalis.

Lacquer – ethyl acetate, amyl acetate, methanol.

Shellac – methanol.

Wood bleach – oxalic acid.

**Pesticides** – moth balls (naphthalene, paradichlorophenol).

## YARD AND GARAGE STORAGE, PET PRODUCTS

**Insecticides, pesticides, herbicides** – Most toxic: aldrin, dieldrin, endrin, endosulfan, paraquat, pentachlorophenol, methyl bromide, arsenic, nicotine, strychnine, thallium.

**Garden plants** (See also Tables 36.1 and 36.2) – Foxglove (digitalis), oleander.

combinations of different drugs or taking drugs with alcohol will increase toxicity. Parents should teach their children the danger of touching, eating, or playing with medicines, pesticides, household chemicals, or plants. They should never refer to flavored drugs as candy, nor should they make the giving of a medication a game.

### References

Boullata JI, Nace AM. Safety issues with herbal medicine. *Pharmacotherapy* 2000;20:257

Brent J. Three new herbal hepatotoxic syndromes. *J Toxicol Clin Toxicol* 1999;37: 715

Fisher AA, *et al.* Toxicity of *Passiflora incarnata* L. *J Toxicol Clin Toxicol* 2000;38:63

Schepens PJ, *et al.* Drugs of abuse and alcohol in weekend drivers involved in car crashes in Belgium. *Ann Emerg Med* 1998;31:633

Shannon M. Alternative medicines toxicology: a review of selected agents. *J Toxicol Clin Toxicol* 1999;37:709

Shannon M. Ingestion of toxic substances by children. *N Engl J Med* 2000;42:186

Woolf A. Essential oil poisoning. *J Toxicol Clin Toxicol* 1999;37:721

Woolf AD, Shaw JS. Nail primer cosmetics: correlations between product pH and adequacy of labeling. *J Toxicol Clin Toxicol* 1999;37:827

## AGRICULTURAL POISONS (insecticides, rodenticides, fungicides, etc.)

Persons exposed to agricultural poisons are divided into two groups – those who work with agricultural poisons during manufacture, preparation for use, storage, or application, and those who come into contact with these chemicals accidentally, either through improper storage, by entering sprayed areas, or by eating sprayed foods from which spray residues have not been removed.

### Storage of poisons

(1) Poisons must be stored in well-marked containers with safety closures, preferably under lock and key.

(2) Mixtures of poisons with flour or cereals must not be stored near food. Sweet mixtures are the most dangerous; warning labels on such mixtures should be designed in such a way as to be obvious even to illiterate persons.

(3)   Emptied containers must be burned immediately to destroy residual poisons; empty cans should be opened before burning.

(4)   Storage in food containers, such as beverage bottles, is extremely dangerous.

## Protective clothing and equipment

(1)   Use masks and exhaust ventilation during dry mixing.

(2)   Wear protective clothing, goggles, and oil-resistant neoprene gloves when prolonged handling of poisons in petroleum oils or other organic solvents is necessary. Remove protective clothing and wash exposed skin thoroughly before eating.

(3)   Wear respirators, goggles, protective clothing, and gloves during preparation and use of sprays, mists, or aerosols when skin contamination or inhalation may occur. Use protective equipment made of rubber in the handling of chlorinated hydrocarbons, and equipment made of neoprene or other oil-resistant materials for handling poisons in organic solvents. The indane derivatives and cholinesterase inhibitors are especially dangerous. Mix pesticides only in totally enclosed systems.

(4)   In work settings, always remove protective (contaminated) clothing before going home. Lead dust on clothing will probably be at toxic levels.

## Other protective measures

(1)   Always spray downwind. If wind velocity is insufficient, discontinue spraying to avoid contact with the mist. Avoid exposure in a closed area when an insecticide vaporizer is being operated for more than 8 h per day. Such vaporizers must be adjusted to release not more than 1 g of lindane per 425 m$^3$ per 24 h at a rate constant within 25%. No other insecticides are safe for use in vaporizers. Never use vaporizers in living quarters or where food is stored, prepared, or served.

(2)   Do not apply chlorinated or phosphate ester insecticides where body contact with residues is likely to occur.

(3)   Food and forage plants should not be sprayed with insecticides unless the procedure used has been clearly shown not to leave a residue above tolerance limits.

(4) For protection of the consumer, the Food and Drug Administration and US Department of Health and Human Services have established specific tolerances that represent levels above which foods cannot be sold. These tolerances are maintained by field inspection, control of pesticide use, and by analysis of samples of foods that will reach the market.

### References

Burgess JL, *et al.* Fumigant-related illnesses: Washington State's five-year experience. *J Toxicol Clin Toxicol* 2000;38:7

*Farm Chemicals Handbook.* Meisterpro, 2000. (Annual publication)

Fenske RA, *et al.* Biologically based pesticide dose estimates for children in an agricultural community. *Environ Health Perspect* 2000;108:515

Klein-Schwartz W, Smith GS. Agricultural and horticultural chemical poisonings: mortality and morbidity in the United States. *Ann Emerg Med* 1997;29:232

Krieger GR. *Handbook of Pesticide Toxicology.* Academic Press, 1998

Landrigan PJ, *et al.* Pesticides and inner-city children: exposures, risks, and prevention. *Environ Health Perspect Suppl* 1999;107:431

Tomlin C, ed. *The Pesticide Manual.* Royal Society of Chemistry, 1994

## INDUSTRIAL CHEMICALS: RESPIRATORY AND SKIN HAZARDS

In many states the department of health or industrial safety has field inspectors who assist in establishing proper safeguards for workers and analyzing air in working areas.

### Environmental controls

(1) Dust-forming operations must be conducted in closed systems with local exhaust ventilation. Ordinary room ventilation is never sufficient to control air contamination.

(2) Hoods for local exhaust ventilation should enclose the process completely to prevent dispersion of contaminants.

(3) Enclosed mechanical conveyors should transport materials.

(4) Areas where hazardous materials are used should have impervious floors and work tables to allow adequate cleaning and to prevent the accumulation of hazardous dusts or liquids. Drains should be provided to allow frequent and thorough flushing.

(5)  Spilled dusts should be removed by sweeping with wet or oiled sweeping compounds. If a vacuum is used, it should have an appropriate filter system to decrease the amount of dust that remains in the exhaust air.

(6)  Spilled liquids should be removed by flushing.

(7)  Room ventilation should be provided by fresh air.

(8)  Substitute with less toxic substances. For example, in many operations toluene or xylene can be substituted for benzene.

(9)  When decomposition to dangerous by-products is possible, control of temperature is necessary.

(10)  Exposure limit values for work or ambient atmospheres have been established as permissible exposure limits (PEL) by the Occupational Safety and Health Administration (OSHA) and the National Institute of Occupational Safety and Health (NIOSH). The American Conference of Governmental Industrial Hygienists (ACGIH) has established workplace exposure guidelines using a threshold limit value (TLV).

(11)  The exposure limit given in this book is the lowest value published by any of these sources. Established concentrations represent an exposure time of 8 h per day for 5 days per week. When exposure is increased, then the safe exposure level is less. The TLV does not separate 'safe' from 'toxic' exposure levels since the degree of toxicity is a function of length of exposure. The TLV-ceiling (TLV-C) is the concentration in air that should not be exceeded during any exposure. TLV-C is used for substances that are so toxic that an 8-hour exposure limit would be inappropriate.

(12)  For gases, these concentrations are ordinarily given in parts per million parts (ppm) or in milligrams per cubic meter ($mg/m^3$) of air. For particulates, concentrations are given only in $mg/m^3$. Since the volume occupied by a given weight of a gas is dependent on its molecular weight, the following formula must be used to convert from ppm to $mg/m^3$ (formula correct at 25°C):

$$mg/m^3 = \frac{ppm \times \text{Molecular weight}}{24.5}$$

For example, the exposure limit of carbon tetrachloride, 5 ppm, represents a concentration of 32 $mg/m^3$ (1 $m^3$ = 35.3 cu ft).

Safe concentrations of substances in air can only be established by analysis, since in many instances the odor threshold is well above the exposure limit value (Table 1.2).

**Table 1.2** Odor thresholds (ppm) for substances with odor thresholds greater than exposure limit

| | | | |
|---|---|---|---|
| Allyl chloride | 25 | Epichlorohydrin | 10 |
| Arsine | 1 | Ethanolamine | 4 |
| Benzene | 100 | Ethylene oxide | 300 |
| Bromine | 3.5 | Isopropyl amine | 10 |
| Carbon dioxide | None | Methanol | 2000 |
| Carbon monoxide | None | Methyl chloroform | 500 |
| Carbon tetrachloride | 79 | Methylene chloride | 300 |
| Chlorine | 5 | Nickel carbonyl | 1 |
| Chlorobromomethane | 400 | Nitromethane | 200 |
| Chloroform | 200 | Propylene oxide | 200 |
| Chloropicrin | 1.1 | n-Propyl nitrate | 50 |
| Diglycidyl ether | 5 | Tolylene 2,4 diisocyanate | 0.4 |
| 1,1 Dimethyl hydrazine | 6 | Turpentine | 200 |
| Dioxane | 200 | Vinyl chloride | 4100 |

**Instructions for and provision of safety equipment**

Simple instructions for the use of safety equipment and of procedures for emergencies should be posted in areas in which hazardous chemicals are in use. Many institutions have departments that monitor hazardous operations and provide instructions for equipment use and for maintaining safe working conditions.

(1) Workers should be trained to:
   (a) evacuate rooms in which spills of hazardous chemicals have occurred;
   (b) understand potential hazards and to properly use safety equipment to avoid exposure;
   (c) disconnect (if possible) electrical equipment if volatile/explosive substances are used;
   (d) decontaminate spills only when trained to do so safely;
   (e) use gloves, goggles, aprons, and protective clothing wherever necessary.

(2) Eye fountains and showers must be provided for rapid removal of corrosive materials.

(3) Protective clothing should be laundered daily.

(4) For operations where local control of contaminants is impractical, supplied air masks, gas masks, or self-contained oxygen helmets should be provided.

(5) Supplied-air masks or gas masks should be available for emergency use wherever dangerous substances are being used. A safety harness and lifeline are necessary to evacuate personnel from areas that may become dangerously contaminated.

(6) Workers handling poisonous substances should be required to wash properly before eating or smoking. A change of clothing after work should be required.

(7) Workers should be instructed to report for examination at the first evidence of illness or injury.

## Adequate medical program

(1) Workers in hazardous occupations should be examined every 6 months to 1 year as a check against failures in control measures. Examinations should be more frequent during periods of exposure to cumulative poisons. They should include complete blood count and urinalysis and, if possible, analysis of blood and urine for the particular hazardous agent. Workers in dusty trades should have a chest X-ray yearly.

(2) Facilities should be inspected weekly or monthly in order to detect failures or inadequacies in control methods. Adequate inspection may require continuous or intermittent sampling of air.

(3) Pre-employment physical examinations should be used to detect chronic respiratory, kidney, liver, or other systemic disease. Individuals with any disease should not be exposed to toxic fumes.

## References

Agency for Toxic Substances and Disease Registry: Toxicological Profiles (300+ titles on industrial chemicals). USDHHS PHS

IARC Monographs. Some Industrial Chemicals. WHO 2000;77

Castegnaro M, *et al.*, eds. Laboratory decontamination and destruction of carcinogens in laboratory wastes: some antineoplastic agents. Lyon: WHO/International Agency for Research in Cancer. IARC Scientific Publication 73, 1985

Chyka PA. How many deaths occur annually from adverse drug reactions in the United States? *Am J Med* 2000;109:122–30

Clayton GD, Clayton FE, eds. *Patty's Industrial Hygiene and Toxicology*, 4th edn. Wiley, 1991, 1995

Consonni D, *et al.* Mortality study in an Italian oil refinery: extension of the follow-up. *Am J Ind Med* 1999;35:287

Dangerous Properties of Industrial Materials Report. Van Nostrand Reinhold. Bimonthly serial

Feldman RG. *Occupational and Environmental Neurotoxicology*. Lippincott-Raven, 1998

Friedman-Jimenez G, *et al.* Clinical evaluation, management, and prevention of work-related asthma. *Am J Ind Med* 2000;37:121

Hansson SE. A case study of pseudo-science in occupational medicine. New Solutions 1998;8:175

Hathaway GJ, *et al. Chemical Hazards of the Workplace*, 4th edn. Van Nostrand Reinhold, 1996

Johnson EG, Janosik JE. Manufacturers' recommendations for handling spilled antineoplastic agents. *Am J Hosp Pharm* 1989;46:318–19

Kilburn KH. Neurobehavioral impairment and symptoms associated with aluminum remelting. *Arch Environ Health* 1999;53:329

Last JM. *Preventive Medicine and Public Health*, 11th edn. Appleton-Century-Crofts, 1980

Lewis RJ Sr. *Sax's Dangerous Properties of Industrial Materials*, 9th edn, 3 vols. Van Nostrand Reinhold, 1996

Lundqvist G, *et al.* A case-controlled study of fatty liver disease and organic solvent exposure. *Am J Ind Med* 1999;35:132

National Institute for Occupational Safety and Health. *Pocket Guide to Chemical Hazards*. DHHS Publication No. 97-140 (NIOSH), 1997

Radon K, *et al.* Lack of combined effects of exposure and smoking on respiratory health in aluminium potroom workers. *Occup Environ Med* 1999;56:468

Sittig M. *Handbook of Toxic and Hazardous Chemicals and Carcinogens*. Noyes, 1992

*Threshold Limit Values for Chemical Substances and Physical Agents*. American Conference of Governmental Industrial Hygienists, 1330 Kemper Meadow Drive, Cincinnati. OH 45240-1634, e-mail: pubs@acgih.org. Annual publication

Tomei F, *et al.* Liver damage among shoe repairers. *Am J Ind Med* 1999;36:541

Vanhanen M, *et al*. Risk of enzyme allergy in the detergent industry. *Occup Environ Med* 2000;57:121

Wallace RB, *et al*. (eds.). *Public Health and Preventive Medicine*, 14th edn. Appleton-Lange, 1998

Xiao JQ, Levin SM. The diagnosis and management of solvent-related disorders. *Am J Ind Med* 2000;37:44

Zenz C, *et al*. *Occupational Medicine: Principles and Practical Applications*. Mosby, 1993

## CANCER

A sizable part of the present incidence of cancer appears to be the result of chemical carcinogenesis; estimates range from 4 to 60% or more. The Occupational Safety and Health Administration (OSHA) has established zero tolerance levels for working atmospheres for the following substances suspected of being carcinogens in humans: 2-acetylaminofluorene, 4-aminodiphenyl, benzidine (and its salts), 3,3′-dichlorobenzidine (and its salts), 4-dimethyl-aminoazobenzene, alpha-naphthylamine, beta-naphthylamine, 4-nitro-biphenyl, *N*-nitrosodimethylamine, beta-propiolactone, bis-chloromethyl ether, methylchloromethyl ether, 4,4′-methylene(bis)-2-chloroaniline, ethyl-eneimine (see NIOSH: Registry of Toxic Effects of Chemical Substances). Table 1.3 lists a number of suspected or confirmed environmental carcinogens. Some substances are considered possible carcinogens based on their structural similarity to vinyl chloride: bromoprene, epibromohydrin, epichlorohydrin, perbromoethylene, perchloroethylene, tribromoethylene, styrene (vinyl benzene), vinyl bromide, vinylidene bromide, and vinylidene chloride.

**Table 1.3** Environmental substances carcinogenic for humans*

| Target organ | Confirmed | Suspected |
|---|---|---|
| Bone | | Beryllium |
| Brain | Vinyl chloride | |
| Endometrium | Estrogens | |
| Esophagus | Alcohol, lye, tobacco smoking | |
| Gastrointestinal tract | Asbestos | Smoked meats |
| Hematopoietic tissue (leukemia) | Alkylating agents: cyclophosphamide, melphalan, busulfan; benzene; styrene butadiene, other synthetic rubbers | |

*Continued*

Table 1.3 (continued)

| Target organ | Confirmed | Suspected |
|---|---|---|
| Kidney | Coke oven emissions, phenacetin | Lead |
| Larynx | Alcohol, asbestos, chromium, mustard gas, tobacco smoking | |
| Liver | Aflatoxin, alcohol, anabolic steroids, contraceptive steroids, vinyl chloride | Aldrin, dieldrin, heptachlor, chlordecone, mirex, DDT, carbon tetrachloride, chloroform, PCBs, trichlorethylene |
| Lung | Arsenic, asbestos, bis(chloromethyl) ether, chloromethyl methyl ether, chromium, coke oven emissions, mustard gas, nickel, polycyclic hydrocarbons, soots and tars, tobacco smoking, uranium, vinyl chloride | Beryllium, cadmium, chloroprene, lead |
| Lymphatic tissue | | Arsenic, benzene |
| Mouth | Alcohol, betel, limes, tobacco | |
| Nasal mucosa | Chromium, formaldehyde, isopropyl alcohol, leather manufacture, nickel, wood dust | |
| Pancreas | | Benzidine, PCBs |
| Peritoneum | Asbestos | |
| Pharynx | Alcohol, tobacco smoking | |
| Pleural cavity | Asbestos | |
| Prostate | Cadmium | |
| Reticuloendothelium | Immunosuppressive drugs | |
| Scrotum | Polycyclic hydrocarbons, soots and tars | Chloroprene |
| Skin | Arsenic, cutting oils, coke oven emissions, polycyclic hydrocarbons, soots and tars | |
| Urinary bladder | Alkylating agents: cyclophosphamide, melphalan; 4-aminobiphenyl; benzidine; chlornaphazine; β-naphthylamine; tobacco smoking | Auramine, magenta, 4-nitrodiphenyl |
| Vagina | Estrogens | |

* Modified from Key MM, *et al.* (eds): *Occupational Diseases, A Guide to Their Recognition*. DHEW Publication No. (NIOSH) 77–181. US Department of Health, Education, and Welfare, 1977

## References

Band PR, *et al*. Identification of occupational cancer risks in British Columbia. *J Occup Environ Med* 2000;42:284

Bardin JA, *et al*. Mortality studies of machining fluid exposure in the automobile industry V: a case-control study of pancreatic cancer. *Am J Ind Med* 1997;32: 240

Brueske-Hohlfeld I, *et al*. Lung cancer risk in male workers occupationally exposed to diesel motor emissions in Germany. *Am J Ind Med* 1999;36:405

CIP Bulletin. Carcinogen Information Program, PO Box 6057, St. Louis, MO 63139

Dinse GE, *et al*. Unexplained increases in cancer incidence in the United States from 1975 to 1994: Possible sentinel health indicators? *Annu Rev Public Health* 1999;20:173

Dossing M, *et al*. Liver cancer among employees in Denmark. *Am J Ind Med* 1997;32:248

Eichholzer M, Gutzwiller F. Dietary nitrates, nitrites, and N-nitroso compounds and cancer risk, a review of the epidemiologic evidence. *Nutr Rev* 1998;56:95–105

Gronbaek M, *et al*. Population based cohort study of the association between alcohol intake and cancer of the upper digestive tract. *Br Med J* 1998;317:884–8

Hunter DJ. Plasma organochlorine levels and the risk of breast cancer. *N Engl J Med* 1997;337:1253–8

IARC Scientific Publications. International Agency for Research on Cancer. Serial monographs

Jahn I, *et al*. Occupational risk factors for lung cancer in women: results of a case-control study in Germany. *Am J Ind Med* 1999;36:90

Laden F, Hunter DJ. Environmental risk factors and female breast cancer. *Annu Rev Public Health* 1998;19:101

Lake BG. Mechanisms of hepatocarcinogenicity of peroxisome-proliferating drugs and chemicals. *Annu Rev Pharmacol Toxicol* 1995;35:483

Langseth H, Andersen A. Cancer incidence among women in the Norwegian pulp and paper industry. *Am J Ind Med* 1999;36:108

Mannetje A, *et al*. Sinonasal cancer, occupation, and tobacco smoking in European women and men. *Am J Ind Med* 1999;36:101

Mannetje A, *et al*. Smoking as a confounder in case-control studies of occupational bladder cancer in women. *Am J Ind Med* 1999;36:75

Miligi L, *et al*. Occupational, environmental, and life-style factors associated with the risk of hematolymphopoietic malignancies in women. *Am J Ind Med* 1999;36:60

Murphy GP, *et al*. *Informed Decisions*. New York: Viking,1997

National Institute of Occupational Safety and Health: *Registry of Toxic Effects of Chemical Substances*. US Government Printing Office. Annual publication

Omenn GS. Chemoprevention of lung cancer: the rise and demise of beta-carotene. *Annu Rev Public Health* 1998;19:73

Straif K, *et al*. Eposure to high concentrations of nitrosamines and cancer mortality among a cohort of rubber workers. *Occup Environ Med* 2000;57:180

Vasama-Neuvonen K, *et al*. Ovarian cancer and occupational exposures in Finland. *Am J Ind Med* 1999;36:83

## AIR POLLUTION AND ENVIRONMENTAL CONTAMINATION

No clear-cut relationship has been found between air pollution and acute, self-limited disease. Air pollution may aggravate pre-existing respiratory and cardiac conditions and is responsible for some of the present incidence of cancer. Conditions most likely to be affected by air pollution are chronic bronchitis, chronic obstructive pulmonary disease/emphysema, asthma, and coronary vascular disease. The chief environmental contaminants are: lead, carcinogens, halogenated hydrocarbons, pesticides, carbon monoxide, hydrogen sulfide, nitrogen oxides, organic compounds, oxidants, particulates, and sulfur oxides.

### References

Eggleston PA, *et al*. The environment and asthma in US cities. *Environ Health Perspect Supp* 1999;107:439

*Environmentally Hazardous Substances on Human Health*. Taylor & Francis, 1996

Giovagnoli MR, *et al*. Carbon and hemosiderin-laden macrophages in sputum of traffic policemen exposed to air pollution. *Arch Environ Health* 1999;54:284

Goren A, *et al*. Respiratory problems associated with exposure to airborne particles in the community. *Arch Environ Health* 1999;54:165

Horner JM. Environmental health implications of heavy metal pollution from car tires. *Rev Environ Health* 1996;11:175

Hughes WW. *The Essentials of Environmental Toxicology*. Taylor & Francis, 1996.

Kumagai S, *et al*. Polychlorinated dibenzo-*p*-dioxin and dibenzofuran concentrations in the serum samples of workers at continuously burning municipal waste incinerators in Japan. *Occup Environ Med* 2000;57:204

Larson TV, Koenig JQ. Wood smoke: emissions and noncancer respiratory effects. *Annu Rev Public Health* 1994;15:133

Selden A, *et al.* Porphyrin status in aluminum foundry workers exposed to hexa-chlorobenzene and octachlorostyrene. *Arch Environ Health* 1999;54:248

Sullivan JB, Krieger GR. *Clinical Environmental Health and Hazardous Materials Toxicology.* Williams & Wilkins, 1997

van der Zee SC, *et al.* Acute effects of urban air pollution on respiratory health of children with and without chronic respiratory symptoms. *Occup Environ Med* 1999;56:802

Wan G, Li C. Indoor endotoxin and glucan in association with airway inflammation and systemic symptoms. *Arch Environ Health* 1999;54:172

Yang C, *et al.* Female lung cancer and petrochemical air pollution in Taiwan. *Arch Environ Health* 1999;54:180

Zmirou D, *et al.* Health effects costs of particulate air pollution. *J Occup Environ Med* 1999;41:847

## SUICIDAL POISONING

### Recognition of suicidal risk

*Symptoms and signs of depression*

(1)  Sleep disturbance – insomnia may be an early symptom of depression. The patient is unable to go to sleep at night or may awaken during the night or early in the morning and be unable to go back to sleep. Others may exhibit hypersomnia.

(2)  Adhedonia or 'lack of interest' – showing little or no interest in friends, occupation or hobbies. The patient may talk about changing jobs or ending a relationship.

(3)  Low mood or sadness.

(4)  Irritability out of proportion to the situation.

(5)  Fatigue – not explained by other medical conditions (sleep apnea, anemia, hypothyroidism, etc.).

(6)  Appetite disturbance – may have a striking history of weight loss and may complain that food no longer 'tastes good'; others may exhibit hyperphagia and overeat.

(7)  Hopelessness about the future (e.g. wants to 'crawl in a hole and hide'), thoughts of death (nobody would miss them if they were gone, they are a burden to their friends/family, would be better off dead, etc.).

(8)  Excessive thoughts of guilt.

(9) Decreased concentration – complaints about not being able to focus on reading, studying, etc. which sometimes is evident at work, home (such as keeping track of expenses), or at school (decline in grades).

(10) Somatic complaints.

(11) Previous history of hospitalization for depression or attempted overdose is a significant risk for further episodes of depression. In addition, patients with chronic conditions (CHF (congestive heart failure), schizophrenia, cancer, etc.), or history of abuse are at increased risk for depression. Patients who make comments about suicide, especially if they indicate a possible plan, are at extremely high risk for suicide.

### *Medical evaluation*

Every patient in whom depression is suspected should be asked about suicidal thoughts and whether they have any desire to live. Ask if the patient feels so hopeless that they might harm themselves. Then ask directly about suicide, including if they have any ideas about how they might harm themselves. In addition, they should be asked about past episodes of depression, psychiatric hospitalizations, substance abuse, past or current physical or sexual abuse and their current source of social support and current life stresses. Family history of psychiatric illness, suicides, or unexplained deaths is important. Refer suicidal patients to a mental health professional for evaluation for hospitalization versus intensive outpatient treatment. Organic etiologies that may present as depression must be considered such as thyroid disease, medication-induced side-effects, etc.

### Prevention

Health professionals should avoid prescribing sedatives or hypnotics for possibly suicidal persons, since these agents are responsible for more than 20% of suicides. When tricyclic antidepressants are prescribed to potentially suicidal patients, the total amount dispensed must be less than a toxic amount in case the patient ingests the entire amount. Tricyclic antidepressants are more toxic in an overdose than the newer selective serotonin reuptake inhibitors (SSRIs). However, when either of these types of agents is taken in combination with alcohol or other CNS acting agents, their toxicity is increased. Excessive amounts of SSRIs can cause serotonin syndrome, which also can be lethal. Relatives should be informed of possible suicidal tendencies in a patient. It may be necessary to prepare a written 'I will not harm' contract with the patient or have a responsible adult with the patient at all times and in possession of the patient's medications. Persons who have made unsuccessful attempts at suicide should have adequate follow-up psychiatric therapy.

### References

Gliatto MF, Rai AK. Evaluation and treatment of patients with suicidal ideation. *Am Family Physician* 1999;59:1500

Johnson JG, *et al*. Psychiatric comorbidity, health status, and functional impairment associated with alcohol abuse and dependence in primary care patients: findings of the PRIME-MD 1000 Study. *J Consult Clin Psychol* 1995;63:133

Post D, *et al*. Teenagers: mental health and psychological issues. *Primary Care* 1998:25:181

## TERATOGENS: DRUG AND CHEMICAL INJURY TO THE FETUS

Before using drugs during pregnancy, evidence for their safety must be established. Self-administration of drugs or chemicals should be discouraged during the childbearing years, since pregnancy may not be recognized during the important first trimester, when fetal injury commonly occurs.

The book *Drugs in Pregnancy and Lactation* (see references) is an excellent resource to have available in the clinic or emergency room. It rates the drugs by level of risk and provides a reference list for each drug.

### Drugs especially to be avoided during pregnancy

All drugs, including prescription drugs, over-the-counter drugs, herbal remedies, alcohol, and tobacco and other drugs of abuse, should be avoided in the first trimester of pregnancy unless maternal need overrides the hazard to the fetus. The following are known to be especially hazardous:

(1) Accutane and other retinoids (oral or topical)
(2) Alcohol
(3) Antineoplastic agents, aminopterin, chlorambucil, melphalan, methotrexate, radio-iodine, cyclophosphamide, 6-azauridine, fluorouracil.
(4) Amphotericin B

(5) Carbamazepine and valproic acid (increased risk of spinabifida). Evaluate risk vs. benefit (as seizures in the mother also increase risk to the fetus). For more information: see Women and Epilepsy Initiative of the Epilepsy Foundation at: http://www.epilepsyfoundation.org.

(6) Lithium

(7) New or incompletely studied drugs: (Check package literature before prescribing.).

(8) Drugs and chemicals dangerous to nursing infants: All drugs and chemicals absorbed by the mother appear in the breast milk. Most of these have little effect on the nursing infant because they appear in relatively small amounts in the milk. Heroin addiction in the mother is associated with withdrawal in the infant whether or not the infant nurses.

**References**

Briggs GG, *et al. Drugs in Pregnancy and Lactation: A Reference Guide to Fetal and Neonatal Risk.* Williams & Wilkins, 1998

Friedman JM, Polifka JE. *The Effects of Neurologic and Psychiatric Drugs on the Fetus and Nursery Infant.* Johns Hopkins University Press, 1998

Kalen B. A register study of maternal epilepsy and delivery outcome with special reference to drug use. *Acta Neurol Scand* 1986;73:253–9

McGrath C, *et al.* Treatment of anxiety during pregnancy: effects of psychotropic drug treatment on the developing fetus. *Drug Safety* 1999;20:171

Nieuwenhuijsen MJ, *et al.* Chlorination disinfection byproducts in water and their association with adverse reproductive outcomes: a review. *Occup Environ Med* 2000;57:73

Olshan AF, Faustman EM. Male-mediated developmental toxicity. *Annu Rev Public Health* 1993;14:159

Shepard TH. *Catalog of Teratogenic Agents.* Johns Hopkins University Press, 1998

## DRUG-INDUCED REACTIONS, FATALITIES, AND INTERACTIONS

Drug-induced reactions can occur with drug abuse or with medical or dental treatment. Prevention of drug reactions due to therapeutic use of drugs is discussed below. Drug abuse is considered in Chapter 3.

Prevention of drug fatalities should be one of the health provider's paramount concerns. Dosage errors due to mistakes in reading or writing decimal places can have devastating effects. Recently the tradenames of some drugs have been changed to reduce the number of similar sounding names in order to reduce potential errors. Physicians, pharmacists, and other health providers should continually evaluate the need for and appropriateness of any drug therapy and should be alert to recognize the early signs of drug reaction. Extreme caution must be exercised when prescribing drugs with a narrow therapeutic index. Laboratory procedures for monitoring a drug or the effects of a drug must be used for maximum safety.

Fatalities from medication errors are not rare. The following data apply to the USA: 7000 patients die each year from medication errors. Therapeutic errors and adverse reactions accounted for 7.5% of all reported human exposures in 1997. A review of 100 case reports of serotonin syndrome, which may be precipitated by drug interactions, found that 40% of patients required admission to an intensive care unit and 25% required ventilator support. The most lethal drugs are those administered intravenously because this route bypasses absorption. Absorption can be decreased or prevented if ingestion is identified early. Depressants (CNS, cardiac, pulmonary), penicillins, heparin/anticoagulants and thrombolytics, cardiac drugs, potassium chloride and other potassium salts, diuretics, and insulin are among the most lethal of IV drugs.

### Risk factors for drug interactions

#### Patient factors

Increased risk is associated with increased number of chronic disorders and number of medications. Other specific patient factors that increase risk include being female, being either very young or elderly, being hypothermic, having decreased renal or hepatic function, hypoalbuminemia, hypotension or having slow acetylator phenotype, or a diagnosis of congestive heart failure.

#### Medication factors

Drugs with a narrow margin of safety: warfarin, digoxin, theophylline, anticonvulsants, antiarrthymics, aminoglycosides, antidepressants, monoamine oxidase inhibitors, and cyclosporine. Monitor these drugs with frequent blood levels.

Drugs that inhibit cytochrome P450 enzymes: amiodarone, cimetidine, ciprofloxacin, clarithromycin, diltiazem, erythromycin, fluconazole, fluoxetine, fluvoxamine, imipramine, isoniazid, itraconazole, ketoconazole, metronidazole, nefazodone, nortriptyline, paroxetine, primaquine, propranolol, ritonavir, valproic acid, verapamil, and others.

Drugs that induce (increase) cytochrome P450 enzymes, chronic alcohol use, barbiturates, carbamazepine, cigarette smoking, griseofulvin, phenytoin, primidone, rifampin, and others.

Drugs metabolized by the same cytochrome P450 isoenzyme(s) may interact. The extent of the interaction will depend on to what extent the enzymes are inhibited and to what extent the other drug is metabolized by the same isoenzyme. In addition, the interaction may depend on the dosages of the two drugs as well as patient-specific factors (such as whether a patient is genetically a fast or slow metabolizer).

Chronic exposure to many drugs and chemicals induces greater production of hepatic microsomal drug-metabolizing enzymes. Consequently, other substances metabolized in the liver are processed more rapidly. Some drugs are metabolized to less active or inactive metabolites and are therefore less active in the presence of an inducer: barbiturates, coumarin anticoagulants, phenytoin, digitoxin, desipramine, aminopyrine, phenylbutazone, amphetamine, adrenocorticosteroids, estrogens, and progestogens. If the dosage of a drug is increased to compensate for the concurrent administration of an inducer and the inducer is later withdrawn, drug toxicity may occur. Rifampin is one of the most potent inducers of liver enzymes. Pregnancy has occurred in women taking estrogen–progestogens who have been given rifampin.

Other drugs and chemicals are metabolized to more active or toxic substances; hence, in the presence of an inducer, the toxicity of these substances is increased. The pesticide azinphos-methyl (Guthion) is not active as a cholinesterase inhibitor until it is metabolized in the body to the active substance. In the presence of induced liver enzymes, Guthion is more toxic. The hepatic toxicity of acetaminophen depends on its metabolism to toxic products. Thus, in the presence of induced liver enzymes, toxicity can occur at lower doses of acetaminophen. Since most environmental carcinogens enter the body as procarcinogens, the possibility exists that in the presence of induced metabolizing enzymes a greater fraction of such procarcinogens will be converted to carcinogens, increasing the carcinogenicity.

An example of altered drug metabolism: any of the following inhibitors – ketoconazole, itraconazole, clarithromycin, erythromycin, troleandomycin, quinine, nefazodone, fluvoxamine, or cimetidine – can produce potentially fatal drug interactions with astemizole, cisapride, or theophylline.

Drug interaction related to distribution can occur when a drug is highly protein bound (>90%) and the other drug displaces the one that is highly bound. This may lead to toxic levels of the drug that had been bound to protein. Example: phenytoin and warfarin may be displaced by sulfa drugs.

Drug effects or interactions related to excretion occur when the substances compete for the same transport mechanism within the kidney (e.g. quinidine inhibits the tubular secretion of digoxin, leading to elevated digoxin levels). It may also occur when one drug changes the urine pH. This occurs because ionized drugs are preferentially excreted. For instance, when the urine is alkalinized, the urinary excretion of amphetamine (a base) decreases because it is in the non-ionized state.

Potential toxicity from both drugs having similar pharmacologic effects occurs when a medicine such as a serotonin reuptake inhibitor (SSRI) is taken with a cough suppressant containing dextromethorphan (which also inhibits serotonin), or when an SSRI is combined with sumatriptan (a serotonin agonist). The result may be serotonergic syndrome. In addition, when a patient taking a monoamine oxidase inhibitor ingests another sympathomimetic amine (ephedrine, ephedra, phenylpropanolamine*), the result may be a hypertensive crisis.

### References

Aronson JK, ed. *Side Effects of Drugs,* vol. 22. Elsevier Science, 1999

Bosse GM, Matyunas NJ. Delayed toxidromes. *J Emerg Med* 1999;17:679

Davies DM. *Textbook of Adverse Drug Reactions*. Edward Arnold, 1999

*Drug Information.* American Hospital Formulary Service, 2000. (Annual publication)

Dukes MNG, ed. *Meyler's Side Effects of Drugs*. Elsevier Science, 1996

---

*Phenylpropanolamide was removed from US market in 2001 due to increased risk of hemorrhagic stroke in women after researchers at Yale University issued a report entitled 'Phenypropanolamine and Risk of Hemorrhagic Stroke: Final Report of the Hemorrhagic Stroke Project'

Goldberg RM, *et al.* A comparison of drug interaction software programs: applicability to the emergency department. *Ann Emerg Med* 1994;24:619

Hansten PD, Horn JR. *Drug Interactions Analysis and Management.* Facts and Comparisons 1997– (www.drugfacts.com)

Mills KC. Serotonin syndrome. *Am Fam Physician* 1995;52:1475

*Mosby's GenRx.* Mosby, 2000. (Annual publication)

*Physician's Desk Reference,* 2000. (Annual publication)

Roberge RJ, *et al.* Dextromethorphan- and pseudoephedrine-induced agitated psychosis and ataxia: case report. *J Emerg Med* 1999;17:285

Tatro DS, ed. *Drug Interaction Facts.* Facts and Comparisons, 2000. (Updated quarterly)

Zucchero FJ, *et al. Evaluations of Drug Interactions.* First Data Bank, 2000. (Updated bimonthly)

# 2 Emergency management of poisoning

With a case of known or suspected poisoning, routine life-support measures – airway establishment, breathing, and cardiac support (ABC) – must be evaluated, and if action is needed it must be started promptly. The time from ingestion or exposure to initial treatment is of the utmost importance in the management of suspected poisoning or overdose. Loss of airway and protective reflexes is a prime contributor to poor outcome or death.

Once life-support measures have been addressed, direct attention to other aspects of the case. Obtain any available historical information; further inquiries may be necessary later. Examine the patient and any materials accompanying the patient for evidence that may clarify the problem. If, for example, an overdose is suspected, and tablets or capsules have been found, the drugs can be identified from the manufacturer's drug imprint.

In order to treat poisoning properly, the physician must possess some special knowledge and equipment. First, knowledge of adequate first-aid treatment is essential. If called by telephone, the physician must decide quickly if first-aid treatment is indicated and be able to give instructions for appropriate measures (see inside front cover), or whether activation of the emergency medical system (EMS) is necessary.

After the type of exposure (inhalation, skin contact, etc.) has been determined and procedures to minimize further absorption instituted, try to identify the poison. If the label does not give the ingredients or if the container is not available, then all possible information (physical state, e.g. liquid, odor, type of container, trade name, manufacturer's drug imprint, use, presence of poison label), must be obtained in an effort to determine the toxic nature of the poison (Table 3.1). To assist in the identification of the poison, the container with its contents, and any vomitus should be brought to the emergency facility.

After first-aid measures (Table 2.1 and inside front and back covers) have been instituted, definitive or supportive treatment must be planned. This usually involves bringing the patient by ambulance to an emergency facility. The emergency room physician should be alerted and given as much information as possible and an expected time of arrival.

While awaiting the arrival of the patient, the physician should try to identify the poison from the information given. For this purpose, thorough familiarity with the index of this book and other information sources is helpful. The telephone number of a functioning poison information center should also be available. The local or regional poison center can supply information about ingredients of the poison, specific toxic consequences, and details of management. If the manufacturer of the product is known, telephoning the company can provide a rapid way to determine all substances contained in the product.

**Table 2.1** Summary of emergency management of poisoning

1. Give first-aid advice (see inside front and back covers of this book). If the substance is not caustic and the patient is alert, induce vomiting with ipecac (if ipecac is not available, liquid detergent may be used).
2. Give instructions to save suspected poison in original container and place vomitus in a clean jar or plastic bag. Bring specimens with patient for possible identification.
3. Provide for transportation to emergency treatment center and alert the center.
4. Maintain respiration and control shock.
5. Remove poison to minimize further absorption (see inside cover).
6. Identify poison if possible, but do not delay adequate control of respiration and blood pressure.

Antidotes, specific therapeutic agents, and necessary equipment are listed in Tables 2.2 and 2.3. If a specific antidote is available, administer it while proceeding with the removal of the poison. Do NOT use antidotes unless positive identification of the poison has been made.

**Table 2.2** List of drugs useful in treatment of poisoning

| Drug | Use |
|------|-----|
| N-Acetylcysteine (Mucosil or Mucomyst Oral) | Acetaminophen |
| Amrinone | For positive ionotrope effect |
| Amyl nitrite | Cyanide |
| Antihistamine (multiple agents), available im/po (intramuscular, oral) | Bee sting |

*Continued*

*Table 2.2 (continued)*

| Drug | Use |
|---|---|
| Anti-snakebite serum, polyvalent, 10 ml* | North American (Crotalidae sp.) snakes |
| Antivenin (*L. mactans*) | *Latrodectus mactans* (black widow spider) |
| Antivenin (*M. fulvius*) | *Micrurus fulvius* (coral snake) |
| Atropine sulfate | Phosphate ester insecticides |
| BAL (see dimercaprol) | |
| Benzodiazepine | Muscle spasm (black widow spider bite) |
| Benztropine | Antipsychotics |
| Beta blockers | Beta-adrenergics, theophylline |
| Botulin antitoxin, available from CDC* | Botulism |
| Bretylium | Cardiac arrhythmias |
| Bromocriptine | Neuroleptic malignant syndrome |
| Calcium chloride or gluconate | Fluoride, Ca-channel drugs and black widow spider |
| Charcoal, activated | Adsorbent |
| Cyanide antidote package (see thiosulphate, amyl nitrate) | |
| Cyanocobalamine | Nitroprusside |
| Dantrolene, sodium | Hyperthermia |
| Deferoxamine, mesylate | Iron |
| Dextrose, 50% | Cerebral edema |
| Dextrose 5% in water or 5% in 0.9% saline | Fluid replacement |
| Diazepam (Valium) | Anticonvulsant, organophosphorus |
| Digoxin immune Fab | Digoxin, digitoxin |
| Dimercaprol (BAL) | Arsenic, mercury |
| Diphenhydramine (Benadryl) | Bee sting, anaphylaxis |
| Distilled water | Diluent |
| DMSA (meso-2,3-dimercapto-succinic acid or succinen) | Lead, mercury, heavy metals |
| Dopamine | For positive ionotropic effect |
| Edetate calcium disodium (EDTA) | Lead |
| Epinephrine | Sensitivity reactions |
| Esmolol | Tachyarrhythmias, hyperthyroid state |
| Ethanol | Methanol |
| Flumazenil | Benzodiazepine overdose |
| Fluorescein solution | Eye contamination |
| Folic acid, 1 mg | Methanol |

*Continued*

*Table 2.2 (continued)*

| Drug | Use |
|------|-----|
| Fomepizole | Methanol, ethylene glycol |
| Fosphenytoin | Arrhythmias |
| Furosemide | Diuretic |
| Glucagon | Beta blocker/myocardial depression |
| Haloperidol | Antipsychotics |
| Hydroxocobalamin, 1 mg/ml | Cyanide |
| Ipecac, syrup of | Emetic |
| Isoproterenol | Bradycardia |
| Labetalol | Stimulant drug overdose |
| Leukovorin | Methotrexate, trimethoprin, pyrimethamine |
| Lidocaine | Ventricular arrhythmias |
| Magnesium sulfate | Convulsions, hypertension |
| Mannitol | Cerebral edema |
| Methylene blue | Methemoglobinemia |
| Metoclopramide | Anti-emetic |
| Milk, evaporated | Acids |
| Milk of magnesia | Acids |
| Morphine sulfate | Pain |
| Nalmefene | Opioid antagonist |
| Naloxone (Narcan) | Opioid antagonist |
| Neostigmine | Curare block |
| Neuromuscular blockers | Stimulant strychnine tetanus |
| Nitroprusside | Ergot, hypertension |
| Norepinephrine bitartrate, 4 mg in 4 ml | Cardiac arrest |
| Octreotide, 1 mg/ml, 5 ml | Sulfonylurea hypoglycemia |
| Ondansetron | Anti-emetic |
| Oxygen | Hypoxia, carbon monoxide |
| Paraldehyde | Acute alcoholic mania |
| Penicillamine, 250-mg capsules | Lead, copper |
| Pentobarbital sodium | Anticonvulsant |
| Phentolamine | Alpha-adrenergics |
| Phenytoin/Fosphenytoin | Arrhythmias |
| Physostigmine | Anti-cholinergic syndrome |
| Potassium chloride | Hypokalemia |
| Pralidoxime | Organophosphate or carbamate insecticide |
| Prednisolone | Cerebral edema |
| Procainamide | Cardiac arrest |

*Continued*

Table 2.2 (continued)

| Drug | Use |
|------|-----|
| Propranolol | Arrhythmias |
| Protamine | Heparin, isoniazid, *Gyromitra* |
| Pyridoxine (Vitamin B$_6$) | Mushrooms, cycloserine |
| Sodium bicarbonate, 8.4%, 50 ml | Acidosis |
| Sodium chloride solution, isotonic 1 liter | Fluid replacement |
| Sodium nitrite | Cyanide |
| Sodium sulfate, magnesium sulfate | Barium |
| Sodium thiosulfate, 25%, 50 ml | Cyanide, bleaching solution |
| Starch, cornstarch or milk | Iodine |
| Succimer (see DMSA) | |
| Succinylcholine chloride | Anticonvulsant |
| Thiopental sodium | Anticonvulsant |
| Thiosulfate | cyanide |
| Urea, 50% | Sulfides |
| Vitamin K$_1$ (phytonadione) | Dicumarol, warfarin |

*Inquire availability at local poison center

## INGESTED POISONS (see inside front cover for administration)

### Precautions

If emesis occurs within 1 hour after ingestion of a poison, 30–60% of the poison may be recovered; emesis after 1 hour may yield less than 20% of the poison. Vomiting may be associated with aspiration of gastric contents, and aspiration of hydrocarbons is dangerous.

*Contraindications*: Do not induce emesis if the patient is drowsy or unconscious. In such cases, if a swallowed poison must be removed, gastric lavage should be performed after insertion of a cuffed endotracheal tube. Do not induce emesis if the patient has ingested acids or alkalis – emesis increases the likelihood of gastric perforation. Do not induce emesis if the patient has ingested a convulsant – vomiting may induce convulsions.

Gastric lavage, like emesis, is most effective if performed immediately after ingestion. While lavage is often performed in emergency rooms, it is invasive and evidence does not support it being superior to ipecac. If 60 minutes have elapsed since the time of ingestion, it has virtually no effect. If patient is unconscious, endotracheal intubation with a secure, cuffed tube must be performed before gastric lavage. Other hazards associated with gastric intubation: perforation of esophagus or stomach, accidental passage of tube into lungs, aspiration from vomiting when lavage performed without a protected airway. See Table 2.3 for equipment used in the treatment of poisoning.

*Contraindications for gastric lavage*: drowsy, unconscious, or convulsing patient. Ingestion of hydrocarbons (gasoline, kerosene, etc.), ingestion of sustained-release (SR) or enteric-coated (EC) tablets is unlikely to be helpful. For SR or EC tablets, whole bowel irrigation should be used. Hydrocarbons are toxic if aspirated; however, once they reach the stomach, systemic toxicity is unusual.

**Method for gastric lavage**

Intubate patient unless patient is fully awake. Position patient in left lateral decubitus position. Select gastric tube: adults 36–40 French for tablets, smaller for liquid poisons, corrosives, or children. Estimate length between teeth and stomach. Pass tube through nose or mouth (neck in flexion assists in avoiding placement in trachea); if an obstruction is met before the mark on the tube reaches the level of the teeth, do not use force. Withdraw tube, reposition patient and attempt procedure again. Check tube position by either placing it in water (bubbling on expiration indicates placement in trachea) or by insufflation of air and listen over patient's stomach. Withdraw stomach contents and either isolate (if toxic to health care team) or save if needed for identification. Administer activated charcoal (1 g/kg) before starting lavage (see p. 31–32) to adsorb a substance that has already reached the bowel. Instill 200–300 ml (less for children) of warm water or 0.9% saline and remove by gravity; if this takes longer than 5 min, assist with gentle suction. Repeat instillation and withdrawal until tablets recovered or 2000 ml has been used (in adults). Large volumes of tap water can cause electrolyte imbalance and/or hypothermia.

After lavage procedure, administer activated charcoal (see p. 31–32), even if toxic substance has not been identified, to further gut decontamination.

If repeated dosages of charcoal are needed, consider use of cathartics.

**Cathartics**

Give magnesium citrate 10% (3–4 ml/kg) or sorbitol 70% (1–2 ml/kg). When substances are ingested that do not adsorb on charcoal (iron tablets), cathartics decrease transit time. However, whether reduced transit time improves

**Table 2.3**  Emergency equipment for treatment of poisoning

Gastric lavage: Mouth gag; gastric tubes (Adult 36–40 French) and syringe to fit
Hypodermic syringes
Oxygen inhaler: Oronasal masks (large, medium, small), rebreathing bag, tubing, regulator, humidifier, and oxygen tank
Oropharyngeal airways and endotracheal tubes
Urethral catheters and suction apparatus
Resuscitation apparatus
Tracheostomy set
Rubber-band tourniquet
Intravenous infusion set (including polyethylene tubing in various sizes)
Transfusion equipment
Sterile cutdown set to expose veins for emergency intravenous injection
Lumbar puncture kit
Cardiac resuscitation supplies and equipment
Chemically clean specimen bottles with screw-top plastic-lined lids for vomitus and excreta
Can opener with canned milk (corrosives)
Laryngoscope

outcome or not is unknown. Cathartics are also used if more than one dose of charcoal is administered. Theoretically, cathartics decrease the risk of intestinal impaction or bezoar.

### *Contraindications*

If the patient has obstruction, ileus, or electrolyte imbalance. Do not use oil-based products: castor oil increases the absorption and toxicity of chlorinated insecticides. Never use irritant cathartics (phenolphthalein, aloes, cascara). Do not give magnesium-containing or hypertonic cathartics to patients with renal disease or those exposed to nephrotoxins, or to any patient in whom myoglobinuria or hemoglobinuria is present or threatened.

### Activated charcoal

Activated charcoal is the most effective adsorbent. It is available, either plain or in sorbitol suspension. If in dry form, shake 50 g activated charcoal in

500 ml polyethylene bottle with 400 ml distilled water until all charcoal is wet and the consistency is like heavy cream.

Initial dose is 1 g/kg administered orally or by gastric tube. Repeat dosages are 0.25–0.5 g/kg every 2–4 h. After 2–3 dosages of charcoal, consider use of cathartic. Charcoal poorly adsorbs boric acid, ferrous sulfate, DDT, cyanide, ethanol, methanol, water-insoluble substances, mineral acids, alkalis, and many metallic compounds. However, it should still be tried because it may adsorb a sufficient amount of the agent to limit toxicity; 60–100 g charcoal will adsorb the usual lethal dose of cyanide.

## SNAKEBITE

Do not apply a tourniquet. Application of cold is too hazardous for emergency use as frostbite will increase tissue damage. Splinting or immobilizing the area may be helpful.

### Incision

Incision and suction removes up to 20% of subcutaneously injected snake venom in the first 10 minutes after bites of some snakes (see p. 596) but damage to underlying structures is common. An extractor may be used, however mouth suction is not appropriate. *Do not delay transport to attempt this.*

### Specific antidote

Obtain specific antidote once identification of the snake is known. Administer according to the directions included with the package. Call Poison Information Center for sources.

## SKIN CONTAMINATION

Flood the contaminated area with copious amounts of water from a hose, shower or poured from a bucket to dilute and remove the poison. Remove the clothing while a continuous stream of water is played on the skin. Protect emergency personnel against contamination by use of rubber gloves and aprons. The rapidity and volume of washing are extremely important in reducing the extent of injury from corrosives or other agents that injure the skin.

*Do not use chemical antidotes.* The heat liberated by a chemical reaction may increase the extent of injury.

Further treatment to involved areas should be the same as for burns of similar severity.

## EYE INJURY DUE TO CHEMICAL IRRITANTS

In industries where eye contamination is liable to occur, foot-operated eye-wash fountains with rubber eye pieces should be available for immediate use. If an eyewash fountain is not available, the victim should be taken to a hose or sink where the eye can be flooded with water under low pressure while the lids are held apart. Washing is continued for a full 15 minutes and the patient is then taken to a first-aid station. Washing must begin immediately, since a delay of a few seconds can greatly increase the extent of injury.

*Do not use chemical antidotes.* These may actually increase the extent of the injury by liberating heat.

At the first-aid station, place the patient in a reclining chair and irrigate the eyes for 15 more minutes with sterile normal saline solution or sterile water. Then instill a few drops of 2% fluorescein solution (which must be sterile) into the eye. (Sterile fluorescein papers or single-dose containers may also be used.) If the fluorescein produces a yellow or green stain, irrigate the eye for another 5 minutes and then send the patient to an ophthalmologist for further examination and treatment. If possible the patient should be seen by an ophthalmologist within 2 h after the injury.

## INHALED POISONS

Remove from exposure, establish an adequate airway, and give $O_2$ and artificial respiration as indicated. Determine blood pressure frequently during the use of positive-pressure resuscitation equipment. A prolonged inspiratory cycle will impair venous return and lower blood pressure. Maintain body temperature.

Use a specific antidote when available (e.g. amyl nitrite for cyanide poisoning).

## RECTALLY ADMINISTERED POISONS

Dilute the poison by giving a tap water enema then allow its expulsion. Catharsis may also be necessary.

## References

Baselt RC, Cravey RH, eds. *Disposition of Toxic Drugs and Chemicals in Man*, 4th edn. Chemical Toxicology Institute, 1995

Brent J, *et al*. Position statement and practice guidelines on the use of multi-dose activated charcoal in the treatment of acute poisoning. *J Toxicol Clin Toxicol* 1999;37:731

Bryson PD. *Comprehensive Review in Toxicology for Emergency Clinicians*, 3rd edn. Taylor & Francis, 1996

Caravati EM, *et al*. Esophageal laceration and charcoal mediastinum complicating gastric lavage. *J Emerg Med* 2001;20:273

Cooney DO. *Activated Charcoal in Medical Applications*. Marcel Dekker, 1995

Goldfrank LR. *Goldfrank's Toxicologic Emergencies*, 6th edn. Appleton & Lange, 1998

Haddad LM, *et al*., eds. *Clinical Management of Poisoning and Drug Overdose*, 3rd edn. WB Saunders, 1998

Moll J, *et al*. Incidence of aspiration pneumonia in intubated patients receiving activated charcoal. *J Emerg Med* 1999;17:279

Position statement: cathartics. *J Toxicol Clin Toxicol* 1997;35:743

Position statement: gastric lavage. *J Toxicol Clin Toxicol* 1997;35:711

Position statement: ipecac syrup. *J Toxicol Clin Toxicol* 1997;35:699

Position statement: single-dose activated charcoal. *J Toxicol Clin Toxicol* 1997;35:721

Position statement: whole bowel irrigation. *J Toxicol Clin Toxicol* 1997;35:753

Pronczuk de Garbino J, *et al*. Antidotes. *J Toxicol Clin Toxicol* 1996;35:333

# 3    Diagnosis and evaluation of poisoning

## PRINCIPLES OF DIAGNOSIS (Table 3.1)

The first responsibility of a physician is to decide whether the poisoning is sufficiently serious to require any treatment. If intervention is necessary, then the physician must decide on the most appropriate treatment plan. Poisoning can usually be categorized as (1) exposure to a known poison, (2) exposure to an unknown substance that may be a poison, and (3) disease of undetermined cause in which poisoning must be considered as part of the differential diagnosis.

## EXPOSURE TO KNOWN POISONS

In many cases of poisoning, the agent responsible is known, and the physician's only problem is to determine whether the degree of exposure is sufficient to require more than first aid or initial emergency treatment. However, sometimes the history is inaccurate. The exact quantity of poison absorbed by the patient will probably be unknown, but the physician may be able to estimate the greatest amount the patient could have absorbed. By examining the container from which the poison was obtained and by questioning relatives or co-workers, it may be possible to determine the amount previously present in the container. The missing quantity is compared to the known fatal dose.

Reported minimum lethal doses may be useful indications of the relative hazards of poisonous substances, but the fatal dose may vary greatly. If the estimated amount of poison is known to have caused serious or potentially fatal poisoning, treatment must be instituted rapidly.

### Lethal dose (LD) and lethal concentration (LC)

To facilitate estimation of the severity of poisoning from substances for which clinical experience does not provide an indication of dangerous doses for humans, lethal doses for experimental animals are given in the tables of toxic substances in this book. Unless otherwise indicated, these constitute the smallest median lethal dose (LD50) that has been reported in any experimental animal by either oral administration or skin application. The LD50 is the amount of chemical that will kill approximately 50% of a group of animals. For some substances, the lethal concentration (LC) is given. This is the lowest concentration, in parts per million parts of air (ppm) or parts per billion parts of air (ppb), that is lethal to any animal species after short or long exposure. When known, the dose that has been fatal to humans is included in the text.

Depending on the steepness of the dose–response curve (the relationship between the smallest dose that will kill any animals and the largest dose that some of the animals will survive), the dangerous dose for humans may be 1–10% or less of the indicated lethal dose. The sources for the lethal doses in the tables are the references listed on pages 8, 11–13, and 49–51. It must be emphasized that there are enormous intraspecies differences in susceptibility to poisons; LD50s can be misleading and must be used with caution.

## EXPOSURE TO SUBSTANCES THAT MAY BE POISONOUS

If a patient has been exposed to a substance the ingredients of which are not known, identification must proceed immediately. This is difficult owing to the large number of trade-named mixtures and the rapidity with which the formulas for such mixtures change. Since some trade-named chemical mixtures do not list the ingredients on the label, it may not be possible to evaluate the significance of exposure without contacting the manufacturer. The sources on page 37 are suggested for evaluating trade-named mixtures.

Note: Physicians should be cautious in incriminating a chemical as the cause of symptoms unless a clear association is obvious or laboratory confirmation has been made, particularly when the symptoms are chronic.

### Index of this book

The index of this book lists the main toxic ingredient of some of the most poisonous trade-named mixtures or indicates the poison that most closely represents the overall effects of the mixture. Many other commercial products are listed according to the nature or use of the product, since it would be impractical to list all trade names. For these general listings, the one ingredient that best represents the toxic potentialities of the product is indicated. Unless further information concerning the toxic ingredients can be obtained, the patient exposed to such a mixture should be treated as if this toxic substance were present. Toxic antidotes should not be given without definite evidence that poisoning has occurred.

**Table 3.1** Summary of diagnosis and evaluation of poisoning

**Acute poisoning**

Speed is essential. Acute poisoning should be considered if the patient: has symptoms that began shortly after exposure to a known poison, has been exposed to a poison known to have caused fatalities, or has been exposed to a substance for which ingredients are not known.

Call poison information center for information on trade names.

**Chronic poisoning**

Consider when a patient has symptoms after a known exposure.

Determine severity of exposure (history, concentration in excreta).

Determine magnitude of organ involvement (see specific poison).

Consider when a patient has symptoms with no known exposure.

Careful history and physical exam with attention to the following poisons: arsenic, carbon monoxide, chlorinated compounds, fluoride, hypnotics and sedatives, lead, mercury, phosphate ester insecticides, analgesics, silica, thallium.

## Poison Information Center

Obtain the telephone number of the nearest poison information center (http://www.aapcc.org). Make certain that 24-hour service is available. Poison information centers are, in most cases, able to identify the ingredients of trade-named mixtures, give some estimate of their toxicity, and suggest the necessary treatment. See also Poisindex under reference below.

## References

Allen LV Jr, *et al.*, eds. *Handbook of Nonprescription Drugs*, 12th edn. American Pharmaceutical Association, 2000

American Hospital Formulary Service. *Drug Information*. American Society of Health-System Pharmacists. (Annual publication)

Billups NF, Billups SM, eds. *American Drug Index*. Facts and Comparisons. (Annual publication)

Kastrup EK, *et al.*, eds. *Drug Facts and Comparisons*. Facts and Comparisons. (Updated quarterly)

*Physicians' Desk Reference*. Medical Economics, Inc. (Annual publication)

*Physicians' Desk Reference for Nonprescription Drugs and Dietary Supplements*. Medical Economics, Inc. (Annual publication)

Rumack BH (ed.) *Poisindex* (computerized poison information system), *Micromedex* Medical Economics, Inc. (Updated quarterly)

## DIFFERENTIAL DIAGNOSIS OF DISEASE THAT MAY BE THE RESULT OF POISONING

In any disease state of unknown origin, poisoning must be considered as part of the differential diagnosis. For example, the high number of cases of lead poisoning that have been discovered in a few medical centers indicates that many cases may go unrecognized. Only when poisoning is considered can the necessary steps to confirm the diagnosis be taken. A small group of poisons accounts for most disabilities that result from unrecognized poisoning: arsenic, carbon monoxide, chlorinated compounds, fluoride, hypnotics and sedatives, lead, mercury, phosphate ester insecticides, analgesics, silica, and thallium. In any patient with a symptom complex of undetermined cause, these poisons should be considered. The diagnostic work-up of a patient who may be a victim of unrecognized poisoning consists of (1) a complete history, (2) complete physical examination, and (3) appropriate laboratory tests.

Table 3.2 on p. 40 provides a list of the most likely poison(s) ingested, given a specific history or physical exam finding.

### History

The history is obtained from parents, friends, or neighbors. For example, in cases of poisoning in children, the parents may not be helpful, whereas a neighbor might have seen the child eating a plant or other poisonous substance. Questioning informants separately helps avoid overlooking important information.

A systematically performed history and physical exam using a list helps prevent omission of essential questions and observations.

### Occupational exposure

Occupational hazards include the following poisons.

**Arsenic** – Smelter workers, refinery workers, gardeners, agricultural workers, pest control operators.

**Asbestos** – Pipe fitters, brake manufacturing, fire barriers.

**Benzene** – Rubber and plastic cement workers and users, dye makers, gasoline blenders, electroplaters, paint and paint remover manufacturers and users, painters, printers, varnishers, dry cleaners.

**Bis(chloromethyl) ether** – Plastic manufacturing.

**Carbon monoxide** – Firefighters, blacksmiths, furnace or foundry workers, brick or cement makers, chimney cleaners, filling-station attendants, parking attendants, garage workers, miners, refinery workers, plumbers, police officers, sewer workers.

**Chloride** – Pool disinfectant and water purification, custodial work, tile cleaners, paper pulp work.

**Chlorinated hydrocarbons** (carbon tetrachloride, etc.) – Rubber cement and plastic cement workers or users, cobblers, leather workers, dry cleaners, painters (including varnish and lacquer painters), furniture finishers, cloth finishers, paint removers, rubber workers.

**Chromium** – Garage mechanics, dye makers, electroplaters, painters, pottery workers, printers, paper makers.

**Cyanide** – Firefighters, metal plating.

**Hydrogen sulfide** – Furnace workers, sewer workers, refinery workers, tannery workers, glass workers, metal degreasing, miners.

**Lead** – Welders, radiator repair, steamfitters, plumbers, painters, ceramic workers, metal workers, battery makers, brass polishers, burners, cable workers, miners, pottery makers, electroplaters, printers, enamel workers, filling-station attendants, junk-metal refiners, individuals remodeling older homes or buildings and who are sanding the paint.

**Mercury** – Amalgam makers, dentists and dental workers, detonator workers, felt hat makers, laboratory workers, jewelers, thermometer manufacturers, radio equipment workers, electroplaters, printers.

**Methanol** – Bookbinders, bronzers, rubber and plastic cement users, dry cleaners, leather workers, printers, painters (including lacquer and shellac painters), wood workers.

**Methylene chloride** – Paint stripping, furniture and woodwork refinishing, old car repair.

**Mustard gas** – Chemical warfare

**Nitro and amino aromatic compounds** – Dye makers, explosives workers, colored pencil makers, rubber workers, tannery workers, vulcanizers.

**Silica** – Sandblasting.

**Sulfur dioxide** – Cement manufacturing, commercial refrigeration.

**Vinyl chloride** – Flame-retardant widely used in industry; parent compound of PVC, plastic resin used in containers, water hoses, electrical insulation, etc.

**Table 3.2** History and physical examination in diagnosis of coma from poisoning

| | *Most likely poison* |
|---|---|
| **History** | |
| Children | Acetaminophen, aspirin, antihistamines, iron tablets |
| Alcohol ingestion | Ethanol, methanol, sedatives, antidepressants, street drugs |
| Suicide | Barbiturates, antidepressants, ethylene glycol, carbon monoxide, acetaminophen, opiates, benzodiazepines |
| Dry cleaning | Chlorinated compounds, petroleum hydrocarbons |
| Spray painting | Chlorinated compounds, petroleum hydrocarbons |
| Lacquering | Chlorinated hydrocarbons, organic solvents |
| Insecticide use | Chlorinated or cholinesterase inhibitor pesticides |
| Epilepsy | Anticonvulsants |
| **Physical findings** | |
| Odor of breath: | |
|   Acetone | Lacquer, alcohol |
|   Alcohol | Phenols, chloral hydrate, alcohols |
|   Acrid | Paraldehyde, chloral hydrate |
|   Carrots | Cicutoxin (water hemlock) |
|   Coal gas | Carbon monoxide |
|   Cyanide | Bitter almonds |
|   Garlic | Arsine, phosphorus, organophosphates, selenium, thallium |
|   Mothballs | Naphthalene, paradichlorobenzene |
|   Rotten eggs | Hydrogen sulfide, stibine, mercaptans |
|   Wintergreen | methylsalicylate |
| Color of skin and mucous membranes: | |
|   Cyanosis | Aniline, nitrobenzene, nitrates, marking ink, phenacetin, dapsone |
|   Hyperemia | Cyanide, alcohol |
|   Jaundice | Mushrooms, quinacrine, nitro compounds, phosphorus, carbon tetrachloride, acetaminophen, halothane, nitrosamine, Penny royal oil, phenol, thallium, valproic acid |
|   Pallor | Benzene, carbon monoxide |
| Temperature: | |
|   Increased | Dinitrophenol, salicylates, atropine, SSRI, stramonium, thyroid hormone |
|   Decreased | Chloral hydrate, opiates, barbiturates, akee, tricyclic antidepressants, phenothiazines, hypoglycemics |
| Pulse: | |
|   Rapid | Theophylline, amphetamines, cocaine, diet aids/ephedrine |
|   Irregular | Insecticides, tricyclic antidepressants |
|   Slow | Morphine |

*Continued*

*Table 3.2 continued*

| | |
|---|---|
| Respiration: | |
| Kussmaul | Salicylates, acetanilid, cinchophen |
| Increased | Salicylates, dinitrophenol, carbon monoxide, cyanide |
| Wheezing | Cholinesterase inhibitor pesticides |
| Convulsions | Alcohol, insecticides, strychnine, isoniazid, theophylline |
| Vomiting | Any poison |
| Neck stiffness/ rigidity | Strychnine, cocaine, black widow spider bite, amphetamine, lysergic acid diethylamide (LSD), MAOI, phencyclidine (PCP), tricyclic antidepressants and amoxapine, maprotiline, bupropion, tetanus |
| Distension and spasticity of the abdomen | Corrosives |
| Muscular twitchings | Cholinesterase inhibitor pesticides |

## Availability of poisons in the home

(1) Search the patient and the patient's home/immediate surroundings for poison containers.
(2) Check ingestion of food, drink, and medicines.
(3) Contact with insecticides or other agricultural chemicals.
(4) Exposures to fumes, smoke, or gases.
(5) Skin contact with liquids such as insecticides or cleaning solvents.

## Review of systems

### *General*

**Breath odor** – Bitter almonds odor: cyanide; garlic odor: arsine, arsenic, phosphorus.

**Decreased blood pressure/orthostasis** – Nitrates, nitrites, nitroglycerin, calcium channel blockers, veratrum, cold wave neutralizer, acetanilid, chlorpromazine, all depressant drugs, antidepressants, quinine, volatile oils, aconite, disulfiram, iron salts, methyl bromide, arsine, arsenic, fluorides, phosphine, nickel carbonyl, stibine, pargyline, ganglionic blocking agents, food poisoning, boric acid, phosphorus, carbon tetrachloride, Cicuta (water hemlock), Goldenseal.

**Elevated blood pressure** – Epinephrine or substitutes, veratrum, ergot, sassafras, ephedra, cortisone, vanadium, lead, nicotine, tranylcypromine, phencyclidine, iproniazid and related drugs.

**Fast pulse** – Potassium bromate, iron salts, atropine, cocaine, theophylline, amphetamines, sassafras (false helebore), ephedra.

**Hyperthermia** – Dinitrophenol or other nitrophenols, jimsonweed (stramonium), deadly nightshade (atropine), boric acid, salicylates, excess serotonin agents (SSRIs) usually with another drug causing increased serotonin levels (e.g. monoamine oxidase inhibitor + SSRI), Hypericum (St. John's wort) is a MAOI, thyroid hormone, PCP, cocaine, any anticholinergic agent, atropine, food poisoning, antihistamines, tranquilizers, camphor, oral podophyllum, ehedra.

**Hypothermia** – Akee, barbiturates, vasodilators, opiates and alcohol.

**Lethargy, weakness** – Lead, arsenic, mercury, chlorinated organic compounds, thiazide diuretics, organic phosphates, nicotine, thallium, nitrites, fluorides, botulism, Kalmia (mountain laurel), selenium, hydrazine sulfate, magnesium.

**Loss of appetite** – Trinitrotoluene.

**Slow or irregular pulse** – Veratrum (false hellebore), Zygadenus (wild onion), Digitalis, mushrooms, oleander, nitrites, Pholfadendron or Viscaceae (mistletoe), Cicuta (water hemlock), Goldenseal

**Weight loss** – Any chronic poisoning, but especially lead, arsenic, dinitrophenol, thyroid, mercury, and chlorinated hydrocarbons.

*Skin*

**Burns** – Lye/alkali, acids, hypochlorite, formaldehyde.

**Corrosion or destruction** – Acids or alkalis, permanganate.

**Cyanosis in the absence of respiratory depression or shock** – Methemoglobinemia from aniline, nitrobenzene, acetanilid, phenacetin, nitrates from well water or food, bismuth subnitrate, cloth marking ink (aniline), chloramine-T, nitrites, chlorates, dapsone.

**Dryness** – Atropine and related compounds.

**Edema** – Irritants, chemical sensitivity.

**Jaundice from hemolysis** – Aniline, nitrobenzene, pamaquine, pentaquine, primaquine, benzene, castor beans, jequirity beans, fava beans, phosphine, arsine, nickel carbonyl, copper

**Jaundice from liver injury** – Carbon tetrachloride, chlorinated compounds, arsenic and other heavy metals, chromates, mushrooms, phenothiazines, sulfonamides, chlorpromazine, trinitrotoluene, aniline, thiazide diuretics, iproniazid and related drugs, phosphorus, acetaminophen, comfrey oral, chaparral.

**Loss of hair** – Thallium, arsenic, selenium, DMEA (dihydroepiandrosterone).

**Pallor** – Lead, naphthalene, chlorates, favism, solanine plant poisons, fluorides.

**Rash** – Bromides, sulfonamides, antibiotics, poison ivy or oak, hair preparations, photo developers, salicylates, trinitrotoluene, chromium, phenothiazines, indomethacin, gold salts, chlorinated compounds, *Fagopyrum esculentum* (buckwheat), Chamomile, Dong Quai or Angelica.

**Redness and flushing** – Atropine, antihistamines, tranquilizers, boric acid, cyanide, selenium.

**Sweating** – Organic phosphate insecticides, muscarine and other mushroom poisons, nicotine, sassafras.

## Central nervous system

**Ataxia** – Lead, organic phosphate insecticides, antihistamines, thallium, barbiturates, Valerian, Tea tree oil (oral).

**Deafness or disturbances of equilibrium** – Streptomycin, neomycin, quinine, salicylates, aminoglycosides.

**Delirium** – Antihistamines, atropine/scopolamine and related drugs, amantidine, bromides, camphorated oil, lead, *Cannabis sativa* (marihuana), carbon monoxide, quinacrine, ergot, santonin, rauwolfia, salicylates, DDT, clordane, barbiturates, boric acid, lithium, 'caines such as lidocaine', lead, salicylates, alcohol withdrawal, disulfiram, cimetidine (especially if renal dysfunction or elderly).

**Depression, drowsiness, or coma** (Table 3.2) – Barbiturates or other hypnotics, alcohols, solvents, kerosene, antihistamines, insecticides or rodenticides, atropine or related drugs, cationic detergents, arsenic, mercury, lead, opium and derivatives, paraldehyde, cyanides, carbon monoxide, phenol, salicylates, chlorpromazine, akee, hypoglycemia from oral hypoglycemic drugs, boric acid, naphthalene, digitalis, mushrooms, metatonin, gamma butyrolactone (multiple brand names) and gamma hydroxybutyrate (GHB), Taxus (yew) *Cicuta maculata* (water hemlock).

**Headache** – Nitroglycerin, nitrates, nitrites, hydralazine, trinitrotoluene, indomethacin, carbon monoxide, organic phosphate insecticides, atropine, lead, carbon tetrachloride, glutamates.

**Mental change or confusion** – Thallium, lead, mercury, alcohol, atropine, nicotine, antihistamines, carbon tetrachloride, digitalis, mushrooms, salicylates, barbiturates, tranquilizers, gamma butyrolactone (multiple brand names) and gamma hydroxybutyrate (GHB).

**Muscular twitchings and convulsions** – Insecticides, strychnine and brucine, camphor, atropine, cyanides, ethylene glycol, nicotine, black widow spider, salicylates, theophylline, amphetamine and other stimulants, boric acid, lead, mercury, phenothiazines, antihistamines, arsenic, kerosene, fluorides, nitrites, barbiturates, digitalis, solanine, thallium.

**Paresthesias** – Lead, thallium, DDT.

**Psychosis (hallucinations) or agitation** – Withdrawal from alcohol, PCP or phencyclidine, LSD, amphetamine, cocaine, SSRIs, adrenal glucocorticoids (steroids), mercury, ephedrine, phenypropanolamine, theophylline, ganglionic blocking agents, Cicuta (water hemlock or cowbane), Peyote cactus, sassafras, hydrazine sulfate.

*Eyes*

**Blurred vision** – Atropine, physostigmine, phosphate ester insecticides, cocaine, solvents, dinitrophenol, nicotine, methanol, indomethacin, botulism.

**Colored vision** – Digitalis.

**Contracted pupils** – Opiates and related drugs, nicotine, clonidine, phenothiazines, physostigmine and related drugs, pilocarpine, organophosphate, carbamate, valproate, insecticides, mushrooms and other plant poisons.

**Dilated pupils** – Atropine and related drugs, amphetamines, cocaine, LSD, glutehimide, nicotine, solvents, depressants, antihistamines, monoamine oxidase inhibitors, tricyclic antidepressants, phenylephrine, mushrooms, thallium, oleander, Abrus (rosary pea) if chewed.

**Double vision** – Alcohol, barbiturates, nicotine, phosphate ester insecticides, botulism.

**Lacrimation** – Organic phosphate insecticides, nicotine, mushrooms.

**Nystagmus** – Barbituratyes, carbamazepine, ethanol, phenytoin, scorpion venom, phencyclidine (PCP).
**Pallor of optic disk** – Quinine, nicotine, carbon disulfide.
**Papilledema** – Lead.
**Pigmented scleras** – Quinacrine, jaundice from hemolysis or liver damage.
**Ptosis** – Botulism, thallium.
**Strabismus** – Botulism, thallium.

*Ears*

**Deafness or disturbances of equilibrium** – Streptomycin, neomycin, quinine, salicylates, aminoglycosides.
**Tinnitus** – Quinine, salicylates, quinidine, indomethacin.

*Nose*

**Anosmia** – Phenol nose drops, chromium.
**Fetornasalis** – Chromium.
**Perforated septum** – Chromium, cocaine.

*Mouth*

**Black line on gums** – Lead, mercury, arsenic, bismuth.
**Dry mouth** – Atropine and related drugs, antihistamines, ephedrine.
**Inflammation of gums** – Lead, mercury, arsenic, bismuth, other heavy metals.
**Loosening of teeth** – Mercury, lead, phosphorus.
**Painful teeth** – Phosphorus, mercury, bismuth.
**Salivation** – Lead, mercury, bismuth, thallium, phosphate ester insecticides, other heavy metals, mushrooms.
**Stomatitis** – Corrosives, thallium, mercury, feverfew.

*Cardiorespiratory system*

**Aspiration pneumonia** – Kerosene, mineral oil, other hydrocarbons.
**Cough** – Smoke, dust, silica, beryllium, hydrocarbons, mercury vapor.
**Palpitations** – Nitrites, nitroglycerin, organic nitrates, potassium bromate.
**Pulmonary edema** – Metal fumes, hydrogen sulfide, irritant gases (e.g. chlorine), morphine and substitutes, methyl bromide, methyl chloride,

beta-blockers, verapamil, paraquat, phosgene, metal fumes, mercury vapor, ethylene glycol, aspirated hydrocarbons.

**Rapid respiration** – Cyanide, atropine, cocaine, carbon monoxide, carbon dioxide, salicylates, chloramine-T, alcohol, amphetamine and other stimulants, mushrooms, oral podophyllum, GHB.

**Respiratory difficulty, including dyspnea on exertion, chest pain, and decreased vital capacity** – Phosphate ester insecticides, salicylates, botulism, nickel carbonyl, black widow spider, scorpion, snakebite, shellfish, fish, tetanus, physostigmine, silicosis, other pneumoconioses, cyanide, carbon monoxide, atropine, strychnine, beryllium, dusts, chloramine-T, alcohol, Goldenseal.

**Slow respiration** – Cyanide, carbon monoxide, barbiturates, opiates, botulism, aconite, magnesium, antihistamines, thallium, fluorides.

**Wheezing** – Phosphate ester insecticides, physostigmine, neostigmine, mushrooms (*Amanita muscaria*), Chamomile.

### Gastrointestinal system

**Activation of peptic ulcer** – Phenylbutazone, salicylates, indomethacin, adrenal corticosteroids.

**Blood in stools** – Coumarin anticoagulants, thallium, iron, salicylates, corrosives, copper.

**Hematemesis** – Corrosive substances, coumarin anticoagulants, aminophylline, fluorides.

**Vomiting, diarrhea, abdominal pain** – Caused by almost all poisons, particularly soaps and detergents, corrosive acids or alkalis, metals, phenols, medicinal irritants, solvents, cold wave neutralizer, food poisoning, black widow spider, boric acid, insecticides, phosphorus, nicotine, fluorides, thallium, solanine and other plant poisons, castor beans, mushrooms, digitalis, oleander, oral podophyllum.

### Genitourinary system

**Anuria** – Mercurials, bismuth, sulfonamides, carbon tetrachloride, formaldehyde, phosphorus, ethylene chlorohydrin, turpentine, oxalic acid, chlordane, castor beans, jequirity beans, trinitrotoluene, chaparral.

**Color of urine** – Coumarin anticoagulants (red), fava beans (red), hepatotoxins (orange).

**Hematuria or hemoglobinuria** – Heavy metals, naphthalene, nitrates, chlorates, favism, solanine and other plant poisons.

**Menstrual irregularities** – Estrogens, lead, bismuth, mercurials, other heavy metals.

**Myoglobinuria** – Phencyclidine (PCP), convulsants, amphetamines.

**Oliguria** – Lead.

**Proteinuria** – Arsenic, mercury, phosphorus.

*Neuromuscular system*

**Muscle cramps** – Thiazide diuretics, lead, black widow spider.

**Muscle fasciculations** – Phosphate ester and other insecticides, nicotine, black widow spider, scorpion, manganese, shellfish.

**Muscular weakness or paralysis (muscle group or single muscle)** – Lead, arsenic, botulism, poison hemlock, organic mercurials, thallium, triorthocresyl phosphate (in gasoline), DDT, chlordane, shellfish, carbon disulfide, other insecticides, arnica.

**Tremors, muscle stiffness** – Phenothiazines.

*Endocrine system*

**Breast enlargement and/or tenderness** – Estrogens, gingseng.

**Decreased libido** – Lead, mercury, other heavy metals, sympathetic blocking agents.

*Laboratory examination of blood*

**Anemia** – Lead, naphthalene, chlorates, favism, solanine and other plant poisons, snakebite.

**Anti-platelet/anticoagulant** – warfarin, arnica, feverfew, garlic, ginseng, ginger, ginkgo, red clover, gamma linoleic acid.

**Cherry-red color** – Carbon monoxide, cyanide.

**Chocolate color (methemoglobin)** – Nitrates, nitrites, aniline, dyes, and chlorates.

### Blood, serum, or plasma chemistry

(See tables at the ends of chapters for toxic blood levels of chemicals and drugs.)

**Bromide** – Serum chloride is spuriously increased in bromism because the standard tests (e.g. AutoAnalyzer) measure total halides.

**Glucose (whole blood)** – Increased after thiazide diuretics or adrenal glucocorticoids; decreased after salicylates, lead, or ethanol.

**Potassium (serum or plasma)** – Decreased after salicylates, thiazide diuretics, adrenal glucocorticoids, excessive rhubarb ingestion, oral podophyllum.

**Uric acid (serum)** – Increased after thiazide diuretics or ethanol.

### Special chemical examinations useful in diagnosis of poisoning

Special chemical examinations for lead or other heavy metals, insecticides, cholinesterase, barbiturates, alkaloids, etc. may be necessary in the differential diagnosis of poisoning. The following laboratories are suggested for the performance of such analyses. (It is wise to make prior arrangements with the laboratory to ensure that it will accept samples for analysis.)

**City, county, or state police laboratory** – Blood alcohol, barbiturates, other poisons.

**County coroner's laboratory** – Heavy metals, blood alcohol, barbiturates, alkaloids.

**County hospital laboratory** – Lead, barbiturates, alkaloids, blood alcohol.

**Federal Bureau of Investigation Laboratory, Washington, DC**

**Private laboratories** – Heavy metals and barbiturates.

**State Departments of Public Health** – These offices usually perform analyses relating only to cases of occupational poisoning (e.g., insecticides, heavy metals).

**State toxicologist's office** – Heavy metals, blood alcohol, barbiturates, alkaloids. Analyses associated with criminal poisonings.

**Toxicology Laboratory, Pesticides Program, Food and Drug Administration, US Public Health Service, Atlanta 30333** – Insecticides in body fat, blood cholinesterase. (They will send sample containers on request by physicians.)

'Toxic screens' should not be requested when evaluating a suspected chronic poisoning. Many such screens are intended only to detect drugs of abuse, and even those with broader coverage may have poor sensitivity and specificity. However, specific laboratory tests for ethanol, methanol, ethylene glycol, acetaminophen, iron, lithium, salicylates, digitalis, theophylline, and methemoglobin may be critical when poisoning with these drugs is suspected, because test results influence therapy. Remember that the most useful test is one whose result is likely to have an impact on therapy.

## SUBSTANCE DEPENDENCY (drugs of abuse)

The most common drug of abuse is alcohol. For other abused drugs see Chapter 28. Another potentially toxic group of products are sold as 'dietary supplements', 'sleeping agents' or as 'body building' agents. These products are CNS and respiratory depressants sold under such names as GHB, Renew, Trient, Revivarant, Blue Nitro, Firewater, and Serenity. They contain chemicals such as gamma-butyrolactone (GBL), gamma-hydroxybutyric acid (GHB), and 1,4 butanediol (BD). GBL and BD have caused at least 145 serious cases, including eight deaths. There have probably been far more toxic reactions to these agents than those known about since many cases go unreported. When taken in combination with other CNS depressants, such as alcohol, they are potentially lethal. GHB has been implicated as a 'date rape' drug, just as flunitrazepam (Rohypnol, Noriel also known as Roofie, La Roche, and the forget pill). These agents cause CNS and respiratory depression in typical doses and death in higher dosages.

The signs and symptoms of drug abuse can be confusing (see index for specific agents), and correct diagnosis depends on a high index of suspicion. Confirmation of the diagnosis can be aided by laboratory tests to detect drugs in urine and blood, but often these tests do not help medical management. In most cases, immediate symptomatic medical management is simple but long-term management to prevent recurrence is far more difficult. Secondary complications, e.g. subacute bacterial endocarditis, hepatic talc granulomatosis, wound botulism, and AIDS in association with intravenous drug abuse present continued challenges for treatment.

## References

Bryson PD. *Comprehensive Review in Toxicology for Emergency Clinicians*, 3rd edn. Taylor & Francis, 1996

Druid H, Holmgren P. A compilation of fatal and control concentrations of drugs in postmortem femoral blood. *J Forensic Sci* 1996;42:79

Ellenhorn MJ, *et al. Ellenhorn's Medical Toxicology,* 2nd edn. Williams & Wilkins, 1997

Goldfrank LR, *et al.*, eds. *Goldfrank's Toxicologic Emergencies.* Appleton & Lange, 1998

Haddad LM, *et al.*, eds. *Clinical Management of Poisoning and Drug Overdose*, 3rd edn. WB Saunders, 1998

Hardman JG, *et al.*, eds. *Goodman and Gilman's The Pharmacological Basis of Therapeutics,* 9th edn. McGraw-Hill, 1996

Jellin JM, ed. *Natural Medicines Comprehensive Database.* Therapeutic Research Faculty, 1999

Jenkins DH. Substance abuse and withdrawal in the intensive care unit. *Surg Clin N Am* 2000;80:1033

Kacew S, Lambert GH, eds. *Environmental Toxicology and Pharmacology of Human Development.* Taylor & Francis, 1997

Kaminski CA, *et al.* Sertraline intoxication in a child. *Ann Emerg Med* 1994;23: 1371–4

Karakayli G, *et al.* Exfoliative dermatitis. *Am Family Physician* 1999;59:625

Klaassen CD, *et al.*, eds. *Casarett and Doull's Toxicology: The Basic Science of Poisons,* 6th edn. Macmillan, 2001

Leikin JB, Paloucek FP, eds. *Poisoning and Toxicology Handbook.* Lexi-Comp, 1995

Li J, *et al.* A tale of novel intoxication: a review of the effects of gamma-hydroxybutyric acid with recommendations for management. *Ann Emerg Med* 1998;31:729

Loomis TA, Hayes AW. *Loomis's Essentials of Toxicology,* 4th edn. Academic Press, 1996

Lu FC. *Basic Toxicology.* Taylor & Francis, 1996

McGuffin M, *et al.*, eds. *Botanical Safety Handbook.* CRC Press, 1997

Miara J. Rohypnol, the 'date rape' drug. *Psychopharmacology Update* 1996;7:3

Mills KC. Serotonin toxicity: a comprehensive review for emergency medicine. *Top Emerg Med* 1993;15:54–73

Olson KR, *et al.*, eds. *Poisoning & Drug Overdose.* Appleton & Lange, 1999

Rea WJ. *Chemical Sensitivity,* 4 vols. CRC Lewis, 1992–1996

Repetto MR, Repetto M. Habitual, toxic, and lethal concentrations of 103 drugs of abuse in humans. *J Toxicol Clin Toxicol* 1997;35:1

Repetto MR, Repetto M. Therapeutic, toxic, and lethal concentrations in human fluids of 90 drugs affecting the cardiovascular and hematopoietic systems. *J Toxicol Clin Toxicol* 1996;35:345

Repetto MR, Repetto M. Therapeutic, toxic, and lethal concentrations of 73 drugs affecting respiratory system in human fluids. *J Toxicol Clin Toxicol* 1998;36:287

Ryan RP, Terry CE. *Toxicology Desk Reference*, 4th edn, 3 vols. Taylor & Francis, 1997–1998

Turner NJ, Szczawinski AF. *Common Poisonous Plants and Mushrooms of North America*. Timber Press, 1991

Wexler P, *et al*., eds. *Encyclopedia of Toxicology*, 3 vols. Academic Press, 1998

# 4    Management of poisoning

Apart from the specific measures directed at the poison itself (emesis, charcoal, antidotes, lavage, etc.), the management of most severe poisonings involves control of the symptoms and effects of poisoning (pain, fluid imbalance, acid/base disturbance, etc.). Equipment, medications, and trained personnel must be readily available to provide supportive care and specific treatment. Emergency care begins with maintaining airway, supporting respiration, and instituting cardiac resuscitation if necessary.

## HYPOXIA AND DEPRESSED RESPIRATION

Hypoxia occurring during coma, unconsciousness, convulsions, or muscular paralysis with depressed or absent breathing requires immediate resuscitation, with the administration of air or $O_2$ until normal respiration returns. Do not wait for the arrival of equipment before beginning artificial respiration. Resuscitation with oxygen equipment is becoming increasingly complex, requiring practice with the available equipment. **Loss of airway or inadequate ventilation is the most common cause of serious morbidity or death in poisoning.**

### Airway

When a patient becomes unconscious from a poison, oropharyngeal muscular relaxation, laryngeal spasm, laryngeal edema, or tracheobronchial secretions frequently impair the airway. Establishing and maintaining an adequate airway is the most critical life-saving intervention.

Place the patient in left side down, head down position so vomitus is less likely to be aspirated.

Aspirate mucus, vomitus, saliva, blood, etc. from nose and pharynx by means of a soft rubber catheter with a syringe, finger sweep, or Magill forceps.

Place head in 'sniffing position – neck extended' (unless neck injury suspected).

Apply 'jaw thrust maneuver', which prevents tongue from obstructing airway.

Insert an endotracheal tube if adequately trained personnel are available. A cuffed endotracheal tube provides the best airway protection and can be used to provide 100% oxygen. However, the procedure has risks, especially for the inexperienced.

## Artificial respiration

Artificial respiration methods vary considerably in their ability to provide adequate tidal air. The simple back-pressure methods may not be effective in deep coma due to drug poisoning because of abdominal muscle paralysis, weakness or rigidity. Direct inflation is superior to other types of artificial respiration.

### Artificial respiration by direct inflation

Direct inflation of the victim's lungs from the operator's mouth is especially useful when there is an obstruction to the free passage of air and no equipment is available. The method requires less effort and allows the operator to watch the patient's chest rise and fall to evaluate effectiveness. Mechanical aids (oropharyngeal airways) may prevent pharyngeal obstruction by the victim's tongue. Inflate at a rate of 15 times per minute in an adult to maintain adequate oxygenation.

If mouth-to-mouth resuscitation fails, check for foreign body obstruction. Roll the victim onto the left side, with head down, and deliver a sharp blow between the shoulder blades. If this measure also fails, use the Heimlich procedure. If an experienced person is available, perform endotracheal intubation.

Give lung inflation by mouth-to-mouth breathing (keeping patient's nostrils pinched/closed) or mouth-to-nose breathing (keeping patient's mouth closed), 15 times per minute – allowing about 2 seconds for inspiration and 3 seconds for expiration – until spontaneous respiration returns. Allow the victim to exhale passively or assist exhalation by pressure on the chest. The operator should be taking their next breath while listening to the sound of the victim's exhalation. Observe rise and fall of the chest, avoiding excessive pressure that may cause gastric distension and subsequent regurgitation. When oxygen is available, always ventilate using 100% oxygen. If equipment is limited to a simple facemask, then high flow (at least 15 l/min) is necessary. For optimum ventilation, use a facemask that has a reservoir (non-rebreather mask and bag).

## Reference

Perkin RM, Van Stralen D. My child can't breathe. *J Emerg Med Serv* 1999;24:43

## Equipment

**Oropharyngeal airway**: This is a curved and flattened plastic or rubber-covered metal device that fits over the curve of the tongue and allows air to pass freely to the pharynx. Small, medium, and large sizes should be available.

**Laryngoscopes**: These are used for exposing the glottis in order to insert an endotracheal airway. They are available in adult, pediatric, and infant sizes. They consist of a handle and a removable blade that can be either straight (Miller) or curved (McIntosh). The handle holds a battery-powered light to visualize the glottis. Always check the battery and make sure the light bulb is not loose before performing intubation.

**Endotracheal airways**: Plain catheters and catheters with inflatable cuffs should be available. Most operators use a malleable stylet within the tube to facilitate insertion of the tube into the larynx and trachea. To avoid injury the stylet must be held in a position so it does not stick out the tracheal end of the tube. While the endotracheal airway is in place, constant supervision is necessary. Foreign bodies must be removed from the mouth and the pharynx before placing the endotracheal airway.

**Suction device**: Use a mechanical suction machine with tubing and traps, or a hand-operated aspirator.

**Syringe and catheter for aspiration**: Use a syringe with a soft rubber catheter for clearing the airway. Aspiration should be done using sterile precautions. Mechanical suction devices can cause tracheal injury.

Emergency use of these procedures requires prior training and familiarity with the equipment.

## PULMONARY EDEMA

Pulmonary edema resulting from poisoning is usually due to the inhalation of irritants, e.g. chlorine gas, with injury to the pulmonary epithelium followed by exudation into the alveoli. Parasympathetic stimulants or cholinesterase inhibitors (phosphate esters) increase bronchial secretion and stimulate pulmonary edema. Overdoses of opiates may cause pulmonary edema.

Pulmonary edema is dangerous because it interferes with $O_2$ exchange in the lungs and patients eventually drown in their own secretions.

### Clinical findings

Symptoms and signs of pulmonary edema include dyspnea, rales (crackles) at the bases of or throughout the lungs, cyanosis, and rapid respiration. In extreme cases gurgling respirations and foaming at the mouth may occur. Patients in respiratory distress often appear anxious, often prefer to be upright, not supine.

### Treatment

#### *Emergency measures*

(1) Relieve anxiety. Give morphine sulfate to decrease rate of rapid, inefficient respiration.
(2) Administer supplemental oxygen to maintain arterial oxygenation of at least 60–70 mmHg.
(3) Intubate patient and use positive end-expiratory pressure (PEEP) ventilation if necessary.
(4) If pulmonary edema is the result of opiate toxicity, give antidote, naloxone.

#### *General measures*

(1) Diuresis (furosemide, 20–80 mg intravenously) is helpful because it reduces fluid volume. Do not inject at a rate faster than 10 mg/min.
(2) Consider a corticosteroid, e.g. IV methylprednisolone (controversial).
(3) If pulmonary edema is the result of heart failure, then pulmonary artery cannulation and wedge pressure may be necessary to guide therapy.
(4) Reassurance and having the patient in a sitting position relieves anxiety.

## CIRCULATORY FAILURE, OR SHOCK

### Clinical findings

**Primary shock**: (Fainting or collapse with low blood pressure.) This type of immediate collapse results from cerebral anoxia and is also termed 'vasovagal reaction'. The initial event, which results in low blood pressure and circulatory insufficiency, may be a painful stimulus, injury, or an unpleasant odor. Medications and chemicals that lower blood pressure (anesthetics, nitrites) can result in collapse. Response to treatment is usually rapid, but unless treatment is prompt, there may be progression into secondary shock.

**Secondary shock (delayed or refractory shock)**: Signs of secondary shock are cold, pale, cyanotic skin; sweating; rapid pulse; and low blood pressure. Secondary shock may develop in almost any type of severe poisoning but is especially common after poisoning with corrosive substances or depressant drugs.

### *Laboratory findings*

The hematocrit may reveal hemoconcentration. Urinalysis may show proteinuria and/or hematuria. Measurement of serum osmolality and osmolar gap helps determine whether acidosis is due to accumulation of lactic acid (as a result of hypoxia, e.g. carbon monoxide poisoning or from agents that cause seizures) or due to agents which result in accumulation of other acid ions (acetone, ethanol, ethylene glycol, diabetic ketoacidosis, mannitol, metaldehyde, methanol, renal failure) an elevated anion gap suggests lactic acidosis. However, a combination elevated anion and osmolar gaps suggests poisoning by ethylene glycol, methanol, salicylate or severe alcohol or diabetic acidosis. Less commonly observed is a narrow anion gap. This may occur with agents that increase sodium chloride levels (e.g. bromide, lithium, nitrate).

### Treatment

### *Emergency measures*

(1)  Place patient in the shock position, i.e. supine with the feet elevated.
(2)  Establish and maintain an adequate airway.
(3)  Establish venous access and begin continuous electrocardiographic (ECG) monitoring. Place a central line once initial resuscitation is completed.

(4)   Restore and maintain adequate circulating blood volume. Estimate fluid requirements from the history and findings of vomiting, diarrhea, sweating, blood loss, and blood pressure. Elevated hematocrit indicates volume depletion. Place an 18-gauge (or larger – 14–16-gauge) venous catheter and start intravenous 0.9% saline. Give a fluid challenge of 10–20 ml/kg over 30–60 min if blood pressure is <80 mmHg. If systolic pressure is >80 mmHg, an infusion rate of 100–200 ml/h is sufficient. Dextrose 5% in saline (D5NS) can be used if 0.9% saline is not available.

(5)   Obtain blood for laboratory studies (can be obtained as soon as initial venous access is established).

(6)   In hypotensive patients, place a Foley catheter to monitor urine output and manage fluid resusitation. Save urine for toxicology studies.

(7)   Blood (packed red blood cells) may be required for volume replacement.

(8)   Maintain body temperature by application of blankets. Do not apply external heat, since this causes peripheral warming resulting in core cooling that aggravates shock.

(9)   Relieve pain. Give morphine sulfate for pain unless the patient is unconscious or stuporous. Do not use morphine in patients with depressed respiration unless personnel and equipment to maintain respiration are immediately available.

(10)   For hypotension not relieved by fluid therapy, give dopamine 5–10 µg/kg/min. As the rate of administration is increased, cardiac output increases and renal blood flow decreases. When the dose exceeds 10 µg/kg/min, the primary effect of dopamine is stimulation of alpha-adrenergic receptors that cause increased vasoconstriction. Adverse effects include tachyarrhythmias and peripheral/renal/splanchnic vasoconstriction at higher doses. Dopamine may be ineffective when patients have depleted catecholamine stores (tricyclic antidepressants, reserpine, disulfiram). Amrinone and milrinone are newer ionotropic drugs.

(11)   Alternatively, use norepinephrine (Levophed) 0.1 µg/kg/min IV. The usual starting dose as infusion is 0.5–1.0 µg/min; average adult dose is 2–12 µg/min; maximum dose is 30 µg/min. Do not administer via a peripheral line, as extravasation will cause tissue necrosis. If the patient has a central line, other inotropic agents such as dobutamine can be used.

*General measures*

(1) Correct anoxia/hypoxia.
(2) Correct or replace inadequate blood circulatory volume.
(3) Correct acidosis.
(4) Observe constantly.

## CONGESTIVE HEART FAILURE (CHF)

Poisons that produce myocardial damage will secondarily cause congestive failure.

### Clinical findings

Symptoms and signs include dyspnea, pulmonary edema, cardiac enlargement, high venous pressure, and dependent edema.

### Treatment

*General measures*

(1) Rest should be in bed or in a chair, with use of a bedside commode rather than a bedpan unless dyspnea is severe.
(2) Sodium restriction aids in reduction of retained fluid. Rapid diuresis may be helpful. Give IV diuretic (furosemide). When converting to the oral dosage, approximately twice the threshold (effective) IV dose is necessary. Hepatic congestion from CHF may necessitate dosage adjustment. If diuretics are given, avoid hyponatremia by restricting free water consumption. Do not institute severe sodium restriction unless the ability of the kidneys to conserve sodium is known.

*Digitalis*

Digitalis does not have a place in the treatment of acute CHF. It is sometimes used to control the ventricular response to atrial fibrillation; however, it does not prevent tachycardia from adrengeric stimulation. Beta-blockers such as esmolol are used to block excess adrenergic activity. Central venous and pulmonary artery pressure can be measured if central IV access can be obtained. Thus, sophisticated treatment of CHF is possible and drugs specific to target the mechanism responsible for CHF can be employed by intensive care physicians (afterload (ACE inhibitors), preload (diuretics), heart rate (beta blockers), etc.).

This book focuses on acute treatment and stabilization; other resources are available to manage chronic conditions.

## CARDIAC ARREST

Cardiac arrest may occur as a result of general anesthesia, asphyxia from carbon monoxide or other gases, inhalation of chlorinated hydrocarbons, injection of local anesthetic agents, accidental ingestion or overdose of cardiac drugs, asphyxia from pulmonary edema following the inhalation of irritants, or drug idiosyncrasy (especially quinidine, procaine or other local anesthetics, procainamide, aminophylline, and iodides). For anyone in the USA involved in emergency medicine, taking the Advanced Cardiac Life Support (ACLS) class (American Heart Association) is a practical method of keeping up to date in the treatment of cardiac arrest.

### Clinical findings

A presumptive diagnosis of cardiac arrest is made when pulse and blood pressure suddenly disappear and no heart sounds are audible on auscultation. The ECG may indicate ventricular fibrillation, classic ST segment changes, or may be normal. Myocardial infarction can occur in the absence of coronary artery disease. Cocaine toxicity can cause a marked disparity between oxygen supply and demand resulting in ischemia and infarction. Most cardiac deaths from poisoning occur suddenly owing to electrical instability. However, if ischemia is suspected and immediately treated, death can be prevented.

### Treatment

Training in the use of cardiac resuscitation is mandatory. When a patient collapses and unresponsiveness is verified, the American Heart Association recommends to 'Call First', get AED (automatic external defibrillation) if available, start basic life support (BLS) – **A**irway, **B**reathing, **C**ardiac (ABCs) etc. However, if the collapse was obviously due to choking/airway obstruction, then the prudent intervention would be to start the airway and breathing interventions of basic first aid. If it was not obviously due to choking, then it most likely represents cardiac/ventricular fibrillation. The critical life-saving intervention is defibrillation. The 'Call First' recommendation reduces the amount of time it takes to get the defibrillator to the patient. If there is no readily available telephone or others to obtain help, then the rescuer must use common sense, give 1–2 precordial thumps, and start CPR (cardiopulmonary resuscitation). The old recommendations of continuing CPR until help arrives or one is exhausted are too stringent, as CPR will not maintain adequate cerebral blood flow for hours. The recommendation is to continue for at least 10–15 minutes.

### References

Ballew KA. Cardiopulmonary resuscitation. *Br Med J* 1997;314:1462

Cummins, RO, ed. *Textbook of Advanced Cardiac Life Support,* 2nd edn. American Heart Association, 1994

Hallstrom A, *et al.* Cardiopulmonary resuscitation by chest compression alone or with mouth-to-mouth ventilation. *N Engl J Med* 2000;342:1546

Hazinski MF, Cummins RO, Field JM, eds. 2000 *Handbook of Emergency Cardiovascular Care for Healthcare Providers*. American Heart Association, 2000

Pertab D. Basic life support techniques in adults. *Prof Nurse* 1999;15:37

Saissy J-M, *et al.* Efficacy of continuous insufflation of oxygen combined with active cardiac compression-decompression during out-of-hospital cardio-respiratory arrest. *Anesthesiology* 2000;92:1523

Zaritsky AL. Recent advances in pediatric cardiopulmonary resuscitation and advanced life support. *New Horizons* 1998;6:201

## CENTRAL NERVOUS SYSTEM INVOLVEMENT

### CONVULSIONS

Drugs and chemicals cause convulsions by direct effect on the central nervous system, in response to the stimulation of peripheral receptors (e.g., the carotid sinus), by oxygen deprivation, by inducing hypoglycemia, and by inducing hyponatremia. Convulsions can be dangerous if accompanied by hypoxia; if hypoxia does not occur, secondary effects are rare. In the case of poisoning, convulsions are a major cause of morbidity and mortality because they can result in anoxia, aspiration, and/or coma and because they can be difficult to treat (due to severe metabolic acidosis). Antidotes that cause central nervous system or respiratory depression must be used cautiously (e.g. phenobarbital). Shorter acting benzodiazepines are preferable. Diazepam and lorazepam are most commonly used. Succinylcholine is also used, but ordinarily only by those trained in anesthesiology and only when absolutely necessary.

Theophylline-induced seizures, are associated with significant metabolic abnormalities, including hypokalemia, hypophosphatemia, hyperglycemia and severe acidosis. In addition to giving anticonvulsants, beta-blockers are useful to treat the beta-adrenergic stimulation. In isoniazid-induced seizures, intravenous pyridoxine (vitamin $B_6$) is a specific antidote. For carbamate- or organophosphate insecticide-induced seizures, pralidoxime or atropine is used.

Substances that act primarily on the cerebrum (e.g. amphetamine, caffeine, and atropine) cause hyperactivity, restlessness, and mania. Substances that act primarily on the brain stem, e.g. pentylenetetrazol and picrotoxin, cause clonic convulsions. Strychnine acts primarily on the spinal cord to produce tonic extensor spasms. Other agents such as veratrum, cyanide, and nicotine may cause convulsions by a combination of reflex, central nervous system, and anoxic effects.

## Emergency treatment

Regardless of etiology, emergency treatment is the same: suppress the convulsion, determine the diagnosis or etiology of the seizure, and institute specific antidote if available.

(1)  Keep the patient in quiet, darkened surroundings and limit unnecessary procedures.

(2)  Do not attempt emesis or gastric lavage while the patient is twitching or hyperirritable unless the airway is controlled and removal of poison is imperative. Remember, if it has been $\geq 60$ minutes from time of ingestion, the benefit of lavage is minimal and focus should be on gut decontamination or facilitating renal excretion.

(3)  Maintain airway, assist ventilation, and protect patient from injury.

(4)  Administer naloxone if seizures are from narcotic-induced hypoxia.

(5)  Administer thiamine 100 mg IV.

(6) Administer 50 ml of 50% dextrose (25 g); in children 2 ml/kg of dextrose 25% unless it is definitely determined that hypoglycemia is not present.

(7) Maintain hydration by oral or intravenous fluid administration. The urine output should be 1–3 l/d.

(8) Reduce elevated temperature by using tepid sponges.

(9) Remove secretions from the pharynx by suction.

(10) Give positive-pressure respiration with $O_2$ during convulsions.

(11) Consider administering an anticonvulsant. Rapid administration of an anticonvulsant can cause hypotension, respiratory or cardiac arrest, therefore close monitoring is necessary.

**Drugs for the control of convulsions**

*Benzodiazepines*

**Diazepam (Valium)**: Give 0.1–0.2 mg/kg IV at 1 mg/min. Less depression of respiration compared to barbiturates. May be given rectally if no IV access. Not effective in all types of convulsions.

**Phenytoin (Dilantin)**: Give 2–5 mg/kg IV over 30 min. Maximum dose, 1 g. Little depression of respiration. Effect lasts 12 h. Does not work for theophylline-induced seizures. Rapid administration dangerous.

**Phenobarbital sodium**: Give 1–1.5 mg/kg IV over 20 min. Maximum dose: 5 mg/kg. Effect lasts 12–24 h. Causes severe persistent respiratory depression in overdoses.

**Midazolam**: Give 0.1–0.2 mg/kg IM or 0.05–0.1 mg/kg IV. IM route an advantage if no IV access and not possible to administer diazepam rectally.

**Lorazepam**: Give 0.05–0.1 mg/kg IV. Less respiratory depression, may be given rectally if no IV access. Not effective in all types of seizures.

**Thiopental sodium (Pentothal sodium)**: Give 2.5% sterile solution IV slowly. Maximum dose: 0.5 ml/kg. Good minute-to-minute control. Can be given during convulsions. Doses larger than recommended may cause persistent respiratory depression.

*Neuromuscular blocking agents*

Succinylcholine is the most powerful anticonvulsant, because it causes complete paralysis. This drug can only be used when the physician is able to completely control respiration and ventilation. For adults, give 10–50 mg IV slowly and maintain adequate oxygenation/ventilation. Pediatric doses are 1.0 mg/kg for children, 2.0 mg/kg for infants. Repeat as necessary; this will control convulsions of any type, but the effect usually lasts only 1–5 minutes. Intubation and placement on a ventilator is commonly done. All equipment for intubation and trained providers must be present before giving the drug. Adverse reactions include vagolytic effects (bradycardia, AV block, asystole), and pediatric patients are more suspect. Other neuromuscular blockers can be used if preferred by the treating physician (atracurium besylate, cisatracurium besylate, pancuronium bromide, rocuronium bromide, vecuronium bromide).

## COMA

Coma due to poisoning results from interference with brain cell function or metabolism. Administering stimulants to treat poison-induced coma is not effective; it is contraindicated. The exact mechanism of action of central nervous system stimulants is unknown, but these drugs presumably act by depressing some inhibiting function in the cell. There is no evidence that any stimulant specifically opposes the cellular effects induced by depressant drugs (barbiturates) or poisons.

### Management of coma

Institute basic and advanced life support: airway, breathing, circulation. The patient must be observed constantly until consciousness returns. The following are specific interventions to perform and items to monitor with accurate, legible documentation. Include in the record measurements, if indicated, and the clock-time of all observations, measurements, treatments, outcomes, etc. This is important, especially if future litigation is a possibility.

(1) Record temperature, pulse, respiration, blood pressure.
(2) Observe state of consciousness – vocalization, laryngeal stridor.
(3) Observe skin color – cyanosis, pallor, and lividity.
(4) Auscultate lungs (pulmonary edema) and suction secretions.
(5) Obtain reflexes (corneal, papillary, gag, patellar, and superficial pain).
(6) Measure urine output – catheterize for accurate measurement to guide fluid resuscitation and monitor renal function. Save specimen for toxicology studies.

(7) Establish intravenous access to administer medications and treat shock. Administer 50 ml of 50% dextrose (in children 2 ml/kg of dextrose 25%) unless hypoglycemia is definitely ruled out. Avoid excessive fluid administration, to prevent cerebral edema.

(8) Treat shock.

(9) After intubation do gastric lavage with activated charcoal (see p. 31–32) if indicated. Gastric lavage performed more than 4 h after poisoning is will not prevent absorption, but may hasten excretion.

(10) Every 30 minutes reposition the patient, massage skin and aspirate airway. Maintain the patient in the horizontal position unless hypotension indicates a need for the shock position.

(11) Monitor for infection; treat with organism-specific antibiotics.

(12) Provide adequate hydration.

(13) If coma continues for more than 48 h and renal function is adequate, then provide nutritional support; external is preferable to intravenous route..

(14) If muscle weakness and electrocardiograph changes suggest hypokalemia, give potassium chloride either via enteral or intravenous supplementation. Do not give potassium in the presence of acute renal failure without laboratory determination of the precise degree of serum potassium deficiency.

### *Special measures*

If coma is a result of poisoning or drug toxicity, consider hemodialysis if the agent is dialyzable.

## HYPERACTIVITY, DELIRIUM, AND MANIA

Hyperactivity and delirium can occur in severe poisoning and complicate treatment. Delirium is characterized by lack of orientation (person, place, time, etc.). In addition, the patient is uncooperative, incoherent and may be hyperactive. Delirious patients may exhibit psychosis, characterized by illusions, delusions, or hallucinations. A manic patient is hyperactive and often psychotic. Their thoughts and speech may be illogical, fast, and hard to follow. Delusions are 'fixed, firm, false beliefs' (thoughts and beliefs or scenarios that the patient absolutely believes are true). A delusion may be entirely plausible (patient is convinced his partner is having an affair). Hallucinations may be auditory (voices heard only by the patient), visual, tactile, or sensory. The patient is absolutely convinced these perceptions are real, therefore history from friends, family, co-workers may be important to determine the facts.

## Treatment

Protect the patient from physical injury. Lock screens, bar windows, and remove furniture. Place in a quiet, dark room with padded walls (if available) and reduce any external stimulation. Reassure the patient. Use calm, quiet language. If relatives and friends remain calm, then their presence may reduce apprehension. Maintain adequate supervision. Monitor vital signs. If hyperthermia exists, only trained personnel should administer wet packs.

## Causes of delirium or psychosis or coma

(1)   Fever or hyperthermia, metabolic derangement, or excess salicylates.

(2)   Anticholinergic and antihistamine drugs (amantidine, antidepressants, phenothiazines etc).

(3)   Neurologic medications, carbamazepine, levodopa, lithium, valproate.

(4)   CNS depressants, barbiturates, benzodiazepines, ethanol/alcohol.

(5)   Substances of recreational abuse, gamma hydroxybutyric acid (GHB), opiates, phencyclidine.

(6)   Disulfiram interaction with alcohol and drugs or chemicals that when taken in combination with ethanol cause a disulfiram reaction. (metronidazole)

(7)   Anti-infective agents: amantidine, cefoperazone, moxalactam, cefotetan, chloramphenicol, diethylthiocarbamate, furazolidone, griseofulvin, metronidazole, quinacrine, nitrofurantoin.

(8)   Oral hypoglycemic agents: acetohexamide, chlorpropamide, glipizide, glyburide, tolazamide, tolbutamide.

(9)   Industrial chemicals: 4-bromopyrazole, carbon disulfide, hydrogen sulfide, tetraethyl lead, pyrogallol.

(10)  Miscellaneous agents: butanol oxime, calcium carbimide, carbon monoxide, clonidine, cyanaide, metyldopa, mushrooms (*Coprinus atramentarius, Clitocybe clavipes*), pargyline, phentolamine, procarbazine, tolazoline.

(11)  Thiamine deficiency, Wernicke–Korsakoff encephalopathy, psychosis.

(12) Withdrawal from alcohol, benzodiazepines, or other sedatives/hypnotics.

## HYPOGLYCEMIA

Coma and convulsions resulting from hypoglycemia occur occasionally from exposure to toxic substances. Since hypoglycemia symptoms are not dependent on the mechanism which decreased blood glucose, the possibility of poisoning should be considered.

The following substances have been reported to induce hypoglycemia:

(1) Alcohol or anesthesia following starvation depresses hepatic gluconeogenesis.
(2) Akee and other plant toxins such as mushrooms are hepatotoxins that depress glycogen storage and gluconeogenesis.
(3) Acetylcholinesterase inhibitors increase parasympathetic release of insulin from the pancreas.
(4) Edetate chelates zinc in slow-release insulin formulations, thus converting the insulin to a quicker-acting product.
(5) In periodic paralysis or after use of sympathomimetic agents, potassium increases the deposition of glycogen in the liver.
(6) Salicylates increase glucose utilization.

### Treatment

Administration of glucose by any route will immediately correct hypoglycemia. In an emergency, give 50% glucose. For prolonged administration, 10–20% glucose should be used. Epinephrine and glucagon can be used.

## GENITOURINARY TRACT INVOLVEMENT

### ACUTE RENAL FAILURE

Acute renal failure with oliguria or anuria may occur in poisoning from (1), chemicals directly toxic to the kidney: aminoglycosides, NSAIDs, *Cortinarius* sp. (mushrooms), cyclosporin, carbon tetrachloride, heavy metals, arsenicals, sulfonamides, ethylene glycol; (2), hemolytic substances:

(naphthalene, benzene, castor bean, etc.); (3), substances that cause myoglobinuria: stimulants, phencyclidine, convulsants, and poisons that cause hyperthermia. Renal failure can occur from prolonged hypovolemia and/or hypotension.

## Clinical and laboratory findings

**Initial period**: The patient may be asymptomatic, with a daily urine output of up to 300–400 ml. Blood pressure may be normal or low. Urine examination reveals hemoglobin, protein, and red blood cells. Serum creatinine increases approximately 1 mg/dl per 24 h after anuria occurs. An accelerated increase should prompt consideration of a toxin that causes rhabdomyolysis.

**Period of renal shutdown**: The patient may continue to be asymptomatic until signs of uremia appear, at which time weight gain, edema, and rales indicate fluid retention from overhydration. During this period, serum creatinine and potassium rise.

**Recovery period**: The diuresis that accompanies recovery from acute renal failure can lead to dehydration and electrolyte imbalance. Monitor for and correct muscle weakness from hypokalemia and tetany from hypocalcemia.

## Treatment

### Emergency measures

(1) Treat shock to prevent acute renal failure.
(2) If ingested poison is a known nephrotoxin and has an antidote, give the specific traetment.
(3) Treat rhabdomyolysis with forced alkaline diuresis (sodium bicarbonate 1–2 mEq/kg every 6–12 h with furosemide); to achieve a urine pH >7.5 and output of about 200 ml/h.

### General measures during period of renal shutdown

(1) Weigh patient daily. Weight gain indicates fluid retention, which must be avoided. Weight loss of 0.3–0.5 kg/d represents tissue catabolism.
(2) Restrict fluids to replacement of insensible water loss. Increase replacement fluid if diarrhea or vomiting occurs.

(3) Prevent infections by reverse isolation.

(4) Monitor blood chemistry (serum sodium and potassium, blood urea nitrogen, blood creatinine, and blood pH) daily and correct deficiencies.

(5) Treat cardiac failure if present. Because digoxin and ACE inhibitors are both used to treat CHF and are both relatively contraindicated in renal dysfunction, consult with nephrologist and cardiologist.

(6) Consider dialysis if the serum creatinine rises above 15 mg/dl or the serum potassium approaches 7–8 mEq/l.

### Measures during period of recovery

During this period, rapid blood electrolyte changes are likely to take place; obtain daily serum electrolytes to manage therapy.

The type of diuresis may vary from one patient to another. The following are examples:

(1) If the return of tubular function is delayed, the patient's urine may be essentially a glomerular filtrate with large volume and low specific gravity. These patients continue to lose large amounts of potassium, sodium, and other ions. Adequate management requires analysis of daily 24-h urine samples for total sodium and potassium losses, and replacement as needed.

(2) The diuresis may be accompanied by retention of sodium and a consequent rapid rise in serum sodium and chloride. Treatment in this case consists of providing sodium-free water.

## URINE RETENTION

Irritant poisons excreted by the kidney may inflame the neck of the bladder sufficiently to cause urine retention. Poisoning can occasionally cause decreased bladder contractility. The size of the bladder and volume of urine retained can be determined by percussion, palpation, or ultrasound. A self-retaining catheter may be advisable. If the patient is retaining urine as a result of spasm, then 'resting' the bladder is appropriate and placement of an indwelling cather is indicated.

# GASTROINTESTINAL TRACT INVOLVEMENT

## VOMITING AND DIARRHEA

Vomiting frequently accompanies poisoning and helps remove toxic substance. Similarly, diarrhea may increase poison excretion. However, if either are prolonged, symptomatic relief is desirable.

### Treatment

**Fluid therapy**: Fluid and nutritional balance must be maintained, although food and fluids must not be given orally until vomiting ceases. Administer IV hydration with 5–10% glucose in 0.3–0.5% saline to maintain hydration until patient tolerates oral liquids.

**Drugs**: Give anti-emetic of choice as necessary every 4–6 h. (Chlorpromazine is contraindicated in central nervous system depression, jaundice, and liver disease; and many pediatricians prefer not to use it in children under 6 years of age.) For diarrhea, use adsorbents (pectin-kaolin, psyllium, colestipol) rather than agents that have a sedative potential (loreramide).

## ABDOMINAL DISTENSION

Intestinal atony is induced by some poisons and may be associated with hypokalemia.

### Treatment

Colonic distension is relieved by passing a rectal or colonic tube (22–32F, 50–75 cm long) and eliminating the cause.

## WATER AND ELECTROLYTE IMBALANCE

Electrolyte imbalance after poisoning may be a result of vomiting, diarrhea, kidney damage, or other processes. An excess or deficit of water can also occur. If renal function is normal and the thirst mechanism is intact, then water and electrolyte imbalances are corrected by giving oral or intravenous fluids. If levels of $Na^+$, $K^+$, $Cl^-$, $HCO_3^-$, etc. are known, then replacements can be calculated. Serum or urine osmolality measurements can be used to evaluate

**Table 4.1** Normal concentrations of electrolytes in plasma and interstitial fluid

| | Traditional measurements | Conversion factor* | SI units |
|---|---|---|---|
| Cations | | | |
| Sodium | 135–147 mEq/l | 1 | 135–147 mmol/l |
| Potassium | 3.5–5 mEq/l | 1 | 3.5–5 mmol/l |
| Calcium | 4.4–5.3 mEq/l | 0.5 | 2.2–2.7 mmol/l |
| Magnesium | 1.6–2.4 mEq/l | 0.5 | 0.8–1.2 mmol/l |
| Anions | | | |
| Bicarbonate | 22–28 mEq/l | 1 | 22–28 mmol/l |
| Chloride | 95–108 mEq/l | 1 | 95–108 mmol/l |
| Phosphate | … | … | 0.8–1.6 mmol/l |
| Miscellaneous | | | |
| Urea nitrogen | 8–18 mg/dl | 0.357 | 3–6.5 mmol/l |
| Creatinine | 0.6–1.2 mg/dl | 88.4 | 50–110 μmol/l |

water status and to make adjustments. Normal concentrations of electrolytes in plasma and interstitial fluid are listed in Table 4.1.

**For emphasis**: Even though $Na^+$ and $Cl^-$ are known to be distributed in the 'extracellular compartment,' which comprises 20% of body weight and 33% of the total body water (total body water = approximately 60% of total body weight), some providers replace $Na^+$ and $Cl^-$ deficits as if these electrolytes occupied the total body water compartment. Other physicians may choose to replenish the extracellular compartment with 0.9% saline (154 mEq/liter of $Na^+$), 10–20 ml/kg body weight, to ensure adequate vascular perfusion, and then administer half of any remaining deficit in the next 8 h and the final amount in the next 16 h.

If the patient has a significant water excess (serum $Na^+ \leq 115$ mEq/l and symptoms are present, e.g. convulsions), 3% NaCl solution (513 mEq/l) should be given until the symptoms stop or the $Na^+$ level exceeds 125 mEq/l. If the serum $Na^+$ level exceeds 155–165 mEq/l, it should not be reduced rapidly by administration of free water; instead, 0.45% saline (77 mEq/l) should be given so that the serum $Na^+$ level does not fall precipitously.

Because most body $K^+$ is confined to the intracellular compartment it is not reflected by the serum $K^+$ level. Thus it is almost impossible to calculate the amount of $K^+$ needed for replacement on the basis of the serum $K^+$ determination alone. To correct a $K^+$ deficit, first re-establish urine flow and then add 30 mEq of $K^+$ to each liter of fluid administered to the patient; with normal kidney function, the $K^+$ level will be corrected.

## ACIDOSIS

Acidosis occurs in association with poisoning by one of two mechanisms: (1) an increase in the production or retention of hydrogen ions, e.g., conversion of methanol to formic acid; or inhibition of respiratory exchange, with retention of $CO_2$; (2) loss of body buffering capacity owing to renal losses or prolonged diarrhea.

Metabolic acidosis from an accumulation of lactic acid occurs during hypoxia. Thus, any agent that causes seizures has the potential to cause hypoxia and resultant lactic acidosis. Treatment is directed at stopping the seizures. Other causes of metabolic acidosis include poisoning with ethylene glycol, methanol, and paraldehyde, since these cause an accumulation of acid anions (oxalate, formate, and acetaldehyde). See also p. 57 Laboratory findings.

### Clinical findings

During respiratory acidosis with $CO_2$ retention, depressed respiratory rate and effort are obvious. The patient may actually become cyanotic.

During metabolic acidosis respiration usually increases in rate and depth in an attempt to correct acidosis; thus, increased respiratory effort is apparent.

### Treatment

The primary goal of therapy should be to eliminate the cause of acidosis. In respiratory acidosis, improved ventilation is necessary to eliminate retained $CO_2$. In metabolic acidosis, the metabolic processes must be altered to reduce the production or retention of excess hydrogen ions. Administration of sodium bicarbonate is only a temporizing step and is unlikely to overcome the basic defect. In acute resuscitation, sodium bicarbonate is administered only when the benefit clearly outweighs the potential risks.

In salicylate poisoning, sodium bicarbonate is given to alkalinize the urine to permit ion trapping. It is not given to correct the acidosis. Salicylate, being an acid, ionizes in alkaline urine; this prevents its reabsorption and allows it to be excreted. In tricyclic antidepressant toxicity, sodium bicarbonate

1–3 mEq/kg is administered, not to overcome any existing acidosis, but to increase the blood pH ; this prevents the development of cardiac arrhythmias.

## BODY TEMPERATURE REGULATION

Maintenance of normal body temperature is important in poisoning because hyperthermia increases the body requirements for $O_2$, food, minerals, water. A temperature rise of 0.8°C increases metabolism by about 10%.

Although hypothermia reduces the metabolic requirements, circulation is impaired and the detoxification and excretion of poisons are correspondingly slowed. Attempts to resuscitate a patient who is hypothermic should continue until their body temperature is normal. Treatment is less effective in the hypothermic state.

### Hyperthermia

Hyperthermia can be caused by: drug side-effects or interactions: muscular overactivity, disrupted thermoregulation or increased metabolic rate.
(1)  Side-effects or interactions:
>  anesthetic or phenothiazine side-effect, serotonin syndrome from drug interactions such as monoamine oxidase inhibitor + selective serotonin reuptake inhibitor (SSRI), monoamine oxidase inhibitor + meperidine, or SSRI + St John's wort, etc.
(2)  Poisons that cause muscular overactivity (seizures) or rigidity:
>  amoxapine, amphetamine, cocaine, LSD, maprotiline, phencyclidine (PCP), tricyclic antidepressants.
(3)  Disrupted thermoregulation:
>  any anticholinergic agent, malignant hyperthermia from some general anesthetics (halothane and succinylcholine), or neuroleptic malignant syndrome (phenothiazines).
(4)  Increased metabolic rate:
>  dinitrophenol, salicylates, thyroid hormone, and pentachlorophenol.

### Treatment of hyperthermia

Body temperatures up to 40°C can be controlled by applying wet towels with adequate air circulation or a cooling blanket. Higher temperatures require the frequent application of wet towels, sponging and fanning. Cooling should not be so rapid as to cause shivering because this generates more heat. Anti-pyretics such as aspirin have no role in the treatment of poison-induced hyperthermia.

Supportive treatment includes monitoring the airway and giving glucose if the patient is hypoglycemic. The etiology of hyperthermia must be determined and treated (seizures, serotonin syndrome, malignant hyperthermia, neuroleptic malignant syndrome, muscular rigidity, etc.).

The most effective treatment for severe hyperthermia is to rapidly lower body temperature by neuromuscular paralysis. Only someone capable of intubating the patient and trained in using a ventilator (usually an anesthesiologist) should do this. If available, give dantrolene for malignant hyperthermia or bromocriptine for neuroleptic malignant syndrome.

### Hypothermia

In many cases hypothermia is caused by exposure to low ambient temperature. The patient may not be aware enough to prevent further exposure, may be unconscious, or may have ingested an agent that causes further heat loss.

Agents cause heat loss by:
(1) Vasodilatation (alcohol, calcium channel blockers).
(2) Decreasing metabolic activity (hypoglycemic agents).
(3) Causing loss of consciousness (barbiturates).

### Treatment of hypothermia

If the body temperature is below 35°C, the patient must be warmed slowly to avoid inducing rewarming arrhythmias. If body temperature is below 30°C, cardiac arrest, and/or ventricular fibrillation may occur and be resistant to treatment. Bradycardia should not be treated, as it will resolve as rewarming occurs. Peripheral warming can lead to pooling of blood and fall in blood pressure. Apply warm blankets to the patient's torso, administer warm IV fluids and humidified 38°C inspired air. In severe cases, if available, use extracorporeal circulation of blood through a bath warmed up to 38°C and use warmed peritoneal/gastric lavage.

Warming by means of heat lamps, heating pads or hot water bottles is dangerous. If the skin temperature exceeds 42°C, local tissue injury with capillary stasis and edema may cause circulatory collapse.

## LIVER DAMAGE FROM DRUGS AND CHEMICALS

Liver toxicity is caused by (1) direct cell injury from the ingested agent or from its toxic intermediate metabolite, (2) delayed cell injury from chronic exposure, (3) agents which cause significant hemolytic anemia, overwhelming hepatic removal of bilirubin (people who genetically have G6PD (glucose-6-phosphate dehydrogenase) deficiency are more susceptible), and (4) hepatic vein thrombosis (pyrrolizidine alkaloids).

### General cell injury

Transaminase values are elevated, but alkaline phosphatase is low. Depending on the extent of damage, this type of injury may not be reversible.

(1) Direct hepatotoxic effects (single dose, effect immediate, all individuals susceptible) – acetaminophen, *Amanita phalloides*, arsenic, carbon tetrachloride, chloroform, phosphorus, stilbamidine, tannic acid, tetracyclines.

(2) Delayed hepatotoxic effect (long exposure, all individuals susceptible) – Ethanol.

(3) Hepatitis reactions (sporadic, possible idiosyncrasy, response delayed) – Chloramphenicol, chlortetracycline, cinchophen, gold salts, halothane, iproniazid, isoniazid, methoxyflurane, novobiocin, penicillins, phenylbutazone, pyrazinamide, streptomycin, sulfamethoxypyridazine, trinitrotoluene, zoxazolamine, valproate.

(4) Chronic hepatitis reactions (slow onset, prolonged or repeated exposure) – acetaminophen, aspirin, chlorpromazine, halothane, isoniazid, methyldopa, nitrofurantoin, oxyphenisatin.

### Cholestatic without inflammatory change

Transaminases and alkaline phosphatase are slightly elevated, and bilirubin markedly increased. Injury is dose-related and follows prolonged administration of methyltestosterone and progestational contraceptives. Individuals with G6PD deficiency are more susceptible to hemolysis and jaundice from poisons that are degraded by this enzyme.

## Cholestatic with portal inflammation

Transaminases are slightly elevated and alkaline phosphatase and bilirubin are significantly elevated. This injury usually occurs after prolonged or repeated administration and may progress to biliary cirrhosis. The following drugs and chemicals have been implicated: aminosalicylic acid, chlorothiazide, chlorpromazine, phenindione, phenylbutazone, prochlorperazine, promazine, sulfadiazine, thiouracil, toluenediamine.

## Clinical findings

**Acute poisoning**: Nausea and vomiting, anorexia, headache, malaise, lethargy, abdominal pain, fever, jaundice, and enlarged, tender liver, hepatic encephalopathy, coma, death.

**Chronic poisoning**: Weight loss, weakness, pallor, hematemesis, palmar erythema, enlarged or atrophic liver, jaundice, ascites, dependent edema, hemorrhoids, pruritus.

**Laboratory findings in hemolytic jaundice due to poisons** (castor beans, naphthalene, methylene blue, primiquine, sulfonamides): Bilirubin is present in the urine. Urinary and fecal urobilinogen are increased. Serum bilirubin is increased, indicating the inability of the liver to remove bilirubin as fast as it is formed. The degree of the accompanying anemia indicates the severity of the process.

**Laboratory findings in hepatic cell injury due to poisons**:

(1) Bilirubin is present in the urine.

(2) Urinary urobilinogen is increased.

(3) Fecal urobilinogen is decreased or unchanged.

(4) Serum bilirubin is increased, indicating the inability of the liver to remove bilirubin as fast as it is formed. A gradual increase in bilirubinemia indicates progression of the lesion; reduction of the bilirubinemia indicates healing of the cellular injury.

(5) Serum levels of liver cell enzymes – aspartate aminotransferase (AST), alanine aminotransferase (ALT), and lactate dehydrogenase (LDH) – are increased.

The synthetic and conjugative functions of the liver can be tested by a variety of methods. While reduced function indicated by these tests is important diagnostically, the presence of severe liver injury cannot be excluded by a normal test.

The following tests are used:

(1) Altered serum albumin–globulin ratio. Serum albumin is decreased and serum globulin is normal or increased. These tests may show little correlation with clinical findings and are poor indicators of prognosis or of overall liver function. However, they are used to monitor the effect of treatment on impaired liver function. Serial values showing trends are more important diagnostically and prognostically than one measurement.

(2) A low plasma prothrombin concentration 24 h after administration of phytonadione, 1 mg/kg intramuscularly, indicates that the liver is unable to synthesize prothrombin from vitamin K. Persistence of low plasma prothrombin in the absence of obstruction indicates a poor prognosis.

**Laboratory findings in bile duct obstruction with cholestasis**:

(1) Serum bilirubin may rise over 30 mg/dl.
(2) Serum alkaline phosphatase activity is increased.
(3) Serum cholesterol is greatly increased.
(4) Urine and fecal urobilinogen are decreased.

**Treatment**

*Emergency measures in acute liver damage*

(1) Discontinue all drugs and chemicals, especially ethanol, barbiturates, sulfonamides, narcotics, salicylates, phenothiazines, steroids, arsenicals and other metals, and antihistamines.
(2) Prevent further injury if toxin is known by giving antidote (chelator for heavy metals) or take measures to alter metabolism to reactive intermediate or to increase excretion.
(3) Avoid anesthesia or surgical procedures.

*General measures in acute or chronic liver damage*

(1) Maintain euvolemia and electrolyte balance.

(2) Vitamin K – Give phytonadione, 2.5 mg daily. If necessary, blood transfusion with fresh frozen plasma for coagulopathy.

(3) Supportive treatment for hypoglycemia, hypoalbuminemia, pulmonary edema, encephalopathy.

## METHEMOGLOBINEMIA

Methemoglobin is formed by oxidation of the ferrous ($Fe^{2+}$) iron of hemoglobin to the ferric ($Fe^{3+}$) form by the action of a number of chemicals. Methemoglobinemia is *not* capable of carrying oxygen. For example, sodium nitrite is used in meat curing; it may be present in excess in home-cured meat, or the meat-curing salt may be used accidentally as table salt. In infants or children, nitrates in well water contaminated from agricultural use of fertilizers or from bismuth subnitrate may be reduced to nitrites in the intestine and absorbed to cause methemoglobinemia. Some agents capable of causing methemoglobin: *analgesics* (phenazopyridine, phenacetin), *anesthetics* (benzocaine, lidocaine), *antimalarials* (choroquine, dapsone), *antibiotics* (primaquine, sulfonamides, trimethoprim), *organic nitrates and nitrites* (ammonium nitrate, amyl nitrite, sodium nitrite, nitrobenzene, nitroglycerin, nitroprusside), and *others* (acetanilid, aniline, dimethylaniline, nitroaniline, aminobenzene, phenols, bromate and chlorate salts.

### Clinical findings

#### Symptoms and signs

Cyanosis occurs when 15% of hemoglobin has been converted to methemoglobin, however the patient may not be symtomatic. Chocolate brown blood occurs when levels exceed 15%. Symptoms of headache, dizziness, weakness, dyspnea, and signs of 'chocolate cyanosis' such as skin, lips, nails aand ear discoloration are not likely to occur until the concentration reaches 30–40%. At levels of 60%, stupor and respiratory depression occur. At levels above 60%, fatalities occur.

#### Laboratory findings

Spectrophotometric analysis will measure the concentration of methemoglobin in the blood. Both the antidote methylene blue and sulfhemoglobin will cause falsely elevated levels. Typical blood gases measure serum $pO_2$ which will imply normal $O_2$ saturation; pulse oximetry is totally unreliable.

## Treatment

### Emergency measures

(1) Give 100% $O_2$ by mask to increase the $O_2$ saturation of plasma and unchanged hemoglobin if the patient shows dyspnea or air hunger.
(2) Remove ingested poison by emesis or gastric lavage; terminate skin contact by removing contaminated clothing and washing the skin thoroughly with soap and water.

*Antidote* Use if methemoglobin concentration is >20% or in presence of symptoms or underlying chronic conditions (such as anemia, angina, pulmonary disease):

(1) Give methylene blue, 1% solution, 0.1–0.2 ml/kg intravenously over a 10-minute period. Cyanosis may disappear within minutes or may persist longer, depending on the degree of methemoglobinemia. Intravenous administration of therapeutic doses of methylene blue may cause a rise in blood pressure, nausea, and dizziness. Individuals who are G6PD deficient may develop hemolysis from methylene blue. Larger doses (>500 mg) cause vomiting, diarrhea, chest pain, mental confusion, cyanosis, and sweating. Hemolytic anemia has also occurred several days after administration. These effects are temporary, and fatalities have not been reported.
(2) If methylene blue is not available, give ascorbic acid, 1 g slowly intravenously.
(3) Consider exchange transfusion.
(4) Without treatment, methemoglobin levels of 20–30% revert to normal within 3 days.

### General measures

(1) Absolute bed rest must be enforced if methemoglobinemia is above 40%.
(2) Continue $O_2$ therapy for at least 2 h after methylene blue has been given.

# AGRANULOCYTOSIS AND OTHER BLOOD DYSCRASIAS

A large number of drugs, chemicals, and metals are capable of causing blood dyscrasias, including agranulocytosis, leukopenia, aplastic anemia, and thrombocytopenia. The incidence of these reactions ranges from one case per 1000 users in patients receiving aminopyrine, phenylbutazone, antineoplastics, apronalide, gold salts, and arsenicals to one to ten cases per 100 000 users of antihistamines, antibiotics, and anticonvulsants.

## Laboratory findings

**Agranulocytosis**: Decrease or disappearance of granulocytes from peripheral blood. Myeloid cells are reduced or absent in bone marrow smears while red cell series and megakaryocytes are normal.

**Aplastic anemia**: Bone marrow is deficient in all cellular elements.

**Thrombocytopenia**: Decrease or disappearance of platelets from blood.

## Treatment

### Emergency measures

Discontinue the offending drug at the first symptom.

### General measures

(1) Chemotherapy – In the presence of fever, sore throat, pulmonary congestion, or other signs of infection, give organism-specific antibiotic therapy until infection is controlled.
(2) Blood transfusion – Give transfusions of specific components needed.
(3) Isolate the patient, if possible, to reduce exposure to infection.

## References

Guest I, Uetrecht J. Drugs that induce neutropenia/agranulocytosis may target specific components of the stromal cell extracellular matrix. *Med Hypothesis* 1999;53:141

Sari R, *et al.* Ticlopidine-induced severe agranulocytosis after the placement of coronary artery stent. *Angiology* 2000;51:591

Wazny LD, Ariano RE. Evaluation and management of drug-induced thrombocytopenia in the acutely ill patient. *Pharmacotherapy* 2000;20:292

## HEMOLYTIC REACTIONS

A number of substances, including arsine, stibine, and dichloromethane, can cause acute hemolytic reactions by a direct effect on red cells. Many other hemolytic reactions occur on the basis of glucose-6-phosphate dehydrogenase (G6PD) deficiency, which occurs in approximately 11% of black American males, in a smaller proportion of the descendants of Mediterranean and Asian ethnic groups, and in about 1% of others. Selected agents that cause hemolysis by this mechanism include: uncooked fava beans, naphthalene, nitrofurantoin, salicylate derivatives such as amino-salicylic acid, sulfa derivatives, primaquine, and water-soluble vitamin K (menadiol and menadione sodium bisulfate).

### Clinical findings

*Symptoms and signs*

Onset is sudden, with chills, fever, nausea and vomiting, abdominal or back pain, jaundice, and dark urine. Hypotension and shock may occur if the onset of anemia is severe and abrupt. Oliguria or anuria indicates acute renal failure as a result of renal ischemia and precipitation of hemoglobin in the renal tubules.

*Laboratory findings*

The anemia is normocytic, but burr cells and red cell fragments are apparent on microscopic examination. Serum may contain hemoglobin or methemalbumin, and urine may contain hemoglobin and hemosiderin. G6PD deficiency can be identified by several tests: glutathione stability, cresyl blue reduction, methemoglobin reduction, and a commercially available dye reduction spot test. The red cell count is lowest several days after onset and then gradually returns to normal.

### Treatment

**Maintain urine output**: In the presence of hemoglobinuria with normal kidney function, maintain urine output at 2–3 ml/kg/h. Furosemide, 20–80 mg orally or intravenously every 4–8 h, may be helpful. Alkalinize the urine by giving sodium bicarbonate, 1–2 mEq/kg every 12 h. Monitor central venous pressure and electrolytes. Mannitol administration has been used to maintain urine output.

**Exchange transfusion**: If serum hemoglobin exceeds 1.5 g/dl, total exchange transfusion may prevent renal failure.

## DERMATITIS DUE TO CONTACT WITH CHEMICALS

Dermatitis due to chemicals may arise as a result of direct contact-sensitization, and from phototoxic reactions. When skin that has come into contact with a certain plant is then exposed to sunlight, a phytophototoxic reaction can occur. Examples of direct contact irritation include various drugs such as local anesthetics, paraben esters (preservatives in some skin care products), ethylenediamine, topical antihistamines such diphenhydramine, mercurials, neomycin, sunscreens, acids, alkalis, soaps, solvents, corrosives, phenol, white phosphorus, and formaldehyde resins in some new clothing.

The most widespread form of allergic contact dermatitis, rhus dermatitis, is triggered by poison ivy, oak, sumac and all members of the genus *Rhu* (*Toxicodendron*). Other forms of sensitization or allergic contact dermatitis include:

- Nickel-containing metal (jewellery, watches, metal studs/snaps in clothing, buckles, etc.)
- Cocamidopropyl betaine, an allergen in some shampoosG
- lyceryl thioglycolate and paraphenylinediamine found in 'hot permanent' hair productsC
- ompounds containing chromium/chromates such as cement, leather, paints, and anti-rust compoundsL
- atex and rubber

Phytophototoxic reactions occur from lime, lemon, bergamot, celery, carrot dill, fennel, and parsley. Photoallergic/irritant dermatitis can result when a person ingests a chemical or drug and then exposes their skin to sunlight. Examples of drugs that interact with ultraviolet rays include sulfa-containing medications (sulfonamides, thiazide diuretics), quinolones, and tetracycline(s).

## Diagnosis

### Primary reactions

Dermatitis due to primary irritants is characterized by the following:
(1) The site of maximal involvement is the site of maximal exposure.
(2) The site of maximal exposure is the site of first appearance.
(3) Other exposed persons have similar involvement.
(4) The time relationship between the beginning of exposure and the onset of dermatitis is similar in all those exposed.

### Allergic reactions

Dermatitis caused by sensitizing materials is characterized by the following:
(1) The site of maximal involvement may be different from the site of maximal exposure.
(2) The time relationship between the onset of exposure and the onset of dermatitis is variable.
(3) Other exposed persons may not have similar eruptions.

## Evaluation of dermatitis due to contact with chemicals

### Contact dermatitis from direct irritants

About 80% of cases of contact dermatitis are due to primary irritants. A primary or direct irritant is an agent that is capable of injuring the skin at the site of the first application if the concentration and duration of exposure are sufficient. Examples of primary irritants are solvents, acids, alkalis, soaps, and other corrosives and irritants (see Chapters 14, 18, 29 and 36).

### Sensitization dermatitis

Dermatitis due to sensitizers occurs only after repeated contact. The site of allergic contact dermatitis is often a clue to the diagnosis; for example, reactions on earlobes or around wrist or neck may be due to jewelry, and scalp reactions may be due to chemicals in hair dyes. However, the dermatitis is not necessarily limited to the site of contact; it may involve larger areas of skin. Patch tests may be helpful in the diagnosis of sensitization to a chemical, but they have serious limitations.

**Patch tests**: Patch testing consists of applying a nonirritating (low) concentration of the suspected contact antigen to the patient's skin and covering it with an occlusive dressing. Sterile, unimpregnated gauze must surround the patch and separate it from the area where the adhesive tape touches the skin (to distinguish reactions to the patch from reactions to adhesive). The dressing is removed after 48 h. An eczematous reaction at the site of the patch test constitutes a positive response. A positive response is more meaningful than a negative one, because false-negative results may occur for many reasons.

## Prevention

Use of impervious gloves, masks, gauntlets, aprons, and clothing if necessary may help to reduce the incidence of dermatitis. Workers should wash frequently with mild soap. The use of degreasing solvents, paint thinner, solvents, and harsh cleaning agents for cleaning the skin should be avoided. Protective creams or ointments may be useful preventives. A high incidence of dermatitis in a factory may require personal inspection of the workplace by an industrial hygiene specialist.

## Treatment

Discontinue contact with any irritating or sensitizing medications. Sensitizers include all mercurial antiseptics, sulfonamides, antibiotics, local anesthetics, phenols, resorcinol, nitrofurazone, adhesive tape, various dyes, and many others. Ointments sometimes contain a mercurial as a preservative.

**Mild wet dressings**: Moist, oozing lesions are treated by application of mild wet dressings, which should be replaced every 2–3 h. Impervious coverings prevent the cooling effects of evaporation and should not be used. The following medications can be used without fear of aggravating the irritation:

(1) Aluminum acetate, 1% solution.
(2) Magnesium sulfate, half-saturated (25%) solution.
(3) Sodium bicarbonate, saturated (10%) or half-saturated (5%) solution.
(4) Starch or oatmeal solution (can be used as a bath and repeated every 2–4 h). A starch bath is prepared by mixing a cup of cornstarch in 2 quarts of water. The mixture is heated to boiling and then poured into a cool bath. The patient then sits in the bath for 10 min and pours the starch solution over the affected areas.

(5) Saline solution (sodium chloride, 10 g/l).
(6) Potassium permanganate, 1:10 000 solution (leaves a stain but otherwise is excellent).

**Mild ointments**: Fissured, thickened, scaling eruptions are treated by mild ointments, of which the following are satisfactory:

(1) Zinc oxide ointment.
(2) Zinc oxide (Lassar's) paste.
(3) Hydrophilic ointment (Aquaphor).

## References

Goskowicz MD, *et al.* Endemic "lime" disease: phytodermatitis in San Diego County. *Pediatrics* 1994;93:828

Blanco C, *et al.* Latex allergy: clinical features and cross-reactivity with fruits. *Ann Allergy* 1994;73:309

Reddy S. Latex allergy. *Am Acad Fam Phys* 1998;57:93

## USEFUL ANTIDOTES AND DRUGS

### Atropine sulfate

Used for excessive salivation from organophosphates and to reverse muscarinic symptoms from mushrooms. Increases heart rate.

Give 1–2 mg (children 0.02 mg/kg) IV or intratracheal. Dilute with 0.9% saline.

May cause angina or infarct in patients with underlying cardiac disease, and decompensate patients with thryrotoxicosis or dysrrhythmias. Precipitates narrow angle glaucoma crisis, myasthenia gravis, and urinary retention.

### Benztropine mesylate

Used to treat acute dystonic reactions caused by antipsychotics, antiemetics, or metoclopramine.

Adults: 1–2 mg, IV, IM or orally every 12 h for 1–3 days; children >3 years old: 0.02–0.05 mg/g/dose every 12 h.

May cause sedation, tachycardia, dry mouth, urinary retention or precipitate narrow angle glaucoma.

**Botulin antitoxin**

Trivalent form contains concentrated equine-derived antibodies directed against toxins formed by three strains (A, B, E) of *Clostridium* botulism. Used to treat clinical botulism, not infant botulism.

See package insert for dosing. Only available from the CDC.

Anaphylaxis, delayed serum sickness may occur 1–2 weeks after administration. Will not reverse already established paralysis

**Calcium**

Used for treating symptomatic hypocalcemia, black widow bite, calcium channel blocker overdose, hydrofluoric acid burns, fluoride ingestion, or severe hyperkalemia.

*Calcium chloride*: 100 mg/ml in 10 ml (27.2 mg/ml elemental calcium). Adults: 8–16 mg/kg (approximately 5–10 ml) slow IV push; children: 10–20 mg/kg (0.1–0.2 ml/kg) slow IV push.

*Calcium gluconate*: 10% = 100 mg/ml (9 mg/ml elemental calcium) 1 g/10 cc = 4.5 mEq calcium. Adults: 10–20 ml slow IV of 10% solution; children: 60–100 mg/kg (0.6–1.0 ml/kg) slow IV push.

**Effects**: Hypotension, bradycardia, arrhythmias, and asystole from rapid IV administration; constipation from oral administration, tissue irritation, or necrosis. May aggravate digitalis-induced dysrhythmias.

**Charcoal (activated charcoal (see pp. 31–32))**

Adsorbent for drugs and poisons.

Initial dose 1 g/kg oral or via gastric tube. 15–30 g (0.25–0.5 g/kg every 2–4 h). Administer a cathartic every 2–3 doses to facilitate charcoal movement through colon. Repeated dosages may increase the rate of elimination of some drugs.

**Effects**: Distension of stomach and possible aspiration, constipation and obstruction. Hypermagnesemia and hypernatremia may occur if cathartics are used with charcoal.

Does not work well for highly ionic substances or small polar substances: boric acid, cyanide, DDT, ferrous sulfate, ethanol, methanol, lithium, water-insoluble substances, mineral acids, alkalis, and many metallic compounds.

**Cyanide antidote** See Nitrite, Thiosulfate

**Cyanocobalamin (hydroxocobalamin, synthetic vitamin B$_{12}$)**

Used for prevention of cyanide toxicity from prolonged nitroprusside infusions. US formulation is too dilute for acute cyanide overdose. A more concentrated product is available in Europe.

Give 0.5 mg/kg/h by IV.

**Effects**: Hypertension, GI disturbance.

**Dantrolene**

Use for malignant hyperthermia, drug-induced hyperthermia and rhabdomyolysis not controlled by cooling or neuromuscular paralysis: serotonin syndrome, cocaine, monoamine oxidase inhibitor, phencyclidine, trichloroacetic acid, etc. Not effective if mechanism of hyperthermia is *not* due to increased cellular activity (heat stroke).

Give 1–2 mg by *rapid* IV injection every 5–10 min, total dosage 10 mg/kg. Use 1–2 mg/kg IV or orally four times per day for 2–3 days to prevent recurrence (100 mg maximum). Note: some products contain the osmotic agent mannitol.

**Effects**: Respiratory arrest; muscle weakness, hepatitis, and sedation. Additive with other CNS depressants.

**Deferoxamine**

Used when serum iron level is >450–500 µg/dl or if patient is in shock, acidosis, or with severe GI symptoms.

Give IV at rate up to 15 mg/kg/h. See package insert for details.

**Effects**: Hypotension or anaphylaxis if given rapidly IV. Can cause adult respiratory distress syndrome (ARDS) and promote growth of *Yersiniia enterocolitica*.

**Digoxin Immune Fab (Digibind)**

See dosage instructions in the package.

Used for digoxin, digitoxin, or digitalis induced cardiac arrhythmias. Also effective against other cardio-active glycosides: oleander, strophanthus, and toad venom. If an asyptomatic patient has known elevated cardiac glycoside *and* a serum potassium $\geq 5$ mEq/l, then treatment is indicated *before* life-threatening arrhythmias occur.

Possible hypersensitivity reactions. Monitor for hypokalemia. Removal of digoxin effect may result in tachycardia and other dysrhythmias. It is *not* indicated for minor elevations of digoxin blood levels.

### Diphenhydramine (Benadryl)

Used for acute, drug-induced, dystonic reactions. Counteracts excessive histamine release from poison ivy, insect bites, scombroid-contaminated fish, too rapid administration of some drugs (acetylcysteine).

For adults, give 50 mg IV or IM and repeat in 30–60 min. For children, give 0.5–1.0 mg/kg IV or IM.

Oral dose in adults: 25–50 mg. For children, give 5 mg/kg/d in divided dosages.

**Effects**: Sedation. Do not give with monoamine oxidase inhibitors or in the presence of anticholinergic delirium or psychosis.

May precipitate narrow angle glaucoma or cause urinary retention.

### Dimercaprol (BAL)

Drug of choice for mercury, arsenic and gold poisoning; second line or adjunctive for lead toxicity. Best given within the first 2 h.

Give 3 mg/kg by deep IM injection every 4 h for the first 2 days and then 2 mg/kg every 12 h. A total of 10 days of treatment may on occasion be necessary. Maintain an alkaline urine during treatment, because the dimercaprol–metal complex is not acid-stable. Monitor patients for central nervous system symptoms. For adjunctive treatment with calcium EDTA when treating *lead* toxicity (blood lead >100 μg/dl), give BAL 4–5 mg/kg by deep IM injection every 4 h for 3–5 days.

**Effects**: Overdose of dimercaprol causes a variety of symptoms depending on the dosage. At doses up to 3 mg/kg, about 20% of patients will have anorexia, restlessness, generalized aches and pains, itching, salivation, and elevation of blood pressure of 10–20 mmHg. At doses up to 5 mg/kg, up to 60% of patients will have, fever, tachycardia, and significant hypertension. Doses over 5 mg/kg cause vomiting, convulsions, and stupor or coma, beginning within 30 min after injection. Such reactions have usually subsided in 1–6 h, even after doses as large as 40 mg/kg. Fatalities have not been reported from these large dosages.

**Contraindications**: Do not use in iron, cadmium, or selenium poisoning or when iron is being administered medicinally; the resulting chelates are more harmful than the metals alone. Do not use in the presence of hepatic insufficiency unless it is due to arsenic poisoning. Discontinue or do not use at all in the presence of acute renal insufficiency.

### Edetate calcium disodium (EDTA)

Primary use is to treat severe lead poisoning. Lead, iron, zinc, manganese, beryllium, and copper form compounds with edetate that cannot be displaced by calcium.

Give 15–25 mg/kg (0.08–0.125 ml/kg) of 20% solution IV in 250–500 ml of 5% dextrose intravenously over a 1- to 2-h period twice daily. For IM administration, give 12.5 mg/kg (20% solution) every 4–6 h and dilute each dose with 1–2 ml of 1% lidocaine. The maximum dose should not exceed 50 mg/kg/d. The drug should be given in 5-day courses with a rest period of at least 2 days between courses. Carefully monitor for nephrotoxicity and lead-induced encephalopathy.

**Effects**: Transient hypotension, hypokalemia, renal tubular damage with oliguria, and large increase in lead excretion on the first day of treatment.

### Epinephrine

Give for severe anaphylaxis or for cardiac arrest.

*Anaphylaxis*: Adults: give 0.05–0.1 mg IV or 0.5–1 ml of 1:10 000 every 5–10 min. Endotracheal route is effective. Dilute dose with 10 cc 0.9% saline and instill into endotracheal tube. Children: 0.01 mg/kg IV or 0.1 ml/kg of 1:10 000. For intratracheal dose in a child, use 0.1 mg/kg or a 0.1 ml/kg of 1:1000.

*Cardiac arrest*: Adults: 1 mg IV bolus or via endotracheal tube, or 10 ml of 1:10 000 solution every 3–5 min.

**Cautions**: Coronary artery disease, peripheral arterial disease, ergot poisoning, narrow angle glaucoma. Severe hypertension due to unopposed alpha effects can occur with beta-blocker, monoamine oxidase inhibitor, digitalis, cocaine, or tricyclic antidepressants. Extravasation causes tissue necrosis.

## Ethanol

For methanol or ethylene glycol poisoning.

Initial dose: 15 ml/kg IV of 5% ethanol in 5% dextrose in water. For oral administration: give 2 ml/kg of a 50% concentration. Maintain ethanol blood level at 1 mg/ml.

**Effects**: Gastritis, hypoglycemia, hypotension, pancreatitis, additive effect with other CNS depressants. Disulfiram-like reactions in presence of drugs such as metronidazole.

## Folic acid

Adjunct to treat ethylene glycol and methanol poisoning as it may increase elimination of formic acid in patients deficient in folic acid. Give 50 mg IV in adults (children 1 mg/kg) every 4 h.

## Fomepizole (4-methylpyrazole, 4MP)

For methanol and ethylene glycol poisoning. Mechanism: inhibits alcohol dehydrogenase.

Initial dose: 15 mg/kg (1 g max.) diluted in at least 100 ml of normal saline or 5% dextrose in water and administered slowly over 30 min. Repeat doses of 10–15 mg/kg every 12 h.

**Effects**: Headache, GI distress, CNS effects, hypotension. Will slow the elimination of drugs that are metabolized by alcohol dehydrogenase.

## Flumazenil (Romazicon)

Reverses benzodiazepine overdose.

Give 0.2 mg IV over 30 seconds. If no response, give 0.3 mg and repeat in 10 min. Maximum dose: 3 mg. For children, give 0.01 mg/kg to maximum dose of 1 mg at no more than 0.1 mg/min.

**Caution**: Short half life, may need repeat dosages or continuous infusion.

## Glucagon

For hypoglycemia or hypotension caused by overdose of beta-blocker or calcium channel blocker. Use empirically to treat patients presenting in stupor or coma when etiology has not yet been identified.

Adults: 5–10 mg IV, then 1–5 mg/h. Children: 0.05–0.1 mg/kg/h.

**Effects**: Hyperglycemia, hyperosmolality, and may cause Wernicke–Korsakoff syndrome if patient is deficient in thiamine; for empiric use, especially in alcoholics, give 100 mg thiamine IM/IV before injecting glucagon.

## Hydroxocobalamin   See cyanocobalamine

## Ipecac syrup

Used immediately for oral poisonings.

Dosage: adults, 30 ml; children 1–12 years old, 15 ml; children 6–12 months old, 5–10 ml. Follow with 120–250 ml water. If no emesis in 30 min, repeat.

**Precautions**: Vomiting can cause reflex bradycardia, esophageal tears, and may delay absorption of oral antidotes; administer charcoal if vomiting persists.

**Contraindications**: If ingested toxin is suspected to be an agent that can cause seizures (TCA, camphor, cocaine, strychnine, INM, etc.); ingestion of petroleum, hydrocarbons, corrosives, and patients who may not be able to protect their airway (decreased conciousness, etc.)

Toxic alkaloids accumulate if used chronically.

## Magnesium sulfate

Used as an anticonvulsant, to control arrhythmias, and for hypomagnesemia.

Give 0.2 ml/kg of 10% (1.7 mEq/ml) over 15 min and not more than 2 ml/kg over 24 h. Serum magnesium should not exceed 3 mEq/l.

**Caution**: Renal disease.

## Methylene blue

Used to treat symptomatic methemoglobinemia (p. 77).

Give 1–2 mg/kg (0.1–0.2 ml/kg of a 1% solution) IV over 5 min. In general, may repeat one time, 30–60 min after initial injection. If toxicity is from dapsone – further dosages may be needed.

**Effects**: Dizziness, headache, and gastrointestinal side-effects.

**Contraindications**: Patients who are G6PD or methemoglobin reductase deficient or have renal failure.

## Nalmefene (Revex)

Reverses opioid intoxication.

Give 0.25 mg IV every 2–5 min. Maximum total dose 1.5 mg. See package insert.

See naloxone (below). More potent, longer duration of action, and more expensive than naloxone.

## Naloxone (Narcan)

Used to reverse opiate toxicity.

Give 0.4–2 mg IV every 2–3 min. May also be used endotracheally, subcutaneously or intramuscularly. Titrate if patient is opiate dependent. Children: same dosage. If no response by 10–15 mg, consider other diagnoses. See package insert for infusion rates.

Rapid reversal precipitates acute withdrawal in opiate-dependent patients. Extremely safe medication(s). Rarely, serious effects have occurred, such as seizures, pulmonary edema, or dysrhythmias.

## Neuromuscular blocking agents

Used for treatment of muscular rigidity from stimulant overdose, serotonin syndrome, neuroleptic malignant syndrome, or tetanus. *Not effective* in malignant hyperthermia; if one of these agents is used and paralysis is not achieved, then evaluate patients for ingestion of agent or other condition which causes malignant hyperthermia.

**Drugs**: A non-depolarizing agent is preferred. Atracurium, cisatracurium, pancuronium, rapacuronium, rocuronium, vecuronium. See package insert for dosages. Personnel who can intubate and are competent in completely managing oxygenation and ventilation must be present before any neuromuscular blocker is given.

**Effects**: Complete paralysis with respiratory depression and bradycardia. Prolonged effects if patient has underlying neuromuscular disorder (myasthenia gravis). See package insert for drug interactions.

Note: Also used to aid intubation; preferred agents are rapid onset (succinylcholine, rocuronium, vecuronium)

**Nicotinamide (Niacinamide or Vitamin B$_3$)** (Note: not to be confused with niacin)

Used to treat ingestion of the rodenticide vacor ($N$-3-pyridylmethyl-$N'$-$p$-nitrophenylurea (PNU) (no longer available in USA).

Give 500 mg IV, then 100–200 mg IV every 4 h for 48 h. IV form not available in USA. Efficacy of oral dosage unknown. Niacin and nicotinic acid are not effective.

**Nifedipine (rapid release)**

Used by oral route to treat hypertension caused by amphetamine, cocaine, phencyclidine (PCP) and phenylpropanolamine. Dose is one capsule of the 10 mg rapid release or short acting form of the drug. The capsule is punctured and the liquid taken sublingually or the capsule is swallowed intact.

**Effects:** Rapid decrease in blood pressure with risk of severe hypotension. This can result in stroke if adequate cerebral perfusion is not maintained. The rate of blood pressure decrease correlates with how fast the drug is absorbed.

**Contraindications:** Some physicians consider the use of the oral, short-acting form of nifedipine contraindicated in patients with underlying aortic/valvular heart disease, obstructive cardiomyopathy, or any underlying condition (even simply 'old age') that predisposes them to complications.

**Nitrite, sodium and amyl**

Nitrites are used to treat *definite*, symptomatic cyanide poisoning; *not* for empiric or suspected poisoning. Nitrites are possibly helpful to treat hydrogen sulfide poisoning.
See package insert in Cyanide Antidote Package.

**Effects:** Symptoms of cyanide poisoning often mask any of the nitrite symptoms.

**Contraindications**: Significant hypotension, patients with carbon monoxide or smoke inhalation, and pre-existing methemoglobinemia >40%.

## Nitroprusside sodium

Used for hypertensive crisis and to treat patients with other cardiovascular disease causing uncontrollable hypertension. Dilute 50 mg to 1 liter 5% dextrose (50 μg/ml). Protect from light. Begin IV administration at 1 μg/kg/min. Maximum rate = 10 μg/kg/min.

**Effects:** Causes hypotension, hyperventilation, vomiting, and tachycardia and results in cyanide poisoning if infusions are maintained over 24 h.

## Octreotide (Sandostatin)

Drug used to treat sulfonylurea hypoglycemia poisoning not responsive to IV dextrose.

Give 50 μg (children 1 μg) IV or SC every 12 h. See package insert for details.

**Effects:** Anaphylaxis, pain at injection site, pancreatitis, cholelithiasis, diarrhea, nausea, bradycardia, hypertension, worsening CHF, prolonged Q-T.

## Ondansetron

Used to stop persistent vomiting in order to perform safe intubation, give oral antidote/charcoal, or perform gastric lavage. Dose is 8 mg or 0.15 mg/kg IV in 50 ml NS or 5% dextrose. Give slowly over at least 30 seconds, optimally 3 min.

## Oxygen, 100%

Oxygen is used to treat carbon monoxide poisoning and in respiratory resuscitation.

To achieve 100% inspired oxygen, the patient must be on a ventilator. By using a non-rebreathing reservoir facemask and a minimum flow rate of 15 l/min 100% oxygen, approximately 60–80% inspired oxygen concentration is achievable.

**Effects:** *Increases* lung toxicity of paraquat and some antineoplastics (adriamycin, bleomycin, daunorubicin). Administration of 100% oxygen >4 h is toxic to the lungs.

**Contraindications:** Pneumothorax or recent thoracic surgery.

## Penicillamine (Cuprimine)

Used for copper, lead, and mercury poisoning.

Give up to 100 mg/kg/d (maximum 1 g/d), divided into four doses, for no longer than 1 week. If a longer administration period is necessary, dosage should not exceed 40 mg/kg/d. Give the drug orally half an hour before meals. For young children, empty capsule into small amount of fruit juice before giving.

**Effects:** Hypersensitivity reactions such as skin rash or purpura, fever, leukopenia, thrombocytopenia. Others include aplastic anemia, purpura, lymph gland enlargement, pyridoxine deficiency, optic neuritis, and nephrotic syndrome. These reactions have occurred when patients have been treated for copper storage disease, cystinuria, or scleroderma. *Such reactions have not been reported in the treatment of lead poisoning.*

**Contraindications:** Penicillin allergy and end-stage renal disease.

## Phentolamine (Regitine)

Used in hypertensive crisis caused by: phenylpropanolamine, ephedrine, amphetamines, cocaine, and when a monoamine oxidase inhibitor interacts with a drug (SSRI), herb (St. John's wort), or tyramine containing food (beer, cheese). In addition, phentolamine is used in cases of sudden clonidine withdrawal and IV extravasation of vasoconstrictors (dopamine, epinephrine, and norepinephrine).

Give 1–5 mg (children 0.02–0.1 mg/kg) IV every 5–10 min to lower blood pressure.

**Effects:** May cause severe hypotension, angina, dysrhythmias; additive effects with other vasodilators.

**Contraindication:** Patients with stroke. Slow infusion may cause transient increase in blood pressure.

### Phenytoin/fosphenytoin

Both used as adjunctive anticonvulsants to treat status epilepticus. After giving 'rapid-onset' benzodiazepines, a loading dose infusion of either agent is initiated. Fosphenytoin must be metabolized in the body to the active compound phenytoin. They are also used to suppress ventricular ectopy; digitalis toxicity arrhythmias. Give IV phenytoin 15–20 mg/kg diluted in 0.9% saline at a rate not to exceed 50 mg/min (children 1 mg/kg/min). The loading dose of fosphenytoin is calculated using the equivalent dosage of phenytoin (750 mg fosphenytoin = 500 mg phenytoin.

**Effects**: Rapid IV injection causes significant hypotension, AV block, or cardiac arrest. Intravenous phenytoin, when extravasated, causes tissue necrosis; fosphenytoin does not. Excessive blood levels of phenytoin cause sedation, ataxia, nystagmus and gastrointestinal side-effects.

**Contraindications:** Known hydantoin hypersensitivity, do not give phenytoin IM.

### Physostigmine (Antilirium)

Used to reverse *severe* anticholinergic poisoning by inhibiting the enzymatic breakdown of acetylcholine; (inhibits acetylcholinesterase). Give 0.05–2 mg (children 0.02 mg/kg) by slow (>1 min) IV injection. Repeat every 5–20 min until anticholinergic symptoms resolve.

**Effects:** Causes muscle weakness, seizures, salivation, bronchospasm, sweating, visual changes, vomiting.

**Contraindications:** Should not be used to counteract anticholinergic side-effects of anti-depressants, neuromuscular blockers, or for anticholinergic toxicity which can be treated with supportive and safer interventions.

### Phytonadione (Vitamin K$_1$)

Used to reverse excess anticoagulation from coumarin and warfarin, and coumarin and indanedione derivatives. Not usually used unless the patient has both an elevated prothrombin time and evidence of, or is at high risk for, bleeding. Empiric use after ingestion of a large dose of these agents is not recommended because inhibition of vitamin K dependent clotting factors takes several days to occur; most one-time overdose situations do not require need treatment with phytonadione. For adults: give 5–10 mg subcutaneously; children: 1–5 mg SQ. Repeat in 6–8 h. Oral dose:adult 10–25 mg/d; children 5–10 mg/d.

**Effects:** Anaphylaxis (more likely if given IV), total reversal of anticoagulation which may be detrimental to a patient whose diagnosis requires chronic, controlled, anticoagulation (atrial fibrillation prophylaxis, valvular heart disease), large hematomas if phytonadione is given IM.

## Pralidoxime (2-PAM)

Used to treat organophosphate cholinesterase inhibitor and carbamate intoxication. Adult dose: 1 g IV over 10 min; children: give 25 mg/kg IV < 4 mg/kg/min. See package insert. Short duration of action necessitates repeated dosages or infusion.

**Effects:** Works mostly on nicotinic receptors to reverse muscular weakness while atropine works more on muscarinic receptors to reverse excessive salivation, sweating, and bradycardia. Most effective if given before the enzyme has been irreversibly bound (some chemical warfare poisons of this class bind within 1–2 min; common insecticides may bind over 24 h). May precipitate myasthenic crisis – rigidity, laryngospasm, and tachycardia – especially if given too quickly.

## Protamine

Used to reverse heparin; generally not needed (heparin has a short half-life). Dose: see package insert.

**Effects:** Hypotension and bradycardia more frequent from rapid injection, anaphylaxis.

**Contraindications**: Because product contains benzyl alcohol, it should not be given to infants; known hypersensitivity to protamine (develops with previous protamine exposure such as protamine insulin),

## Pyridoxine (Vitamin B$_6$)

Used for acute seizures caused by isoniazid, ethylene glycol, cycloserine and mushroom poisoning (*Gyromitra* and *Helvella* species contain methylhydrazine and monomethylhydrazine).

Dose is 1 g IV for each gram of isoniazid ingested. Dilute in 50 ml 5% dextrose or 0.9% saline; give over 5 min. For unknown amounts, begin with 5 g

IV. For mushroom methylhydrazine poisoning, use 25 mg/kg IV. For ethylene glycol poisoning, use 50 mg IV or IM every 6 h. For cycloserine toxicity use 300 mg/24 h.

**Effects:** Acute: rare, however, anaphylaxis and vagal reaction can occur if given by rapid injection; chronic: if dose excessive it can cause peripheral neuropathy.

## Sodium bicarbonate

Used in the treatment of acidosis from methanol, ethylene glycol, salicylates, to alkalinize urine, and in the treatment of polycyclic antidepressant and cocaine cardiac toxicity.

Give 1–3 ml/kg of 1 M sodium bicarbonate (8.4%) diluted in 5% dextrose in water over 1 h. For maintenance, give up to 0.3 ml/kg/h. Maintain serum pH at 7.2 or above, or urine pH above 7.

**Effects**: Hypokalemia, alkalemia, hypocalcemic tetany, hypernatremia, tissue damage from extravasation.

## Sodium thiosulfate

Used to treat acute cyanide poisoning and to prevent cyanide accumulation in patients on prolonged nitroprusside infusions. It is one of the chemicals contained in the Cyanide Antidote Package. Because it does *not* cause significant adverse effects (contrast to amyl nitrite), it is also available separately and is safe to give empirically before cyanide poisoning is confirmed.

*Treatment dose – cyanide poisoning*: in adults give 12.5 g (50 ml of 25%) IV at 2.5–5.0 ml/min, and in children give 400 mg/kg (1.6 ml/kg of 25% solution up to maximum of 50 ml). If symptoms persist, repeat dose in one hour.

*Preventive dose – for prolonged nitroprusside infusion*: 10 mg thiosulfate sodium for each mg of nitroprusside in the solution

**Effects**: nausea, vomiting, muscle spasms or twitching, and pain at the injection site.

## Succimer or DMSA (meso-2,3-dimercaptosuccinic acid)

Used as a chelator to treat lead and mercury poisoning.

Give 10 mg/kg PO every 8 h for 5 days then every 12 h for 14 days. Re-evaluate lead level approximately 2 weeks later, and if necessary, may need further chelation.

**Effects:** Nausea, vomiting, and diarrhea are most common. Other reactions include rashes, neutropenia, elevated liver enzymes, hyperglycemia, and increased excretion of copper and zinc which is minimal and has no clinical significant effect.

**Contraindication:** Hypersensitivity.

## OSMOTIC DIURESIS

Forced diuresis has been considered useful in increasing the excretion of some drugs, but it can be hazardous, and there is limited evidence that it is significantly effective. Intravenous infusions of hypertonic solutions of dextrose, urea, and mannitol increase extracellular fluid volume, resulting in temporary diuresis. Osmotic diuretics are used as an aid in the treatment of cerebral edema resulting from lead poisoning.

### Reference

Better D. Mannitol therapy revisited (1940–1997). *Kidney Int* 1997;51:886

## HEMODIALYSIS, HEMOPERFUSION, AND PERITONEAL DIALYSIS

Hemodialysis and peritoneal dialysis are used to removing certain poisons from the body, especially if kidney function is impaired (Table 4.2). These procedures are not necessary if safer, equally effective or more effective interventions are available. For example, supportive care to treat/manage barbiturate overdose or urine alkalinization to treat salicylate intoxication can be employed. However, dialysis is used when these interventions fail. In addition, dialysis is used to remove excess drugs, etc. that are known to cause significant detrimental outcomes. For example, a patient may have an elevated theophylline level with absolutely no symptoms. However, if they were to suddenly develop seizures, it is known that seizures from theophylline toxicity are difficult to treat and the outcome is often fatal. Therefore, it is prudent to remove the excess drug by dialysis. Indications for dialysis include deep coma with low blood pressure, anuria, and apnea following severe poisoning

**Table 4.2** Toxic agents for which peritoneal dialysis or hemodialysis may be indicated*

| Sedative-hypnotics | Heavy metals | Quinine |
|---|---|---|
| Alcohols | Arsenic (after | Strychnine |
| Chloral hydrate | dimercaprol) | **Miscellaneous** |
| Ethanol | Arsenicals | Anilines |
| Ethchlorvynol | Arsine | Antibiotics |
| (Placidyl) | Iron (after deferoxamine) | Borates |
| Ethylene glycol | Lead (after edetate) | Boric acid |
| Methanol | Mercury (after | Carbon tetrachloride |
| Barbiturates | dimercaprol) | Chlorates |
| Carbamates | **Other metals** | Dichromate |
| Ethinamate (Valmid) | Calcium | Ergotamine |
| Meprobamate | Lithium | Isoniazid |
| (Equanil, Miltown) | Magnesium | Mushroom (*Amanita* |
| Paraldehyde | Potassium | *phalloides*) |
| **Non-narcotic analgesics** | **Halides** | Nitrobenzenes |
| Acetaminophen | Bromides | Nitrofurantoin |
| Aspirin | Fluorides | Phenytoin (Dilantin) |
| Methyl salicylate | Iodides | Sulfonamides |
| Phenacetin | **Alkaloids** | Theophylline |
| **Amphetamines** | Quinidine | Thiocyanates |

**\*Dialysis is not usually useful for the following compounds**

| Amitriptyline (Elavil) | Digitalis | Methyprylon (Noludar) |
|---|---|---|
| Anticholinergics | Diphenoxylate (Lomotil) | Nortriptyline (Aventyl) |
| Antidepressants | Glutethimide (Doriden) | Oxazepam (Serax) |
| Antihistamines | Hallucinogens | Phenelzine (Nardil) |
| Atropine | Heroin, other opiates | Phenothiazines |
| Chlordiazepoxide | Imipramine (Tofranil) | Propoxyphene (Darvon) |
| (Librium) | Methaqualone | |
| Diazepam (Valium) | (Quaalude) | |

with any agents for which dialysis is effective. Lipid dialysis has been successfully used to remove the lipid-soluble agent camphor. Hemoperfusion through resin or coated charcoal columns is another method used to remove toxins. Peritoneal dialysis was originally used to cleanse the bowel before colon surgery. This 'flushing of the intestine' is performed with a hypotonic electrolyte-containing solution administered. It has been tried in the treatment of paraquat ingestion, but its effectiveness is unknown.

## PHARMACOKINETICS AND TOXIC CONCENTRATIONS
(See tables at end of Chapters 21, 22, 23, 24, 26, 27, 28, 31, and 32)

Data concerning the distribution, metabolism, and elimination of drugs and chemicals is useful to in the management of an overdose or poisoning. For example, if a pH gradient exists across a membrane, drugs and chemicals tend to be 'trapped' in the compartment in which they are more ionized. Thus, aspirin, for which the dissociation constant ($pK_a$) of the carboxyl group is $3.16 \times 10^{-4}$, is half ionized at pH 3.5 ($pK_a = 3.5$) and even more ionized with higher pHs. Thus it is trapped on the more alkaline side of membranes. By alkalinizing the urine, the excretion of aspirin can be increased by a factor of 10–20. The excretion of phencyclidine, which has a $pK_a$ around 9.0, can be increased 200-fold by acidifying the urine to pH <5.0. However, excretion of phencyclidine in urine, unlike that of aspirin, only accounts for a small fraction of PCP elimination.

The volume of distribution ($V_d$ in l/kg) estimates body volume into which a substance is distributed after absorption. The $V_d$ in l/kg is calculated by dividing the amount of a substance absorbed (mg/kg) by the plasma or serum level of the substance in mg/l.

$$V_d \text{ (l/kg)} = \frac{\text{Dose absorbed (mg/kg)}}{\text{Plasma concentration (mg/l)}}$$

Substances that have volumes of distribution appreciably greater than 1 liter/kg ( i.e. that are deposited in fat such as tricyclic antidepressants and digitalis, or that are >90% bound to plasma proteins, are not effectively dialyzable in practice.

For some drugs, such as salicylate and acetaminophen, the 'zero time' concentration is most indicative of the toxic effect to be expected. Serial blood concentrations can be used to estimate zero time concentration by extrapolation ($t_{1/2}$).

Disappearance half-life ($t_{1/2}$) indicates the length of time (in hours) required to reduce the plasma concentration of a substance by one-half. By graphing the serial plasma concentration on semi-logarithmic paper, the resulting straight line can be used to determine the disappearance half-time in any particular patient. The rate of disappearance from plasma is often dose-dependent or varies depending on the concentration; this is referred to as 'first-order' kinetics. Some compounds, such as ethanol, rapidly saturate the metabolic enzymes resulting in a constant rate of elimination regardless of the drug concentration serum level (ethanol $t_{\frac{1}{2}}$ = 15 mg %/h); this is called 'zero-order' kinetics. In other instances, metabolism of a given drug will follow 'first-order' kinetics when the drug is present in low concentrations but will revert to 'zero-order' kinetics as the serum concentration of the drug rises. This situation is called Michaelis–Menten or saturation kinetics.

## References

Baselt RC, Cravey RH, eds. *Disposition of Toxic Drugs and Chemicals in Man,* 4th edn. Chemical Toxicology Institute, 1995

Bjerneroth G. Tribonat – A comprehensive summary of its properties. *Crit Care Med* 1999;27:1009

de Garbino JP, *et al.* Evaluation of antidotes: activities of the International Programme on Chemical Safety. *J Toxicol Clin Toxicol* 1997;35:333

Hallstrom A, *et al.* Cardiopulmonary resuscitation by chest compression alone or with mouth-to-mouth resuscitation. *N Engl J Med* 2000;342:1546

Hochhaus G, *et al.* Evolution of pharmacokinetics and pharmacokinetic/dynamic correlations during the 20th century. *J Clin Pharmacol* 2000;40:908

Stork CM, *et al.* Propoxyphene-induced wide QRS complex dysrhythmia responsive to sodium bicarbonate – a case report. *J Toxicol Clin Toxicol* 1995;33:179

Wright RO, *et al.* Methemoglobinemia: etiology, pharmacology, and clinical management. *Ann Emerg Med* 1999;34:646

# 5 Legal and medical responsibility in poisoning

Responsibility for the consequences of poisoning has been shifting in recent years with the advent of legal action by consumers and workers against producers and sellers of toxic materials. For example, a class action suit on behalf of asbestos workers in one company was settled for $20 million, and thousands of other legal claims involving asbestos are still pending. Workers and consumers are beginning to assert their right to know what poisons are present in products they are exposed to.

Legal action for alleged mismanagement of poisoning cases has been taken against physicians and against at least one poison information center.

## WRITTEN RECORDS

In any case of poisoning in which there is a possibility of legal action at a later date, the physician must keep careful written records of all relevant observations and findings. A history obtained from another party must be carefully noted as such in the records. Since court action may begin several years later, written records are essential to maintain the physician's position as an accurate and unbiased observer.

## PRESERVATION OF EVIDENCE

If the physician suspects poisoning in any patient, care must be used to save evidence that may be important for identification of the poison. The bottles used for storing specimens should be clean and free from contamination by chemicals or metals. It is best not to use bottles that have been previously used for chemicals or for pathologic specimens. A clear glass bottle with a plastic or metal cap with a heavy waxed paper liner is adequate. The container should be sealed with a glue-paper label extending over the cover and down onto the jar. The physician's signature should be affixed to the label at the juncture between cap and bottle. Avoid using a seal such as adhesive tape, which can be removed and replaced. If analysis cannot be done immediately the material should be stored in a freezer. Preservatives should not be used, since they may mask chemicals of toxicologic importance. If shipping is necessary, containers should be wrapped with paper and placed in cartons with dry ice.

### Evidence to be saved in non-fatal poisoning

(1) Prescription containers or other containers from which the poison was obtained.
(2) Urine (24-h specimen).
(3) Blood (10–50 ml).
(4) Vomitus and first two gastric washings. (Indicates ingestion of poison but not necessarily systemic poisoning.)
(5) Feces.
(6) Body fat (obtained by biopsy).
(7) Hair clippings.
(8) Clippings of fingernails and toenails.
(9) Food.

### Evidence to be saved in fatal poisoning

Autopsy must be performed prior to embalming because blood collected at the time of embalming will be contaminated by embalming fluid. In taking pathologic specimens, be certain that gloves and instruments are not contaminated by disinfectants or chemicals which may be transferred to specimens. Specimens should be placed directly in containers known to be clean; do not allow them to become contaminated on a table or sink. Store the specimens in a frozen state without any chemical preservatives. In addition to the items listed above, the following should be collected and stored:

(1) The stomach and contents
(2) Liver (at least one-half)
(3) Kidneys (at least one)
(4) Blood (50–100 ml; should completely fill container)
(5) Bone (100 g)
(6) Lung (at least one)
(7) Brain (at least one half).

## Legal chain of custody

In cases of poisoning in which specimens are of medico-legal importance, the physician must use care to establish a legal chain of custody so that each person having responsibility for the material can state under oath that it has not been contaminated or tampered with.

## SPECIAL PROBLEMS

### Attempted suicide

In treating a patient who has attempted suicide, the physician's main responsibility is to give immediate medical care and to prevent further attempts. The patient must be placed in quiet, protected surroundings, preferably away from the family. Hospitalization is frequently necessary. After the patient recovers from the immediate symptoms, a careful evaluation should be made, preferably by a psychiatrist, to minimize the possibility of further suicide attempts.

### Successful suicide

If a patient commits suicide, the physician is legally responsible for reporting the death to the police and to the coroner. Proof of suicide may have considerable legal importance, and the physician will be called upon to justify all statements by careful observations and written records.

### Homicidal poisoning

Although homicidal poisoning appears to be rare, in view of the frequent newspaper accounts of poisoners being discovered only after they have successfully poisoned as many as 6 or 8 of their relatives, many cases must go unrecognized even today. If attempted homicidal poisoning is considered as a possible cause of unexplained illness, the patient must be hospitalized until recovery. The circumstances should be reported to the police. Further proof of attempted homicidal poisoning must be left to the police. If a patient dies as a result of a suspected homicidal poisoning, the physician is legally bound to report the death to the police and to the coroner. Carefully written records of all observations will aid the physician in court appearances.

In recent years poisoning has been increasingly recognized as a form of child abuse. Both acute poisoning from single overdoses and chronic poisoning from multiple doses have been reported. The physician is required by law to report suspected cases of child abuse by poisoning or other means to the appropriate protective services agency.

## Accidental poisoning

In accidental poisoning the first responsibility of the physician is to give proper treatment. The frequency of litigation involving poisoning indicates that treatment must be thorough and personal; instructions given over the telephone may not be sufficient even if the poisoning appears to be inconsequential. The physician may have to see the patient immediately, carry out the necessary emergency measures – even if these seem superfluous – and continue observing the patient during the time when the maximum effects of the poison are calculated to occur. This may require 24 hours of observation. Absence of symptoms or presence of mild symptoms an hour or more after ingestion is not necessarily an indication for complacency.

Of all non-occupational poisonings, food poisoning resulting from eating in a public restaurant or from eating contaminated commercial food is the only type that must be reported. Such cases must be reported to the local public health officer.

Fatalities from suspected accidental poisonings must be reported to the police and to the coroner.

## Occupational poisoning

If poisoning has resulted from occupational exposure, a report must be sent to the proper authorities if the poisoning is reportable. The local health department will have the name and address of the agency to which these reports should be sent.

## References

Ferner RE. *Forensic Pharmacology.* Oxford University Press, 1996

Stever DW. *Law of Chemical Regulation and Hazardous Waste,* 3 vols. Clark Boardman Callaghan, 1986

# II. Agricultural poisons

# 6 Halogenated insecticides

## HALOBENZENE DERIVATIVES AND ANALOGS

Halobenzene derivatives (Table 6.1) are synthetic chemicals that are stable for weeks to years after application. They are soluble in fat but not in water. Some of these chemicals decompose at high temperatures and possibly in the environment to 2,3,7,8-tetrachlorodibenzodioxin (TCDD, dioxin) or similar compounds (see p. 117). Commercial insecticide formulas consist of, variously, insecticides in technically pure form, dry mixtures of several insecticides, or solutions of one or more insecticides in various organic solvents, especially kerosene, toluene, or other petroleum derivatives. These organic solvents are themselves toxic (see Chapter 13).

Dichlorodiphenyl trichloroethane (DDT) seems to be one of the most toxic of these chemicals, at least in experimental animals. In humans, ingestion of 20 g of DDT in the form of a 10% dry mixture with flour has induced severe symptoms that persisted for more than 5 weeks, with gradual recovery. Virtually all fatalities reported in the literature have resulted from intentional ingestion of DDT in various solvents. The toxicity of these solutions is greater than that of either DDT or the solvent alone.

The tolerance of chlorobenzene derivatives in most foods is 0.05–7 ppm, with the exception of methoxychlor (14 ppm). Fatal doses of the various halobenzene derivative insecticides as estimated on the basis of animal experiments are shown in Table 6.1.

The mechanism of poisoning by these agents is not known. The toxic action does not require metabolic alteration of their chemical structure. DDT acts chiefly on the cerebellum and motor cortex of the central nervous system, causing a characteristic hyperexcitability, tremors, muscular weakness, and convulsions. The myocardium becomes sensitized so that, at least in experimental animals, injection of epinephrine may induce ventricular fibrillation. DDD and Perthane specifically depress the function of the adrenal cortex, and they have been used for this purpose in humans. Ovotran has caused skin irritation or skin sensitization in humans.

**Table 6.1** Halobenzene derivative pesticides

| | *LD50* (g/kg) |
|---|---|
| Acifluorfen, Blazer | 1.4 |
| Amiben (3-amino-2,5-dichlorobenzoic acid) | 5+ |
| Bromopropylate, Acarol | 5+ |
| Chlomethoxyfen | 10+ |
| Chlorflurenol, Maintain | 12+ |
| Chlorobenzilate (ethyl-4,4'-dichlorobenzilate) | 2.7 |
| Chloroneb, Demosan | 11+ |
| Chlorothalonil, Bravo, Daconil | 10+ |
| Chlorotoluron, Dicuran | 10+ |
| Chlorpropham, ChloroIPC | 5 |
| Chlorsulfuron | 5.5 |
| Clofentezine | 5+ |
| Clopyralid | 5+ |
| Dacthal, chlorthal | 12+ |
| DDT, dichlorodiphenyltrichloroethane (exposure limit, 1 mg/m$^3$) | 0.1 |
| Dicamba, Banvel | 1.7 |
| Dicloran, DCNA | 1.5 |
| Dicofol | 0.4 |
| Dienochlor | 1.2 |
| Diflubenzuron, Dimilin | 4.6+ |
| Fenarimol, Rubigan | 2.5 |
| Fenoxaprop, Furore, Whip | 2.3 |
| Fenvalerate | 0.45 |
| Figaron, Ethychlozate | 1.6 |
| Flamprop-isopropyl, Barnon, Suffix BW | 4+ |
| Flamprop-methyl, Mataven | 0.7 |
| Flutriafol | 1.1 |
| Fomesafen, Flex | 1.2 |
| Fthalide, Rabcide, phthalide | 10+ |
| Fusarex, Tecnazene | 1.2 |
| Imazalil, Bromazil | 0.2 |
| Ioxynil, Actril, Bantrol | 0.1 |
| Kelthane, Dicofol | 0.5 |
| Lactofen, Cobra | 5+ |
| Methoxychlor (exposure limit, 10 mg/m$^3$) | 0.6 |
| Nuarimol, Trimidal | 1.25 |
| Penconazole, Topaz | 2 |
| Ronilan, Vinclozolin | 10+ |
| Tetradifon, Tedion (tetrachlorodiphenylsulfone) | 14+ |
| Triclopyr, Garlon | 0.6 |
| Triflumizole, Trifmine | 0.7 |
| Triflumuron, Alsystin | 5+ |

Since most deaths from DDT are complicated by the presence of other insecticides and of solvents, data obtained at autopsy are not reliable. In DDT-poisoned animals, the findings are centrilobular necrosis of the liver, vacuolization around large nerve cells of the central nervous system, fatty change of the myocardium, and renal tubular degeneration. The most characteristic finding in experimental animals exposed to the other halobenzene derivatives is liver damage.

**Clinical findings**

The principal manifestations of poisoning with these agents are vomiting, tremors, and convulsions.

*Acute poisoning* (Results only from ingestion)

(1) Ingestion of 5 g or more of dry DDT – Severe vomiting begins within 30 min to 1 h; weakness and numbness of the extremities have a more gradual onset. Apprehension and excitement are marked, and diarrhea may occur.

(2) Ingestion of more than 20 g of dry DDT – Twitching of the eyelids begins within 8–12 h; this is followed by muscular tremors, first of the head and neck and then more distally, involving the extremities in severe clonic convulsions similar to those seen in strychnine poisoning. The pulse is normal; respiration is accelerated early and slowed later.

(3) Effects of solvents – The organic solvents present in many commercial insecticides decrease the convulsive effects of DDT and increase the depression of the central nervous system. Onset of slow, shallow breathing within 1 h after inhaling, ingesting, or absorbing a DDT solution through the skin implicates the solvent rather than the DDT.

*Chronic poisoning*

Workers with a history of many months' exposure to DDT and having up to 648 ppm of DDT in their body fat have remained completely well, whereas most persons have body fat levels of halogenated insecticides below 15 ppm. These insecticides are all stored for long periods in body fat, but not in sufficient quantity to induce symptoms on starvation. Liver damage from exposure to DDT might be expected from evidence obtained in experimental animals, but no such reports have appeared.

### Laboratory findings

(1) A high urine level of organic chlorine or especially of bis(*p*-chlorophenyl)acetic acid (DDA) indicates exposure to DDT or to one of the analogous compounds and is indicative of the severity of the exposure.

(2) In suspected poisoning analysis of serum or a fat biopsy is useful for diagnosis. A sample of fat can be taken from subcutaneous tissue by means of an 18-gauge disposable needle and disposable syringe. The sample should weigh at least 50 mg. Place sample in previously weighed glass-stoppered vial or vial with Teflon-lined cap and weigh to the nearest 0.1 mg. Prepare at least 5 ml of serum from blood taken after an overnight fast. The container should be carefully labeled with the patient's name, weight of sample, date of collection, and name and address of physician. Send frozen sample to Toxicology Laboratory, Pesticides Program, Food and Drug Administration, US Public Health Service, Atlanta 30333. Containers and further directions are obtainable from the same source. The local health department may also be able to arrange for analysis.

**Prevention** (See p. 6)

**Treatment of halogenated insecticide poisoning (acute)**

### Emergency measures

(1) Emesis – Give syrup of ipecac (see p. 90).

(2) Give activated charcoal (see pp. 31–32) followed by gastric lavage with 2–4 liters of tap water. Follow with saline cathartic. Do not give fats or oils. Intestinal lavage with 20% mannitol (200 ml) by stomach tube is also useful.

(3) Scrub skin with soap and water to remove skin contamination.

(4) Give artificial respiration with $O_2$ if respiration is slowed.

### General measures

(1) Anticonvulsants – Give diazepam, 10 mg slowly intravenously. If convulsions persist, use a neuromuscular blocking agent and controlled respiration. For hyperactivity or tremors, give phenobarbital sodium, 100 mg subcutaneously hourly until convulsions are controlled or until 0.5 g has been given. Thiopental administration may be necessary.

(2) *Do not give stimulants*, especially epinephrine, since they sometimes induce ventricular fibrillation. Give propranolol for cardiac irritability.

### Prognosis

Recovery has occurred except when DDT was ingested dissolved in an organic solvent. If convulsions are severe and protracted, recovery is questionable. If symptoms progress only to tremors, recovery is complete within 24 hours. After convulsions, recovery may require 2 weeks.

## BENZENE HEXACHLORIDE (Gamma Isomer = Lindane)

Benzene hexachloride (hexachlorocyclohexane) is stable for 3–6 weeks after application. It is soluble in fat but not in water. Wettable powders, emulsions, dusts, and solutions in organic solvents are available for use as insecticides. Both the technical preparation and the gamma isomer (lindane) are used in vaporizers, and serious poisoning has occurred from exposure to vapor. Ingestion of 20–30 g of technical benzene hexachloride will produce serious symptoms, but death is unlikely unless this amount was dissolved in an organic solvent. In the case of lindane, 3.5 g/70 kg is considered a dangerous dose. In a 2.5-year-old girl, ingestion of 50–100 mg/kg caused convulsions, with recovery in 24 hours. The tolerance of benzene hexachloride or lindane in food is 10 ppm or less. The exposure limit for lindane is 0.5 mg/m$^3$. Reported instances of serious poisoning have been rare and have resulted from accidental or suicidal ingestion.

Technical benzene hexachloride and lindane stimulate the central nervous system, causing hyperirritability, ataxia, and convulsions. Pulmonary edema and vascular collapse may also be of neurogenic origin. Effects of lindane on experimental animals have their onset within 30 minutes and last up to 24 hours; with the technical product, onset of effects may be delayed for 1 to 6 hours and then persist for up to 4 days. Benzene hexachloride is stored in the body fat and slowly lost through metabolism or excretion in urine, feces, or milk. Of the various isomers of benzene hexachloride, lindane is excreted most rapidly.

The most prominent feature of benzene hexachloride or lindane poisoning in animals is liver necrosis. Other changes seen in experimentally-poisoned animals are hyaline degeneration of renal tubular epithelium and histologic changes in the brain, adrenal cortex, and bone marrow. Benzene hexachloride is a carcinogen in animals.

## Clinical findings

The principal manifestations of poisoning with benzene hexachloride or lindane are vomiting, tremors, and convulsions.

*Acute poisoning* (from ingestion or massive skin contamination with a concentrated solution in an organic solvent)

Symptoms begin 1–6 h after exposure. Vomiting and diarrhea appear first and convulsions later. Recovery is likely unless the material contains an organic solvent, in which case dyspnea, cyanosis, and circulatory failure may progress rapidly. Exposure to smaller amounts by skin contamination or by ingestion leads to dizziness, headache, nausea, tremors, and muscular weakness. In addition to these symptoms, exposure to vaporized benzene hexachloride or lindane produces irritation of the eyes, nose, and throat. Such symptoms disappear rapidly upon removal from exposure.

*Chronic poisoning*

True systemic chronic poisoning has not been reported from any of the isomers of benzene hexachloride. Dermatitis from skin contamination with benzene hexachloride has occurred but has improved rapidly upon elimination of exposure.

*Laboratory findings*

Liver function may be impaired. Specific examination of feces, urine, or fat may reveal the presence of benzene hexachloride. For method of collection and analysis of fat specimens, see p. 112.

**Treatment**

Treat as for halogenated insecticide poisoning (see p. 112).

**Prognosis**

*Acute poisoning*

In acute poisoning not complicated by ingestion of an organic solvent, complete recovery occurs in 1–2 weeks. Progression of symptoms to pulmonary edema and vascular collapse following ingestion of benzene hexachloride or lindane in an organic solvent may make recovery unlikely.

*Mild exposure*

Symptoms from slight exposure to benzene hexachloride or lindane vaporizers or ingestion of small amounts of benzene hexachloride have lasted not more than 2 weeks.

## TOXAPHENE (Chlorinated camphenes)

Toxaphene consists of chlorinated terpenes, with chlorinated camphene predominating. It is stable for 1–6 months after application and is fat-soluble and water-insoluble. Toxaphene is available for insecticidal use in the form of wettable powders, dusts, emulsion concentrates, and concentrated solutions in oil. The fatal dose of toxaphene for an adult is estimated to be around 2 g. Several members of one family were non-fatally poisoned after eating greens contaminated with toxaphene to the extent of 3 g/kg of greens. The maximum dose ingested by one person was thought to be approximately 1 g. Several fatalities in children have followed ingestion of larger but undetermined amounts. The tolerance of toxaphene in foods is 7 ppm. At least three fatalities from toxaphene ingestion have been reported. The exposure limit for toxaphene is 0.5 mg/m$^3$.

Toxaphene induces convulsions by diffuse stimulation of the brain and spinal cord. These are clonic in character; salivation, vomiting, and auditory reflex excitability indicate medullary stimulation comparable to that induced by camphor. Pathologic findings in acute poisoning are petechial hemorrhages and congestion in the brain, lungs, spinal cord, heart, and intestines. Pulmonary edema and focal areas of degeneration in the brain and spinal cord are also present. In experimentally-induced chronic poisoning, degenerative changes were found in the liver parenchyma and renal tubules of animals.

### Clinical findings

The principal manifestations of toxaphene poisoning are vomiting and convulsions.

*Acute poisoning* (from ingestion or skin absorption)

Convulsions frequently begin without premonitory symptoms but may be preceded by nausea and vomiting. In fatal poisoning convulsions occur at decreasing intervals until respiratory failure supervenes, almost always within 4–24 h after poisoning. In non-fatal poisoning cessation of convulsions is followed variably by a period of weakness, lassitude, and amnesia.

*Chronic poisoning* (from ingestion, inhalation, or skin absorption)

Instances of chronic poisoning have not appeared in the literature. Experiments in animals indicate that toxaphene is less apt to cause chronic toxicity than DDT but that similar changes in the liver and kidneys are possible.

*Laboratory findings*

Liver function may be impaired. Analysis of body fat or serum for toxaphene indicates severity of exposure (see p. 112).

### Treatment

Treat as for halogenated insecticide poisoning (see p. 112).

### Prognosis

In acute poisoning recovery is likely unless convulsions are progressive and cannot be controlled. The interval from 4 to 24 h after poisoning is the most dangerous.

## 2,4-DICHLOROPHENOXYACETIC ACID AND RELATED PESTICIDES

2,4-Dichlorophenoxyacetic acid (2,4-D) and its esters, 2,4,5-trichloro-phenoxyacetic acid (2,4,5-T) and its esters, and 2-methyl-4-chlorophenoxy-acetic acid (MCPA) and its salts and esters are used as herbicides. The propanoate or butanoate esters are known as MCPB, MCPP, 2,4-DB, Butyrac, Butoxone, Embutox, Silvex, and Tropex. Other herbicides that would be expected to have similar toxicities include erbon, Natrin, dichlorprop, Diphenex (chlomethoxynil), diclofop methyl, mecoprop, Methoxone, phenothiol, bifenox (Modown), fenac, and sesone (2,4-dichlorophenoxyethyl sulfate). Tetrachlorodibenzo-*p*-dioxin (TCDD, dioxin), a contaminant and degradation product of 2,4,5-T and other chlorophenoxy herbicides, is a potent mutagen in experimental systems and is suspected of being mutagenic in humans at extremely low doses.

One fatality has occurred from an amount of 2,4-D not less than 6.5 g. Other fatalities have occurred from varying amounts up to 120 g. The LD50 for these compounds in animals ranges from 300 to 700 mg/kg. The exposure limit for 2,4,5-T and 2,4-D is 10 mg/m$^3$ and the exposure limit for sesone is 0.1 mg/m$^3$.

The mechanism of poisoning has not been elucidated; no specific patho-logic changes have been reported.

### Clinical findings

The principal manifestations of 2,4-D poisoning are weakness and fall in blood pressure.

*Symptoms and signs* (from ingestion or skin absorption)

Ingestion of amounts near the lethal dose causes burning pain in the tongue, pharynx, and abdomen; flushing of the skin; vomiting; painful and tender muscles with fibrillary twitching; fever or subnormal temperature; lethargy, weakness, absent reflexes, peripheral neuropathy; intercostal paralysis; coma. Skin absorption has also caused muscle weakness. After a delay of a week, urine may become dark. Patients ingesting massive doses have had persistent irreversible fall in blood pressure. Convulsions and disturbances in cardiac rhythm have been reported but have not been a constant finding.

Effects of exposure to 2,3,7,8-tetrachlorodibenzodioxin (TCDD, dioxin) include a burning sensation in the eyes, nose, and throat followed by headache, dizziness, and nausea and vomiting. One to several days later, itching, redness, and swelling of the face that is more marked over the eyelids, nose, and lips develop. Within weeks, nodules as well as pustules appear on the face, forearms, shoulders, neck, and trunk, progressing to comedones and cysts. Acneiform eruptions appear after a month or more, and the skin becomes hyperpigmented. At the same time, aching muscles – mainly in the thighs and chest – are evident. The muscle pain is aggravated by exertion. Insomnia, extreme irritability, and loss of libido also occur. There may also be neuromuscular symptoms of weakness and pain with nerve conduction abnormalities. Porphyria cutanea tarda, hepatic dysfunction, hyperlipidemia, hirsutism, chronic eye irritation, emotional disorders, and neuropsychiatric syndromes have been observed. Personality changes may persist for years.

### Laboratory findings

Myoglobin and hemoglobin may be found in the urine. Elevations in levels of lactate dehydrogenase (LDH), SGOT, SGPT, and aldolase indicate the extent of muscle damage. The ECG should be monitored for cardiac rhythm abnormalities.

## Treatment

### Emergency measures

(1) Give syrup of ipecac (see p. 90). After emesis, perform gastric lavage with activated charcoal (see p. 85). Follow with saline cathartic.

(2) Remove skin contamination by scrubbing with soap and water.

### Antidote

For muscle and cardiac irritability, give lidocaine 50–100 mg intravenously, followed by 1–4 mg/min by intravenous infusion as necessary to control cardiac rhythm abnormalities.

### General measures

(1) Treat convulsions or coma. Maintain respiration.

(2) Reduce fever by cool (10°C) applications. Raise subnormal temperature by applying warm packs at not more than 40°C.
(3) Replace electrolyte losses due to vomiting.
(4) For alkaline diuresis, maintain urine above pH 8.0 and urine volume above 500 ml/h by the administration of sodium bicarbonate and fluids.
(5) Hemodialysis and hemoperfusion are effective.

**Prognosis**

Survival for more than 48 hours has been followed by complete recovery. Impotence and muscle weakness may persist for several months.

## POLYCYCLIC CHLORINATED INSECTICIDES: CHLORDANE, HEPTACHLOR, ALDRIN, DIELDRIN, ENDRIN, MIREX, THIODAN, AND CHLORDECONE

These compounds are synthetic fat-soluble but water-insoluble chemicals. Aldrin is stable for 1–3 weeks after application. The others are stable for months to a year or more. These chemicals, either singly or in mixtures in the form of dusts, wettable powders, or solutions in organic solvents, are used as insecticides for the control of flies, mosquitoes, and field insects.

The toxicity of these polycyclic derivatives for rodents is considerably greater than that of the chlorobenzene derivatives. For example, the experimental fatal dose (LD50; see p. 35) in rats for aldrin or endrin is 5 mg/kg; for dieldrin, it is 40 mg/kg; for heptachlor, 90 mg/kg; for chlordecone (Kepone), 65 mg/kg; for chlordane, 200 mg/kg; for mirex, 300 mg/kg; and for endosulfan (Thiodan), 30 mg/kg. In an average adult human, severe symptoms follow ingestion of or skin contamination with 15–50 mg/kg or 1–3 g of chlordane. Other indane derivatives are probably more toxic. In one instance, accidental skin contamination with 30 g of chlordane as a 25% solution in an organic solvent was fatal to an adult in 40 minutes.

Allowable residual tolerances of these indane chemicals in food range from 0 to 0.1 ppm. The exposure limit for chlordane and heptachlor is 0.5 mg/m$^3$; for dieldrin and aldrin, 0.2 mg/m$^3$; for endrin, 0.1 mg/m$^3$; and for endosulfan, 0.1 mg/m$^3$. No safe level has been established for chlordecone or mirex.

Pathologic changes include congestion, edema, and scattered petechial hemorrhages in the lungs, kidneys, and brain. The kidneys also show damage to tubular cells. In the liver, hepatic cell enlargement and peripheral margination of basophilic granules are induced by feeding experimental animals the various indane derivatives at levels of 10–200 ppm. At higher doses, degenerative changes are found in the hepatic cells and renal tubules.

### Clinical findings

The principal manifestations of poisoning with the indane derivatives are tremors and convulsions.

*Acute poisoning* (from ingestion or inhalation of or skin contamination by any indane derivative, even in the absence of solvent)

Symptoms of hyperexcitability, tremors, ataxia, and convulsions begin within 30 min to 6 h and are followed by central nervous system depression that may terminate in respiratory failure. In one person who ingested chlordane, 25 mg/kg, evidence of renal damage was indicated by proteinuria, hematuria, and anuria. Liver damage and rhabdomyolysis have also been reported. Two years after exposure to endosulfan while cleaning vats, a patient had cognitive and emotional deterioration, severe impairment of memory, gross impairment of visual motor co-ordination, and inability to perform any but the simplest tasks.

*Chronic poisoning* (from ingestion, inhalation, or skin contamination)

Prolonged exposure to chlordecone has caused neurologic symptoms. Both chlordecone and mirex have been shown to be carcinogenic in animal experiments. Occasional epileptiform convulsions of the grand mal or petit mal type have occurred in workers from dermal absorption of endosulfan in powder form. Electroencephalographic findings in poisoning have been suggestive of epilepsy but have reverted to normal when exposure was discontinued. Symptoms may persist for more than 1 week after exposure is discontinued or after acute poisoning.

### Laboratory findings

Liver function may be impaired as revealed by appropriate tests (see p. 75). A fat biopsy or serum test may reveal the presence of indane derivatives (see p. 112 for method of collection).

## Treatment

(1) Treat as for halogenated insecticide poisoning (see p. 112). Cholestyramine resin (Questran) can be administered to increase the elimination of chlordecone up to 7-fold. Personnel involved in therapy should wear neoprene gloves as protection against contamination.

(2) Maintain alkaline urine to prevent myoglobin precipitation in the kidneys.

## Prognosis

If the liver has previously been damaged the toxicity of the polycyclic halogenated insecticides is greatly increased. Recovery is likely if onset of convulsions is delayed more than 1 hour and if convulsions are readily controlled.

## References

Boereboom FTJ, *et al.* Nonaccidental endosulfan intoxication: a case report with toxicokinetic calculations and tissue concentrations. *J Toxicol Clin Toxicol* 1998;36:345

Bradberry SM, *et al.* Mechanisms of toxicity, clinical features, and management of acute chlorophenoxy herbicide poisoning: a review. *J Toxicol Clin Toxicol* 2000;38:111

Fontana A, *et al.* Incidence rates of lymphomas and environmental measurements of phenoxy herbicides: ecological analysis and case-control study. *Arch Environ Health* 1999;53:384

Grimmett WG, *et al.* Intravenous thiodan (30% endosulfan in xylene). *J Toxicol Clin Toxicol* 1996;34:447

Guallar MIS-G, *et al.* Determinants of *p,p'*-Dichlorodiphenyldichloroethane (DDD) concentration in adipose tissue in women from five European cities. *Arch Environ Health* 1999;54:277

Longnecker MP, *et al*. The human health effects of DDT (dichlorodiphenyl-trichloroethane) and PCBs (polychlorinated biphenyls) and an overview of organochlorines in public health. *Annu Rev Public Health* 1997;18:211

Nordt SP, Chew G. Acute lindane poisoning in three children. *J Emerg Med* 2000;18:51

Sim M, *et al*. Termite control and other determinants of high body burdens of cyclodiene insecticides. *Arch Environ Health* 1998;53:114

Torres-Arreola L, *et al*. Levels of Dichloro-Diphenyl-Trichloroethane (DDT) metabolites in maternal milk and their determinant factors. *Arch Environ Health* 1999;54:124

# 7 Cholinesterase inhibitor pesticides

Cholinesterase inhibitors are mostly used in agriculture for the control of soft-bodied insects. They consist of 2 distinct chemical groups of compounds: organophosphorus derivatives and carbamates (Figure 7.1). In both groups there are widely varying toxicities. The chemical difference is of interest, since antidotes useful in treating the organophosphorus type may not work or may be contraindicated in poisoning by carbamate-type insecticides. Formulations containing from less than 1% to more than 95% of pure material are commonly available. The highest concentrations are mostly used to prepare dusts and wettable powders in factories, although TEPP and malathion concentrates have been available to the general public.

Tables 7.1 and 7.2 give fatal doses in experimental animals, and the data can be used as an indication of hazard to humans. Thus, exposure to methylchlorothion, DEF, malathion, or Phostex is unlikely to cause fatal poisoning, whereas EPN, parathion, Di-Syston, and Bidrin can be dangerous

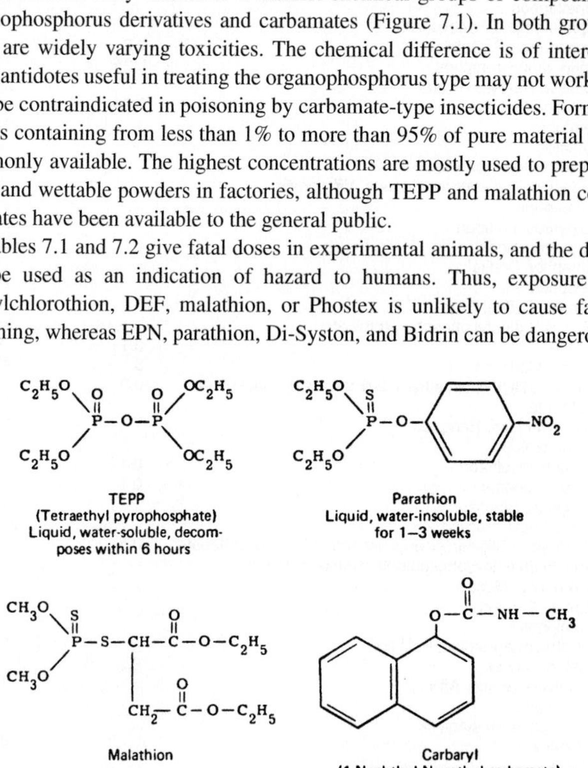

TEPP
(Tetraethyl pyrophosphate)
Liquid, water-soluble, decomposes within 6 hours

Parathion
Liquid, water-insoluble, stable for 1–3 weeks

Malathion

Carbaryl
(1-Naphthyl-N-methyl carbamate)

**Figure 7.1** Cholinesterase inhibitors

**Table 7.1** Organic phosphate pesticides

| | Exposure limit (mg/m³) | LD50 (mg/kg) |
|---|---|---|
| Abate, temophos | 10 | 4204 |
| Acephate, Orthene | | 361 |
| Anilofos | | 360 |
| Azamethiphos | | 1180 |
| Azinphos-ethyl, Gusathion-A | | 12 |
| Azinphos-methyl, Guthion | 0.2 | 6 |
| Azodrin, monocrotophos | 0.25 | 18 |
| Bensulide, Betasan, Prefar | | 271 |
| Bidrin, dicrotophos | 0.25 | 15 |
| Butamiphos | | 845 |
| Cadusafos | | 37 |
| Chlorethoxyfos, Fortress | | 10 |
| Chlorfenvinphos, Birlane, Supona, Vinylphate | | 24 |
| Chlormephos | | 7 |
| Chlorpyrifos, Lorsban | | 135 |
| Chlorpyrifos-methyl | | 1000 |
| Coumaphos Co-Ral | | 15 |
| Cyanophos | | 710 |
| Cythioate, Cyflee, Proban | | 107 |
| DEF, S,S,S-tributyl phosphorotrithioate | | 250 |
| Diazinon | 0.1 | 80 |
| Dibrom, naled | 3 | 430 |
| Dichlorvos, DDVP, dimethyl-2,2-dichlorovinyl phosphate | 0.9 | 50 |
| Dimethoate | | 160 |
| Dimethylvinphos, Rangado | | 155 |
| Dioxabenzofos | | 125 |
| Di-Syston, disulfoton | 0.1 | 2 |
| Dyfonate, fonofos | 0.1 | 5 |
| Edifenphos, Hinosan | | 100 |
| Efosite, Aliene, Fosetyl | | 3700 |
| EPN, O-ethyl-O-*p*-nitrophenyl benzenethionophosphonate* | 0.5 | 24 |
| Ethion, bis(diethoxyphosphinothioylthio)methane | | 40 |
| Ethoprophos, Mocap | | 55 |
| Famphur, Famfos | | 27 |
| Fenamiphos | | 6 |
| Fenitrothion, Agrothion, Folithion | | 250 |
| Fenthion, Baytex | 0.2 | 88 |
| Formothion, Anthio, Aflix | | 102 |
| Fosthioazate | | 57 |
| Heptenophos, Hostaquick | | 96 |
| Iprobenfos | | 490 |
| Isazofos | | 40 |
| Isophenphos, Oftanol, Amaze | | 20 |
| Isophamfos | | 1700 |
| Isoxathion, Karphos | | 112 |

*Continued*

*Table 7.1 (continued)*

| | Exposure limit (mg/m³) | LD50 (mg/kg) |
|---|---|---|
| Krenite, fosamine | | 5000+ |
| Malathion | 10 | 1375 |
| Mecarbam, Murfotox | | 36 |
| Mephosfolan, Cytrolane | | 4 |
| Metasystox-R, oxydemeton-methyl | | 50 |
| Methacrifos | | 678 |
| Methamidophos, Monitor | | 20 |
| Methidathion, Supracide, Ultracide | | 25 |
| Methylchlorothion | | 625 |
| Methyl demeton | 0.5 | 30 |
| Methyl parathion, Metacide | 0.2 | 6 |
| Miral, isazophos | | 40 |
| Nemacur, Fenamiphos | 0.1 | 6 |
| Omethoate, Folimat | | 25 |
| Parathion* | 0.1 | 2 |
| Phenthoate, Cidial, Papthion | | 300 |
| Phorate, Thimet | 0.05 | 1.6 |
| Phosalone, Zolone | | 120 |
| Phosdrin, mevinphos | 0.09 | 3.7 |
| Phosmet, Imidan | | 113 |
| Phosphamidon, Dimecron | | 17 |
| Phostex | | 265 |
| Phoxim, Baythion | | 2000+ |
| Piperophos | | 324 |
| Pirimiphos-ethyl, Primicid | | 25 |
| Pirimiphos-methyl | | 1180 |
| Profenofos, Curacron | | 358 |
| Propaphos | | 70 |
| Propetamphos, Safrotin | | 60 |
| Prothiofos, Tokuthion | | 1500 |
| Pyraclofos | | 237 |
| Pyrazophos, Afugan | | 151 |
| Pyridaphenthion, Ofunack | | 459 |
| Quinalphos, Bayrusil | | 71 |
| Sulfotepp, Bladafume, tetraethyl dithionopyrophosphate | 0.2 | 10 |
| Sulprofos, Bolstar | 1 | 200 |
| Systox, Demeton | 0.01 | 30 |
| TEPP, tetraethyl pyrophosphate† | 0.05 | 1 |
| Terbuphos, Counter | | 1.6 |
| Tetrachlorvinphos, Gardona, Rabon | | 2500 |
| Thiometon, Ekatin | | 88 |
| Triazophos, Hostathion | | 57 |
| Trichlorfon, Dipterex, Dylox | | 250 |
| Vamidothion | | 34 |

*May cause delayed paralysis of extremities; †TEPP decomposes in about 6 hours in the presence of moisture. The rest of these compounds are stable for from 1 week to 1 month after spraying

**Table 7.2** Carbamate pesticides

| | Exposure limit (mg/m³) | LD50 (mg/kg) |
|---|---|---|
| Alanycarb | | 440 |
| Aldicarb, Temik | | 0.9 |
| Aldoxycarb | | 26 |
| Allyxycarb, Hydrol | | 90 |
| Bendiocarb, Ficam | | 40 |
| Benfuracarb | | 138 |
| Benomyl, Benlate | 10 | 10 000 |
| Butacarb | | 4000+ |
| Butocarboxim | | 153 |
| Butoxycarboxim | | 275 |
| Butylate, Diisocarb | | 3500 |
| Carbaryl, Sevin | 5 | 246 |
| Carbendazime | | 15 000+ |
| Carbetamide | | 1000 |
| Carbofuran, Furadan | 0.1 | 8 |
| Carbosulfan, Advantage | | 185 |
| Chlorbufam | | 2380 |
| Chlorpropham | | 5000 |
| Cloethocarb, Lance | | 35.4 |
| Cosban, Macbal, XMC | | 245 |
| Dacamox, Thiofanox | | 8.5 |
| Desmedipham, Betanex | | 5000+ |
| Diethofencarb | | 5000+ |
| Ethiofencarb, Croneton | | 50 |
| Etrofol, Hopcide, CPMC | | 648 |
| Fenobucarb, BPMC, Osbac | | 425 |
| Fenoxycarb | | 10 000+ |
| Formetanate, Carzol | | 13 |
| Furathiocarb | | 53 |
| Isocarbamide | | 3500 |
| Isoprocarb, Etrofolan, MIPC | | 450 |
| Mesurol, methiocarb | | 20 |
| Methomyl, Lannate | 2.5 | 17 |
| Metocarb, MTMC, Metacrate | | 109 |
| Mexacarbate, Zectran | | 24 |
| Orbencarb, Lanray | | 1010 |
| Oxamyl, Vydate | | 5 |
| Pirimicarb, Pirimor | | 107 |
| Propamocarb | | 1450 |
| Propham | | 3000 |
| Propoxur, Baygon | 0.5 | 50 |
| Swep | | 4197 |
| Tandex, karbutilate | | 3000 |
| Thiobencarb | | 560 |
| Thiodicarb, Darvin | | 66 |
| Thiofanox | | 8.5 |
| Trimethacarb, Broot | | 130 |
| Xylylcarb | | 325 |
| Xylylcarb, Meobal, MPMC | | 325 |

to life. Humans may also be more sensitive to some of the cholinesterase inhibitors than are experimental animals.

Among the organic phosphates fatalities have resulted from 2 mg (0.1 mg/kg) of parathion in 5- and 6-year-olds and 120 mg in a man. Five grams of malathion were fatal to a 75-year-old man, but ingestion of 4 g by a child was followed by recovery. Fatalities have also occurred following exposure to concentrated preparations of Diazinon, DDVP, Systox, TEPP, and carbophenothion. Among the carbamates a single dose of carbaryl, 2.8 mg/kg, caused moderate symptoms with recovery in 2 h. Carbofuran in dust has also caused mild symptoms with recovery in 2 h.

Organophosphorus derivatives act by combining with and inactivating the enzyme acetylcholinesterase (AChE). For example, the phosphate esters appear to combine as follows:

The rapidity of the reaction and the stability of the final cholinesterase-phosphate combination are influenced markedly by the structure of the phosphate ester. Pralidoxime, a substance capable of reversing the phosphate ester–cholinesterase combination, is available. The carbamate insecticides combine similarly with cholinesterase, but the combination is reversible with time. Thus, the hazard is not increased by daily exposure to amounts less than those required to produce immediate symptoms. If symptoms develop, they do not persist for more than 8 hours. Pralidoxime increases the hazard from carbaryl but apparently not from other carbamates.

The inactivation of cholinesterase by cholinesterase inhibitor pesticides allows the accumulation of large amounts of acetylcholine, with resultant widespread effects that may be conveniently separated into four categories:

(1) Potentiation of postganglionic parasympathetic activity. The following structures are affected: pupil (constricted), intestinal muscle (stimu-

lated), salivary and sweat glands (stimulated), bronchial muscles (constricted), urinary bladder (contracted), cardiac sinus node (slowed), and atrioventricular node (blocked).

(2) Persistent depolarization of skeletal muscle, resulting in initial fasciculations followed by neuromuscular block and paralysis.

(3) Initial stimulation followed by depression of cells of the central nervous system, resulting in inhibition of the inspiratory center (depression of phrenic discharge) and convulsions of central origin.

(4) Variable ganglionic stimulation or blockade, with rise or fall in blood pressure and dilation or constriction of pupils.

No specific anatomic changes are found in acute poisoning. The usual postmortem findings are pulmonary edema and capillary dilatation and hyperemia of lungs, brain, and other organs. Parathion, DFP, EPN, malathion, and mipafox cause paralysis in the extremities of chickens.

## Clinical findings

The principal manifestations of poisoning with the cholinesterase inhibitor pesticides are visual disturbances, respiratory difficulty, and gastrointestinal hyperactivity.

*Acute poisoning* (from inhalation, skin absorption, or ingestion)

The following symptoms and signs, listed in approximate order of appearance, begin within 30–60 minutes and are at a maximum in 2–8 hours:

(1) Mild – Anorexia, headache, dizziness, weakness, anxiety, substernal discomfort, tremors of the tongue and eyelids, miosis, and impairment of visual acuity.

(2) Moderate – Nausea, salivation, tearing, abdominal cramps, vomiting, sweating, slow pulse, and muscular fasciculations.

(3) Severe – Diarrhea, pinpoint and non-reactive pupils, respiratory difficulty, pulmonary edema, cyanosis, loss of sphincter control, convulsions, coma, and heart block. Neuropathy, hyperglycemia, and acute pancreatitis have occurred.

*Chronic poisoning*

The cholinesterase inhibition from organophosphorus cholinesterase inhibitors sometimes persists for 2–6 weeks. Thus, an exposure that would not produce symptoms in a person not previously exposed might produce severe symptoms in a person previously exposed to smaller amounts. Phosvel, Dipterex, and Divipan are reported to cause peripheral nerve damage with persistent muscular weakness.

*Laboratory findings*

(1) The usual clinical laboratory tests are noncontributory.
(2) Cholinesterase levels of red blood cells and plasma are reduced markedly. Levels 30–50% of normal indicate exposure, although symptoms may not appear until the level falls to 20% or less. Because the normal variation of the cholinesterase level is wide, a determination should be made upon all individuals prior to occupational exposure. Repeated determinations should then be made at weekly intervals during exposure.
(3) Elevated serum lipase and amylase are indicators of pancreatitis.

Samples for cholinesterase level determination may be sent after inquiry to the Toxicology Laboratory, US Public Health Service, Atlanta 30333.

## Treatment

*Acute poisoning*

(1) Emergency measures:
  (a) Establish airway (see p. 52).
  (b) Artificial respiration and $O_2$ – Treat convulsions and respiratory difficulty by mouth-to-mouth insufflation. When equipment is available this type of ventilation can also be carried out by applying intermittent compression to a rubber rebreathing bag attached to a tight fitting face mask of the anesthesia type. Air or $O_2$ must be supplied continuously. A resuscitator, bellows respirator, or face mask and demand flow regulator may also be used. All such equipment must be fitted with a safety valve limiting the maximum pressure developed to 20 mmHg. Be prepared to maintain artificial respiration for many hours. The patient must be watched constantly so that

artificial respiration may be administered when necessary. Necessary equipment must be at hand for the first 48 h after poisoning.

(c) Give atropine in large doses (see Antidote, below).

(d) Wash skin – Before symptoms appear or after they are controlled by atropine, the skin and mucous membranes are decontaminated by washing with copious amounts of tap water and soap. Emergency care personnel should wear gloves and avoid contamination.

(e) Lavage or emesis – If symptoms have not appeared, remove ingested material by lavage with tap water or emesis induced by syrup of ipecac (see pp. 29–32 and 90).

(2) Antidote:

(a) Atropine – In the presence of symptoms give atropine sulfate, 2 mg intramuscularly, and repeat every 3–8 min until signs of parasympathetic toxicity are controlled: eyelid and tongue tremors, miosis, salivation, sweating, slow pulse, muscular fasciculations, respiratory difficulty, pulmonary edema, heart block. Repeat dose of 2 mg of atropine frequently to maintain control of symptoms. As much as 12 mg of atropine has been given safely in the first 2 h. Interruption of atropine therapy may be rapidly followed by fatal pulmonary edema or respiratory failure.

(b) Cholinesterase reactivator – Do not use in the presence of carbaryl intoxication. Use only with maximum atropine administration. Give pralidoxime (Protopam, pyridine-2-aldoxime methochloride, 2-PAM), 1 g in aqueous solution, intravenously and slowly. Repeat after 30 min if respiration does not improve. This dose may be repeated twice within each period of 24 h. Obidoxim (Toxogonin) is available in some countries and is used similarly.

(3) General measures:

Pulmonary secretions are removed by postural drainage or by catheter suction. Avoid morphine, aminophylline, barbiturates, phenothiazines, and other respiratory depressants. Treat hyperglycemia in acute pancreatitis with insulin. Treat convulsions.

## *Chronic poisoning*

Absorption of phosphate esters as detected by a decrease in blood cholinesterase (see above) indicates the need to avoid further exposure until the
cholinesterase level is normal.

## Prognosis

The first 4–6 h are most critical in acute poisoning. Improvement of symptoms after treatment is instituted means that the patient will survive if adequate treatment is continued. Combined therapy with atropine and artificial
respiration is theoretically capable of protecting a patient against 50–100
times the dose that would be fatal without treatment.

## References

Chuang F-R, *et al*. $QT_c$ prolongation indicates a poor prognosis in patients with
  organophosphate poisoning. *Am J Emerg Med* 1996;14:451

Emerson GM, *et al*. Organophosphate poisoning in Perth, Western Australia
  1987–1996. *J Emerg Med* 1999;17:273

Guadarrama-Naveda M, *et al*. Intermediate syndrome secondary to ingestion of
  chlorpiriphos. *Vet Human Toxicol* 2001;43:34

Hsiao C-T, *et al*. Acute pancreatitis following organophosphate intoxication. *J
  Toxicol Clin Toxicol* 1996;34:343

Kalabalakis P, *et al*. Paraquat poisoning in a family. *Vet Human Toxicol* 2001;43:
  31

Kamijo Y, *et al*. A case of serious organophosphate poisoning treated by percutaneous cardiopulmonary support. *Vet Human Toxicol* 1999;41:326

Kingston RL, *et al*. Chlorpirifos: a ten-year US poison center exposure experience.
  *Vet Human Toxicol* 1999;41:87

Lee W-C, *et al*. The clinical significance of hyperamylasemia in organophosphate
  poisoning. *J Toxicol Clin Toxicol* 1998;36:673

Leng G, Lewalter J. Role of individual susceptibility in risk assessment of pesticides. *Occup Environ Med* 1999;56:449 (organoP)

Lifshitz M, *et al*. Carbamate poisoning in early childhood and in adults. *J Toxicol
  Clin Toxicol* 1996;35:25

Ohayo-Mitoko GJ, *et al*. Self reported symptoms and inhibition of acetylcholinesterase activity among Kenyan agricultural workers. *Occup Environ Med*
  2000;57:195

Okudera H, *et al*. Unexpected nerve gas exposure in the city of Matsumoto: report of rescue activity in the first sarin gas terrorism. *Am J Emerg Med* 1997;15:527

Rolfsjord LB, *et al*. Severe organophosphate (demeton S-methyl) poisoning in a two-year-old child. *Vet Human Toxicol* 1998;40:222

Saadeh AM, *et al*. Clinical and sociodemographic features of acute carbamate and organophosphate poisoning: a study of 70 adult patients in North Jordan. *J Toxicol Clin Toxicol* 1996;34:45

Sakata M, *et al*. Prothiofos metabolites in human poisoning. *J Toxicol Clin Toxicol* 1999;37:327

Schexnayder S, *et al*. The pharmacokinetics of continuous infusion pralidoxime in children with organophosphate poisoning. *J Toxicol Clin Toxicol* 1998;36:549

Seno H, *et al*. Quantitation of postmortem profenofos levels. *J Toxicol Clin Toxicol* 1998;36:57

Sudakin DL, *et al*. Intermediate syndrome after malathion ingestion despite continuous infusion of pralidoxime. *J Toxicol Clin Toxicol* 2000;38:47

Yang P-Y, *et al*. Carbofuran-induced delayed neuropathy. *J Toxicol Clin Toxicol* 2000;38:43

Yokoyama K, *et al*. Chronic neurobehavioral effects of Tokyo subway sarin poisoning in relation to posttraumatic stress disorder. *Arch Environ Health* 1998;53:249

Zoppellari R, *et al*. Isofenphos poisoning: prolonged intoxication after intramuscular injection. *J Toxicol Clin Toxicol* 1996;35:401

# 8   Miscellaneous pesticides*

## BARIUM

Absorbable compounds of barium such as the carbonate, hydroxide, or chloride are used in pesticides. The sulfide is sometimes used in depilatories for external application. A soluble barium compound such as the nitrate or hydroxide may be present as a contaminant in the insoluble barium sulfate used as a radio-opaque contrast medium. The fatal dose of absorbed barium is approximately 1 g. The exposure limit for barium and its soluble or insoluble salts is $0.5\,\text{mg/m}^3$.

Barium ion presumably induces a change in permeability or polarization of the cell membrane that results in stimulation of all muscle cells indiscriminately. This effect is not antagonized by atropine but is antagonized by magnesium ions. No specific histologic changes are seen.

### Clinical findings

The principal manifestations of barium poisoning are tremors, convulsions, and cardiac arrhythmias plus hypokalemia.

*Symptoms and signs* (from ingestion or, rarely, from inhalation)

Symptoms and signs include tightness of the muscles of the face and neck, vomiting, diarrhea, abdominal pain, fibrillary muscular tremors, anxiety, weakness, difficulty in breathing, cardiac irregularity, convulsions, and death from cardiac and respiratory failure. Inhalation of barium sulfate or barium oxides has caused benign pneumoconiosis.

*Laboratory findings*

The ECG shows ectopic beats. The red blood cell count may be increased as a result of dehydration from vomiting and diarrhea. Serum potassium may be reduced, and respiratory acidosis may be present.

---

*See also Table 8.1

## Prevention

Orders for radiologic barium sulfate should never use abbreviated terms. Users must be certain that barium sulfate is not contaminated by soluble barium salts. A convenient test is to shake up a portion with water and, to the clear supernatant portion, add a small amount of a solution of magnesium sulfate or sodium sulfate in water. Appearance of a precipitate indicates the presence of a soluble barium salt.

## Treatment of acute poisoning

### Emergency measures

(1) Give soluble sulfates orally (see Antidote).
(2) If respiration is affected give artificial respiration, using $O_2$ if available, until a sulfate antidote can be given and normal respiration has resumed.

### Antidote

Give 30 g of sodium sulfate in 250 ml of water orally and repeat in 1 h. Give by gastric tube if symptoms have appeared. The administration of sulfate salts intravenously is hazardous, since they induce the precipitation of barium sulfate in the kidney, with subsequent renal failure. Administration of potassium is critical.

### General measures

(1) In persistent paralysis that does not respond to sulfate administration, begin infusion of normal saline at a rate of 1 liter every 4 h to induce saline diuresis. Give furosemide, 10–40 mg intravenously every 4–6 hours or as necessary to maintain diuresis for 24 hours.
(2) In the presence of hypokalemia potassium should be supplemented. Give 1–2 mEq/kg body weight intravenously initially; if hypokalemia persists, give additional potassium.
(3) Give morphine, 5–10 mg subcutaneously, for severe colic.

**Prognosis**

If a soluble sulfate (e.g. magnesium sulfate or sodium sulfate) is given before symptoms become severe, the patient will recover. Patients who have survived for more than 24 hours have always recovered.

# DINITROPHENOL, DINITRO-*o*-CRESOL

Dinitro derivatives of phenol and cresol are used as insecticides and herbicides. Dinitrophenol was formerly used medically as a metabolic stimulator to aid in weight reduction. The acute fatal dose of dinitrophenol is approximately 1 g; the acute fatal dose of dinitro-*o*-cresol (DNOC) is 0.2 g. Other compounds with similar toxicities include dinitro-6-sec-butylphenol (dinoseb), binapacryl (Morocide), dinitrocyclohexylphenol, dinitramine (Cobex), dinobuton (Acrex), Amex, dinoprop, dinoterb, and dinocap (Karathane). Danger is greatest during hot weather, when loss of body heat is impaired. The exposure limit for dinitro-*o*-cresol and dinitrophenol is 0.2 mg/m$^3$.

The dinitro derivatives of various phenols apparently act by inhibiting the synthesis of certain phosphate bonds that are important in conserving energy utilization in the cell. In the absence of this mechanism, cellular respiration is markedly increased. In patients who die from exposure to dinitro derivatives postmortem examination reveals degenerative changes of the heart, liver, and kidneys.

**Clinical findings**

The principal manifestation of poisoning with the dinitro derivatives is fever.

*Acute poisoning* (from skin contamination, ingestion, or inhalation)

Symptoms are frequently of sudden onset up to 2 days after cessation of exposure and include high fever, prostration, thirst, nausea and vomiting, excessive perspiration, and difficulty in breathing. Later, symptoms progress to anoxia with cyanosis and lividity, and finally muscular tremors and coma. Oliguria, hematuria, and jaundice may appear later from kidney and liver injury.

## Chronic poisoning

Chronic poisoning has not been reported following agricultural exposure. Medicinal use to induce weight loss has been accompanied by the following toxic reactions: skin eruptions, peripheral neuritis, liver damage, kidney damage, granulocytopenia, and, rarely, cataract formation.

## Laboratory findings

In exposed workers blood concentrations of dinitro derivatives should not exceed 10 μg/g. (See Harvey: *Lancet* 1962;1:796). Take a white blood count if the exposed person has unexplained persistent fever.

## Prevention

Persons who show decreases in the white blood count should avoid further exposure.

## Treatment

### Emergency measures

Remove ingested poison by thorough gastric lavage with saturated sodium bicarbonate solution. If gastric lavage cannot be accomplished immediately, give syrup of ipecac to induce emesis (see p. 90), and follow with saline cathartic (see p. 31). Remove skin contamination by scrubbing with soap and water after removal of clothing. If body temperature is elevated, reduce to 37°C by immersion in cool water or by applying cooling blanket. If body temperature is above 40°C, ice water is necessary. In respiratory distress or cyanosis, maintain airway and respiration (see p. 52).

### General measures

(1) Glucose – Administer 5% glucose in saline intravenously or orally at the rate of 1 liter every 2 hours until body temperature is controlled.
(2) Feeding – Administer readily digested food frequently to aid in maintaining an adequate source of energy for the increased metabolism.

**Prognosis**

Recovery from severe poisoning is likely if the body temperature can be kept below 40°C and if adequate nutrition is supplied.

## FLUOROACETATE

The sodium salt of fluoroacetic acid ($CH_2FCOONa$; 1080) is a water-soluble, synthetic chemical used in the past as a rodenticide. Fluoroacetate is no longer marketed in the USA, but fluoroacetamide is still available.

The fatal dose is estimated to be 50–100 mg. At least 13 deaths from sodium fluoroacetate have occurred. Fluoroacetamide and fluoroacetanilide have similar toxicities. The LD50 of fluoroacetic acid in rats is 0.22 mg/kg; that of fluoroacetamide is 15 mg/kg. The relative toxicity in humans is not known. The exposure limit for sodium fluoroacetate is 0.05 mg/m$^3$.

Fluoroacetate in the body forms fluorotricarboxylic acid, which blocks cellular metabolism at the citrate stage. The relationship between this metabolic effect and poisoning has not been elucidated. All body cells, and especially those of the central nervous system, are affected by fluoroacetate as shown by depression of $O_2$ consumption of isolated tissues. No specific histologic changes are seen in fluoroacetate poisoning. Findings include pulmonary and cerebral edema, congestion of the kidneys and lungs, and mediastinal emphysema.

### Clinical findings

The principal manifestations of acute fluoroacetate poisoning from ingestion or inhalation are vomiting and convulsions. Chronic poisoning does not occur. Symptoms begin within minutes to 4–5 hours, with vomiting, excitability, tonic-clonic convulsions, irregular heartbeat and respiration, exhaustion, coma, and respiratory depression. Death is from respiratory failure associated with pulmonary edema and bronchial pneumonia.

### Prevention

Fluoroacetate is too toxic for use as a rodenticide.

**Treatment**

*Emergency measures*

(1) Lavage – Remove ingested poison by thorough gastric lavage with tap water. Follow with saline catharsis (see pp. 29–32).
(2) Emesis – Give syrup of ipecac (see inside front cover and p. 90).

*General measures*

Control convulsions (see p. 58).

**Prognosis**

Complete recovery may follow repeated convulsions. Rapid progression of symptoms within 1–2 hours after poisoning is likely to result in death. Survival for more than 24 hours indicates a favorable outcome.

## TOBACCO AND NICOTINE

Exposure to nicotine occurs during processing or extraction of tobacco; during the mixing, storage, or application of insecticides containing nicotine; or during smoking. Nicotine is available in concentrates as a free base, which is volatile, or as the sulfate. Both are liquids, even in pure form. In addition to concentrates, nicotine is also present in a large number of insecticide mixtures in concentrations of 1% or more. Additional less toxic compounds with similar actions are anabasine, nornicotine, and lobeline. The less toxic nicotine polacrilex (Nicorette) is used as a tobacco substitute.

The fatal dose of pure nicotine is about 40 mg (0.6 mg/kg, 1 drop), the quantity contained in 2 g of tobacco (two cigarettes). However, because of diminished bioavailability, tobacco is much less poisonous than would be expected on the basis of its nicotine content. When tobacco is smoked most of the nicotine is burned, but a number of carcinogens are produced. After ingestion of tobacco, nicotine is poorly absorbed. The exposure limit for nicotine is 0.5 mg/m$^3$. The fatal dose of lobeline, which is used in tobacco substitutes, could be as low as 5 mg/kg. Nicotine first stimulates, then depresses and paralyzes the cells of the peripheral autonomic ganglia, brain (especially midbrain), and spinal cord. Skeletal muscle, including the diaphragm, is paralyzed. No specific histologic changes are found after nicotine poisoning.

After ingestion the mouth, pharynx, esophagus, and stomach may show evidence of the caustic effect of nicotine.

## Clinical findings

The principal manifestations of nicotine poisoning are respiratory stimulation and gastrointestinal hyperactivity.

### Acute poisoning

(1) Small doses – (from skin contamination or inhalation of tobacco smoke, tobacco dust, or insecticide sprays.) Respiratory stimulation, nausea and vomiting, dizziness, headache, diarrhea, tachycardia, elevation of blood pressure, sweating, and salivation. Gradual recovery follows a period of weakness.

(2) Large doses – (from ingestion or skin contamination with insecticide concentrates.) Initially there is burning of the mouth, throat, and stomach, followed by rapid progression of the above symptoms, proceeding to prostration, convulsions, respiratory slowing, cardiac irregularity, and coma. Death occurs within 5 minutes to 4 hours.

### Chronic poisoning

No cumulative effect from exposure to small amounts of nicotine insecticides has been noted. Tobacco smoking increases the incidence of coronary heart disease and oral, urinary bladder, and respiratory tract cancer.

## Treatment

### Acute poisoning

(1) Emergency measures:
   (a) Wash skin – Remove nicotine from the skin by flooding with water and scrubbing vigorously with soap.
   (b) Emesis – Patient is likely to be already vomiting. If possible give activated charcoal orally to adsorb any nicotine not expelled (see pp. 31–32).

    (c)  Lavage – Remove ingested nicotine by thorough gastric lavage with tap water containing activated charcoal, if readily available (see pp. 29–32).

    (d)  Give artificial respiration, using $O_2$ if available.

(2)  Antidote – Give atropine in maximum doses (see p. 130) to control the signs of parasympathetic overstimulation, or give phentolamine, 1–5 mg intramuscularly or intravenously, to control signs of sympathetic hyper-activity, such as hypertension.

(3)  General measures – Control convulsions (see p. 62).

***Chronic poisoning***

Remove from further exposure to dust or smoke.

**Prognosis**

Survival for more than 4 hours is usually followed by complete recovery.

## THALLIUM

Thallium has been used as a rodenticide and an ant killer. Its use as a pesticide is now prohibited in some countries. Poisoning has most frequently resulted from the accidental ingestion of thallium rodent or ant baits, which consisted of thallium sulfate or acetate mixed with grain, cookie crumbs, cracker crumbs, honey, or sweetened water. The most commonly available salts of thallium are the sulfate, acetate, and carbonate. Thallium sulfide and iodide are appreciably less soluble than the other salts.

    The fatal dose is approximately 1 g of absorbed thallium. The exposure limit for thallium and its compounds is 0.1 mg/m³. Pathologic findings include pneumonitis and vacuolization and degenerative changes in the cells of the hair follicles, adrenal cortex, thyroid, and central nervous system.

**Clinical findings**

The principal manifestations of thallium poisoning are loss of hair and pains in the extremities.

*Acute poisoning* (from ingestion or skin absorption)

Evidence of poisoning appears in 1–10 days and includes pains and paresthesias of the extremities, bilateral ptosis, ataxia, loss of hair, fever, coryza, conjunctivitis, abdominal pain, and nausea and vomiting. Progression of poisoning is indicated by the appearance of lethargy, jumbled speech, tremors, choreiform movements, convulsions, and cyanosis. Signs of pulmonary edema and bronchopneumonia may precede death in respiratory failure. Anuria with renal damage has also been reported.

*Chronic poisoning* (from ingestion or skin absorption)

If absorption of thallium occurs over an extended period, the earliest indications of poisoning are alopecia, atrophic changes in the skin, and occasionally salivation and a blue line on the gums. Gastrointestinal symptoms are also common. If absorption continues, renal damage and functional changes of the endocrine system (amenorrhea and aspermia) may appear along with symptoms and signs as in acute poisoning.

### Laboratory findings

Examination of urine may reveal proteinuria and an increase in red cells and cellular casts. Increase in eosinophils, lymphocytes, or polymorphonuclear leukocytes may occur.

## Prevention

The sale of thallium for any household purpose should be banned.

## Treatment

### Acute poisoning

(1) Emergency measures:
   (a) Remove ingested thallium by prompt emesis with syrup of ipecac (see p. 90). Follow by gastric lavage with activated charcoal (see pp. 29–32). Leave 50 g of activated charcoal in the stomach. Intestinal lavage with activated charcoal will interrupt enterohepatic circulation of thallium.

(b) Consider oral administration of a cathartic.

(c) Remove skin contamination by scrubbing with soap and water.

(2) Antidote – No specific antidote is known to be effective.

(3) General measures:

(a) Forced diuresis with furosemide and mannitol, hemoperfusion using activated charcoal (see pp. 31–32), and hemodialysis can remove up to 40% of absorbed thallium.

(b) Maintain blood pressure by administering 5% glucose in saline intravenously.

(c) Maintain warmth and adequate fluid intake and nutrition.

(d) Maintain urine output at 1000 ml or more daily. If renal insufficiency appears give only enough fluid to replace losses (see p. 67).

*Chronic poisoning*

Remove from further exposure.

**Prognosis**

If the progression of signs of cerebral damage (lethargy, delirium, and muscular twitchings) can be halted, recovery is possible. Complete recovery may require 2 months or more.

## THIOCYANATE INSECTICIDES: THANITE, LETHANE

Thiocyanate insecticides are ordinarily available in mixtures as concentrated solutions in an organic solvent, as emulsion concentrates, or in combination with other insecticides. The toxicity of these compounds is moderate compared with that of nicotine. One adult died after ingesting a mixture containing approximately 5 g of Lethane-384 and 14 g of lauryl thiocyanate. Other fatalities have been reported following ingestion of similar quantities. The toxicities of ethyl and methyl thiocyanate are considerably greater, reaching 10 mg/kg in experimental animals, because they are converted to cyanide in the body. In rats Thanite has an LD50 of 1600 mg/kg.

The thiocyanate insecticides induce coma, cyanosis, dyspnea, and tonic convulsions in rats at doses ranging from 90 mg/kg (Lethane-384) to 1 g/kg (Thanite). Pathologic examination of animals poisoned by thiocyanate insecticides has not revealed organ damage.

## Clinical findings

The principal manifestation of acute poisoning with the thiocyanate insecticides is convulsions. Chronic poisoning does not occur.

*Symptoms and signs* (from ingestion or excessive skin contamination)

Convulsions with respiratory difficulty.

*Laboratory findings*

The blood thiocyanate level is likely to be high.

## Treatment

*Emergency measures*

Remove skin contamination by scrubbing with soap and water. Remove swallowed poison by thorough gastric lavage with tap water. If gastric lavage cannot be accomplished immediately, give syrup of ipecac (see p. 90), 15 ml, and 250 ml of tap water or milk. Maintain artificial respiration during convulsions or respiratory difficulty.

*Antidote*

Treat methyl and ethyl thiocyanate as for cyanide (see p. 315).

*General measures*

Give anticonvulsants (see p. 62).

## Prognosis

If adequate gastric lavage and catharsis can be accomplished before onset of symptoms, recovery is likely. Progression of symptoms after gastric lavage indicates a poor outcome.

## VACOR

Vacor – $N$-3-pyridylmethyl-$N'$-$p$-nitrophenylurea (PNU) – is used as a rodenticide. No longer commercially available in the USA, it was formerly marketed in 39-g packets containing 2% vacor in a dry bait. Fatalities have occurred following ingestion of 0.78 g of vacor, the amount contained in one packet. Most deaths have been the result of suicidal ingestion. The chief pathologic finding is destruction of the B islet cells of the pancreas. Vacor may interfere with nicotinamide metabolism.

## Clinical findings

The principal manifestations of poisoning with vacor are hypotension and hyperglycemia.

### Symptoms and signs (from ingestion)

Nausea and vomiting, diffuse abdominal pain, lightheadedness, chest pain, weakness, blurred vision, polyuria, thirst, numbness of the legs, lethargy, ataxia, hypotension, tremor, muscle cramps, sluggish papillary responses, areflexia, loss of muscle stretch reflexes, dysphasia, postural hypotension, gastrointestinal hypomotility, bladder atony, impaired intellect, disturbances of balance, and delirium or stupor.

### Laboratory findings

The ECG shows ischemic changes in the myocardium. Blood analysis reveals hyperglycemia and hyponatremia. Ketotic acidosis may be present.

## Prevention

Vacor is too dangerous for use as a household rodenticide. It has far more serious effects on humans than on rodents.

## Treatment of acute poisoning

### Emergency measures

Remove vacor by emesis induced by syrup of ipecac (see p. 90) followed by gastric lavage with activated charcoal (see p. 29). Follow with a saline cathartic.

*Antidote*

Give nicotinamide parenterally within 30 minutes after vacor ingestion. Nicotinamide may not be effective if given several hours after ingestion of vacor.

*General measures*

(1) Treat hyperglycemia with insulin.
(2) Control orthostatic hypotension with elastic stockings.

**Prognosis**

Removal within the first 30 minutes has been followed by recovery. If symptoms develop, diabetes mellitus caused by vacor is permanent. Spontaneous recovery from orthostatic hypotension after a year or more is possible. The peripheral neuropathy also improves gradually for at least one year.

## PARAQUAT AND DIQUAT

Paraquat or methyl viologen (1,1′-dimethyl-4,4′-dipyridylium dichloride), diquat, chlormequat (Cycocel), mepiquat (Pix), morfamquat, and difenzoquat (Avenge) are water-soluble quaternary ammonium herbicides supplied in concentrations of 20–50%. They are inactivated by contact with soil, presumably as a result of combination with clay particles in the soil, and are also subject to rapid photodecomposition.

More than 80 fatalities from paraquat have been reported in the literature. One individual died after ingesting 3 ml of 19% solution, or an amount less than 10 mg/kg. The fatal dose for humans has been estimated to be as small as 4 mg/kg, although the oral LD50 in rats is 120 mg/kg. At least 4 fatalities have occurred following diquat ingestion. The smallest fatal dose was 30 mg/kg. The oral LD50 for diquat in rats is 200–300 mg/kg; for difenzoquat it is 270 mg/kg; for chlormequat it is 670 mg/kg; and for mepiquat it is 1420 mg/kg. The exposure limit for paraquat is 0.1 mg/m$^3$; for diquat it is 0.5 mg/m$^3$. Contaminated marihuana has contained from 3 to 2264 mg of paraquat per kilogram, and 0.03% of paraquat from burned marihuana appears in the smoke (0.6 µg of paraquat inhaled from 1 g of marihuana containing 2 mg of paraquat). Rabbits develop lung fibrosis from 10 µg of paraquat instilled into the lung. Morfamquat causes reversible renal tubular damage in dogs and rats.

Although the mechanism of poisoning has not been fully elucidated, it is believed to involve inhibition of superoxide dismutase in the lungs, making the lungs particularly susceptible to oxygen toxicity. Pathologic findings after paraquat fatalities include focal myocardial necrosis, pulmonary hemorrhages and edema, eosinophilic alveolar hyaline membrane formation, proliferation of fibroblasts in alveolar septa, necrosis of the adrenal cortex (mostly in fasciculata and reticularis), renal tubular necrosis, and centrilobular biliary stasis. In experimental studies diquat has not produced the lung lesion found with paraquat. Pathologic findings after death from diquat include hemorrhagic necrotic areas in the brain, distension of the intestines, severe renal tubular necrosis, pulmonary edema and congestion, and bronchopneumonia.

## Clinical findings

The principal manifestations of paraquat poisoning are gastrointestinal distress (nausea, vomiting, and pain) and respiratory distress and cyanosis.

*Symptoms and signs* (from ingestion, skin contamination, or inhalation)

Ingestion of paraquat causes burning in the mouth and throat and vomiting. After 2–5 days hemoptysis, oliguria, and ulceration of the tongue, pharynx, and esophagus appear. After 5–8 days severely poisoned patients show jaundice, fever, tachycardia, respiratory distress, and cyanosis. Heavy skin contamination has caused corrosive damage and subsequent fatal lung damage. Inhalation of $1–100\,\mu g$ of paraquat could cause delayed fibrosis of the lungs without immediate symptoms. Ingestion of diquat has caused corrosive damage, abdominal cramps, vomiting, diarrhea, coma, oliguria and progressive renal failure, ventricular arrhythmias including fibrillation, and impaired pulmonary diffusion. Corrosive damage to skin has occurred.

*Laboratory findings*

A urinary paraquat excretion rate above 1 mg/h or a plasma paraquat level above $0.1\,\mu g/ml$ indicates severe poisoning. Paraquat may continue to appear in the urine for more than a month after poisoning. The alveolar/arterial $O_2$ gradient is markedly increased. Elevation of blood urea nitrogen, serum alkaline phosphatase, and serum bilirubin indicates the severity of damage to liver and kidneys. A decrease in the level of serum trypsin inhibitor has been found; this may be an indicator of the extent of damage to the lungs.

## Treatment

### Emergency measures

Give activated charcoal (see pp. 31–32)followed by gastric lavage with repeated 200-ml volumes of 1% bentonite solution (1 part of bentonite magma diluted with four parts of water). The administration of bentonite should be repeated twice daily for the first 48 h. The addition of a saline cathartic to bentonite is also useful. If bentonite is not available, activated charcoal should be given.

### General measures

(1) Whole gut lavage with a solution containing 6 g of sodium chloride, 0.75 g of potassium chloride, and 3 g of sodium bicarbonate per liter at a rate of 1 ml/kg/min by gastric tube has been suggested. Administer 200 ml of 20% mannitol into the gastric tube hourly and 100 g of activated charcoal in 200 ml of water into the gastric tube every 2 h. Continue gut lavage until only charcoal is passed, usually 2–6 h.

(2) Maintain urine output at 200 ml/h by giving 4–8 l of fluid intravenously daily if renal function is not impaired. Furosemide, 20 mg intravenously every 4–8 h, may be necessary.

## Prognosis

Patients have died of lung dysfunction up to 3 weeks after poisoning.

## AVERMECTINS: ABAMECTIN, IVERMECTIN

The avermectins are microbial products (*Streptomyces avermitilis*) used as pesticides in agriculture and as antihelminthic agents in medicine. They are supplied for agricultural use as 1–2% solutions. Ivermectin is supplied as 3- or 6-mg tablets for medical use. Doses up to 67 mg/kg of abamectin have produced only minor symptoms while one person died from 88 mg/kg. Ingestion of 15 mg/kg ivermectin caused severe symptoms.

## Clinical findings

Exposure to ivermectin causes rash, headache, dizziness, weakness, nausea and vomiting, diarrhea, convulsions, paresthesias, coma, aspiration with respiratory failure, and hypotension. One fatality from multiple organ failure has been reported.

## Treatment

### Emergency measures

Remove by emesis induced by syrup of ipecac (see p. 90) followed by gastric lavage with activated charcoal (see pp. 31–32). Follow with a saline cathartic.

### General measures

Maintain respiration and blood pressure. Prevent aspiration if respiration is depressed.

## Prognosis

Death from doses less than 200 mg/kg of abamectin or 20 mg/kg of ivermectin is unlikely.

## References

Arbuckle TE, Sever LE. Pesticide exposures and fetal death: a review of the epidemiologic literature. *CRC Crit Rev Toxicol* 1998;28:229

Bateman DN. Management of pyrethroid exposure. *J Toxicol Clin Toxicol* 2000;38:107

Benowitz NL. Pharmacology of nicotine: addiction and therapeutics. *Annu Rev Pharmacol Toxicol* 1996;36:597

Benowitz NL. *Nicotine Safety and Toxicity.* Oxford University Press, 1998

Brownson RC, *et al.* Environmental tobacco smoke: health effects and policies to reduce exposure. *Annu Rev Public Health* 1997;18:163

Chi C-H, *et al.* Clinical presentation and prognostic factors in sodium monofluoro-acetate intoxication. *J Toxicol Clin Toxicol* 1996;34:707

Chuang C-C, *et al.* Clinical experience with pendimethalin (STOMP) poisoning in Taiwan. *Vet Human Toxicol* 1998;40:149. (dinitrobenzene)

Chung K, *et al*. Agricultural avermectins: an uncommon but potentially fatal cause of pesticide poisoning. *Ann Emerg Med* 1999;34:51. (abamectin, ivermectin)

Dalvie MA, *et al*. Long term respiratory health effects of the herbicide paraquat among workers in the Western Cape. *Occup Environ Med* 1999;56:391

Eisenman A, *et al*. Nitric oxide inhalation for paraquat-induced lung injury. *J Toxicol Clin Toxicol* 1998;36:575

Fielding JE. Smoking control at the workplace. *Annu Rev Public Health* 1991;12:209

Fisher MH, Mrozik H. The chemistry and pharmacology of avermectins. *Annu Rev Pharmacol Toxicol* 1992;32:537

Floyd RL, *et al*. A review of smoking in pregnancy: effects on pregnancy outcomes and cessation efforts. *Annu Rev Public Health* 1993;14:379

Fuortes L. Urticaria due to airborne permethrin exposure. *Vet Human Toxicol* 1999;41:92

Gotoh Y, *et al*. Permethrin emulsion ingestion: clinical manifestations and clearance of isomers. *J Toxicol Clin Toxicol* 1998;36:57

Hantson P, *et al*. A case of fatal diquat poisoning: toxicokinetic data and autopsy findings. *J Toxicol Clin Toxicol* 2000;38:149

Jones GM, Vale JA. Mechanisms of toxicity, clinical features, and management of diquat poisoning: a review. *J Toxicol Clin Toxicol* 2000;38:123

Lee H-L, *et al*. Acute poisoning with a herbicide containing imazapyr (Arsenal): A report of six cases. *J Toxicol Clin Toxicol* 1999;37:83

Legras A, *et al*. Herbicide: Fatal ammonium thiocyanate and aminotriazole poisoning. *J Toxicol Clin Toxicol* 1996;34:441

Malbrain MLNG, *et al*. Treatment of severe thallium intoxication. *J Toxicol Clin Toxicol* 1996;35:97

Osimitz TG, Murphy JV. Neurological effects associated with use of the insect repellent *N,N*-diethyl-*m*-toluamide (DEET). *J Toxicol Clin Toxicol* 1996;35:435

Ray DE, Forshaw PJ. Pyrethroid insecticides: poisoning syndromes, synergies, and therapy. *J Toxicol Clin Toxicol* 2000;38:95

Rose JE: Nicotine addiction and treatment. *Annu Rev Med* 1996;47:493

Rudez J, *et al*. Vaginally applied diquat intoxication. *J Toxicol Clin Toxicol* 1999;37:877

Schmidt DM, *et al*. Clinical course of a fatal ingestion of diquat. *J Toxicol Clin Toxicol* 1999;37:881

Schmoldt A, *et al*. Massive ingestion of the herbicide 2-methyl-4-chlorophenoxyacetic acid (MCPA). *J Toxicol Clin Toxicol* 1996;35:405

Shiffman S, *et al*. Tobacco dependence treatments: review and prospectus. *Annu Rev Public Health* 1998;19:335

Tanaka J, *et al*. Two cases of glufosinate poisoning with late onset convulsions. *Vet Human Toxicol* 1998;40:219

Takahashi H, *et al*. A case of transient diabetes insipidus associated with poisoning by a herbicide containing glufosinate. *J Toxicol Clin Toxicol* 2000;38:153

Tominack RL. Herbicide formulations. *J Toxicol Clin Toxicol* 2000;38:129

Wilks MF. Pyrethroid-induced paresthesia – A central or local toxic effect? *J Toxicol Clin Toxicol* 2000;38:103

Woolf A, *et al*. Self-poisoning among adults using multiple transdermal nicotine patches. *J Toxicol Clin Toxicol* 1996;34:691

Woolf SH, *et al*. Is cigarette smoking associated with impaired physical and mental functional status? An office-based survey of primary care patients. *Am J Prev Med* 1999;17:134

**Table 8.1** Miscellaneous pesticides

| | Possible symptoms and signs* | | | | | |
| | Skin sensitivity reactions | Convulsions or coma | Irritation: GI–skin–respiratory tract | Liver and/or kidney damage | Blood pressure fall | LD50 (mg/kg) |
|---|---|---|---|---|---|---|
| **Rodenticides** | | | | | | |
| Castrix (see Strychnine, p. 513) | | + | | | | 1 |
| α-Naphthylthiourea, ANTU (0.3 mg/m$^3$)$^†$ | | | | + | | 10 |
| Norbormide | | | | | + | 1000+ (dog) |
| **Repellents** | | | | | | |
| 9,10-Anthraquinone, Corbit | | | | | | 5000 |
| Deet, N,N-diethyl-m-toluamide | | + | + | | | 2000 |
| Dibutyl phthalate (5 mg/m$^3$)$^†$ | | + | + | + | | 8000 |
| Dibutyl succinate, Tabatrex | | + | | + | | 8000 |
| Dimethyl carbate, Dimelone | | + | | | | 1000 |
| Dimethylphthalate (5 mg/m$^3$)$^{†‡}$ | | + | + | + | | 8000 |
| 2-Ethylhexanediol-1,3; 612 | | + | + | + | | 6500 |
| MGK-11 | | | | | | 2500 |
| 2-Octylthioethanol, MGK-874 | | | | | | 8530 |
| **Herbicides and fungicides** | | | | | | |
| Alanap, naptalam | | | | | | 820 |
| Alloxydim, Clout | | | | | | 2322 |
| Ametryn, Evik | | | | | | 1950 |
| 3-Amino-1,2,4-triazol, amitrole (0.2 mg/m$^3$)$^{†‡}$ | + | | | | | 10 000 |
| Arsenal | | | + | | | 5000+ |
| Asulam, Asulox | | | | | | 5000 |

*Continued*

*Table 8.1 (continued)*

| | Possible symptoms and signs* | | | | | |
|---|---|---|---|---|---|---|
| | *Skin sensitivity reactions* | *Convulsions or coma* | *Irritation: GI–skin–respiratory tract* | *Liver and/or kidney damage* | *Blood pressure fall* | *LD50* (mg/kg) |
| Atrazine, Aatrex (5 mg/m$^3$)† | | + | | + | | 1869 |
| Azide, sodium salt | | | | | | 27 |
| Benalaxyl, Galben | | | | | | 680 |
| Benazolin | | | | | | 4800 |
| Benefin, Balan | | | | | | 10 000 |
| Benodanil, Calirus | | | | | | 6400+ |
| Bentazone, Basagran | | | + | | | 1000 |
| 2-Benzanilide, Benodenil | | | | | | 6400+ |
| Bitertanol, Baycor | | | | | | 5000+ |
| Bladex, cyanazine | | + | | | | 141 |
| Blasticidin-S | | | | | | 50 |
| Bromacil (1 ppm)† | | | | | | 5200 |
| Bromofenoxim, Faneron | | | | | | 1217 |
| Bromoxynil, Brominal | | | | | | 190 |
| Bronopol | | | | | | 180 |
| Bupirimate, Nimrod | | | | | | 4000+ |
| Butachlor, Machete | | + | + | | | 2000 |
| Captafol, Difolatan (0.1 mg/m$^3$)† | + | | + | | | 5000 |
| Carbendazim, Derosal | | | | | | 15 000 |
| Carbetamide | | | | | | 11 000 |
| Carboxin, Vitavax | | + | | + | | 3280 |

*Continued*

*Table 8.1 (continued)*

| | Possible symptoms and signs* | | | | | |
|---|---|---|---|---|---|---|
| | Skin sensitivity reactions | Convulsions or coma | Irritation: GI–skin–respiratory tract | Liver and/or kidney damage | Blood pressure fall | LD50 (mg/kg) |
| Chinosol, 8-hydroxyquinoline | | | + | | | 1200 |
| Chloridazone, Pyramin | | | | | | 2140 |
| Chlorthiamid, Prefix | | | | | | 500 |
| Cycloheximide, Actidione | | + | + | | | 2.5 |
| Cymoxanil, Curzate | | | | | | 1100 |
| Cyprazine, Outfox | | | | | | 1200 |
| Cyprofuram | | | | | | 174 |
| Cyprex, dodine | | + | + | | | 660 |
| Dazomet, Mylone | + | + | | | | 519 |
| Desmetryn, Semeron | | | | | | 1390 |
| Devrinol, napropamide | | | + | | | 500+ |
| Dichlobenil, Casoron | | | | | | 1014 |
| Dichlofluanid, Euparen | | | | | | 5000+ |
| Dimefuron | | | | | | 1000 |
| Dimethachlor, Ohric, Teridox | | | | | | 1600 |
| Dimethametryn | | | | | | 3000 |
| Dimethenamid | | | | | | 1570 |
| Dimethipin | | | | | | 500 |
| Dimethirimol, Milcurb | | | | | | 800 |
| Dimethomorph | | | | | | 3700 |
| Diphenamid, Dymid | | + | + | | | 1000 |

*Continued*

*Table 8.1 (continued)*

| | Possible symptoms and signs* | | | | | |
|---|---|---|---|---|---|---|
| | Skin sensitivity reactions | Convulsions or coma | Irritation: GI–skin–respiratory tract | Liver and/or kidney damage | Blood pressure fall | LD50 (mg/kg) |
| Dithianon, Delan | | | | | | 610 |
| Diuron, Dynex, Vonduron (10 mg/m³)† | | | | | | 5000+ |
| Dodemorph, Meltatox | | | | | | 4180 |
| Dymron | | | | | | 4000+ |
| Dyrene, anilazine | | | + | | | 4000+ |
| Endothall | | + | + | | | 50 |
| Etaconazole, Vangard | | | | | | 1343 |
| Ethirimol, Milcurb Super | | | | | | 6340 |
| Ethofumesate, Nortron | | | | | | 1200 |
| Etridazole, Terrazole, Truban | | | | | | 779 |
| Fenpropimorph, Corbel, Mistral | | | | | | 1400+ |
| Fenuron, Dybar | | | | | | 6400 |
| Fluazifop-butyl, Fusilade | | | | | | 621 |
| Fluchloralin, Basalin | | | | | | 730 |
| Fluometuron, Cotoran, Lanex | | + | + | | + | 6400 |
| Fluridone, Sonar | | | | | | 10 000+ |
| Fuberidazol, Voronit | | | | | | 500 |
| Furalaxyl, Fongarid | | | | | | 603 |
| Glyodin | | | | | | 4600 |
| Glyphosate, Roundup | | + | + | | | 5600 |
| Guazatine, Panoctine | | | | | | 227 |

*Continued*

Table 8.1 (continued)

| | Possible symptoms and signs* | | | | | |
|---|---|---|---|---|---|---|
| | Skin sensitivity reactions | Convulsions or coma | Irritation: GI–skin–respiratory tract | Liver and/or kidney damage | Blood pressure fall | LD50 (mg/kg) |
| Herbisan, ethyl xanthic disulfide | | + | + | | | 600 |
| Hexazinone, Velpar | | | | | | 860 |
| Hymexazol, Tachigaren | | | | | | 1968 |
| Isocarbamid, Merpelan | | | | | | 3500 |
| Isoprothiolane, Fuji-One | | | | | | 1190 |
| Isoproturon | | | | | | 1800 |
| Kasugamycin, Kasumin | | | | | | 5000 |
| Lasso, alachlor | | | | | | 930 |
| Lenacil, Venzar | | | | | | 11 000+ |
| Linuron, Lorox | | | | | | 4000 |
| Mepronil, Basitac | | | | | | 10 000 |
| Metalaxyl, Ridomil | | | | | | 669 |
| Metamitron, Goltix | | | | | | 1450 |
| Metazaclor, Butisan-S | | | | | | 2150 |
| Metobromuron, Patoran | | | | | | 2000 |
| Metolachlor, Dual | | | | | | 2780 |
| Metoxuron, Dosanex | | | | | | 3200 |
| Metribuzin, Sencor (5 mg/m$^3$)† | | | | | | 1936 |
| Molinate, Ordram | | + | + | + | | 5000+ |
| Monolinuron, Aresin | | | | | | 2100 |
| Monuron | | + | | | + | 3600 |

Continued

*Table 8.1 (continued)*

| | Skin sensitivity reactions | Convulsions or coma | Irritation: GI–skin–respiratory tract | Liver and/or kidney damage | Blood pressure fall | LD50 (mg/kg) |
|---|:---:|:---:|:---:|:---:|:---:|:---:|
| | Possible symptoms and signs* | | | | | |
| Naproanilide, Uribest | | | | | | 15 000+ |
| Neburon, Kloben, Neburex | | | | | | 11 000 |
| Nitrofen, TOK | | | | | | 2630 |
| Norflurazon, Evital, Zorial | | | | | | 8000+ |
| Ofurace | | | | | | 3500 |
| Oryzalin, Surflan | | | | | | 10 000+ |
| Oxadiazon, Ronstar | | | | | | 5000+ |
| Oxadixyl | | | | | | 3480 |
| Oxycarboxin, Plantvax | | | | | | 2000 |
| Oxyfluorfen, Goal | | | | | | 5000+ |
| Panoram, fenfuram | | | + | | | 2450 |
| Pendimethalin, Prowl | | | | | | 1050 |
| Perfluidone, Destun | | | | | | 920 |
| Phaltan, captan, folpet (5 mg/m$^3$)[†] | + | | + | | | 9000 |
| Phenmedipham, Betanal | | | | | | 4000+ |
| Picloram, Tordon (10 mg/m$^3$)[†] | | | | | | 8200 |
| Piperalin, Pipron | | | | | | 2500 |
| Prometon, Pramitol | | + | | | | 2950 |
| Prometryne, Caparol | | + | | + | | 3750 |
| Pronamide, Kerb, propyzamide | | | | | | 5620 |
| Propachlor, Ramrod, Bexton | | + | + | | | 500 |

*Continued*

*Table 8.1 (continued)*

| | Possible symptoms and signs* | | | | | |
| --- | --- | --- | --- | --- | --- | --- |
| | Skin sensitivity reactions | Convulsions or coma | Irritation: GI–skin–respiratory tract | Liver and/or kidney damage | Blood pressure fall | LD50 (mg/kg) |
| Propanil, Rogue | | | | | | 1384 |
| Propazine, Gesamil, Milogard | | + | | + | | 5000 |
| Propham, IPC | | | | | | 3000 |
| Pyridate | | | | | | 2000 |
| Scepter | | | | | | 3078 |
| Sethoxydim, Poast | | | | | | 2676 |
| Siduron, Tupersan | | | + | | | 5000+ |
| Simazine, Princep | | + | | + | | 5000+ |
| Simetryn | | | | | | 1830 |
| Sonalan, ethalfluralin | | | | | | 10 000+ |
| Sulfamate, Ammate (10 mg/m³)† | | + | + | | | 3900 |
| Sumilex, procymidone | | | | | | 6800 |
| Tebuthiuron, Spike | | | | | | 644 |
| Terbacil, Sinbar | | | | | | 5000 |
| Terbumeton, Caragard | | | | | | 485 |
| Terbuthylazine, Gardoprim | | | | | | 2160 |
| Terbutryn, Igran | | + | + | | | 2500 |
| Thiophanate, Cercobin, Topsin | | | | | | 15 000+ |
| Tilt, propiconazole | | | | | | 1517 |
| Tolylfluanid, Euparen M | | | | + | | 22 |
| Triadimefon, Bayleton | | | | | | 400 |

*Continued*

*Table 8.1 (continued)*

| | Possible symptoms and signs* | | | | | |
|---|---|---|---|---|---|---|
| | *Skin sensitivity reactions* | *Convulsions or coma* | *Irritation: GI–skin–respiratory tract* | *Liver and/or kidney damage* | *Blood pressure fall* | *LD50* (mg/kg) |
| Triadimenol, Baytan | | | | + | | 22 |
| Tribunil | | | | | | 5000+ |
| Triclopyr | | | | | | 577 |
| Tricyclazole, Bim | | | | | | 250 |
| Tridemorph, Calixin | | | | | | 480 |
| Trietazine, Gesafloc | | | | | | 594 |
| Trifluralin, Treflan | | + | + | | | 10 000+ |
| Triforine, Saprol, Funginex | | | | | | 2000+ |
| Validamycin, Validacin | | | | | | 20 000+ |
| **Insecticides** | | | | | | |
| Allethrin | + | + | | | | 920 |
| Amitraz, Baam | | | | | | 650 |
| Azacyclotin, Peropal | | | | | | 261 |
| Benzoxinate, Benzomate | | | | | | 15 000+ |
| Bensultap, Bancol | | | + | | | 484 |
| Buprofezin, Applaud | | | | | | 2188 |
| Cartap, Padan | | | | | | 250 |
| Cyfluthrin, Baythroid | | | | | | 590 |
| Cyhexatin, Plictran (5 mg/m$^3$)$^{†)}$ | | | | | | 540 |
| Cypermethrin, Ripcord | | | | | | 250 |
| Cyromazine | | | | | | 3387 |

*Continued*

Table 8.1 (continued)

| | Possible symptoms and signs* | | | | | |
|---|---|---|---|---|---|---|
| | Skin sensitivity reactions | Convulsions or coma | Irritation: GI–skin–respiratory tract | Liver and/or kidney damage | Blood pressure fall | LD50 (mg/kg) |
| Dalapon, Dowpon | | | + | | | 9330 |
| Deltamethrin, Decis | | | | | | 128 |
| Fenbutatin, Vendex | | | | | | 2631 |
| Hexythiazox, Nissorun | | | | | | 5000+ |
| Hydromethylnon, Amdro | | | | | | 1131 |
| Iprodione, Rovral | | | | | | 2000+ |
| Kinoprene, Enstar | | | | | | 3083 |
| Oxythioquinox, Morestan | | | | | | 1095 |
| Pentac, dienochlor | | | | | | 3160+ |
| Permethrin, Ambush, Talcord | | | | | | 430 |
| Phenothiazine$^§$ (5 mg/m$^3$)$^†$ | | | + | + | | 300 |
| Piperonyl butoxide | | + | | | | 7500 |
| Propargite, Omite, Comite | | | | | | 2200 |
| Pyrethrin (5 mg/m$^3$)$^†$ | + | + | | | | 1500 |
| Resmethrin, Chryson, Synthrin | | | | | | 4240 |
| Rotenone (5 mg/m$^3$)$^†$ | + | + | | | | 132 |
| Ryania | | + | + | | | 1200 |
| S-bioallethrin, Esbiol | | | | | | 680 |
| Sumithrin (D-phenothrin) | | | | | | 10 000+ |
| Tetramethrin, Phthalthrin | | | | | | 4640 |
| Thiocyclam | | | | | | 310 |

*Continued*

*Table 8.1 (continued)*

| | Possible symptoms and signs* | | | | | |
|---|---|---|---|---|---|---|
| | *Skin sensitivity reactions* | *Convulsions or coma* | *Irritation: GI–skin–respiratory tract* | *Liver and/or kidney damage* | *Blood pressure fall* | *LD50* (mg/kg) |
| Thiophanate-methyl | | | | | | 7500 |
| **Fish, worm, and mollusk toxicants** | | | | | | |
| Niclosamide, Yomesan, Bayluscid | | | | | | 5000 |
| **Plant growth regulators** | | | | | | |
| Ancymidol, A-Rest | | | | | | 4500 |
| Atrinol, dikegulac | | | | | | 18 000 |
| 6-Benzylaminopurine, Bap | | | | | | 3980 |
| Butralin, Amex | | | | | | 1540 |
| Daminozide, Alar | | | | | | 8400 |
| Dimethepin, Harvade | | | | | | 500 |
| Ethephon, Florel | | | | | | 3030 |
| Gibberellic acid | + | | | | | 1500 |
| Maleic hydrazide | | + | | | | 3800 |
| Mefluidide, Embark | | | | | | 1920 |
| Nitrapyrin, N-Serve (10 mg/m$^3$)† | | | | | | 500 |
| $\alpha$-Naphthalene acetic acid, NAA | | | + | + | | 1000 |
| Thidiazuron, Dropp | | | | | | 4000+ |
| TIBA, Floraltone | | | | | | 813 |
| Tomaset, Duraset | | | | | | 5230 |

*Treatment: lavage and catharsis; artificial respiration if respiration is depressed; †exposure limit; ‡teratogen in animals; §for phenothiazine poisoning, also force fluids to 2–4 l/d;

# III.  Industrial hazards

# 9 Nitrogen compounds

## ANILINE, DIMETHYLANILINE, NITROANILINE, TOLUIDINE, AND NITROBENZENES

Aniline is used in printing inks, cloth-marking inks, paints, and paint removers and in the synthesis of dyes. Dimethylaniline, nitroaniline, toluidine, and nitrobenzene are used in the synthesis of other chemicals.

Ingestion of 1 g of aniline has caused death, although recovery has followed ingestion of 30 g. The toxicity of nitrobenzene is similar. The fatal dose (LD50) in animals for aniline is 400 mg/kg, and for nitrobenzene it is 700 mg/kg. The toxicities of aniline derivatives are given in Table 9.1. Infant deaths have been caused by absorption of aniline from diapers stenciled with cloth-marking ink containing aniline as the vehicle for dyes. The residual pigment is safe after washing.

Aniline and nitrobenzene act through an intermediate to change hemoglobin to methemoglobin. In one subject, 65 mg of aniline increased the methemoglobin level by 16% within 2 h. The intense methemoglobinemia produced by all these chemicals may lead to asphyxia severe enough to injure the cells of the central nervous system. These compounds sometimes cause hemolysis.

Pathologic findings in acute fatalities from aniline and nitrobenzene derivatives include chocolate color of the blood; injury to the kidney, liver, and spleen; and hemolysis. Bladder wall ulceration and necrosis may also occur. $\beta$-Naphthylamine, which contaminates commercial aniline, causes bladder papillomas after 1–30 years' exposure. These papillomas become malignant if not removed.

### Clinical findings

The principal manifestations in poisoning with these compounds are cyanosis and jaundice.

*Acute poisoning* (from inhalation, skin absorption, or ingestion)

Symptoms and signs include cyanosis at methemoglobin levels above 15%; headache, shallow respiration, and dizziness at methemoglobin levels of 40–50%; confusion, blood pressure fall, lethargy, and stupor at 60%; and convulsions, coma, blood pressure fall, and possibly death at methemoglobin levels of 70% or higher. Jaundice, pain on urination, and anemia may appear later.

**Table 9.1** Nitro and amino compounds and miscellaneous nitrogen compounds (For treatment, see p. 169)

| | Exposure limit (ppm) | LD50 (mg/kg) or LC (ppm, ppb) | Forms methemoglobin | Sensitization | Irritation, corneal damage | Bladder irritation | Kidney and liver damage | CNS effects | Carcinogen | Other adverse clinical effects |
|---|---|---|---|---|---|---|---|---|---|---|
| Acetamide | | 7000 | | | + | | | | + | |
| 2-Acetylaminofluorene | 0 | 5240 | | | | | | | + | |
| Acridine | 0.2 | 500 | | | + | | | | | |
| Acrylamide | 0.03* | 126 | | | | | | | | Neuropathy |
| 2-Aminoanthraquinone | | 225 g | | | | | | | + | |
| 3-Amino-9-ethylcarbazole | | 33 g | | | | | + | | + | |
| 4-Aminodiphenyl | 0 | 205 | | | + | + | + | + | + | Debility |
| *p*-Aminophenol | | 375 | + | + | + | | + | + | | |
| 1-Amino-2-propanol | | 4000 | | | | | | | | |
| 2- or 4-Aminopyridine | 0.5 | 20 | + | | | | | + | | Convulsions |
| 2-Aminothiazole | | 120 | | + | + | | | + | | |
| Aniline | 2 | 250 | + | | + | | | | | |
| Anisidine, *o*- or *p*- | 0.1 | 870 | + | + | + | | + | | | |
| Azobenzene | | 300 | | | | | + | | + | |
| Benzidine | 0 | 75 | | + | | + | | | + | |
| Bone oil | | 800 | + | | | | | + | | |

*Continued*

Table 9.1 (continued)

| | Exposure limit (ppm) | LD50 (mg/kg) or LC (ppm, ppb) | Forms methemoglobin | Sensitization | Irritation, corneal damage | Bladder irritation | Kidney and liver damage | CNS effects | Carcinogen | Other adverse clinical effects |
|---|---|---|---|---|---|---|---|---|---|---|
| ε-Caprolactam | 5, 1* | 930 | | + | + | | | + | | Convulsions |
| p-Chloroaniline | | 100 | + | + | | | | | | |
| Chloronitrobenzenes | | 135 | + | + | + | | + | + | | Hyperthermia |
| 1-Chloro-1-nitropropane | 2 | 50 | | | + | | + | | | |
| Chloropicrin | 0.1 | 250 | | | + | | | | | Heart damage |
| Chlorotoluidines | | 1 | + | | | | + | | | |
| Clopidol | 10* | 8000 | | | | | | | | |
| Cyclohexylamine | 10 | 156 | | | + | | | + | | |
| Diallylamine | | 280 | | | + | | | + | | |
| Diaminodiphenyl-methane | 0.1 | 8 | | | | | + | | + | |
| Diazomethane | 0.2 | 100 | | | + | | | + | + | Lung damage |
| 3,3′-Dichlorobenzidine | 0 | 5100 | | | | | | | + | |
| Dichloronitrobenzene | | 643 | + | + | + | + | | | | |
| 1,1-Dichloro-1-nitroethane | 2 | 150 | | | + | + | + | | | |
| Dimethylacetamide | 10 | 4620 | | | + | | + | + | | Teratogen |
| Dimethylamino-azobenzene | 0 | 200 | | | | | | | + | |
| N,N-Dimethyl aniline | 5 | 200 | + | | + | | | | | |
| 3,3′-Dimethylbenzidine | 0? | 1120 | | | | + | | | + | |
| Dimethylcarbamoyl chloride | 0? | 1 ppm | | + | + | | | | + | |
| Dimethylformamide | 10 | 2850 | | | + | | + | + | | Ethanol intolerance |
| Dimethylhydrazines | 0.01 | 36 | | | + | | + | | + | Convulsions |
| Dimethylnitrosamine | 0 | 20 | | | + | | + | | + | |
| Dinitrobenzenes | 0.15 | 30 | + | | + | | | | | |

Continued

*Table 9.1 (continued)*

| | Exposure limit (ppm) | LD50 (mg/kg) or LC (ppm, ppb) | Forms methemoglobin | Sensitization | Irritation, corneal damage | Bladder irritation | Kidney and liver damage | CNS effects | Carcinogen | Other adverse clinical effects |
|---|---|---|---|---|---|---|---|---|---|---|
| Dinitrotoluamide | 5* | 560 | + | | + | | + | | | |
| Dinitrotoluene | 0.2* | 200 | + | | | | + | + | + | Anemia |
| *N,N*-Diphenylamine | 10 | 2000 | | + | + | + | + | | | Heart damage |
| 1,2-Diphenylhydrazine | 0? | 2600 | | | | | | | + | |
| Diphenylnitrosamine | | 1800 | | | + | | | | + | |
| 2,4-Dithiobiuret | | 5 | | | | | | + | | |
| Ethylene diamine | 10 | 500 | | + | + | | | | | |
| Ethylenimine | 0.5 | 15 | | + | + | | | | + | Lung damage |
| *N*-Ethylmorpholine | 5 | 1200 | | | + | | | | | Corneal damage |
| Formamide | 10 | 3150 | | | + | | + | + | | |
| Hexamethyl phosphoramide | 0? | 50 ppb | | | | | + | | + | |
| Hydrazine | 0.01 | 60 | | | + | | + | + | + | Hemolysis |
| Hydrazoic acid | 0.1 | 300 ppb | | | | | | + | | Hypotension |
| Hydroxylamine | | 175 | + | + | + | | | | | Teratogen |
| Imidazolidinethione | | 1832 | | | | | | | + | Teratogen |
| Isophorone diisocyanate | 0.005 | 260* | | + | + | | | | | |
| *N*-Isopropyl aniline | 2 | 560 | + | | + | | | | | |
| *N*-Methyl aniline | 0.5 | 280 | + | | + | | + | | | |
| 4,4′-Methylene-bis (2-chloroaniline) | 0.01 | 1140 | | | | | | | + | |
| Methylene bis-(4-cyclo hexyl) isocyanate | 0.005 | 20 ppm | | + | + | | | | | |
| Methylene bisphenyl isocyanate (MDI) | 0.005 | 130 ppb | | + | + | | | | | |
| Methyl hydrazine | 0.01 | 33 | + | | + | | | | + | Convulsions |

*Continued*

Table 9.1 (continued)

| | Exposure limit (ppm) | LD50 (mg/kg) or LC (ppm, ppb) | Forms methemoglobin | Sensitization | Irritation, corneal damage | Bladder irritation | Kidney and liver damage | CNS effects | Carcinogen | Other adverse clinical effects |
|---|---|---|---|---|---|---|---|---|---|---|
| Methyl isothiocyanate | | 72 | | | + | | + | | | |
| N-Methyl-N′-nitro-N-nitrosoguanidine | | 90 | | | | | | | + | |
| N-Methyl-N-nitrosourea | | 6 | | | + | | | | + | Pancreatic damage |
| N-Methyl-2-pyrrolidone | | 3914 | | | + | | | | | |
| Morpholine | 20 | 1000 | | | + | | + | | | |
| α- or β-Naphthylamine | 0 | 700 | | | + | + | + | | + | |
| Naphthylamine mustard | 0? | 2468 | | | | | | | + | |
| Nitrilotriacetate (NTA) | | 680 g | | | + | | | | | |
| Nitroanilines | 3* | 75 | + | + | | + | | | | |
| Nitrobenzene | 1 | 200 | + | + | + | | | | | |
| 4-Nitrodiphenyl | 0 | 1970 | | | + | | + | | + | |
| Nitroethane | 100 | 500 | | | + | | + | + | | |
| Nitromethane | 20 | 125 | | | + | | + | + | | Convulsions |
| Nitrophenols | | 328 | + | | + | | + | + | | Hyperthermia |
| Nitropropanes | | 20 ppm | + | | + | | | + | | |
| N-Nitrosodimethylamine | 0 | 23 | | | | | + | | + | |
| Nitrotoluenes | 2 | 890 | + | | + | | + | | | Anemia |
| Pentachloronitrobenzene | 0.5* | 1100 | | + | + | | + | | + | |
| p-Phenylenediamine | 0.1* | 100 | + | + | + | | + | + | | |
| Phenylhydrazine | 0.1 | 80 | | + | + | | + | + | + | Anemia |
| Phenylhydroxylamine | | 30 | + | + | + | | + | | | |
| p-Phenyl-β-naphthylamine | 0 | 208 | | | | | | | + | |
| 2-Picoline | | 674 | | | + | | + | | | Lymph nodes |
| Picric acid | 0.1* | 100 | | + | + | | + | + | | Hyperthermia |

Continued

*Table 9.1 (continued)*

| | Exposure limit (ppm) | LD50 (mg/kg) or LC (ppm, ppb) | Forms methemoglobin | Sensitization | Irritation, corneal damage | Bladder irritation | Kidney and liver damage | CNS effects | Carcinogen | Other adverse clinical effects |
|---|---|---|---|---|---|---|---|---|---|---|
| Piperidine | | 30 | | | | | | + | | Vomiting |
| Polyamines | | 1500 | | | + | | | | | Caustic |
| Propylene imine | 2 | 19 | | | + | | | + | + | |
| n-Propyl nitrate | 25 | 100 iv | + | | + | | | + | | Hypotension |
| Pyridine | 5 | 891 | | | + | | + | + | | Heart damage |
| Quinoline | | 331 | + | | + | | + | | | |
| Sulfanilic acid | | 6 g | + | | + | | | | | |
| Tetrachloronitrobenzene | | 250 | + | + | + | | + | | + | |
| Tetramethylsuccinonitrile | 0.5 | 39 | | | + | | | + | | Convulsions |
| Tetranitromethane | 0.005 | 18 ppm | + | | + | | | + | | Heart damage |
| Tetryl | 1.5* | 500 sc | | | + | | | | | |
| o-Toluidine | 0.02* | 4500 | | | + | | | + | + | |
| Toluenediamine | | 100 | + | + | + | | + | + | | |
| Toluene diisocyanate | 0.005 | 50 ppb | | + | + | | | | | Asthma |
| Toluidines | 2 | 42 | + | | + | | | | + | |
| Triallylamine | | 492 | | | + | | + | | | |
| Triphenylamine | 5* | 1600 | | | | | | | | |
| Tris (hydroxymethyl)-aminomethane | | 1000 | | | + | | | | | |
| m-Xylene α,α'-diamine | 0.1* | 930 | + | + | + | | + | | | |
| Xylidines | 0.5 | 250 | + | | | | | + | + | |

*mg/m$^3$

*Chronic poisoning* (from inhalation or skin absorption)

Nervous system, liver, kidneys, and bone marrow may be affected. Weight loss, anemia, weakness, and irritability occur.

*Laboratory findings*

(1) Blood methemoglobin, determined photometrically, is the best measure of the seriousness of poisoning with these substances.

(2) Red blood cells may be reduced to 20–30% of normal, with accompanying poikilocytosis and anisocytosis. Erythrocyte inclusion (Heinz) bodies are common.

(3) Hepatic cell function impairment may be indicated by the appropriate tests (see p. 75).

(4) *N*-Acetyl-*p*-aminophenol in urine indicates chronic exposure. Gross or microscopic hematuria may be present as a result of bladder or kidney irritation or hemolysis. Renal function may also be impaired.

## Treatment

*Acute poisoning*

(1) Emergency measures:
   (a) Remove poison from skin by washing thoroughly with soap and water.
   (b) If poison was swallowed remove by emesis or gastric lavage and consider using activated charcoal (see pp. 31–32).
   (c) Give $O_2$ if respiration is shallow or anoxia is present.

(2) Antidote – For severe methemoglobinemia, give methylene blue, 1% solution, 0.1 ml/kg (1 mg/kg) slowly intravenously, to reduce methemoglobin to normal hemoglobin (see p. 78).

(3) Other measures – If methemoglobinemia does not respond to methylene blue, hemodialysis or exchange transfusion is useful.

*Chronic poisoning*

(1) Remove from exposure.

(2) Treat liver damage (see p. 76).

## Prognosis

Survival for 24 hours is usually followed by complete recovery.

# TRINITROTOLUENE AND TRINITROBENZENE

Trinitrotoluene (TNT) and trinitrobenzene are used as explosives. The acute fatal dose is estimated to be 1–2 g. The exposure limit is 0.5 mg/m³. At least 22 fatalities from trinitrotoluene absorption occurred in the USA during World War II.

Trinitrotoluene and trinitrobenzene injure almost all cells, especially those of the liver, bone marrow, and kidney. Trinitrobenzene damages the central nervous system. Pathologic findings are acute yellow atrophy of the liver, bone marrow aplasia, petechial hemorrhages, and toxic nephritis.

## Clinical findings

The principal manifestation of trinitrotoluene poisoning is jaundice.

*Acute or chronic poisoning* (from inhalation, skin absorption, or ingestion)

Jaundice, dermatitis, cyanosis, pallor, nausea, loss of appetite, aplastic or hemolytic anemia, and oliguria or anuria occur variably. The liver may be enlarged early or atrophic later. Convulsions or coma may occur.

## Laboratory findings

(1) The blood methemoglobin level is the best measure of the seriousness of poisoning (see p. 164).
(2) In chronic poisoning hepatic cell injury will be revealed by appropriate tests (see p. 75).
(3) The red blood cell count may be depressed, with anisocytosis and poikilocytosis. There may be relative lymphocytosis.
(4) Urine may show protein and casts prior to the onset of anuria.

## Treatment

*Emergency measures*

Terminate skin contamination by thorough washing with soap and water. Remove swallowed trinitrotoluene by gastric lavage or emesis (see pp. 29–32).

*Other measures*

Treat failure of liver function (see p. 76). Treat hemolytic reactions (see p. 80).

## Prognosis

Approximately 50% of patients with severe liver damage die of acute yellow atrophy. The others recover completely.

## References

Aitio A, *et al*. 2,4,6-Trinitrotoluene. *IARC Monographs on the Evaluation of Carcinogenic Risks to Humans* 1996;65:449

Bernstein DI, Jolly A. Current diagnostic methods for diisocyanate induced occupational asthma. *Am J Ind Med* 1999;36:459

Fiorito A, *et al*. Liver function alterations in synthetic leather workers exposed to dimethylformamide. *Am J Ind Med* 1997;32:255

Mullins ME, Hammett-Stabler CA. Intoxication with nitromethane-containing fuels: don't be 'fueled' by the creatinine. *J Toxicol Clin Toxicol* 1998;36:315

Ott MG, *et al*. Respiratory health surveillance in a toluene di-isocyanate production unit, 1967–97: clinical observations and lung function analyses. *Occup Environ Med* 2000;57:43

Sheperd G, *et al*. Prolonged formation of methemoglobin following nitroethane ingestion. *J Toxicol Clin Toxicol* 1998;36:613

Siribaddana SH, *et al*. Toluene diisocyanate exposure in a glove manufacturing plant. *J Toxicol Clin Toxicol* 1998;36:95

Straif K, *et al*. Elevated mortality from nonalcohol-related chronic liver disease among female rubber workers: is it associated with exposure to nitrosamines? *Am J Ind Med* 1999;35:264

Su T-C, *et al*. Dimethylacetamide, ethylenediamine, and diphenylmethane diisocyanate poisoning manifest as acute psychosis and pulmonary edema: treatment with hemoperfusion. *J Toxicol Clin Toxicol* 2000;38:429

Testud F, *et al*. Acute hexogen poisoning after occupational exposure. *J Toxicol Clin Toxicol* 1996;34:109. (Trinitrotriazine).

Tillmann HL, *et al*. Accidental intoxication with methylene dianiline-*p,p'*-diaminodiphenyl methane: acute liver damage after presumed ecstasy consumption. *J Toxicol Clin Toxicol* 1996;35:35

Williams NR, *et al*. Biological monitoring to assess exposure from use of isocyanates in motor vehicle repair. *Occup Environ Med* 1999;56:598

# 10 Halogenated hydrocarbons

## CARBON TETRACHLORIDE

**Formula:** $CCl_4$; bp: 76.7°C; vapor pressure at 20°C: 91 mmHg. Carbon tetrachloride decomposes to phosgene ($COCl_2$) and hydrochloric acid on heating.

Carbon tetrachloride is metabolized to a trichloromethyl free radical ($CCl_3$) which then forms chloroform, hexachloroethane, carbon monoxide, trichloromethanol, and eventually forms phosgene and carbon dioxide.

Carbon tetrachloride is a clear, nonflammable liquid that produces a sweet odor when it evaporates. It is consumed in the synthesis of chlorofluoro-carbons that are heat transfer agents in refrigeration equipment and as aerosol propellants. $CCl_4$ has been used as an industrial solvent, as an extracting agent for removing stains from furniture, as a component in fire extinguishers, and prior to 1969, was used as a waterless shampoo. The largest source of its release was when it was used to fumigate grains. However, in 1986 its use for fumigation was banned except for preservation of museum artifacts. There have been attempts to restrict the use of chlorofluorocarbons because they are thought to deplete the ozone layer; however, carbon tetrachloride is still used for many purposes in European and Third World countries.

While acute exposure has declined, it is most likely to occur in those who work in industries that manufacture carbon tetrachloride or in those who work or live near chemical waste sites. Other occupations at higher risk are auto-mobile mechanics*, workers in dry cleaning*, pesticide applicators*, grain workers*, museum employees, tin waste-recovery workers, steel mill and blast furnace workers, air transportation employees, and those who work in the pharmaceutical and in the telegraph equipment industries.

Chronic exposure can occur if carbon tetrachloride is present in ambient air. Indoor concentrations are higher than outdoor levels because pesticides and cleaning agents inside the home may be sources of airborne carbon tetra-chloride.

---

*Carbon tetrachloride is no longer used in these industries in the United States

The adult fatal dose by ingestion or inhalation is 3–5 ml. The exposure limit is 5 ppm (NIOSH 2 ppm) or 30 mg/m$^3$ (1.5 g evaporated in a room 10 × 10 × 8 ft gives 10 ppm). Carbon tetrachloride depresses and injures almost all cells of the body, including those of the central nervous system, liver, kidney, and blood vessels. Toxicity appears to result from the intracellular breakdown of carbon tetrachloride to more toxic intermediates, including epoxides, particularly in the liver. The heart muscle may be depressed, and ventricular arrhythmias may occur. Concomitant ethanol ingestion increases the effect of carbon tetrachloride on all organs. On postmortem examination the kidneys show marked edema and fatty degeneration of the tubules. The liver shows centrilobular necrosis and fatty degeneration and may be enlarged. The heart may also show fatty degeneration. The endothelium of blood vessels may be injured, with resultant petechiae or larger hemorrhages. At a level of 79 ppm, the sweet odor of carbon tetrachloride is evident.

See Table 10.2 for halogenated hydrocarbons not otherwise discussed. Many of these produce poisoning like carbon tetrachloride. Treatment of poisoning is the same as for carbon tetrachloride.

**Clinical findings**

The principal manifestations in poisoning with carbon tetrachloride are coma, oliguria, and jaundice.

*Acute poisoning* (from inhalation, skin absorption, or ingestion)

The immediate effects are abdominal pain, nausea and vomiting, dizziness, and confusion, progressing to unconsciousness, respiratory slowing, slowed or irregular pulse, and fall in blood pressure. If consciousness is regained, the patient may have mild symptoms of nausea and anorexia or be free of symptoms for 1 day to 2 weeks until evidence of liver or kidney damage appears. Liver damage is indicated by nausea and vomiting, jaundice, and a swollen, tender liver; kidney damage is indicated by decreased urine output, edema, sudden weight gain, and azotemia progressing to uremia. Coma, liver damage, or kidney damage may appear independently, or all may occur in the same individual at different times.

*Chronic poisoning* (from inhalation or skin absorption)

The above symptoms occur after repeated exposures to low concentrations but are less severe. Vague symptoms suggestive of poisoning include fatigue, anorexia, occasional vomiting, abdominal discomfort, anemia, weakness, nausea, blurring of vision, memory loss, paresthesias, tremors, and loss of peripheral color vision. Dermatitis follows repeated skin exposure. Carbon tetrachloride is a potential carcinogen.

*Laboratory findings*

(1) Increased liver functions tests (ALT, AST) and later increased protime due to liver damage (with resultant bleeding abnormalities).
(2) Urine may show red cells, protein, and casts.
(3) Elevated blood urea nitrogen and serum creatinine that can progress to acute and/or chronic renal failure.
(4) White blood count elevation in response to hepatic necrosis.
(5) Chest radiograph may show congestion. Fluid overload and decreased albumin synthesis contributes to pulmonary edema.

**Prevention**

Carbon tetrachloride workers must not drink alcoholic beverages and should have a twice-yearly physical examination, including laboratory evaluation of liver function. There has been a report of toxicity in a male after 3–4 hours of exposure despite full protective gear and respiratory mask. Clinical signs were initially CNS as one would expect (ataxia and trouble concentrating).

Carbon tetrachloride should not be used as a fire extinguisher, since heat decomposes it to phosgene.

**Treatment**

*Acute poisoning*

(1) Emergency measures:
    (a) If carbon tetrachloride is inhaled, give artificial respiration until consciousness returns.
    (b) Because $CCl_4$ is very lipid soluble and penetrates intact skin, clothing must be removed and skin cleansed with copious amounts of water.

(c) If carbon tetrachloride is ingested, perform gastric lavage followed by giving activated charcoal (see pp. 31–32). Do NOT induce vomiting (increased risk of aspiration).

(2) General measures:

(a) Maintain blood pressure by giving 5% glucose intravenously.

(b) *Do not give stimulants.* Epinephrine or ephedrine may induce ventricular fibrillation.

(c) If urine output is normal, maintain it at 1–2 liters daily by osmotic diuresis or by giving fluids orally. Do not give diuretics.

(d) Give a high-carbohydrate diet to attempt to restore optimal liver function.

(3) Special problems:

(a) Acute renal shutdown is treated as described on p. 67. The oliguric phase of carbon tetrachloride intoxication is likely to last 7–10 days and is followed by a diuretic phase that may last up to 3 weeks before normal kidney function returns.

(b) Treat hepatic coma by controlling blood ammonia levels. Useful measures include reducing protein intake to 20–30 g daily, preventing ammonia absorption from stool by daily administration of milk of magnesia or sodium sulfate, giving 8 g of neomycin daily to reduce ammonia formation in the bowel, avoiding chlorothiazide and acetazolamide, and using peritoneal dialysis.

(c) Hemodialysis may be necessary to control blood electrolytes.

### Chronic poisoning

Remove from exposure and treat as indicated for acute poisoning.

### Prognosis

In anuria, spontaneous return of kidney function may begin 2–3 weeks after poisoning. Complete return of liver and kidney function requires 2–12 months.

# METHYL BROMIDE, METHYL CHLORIDE, AND METHYL IODIDE

**Formulas**: Methyl bromide, $CH_3Br$; methyl chloride, $CH_3Cl$; methyl iodide, $CH_3I$; all are gaseous or have high vapor pressure at ordinary temperatures.

Methyl bromide, methyl chloride, and methyl iodide are used as refrigerants, in chemical synthesis, and as fumigants. Methyl bromide is used with carbon tetrachloride in fire extinguishers. The exposure limit is 5 ppm for methyl bromide, 50 ppm for methyl chloride, and 2 ppm for methyl iodide. The fat-soluble methyl bromide, methyl chloride, and methyl iodide enter cells, where hydrolysis to methanol and halogen ions occurs.

Pathologic findings are congestion of the liver, kidneys, brain, and lungs, with degenerative changes in the cells. Bronchial pneumonia and pulmonary edema are common. These substances damage almost all body cells.

## Clinical findings

The principal manifestations of poisoning with these agents are coma and convulsions.

*Acute poisoning* (from inhalation or skin absorption)

If the concentration of methyl bromide, iodide, or chloride is high, nausea and vomiting, blurred vision, vertigo, weakness or paralysis, oliguria or anuria, drowsiness, confusion, hyperactivity, fall in blood pressure, coma, convulsions, and pulmonary edema progress over 4–6 h after a latent period of 1–4 h. After exposure to lower concentrations, symptoms may not appear for 12–24 h. Pulmonary edema and bronchial pneumonia are most often the cause of death. Skin contact causes irritation and vesiculation.

*Chronic poisoning* (from inhalation or skin absorption)

Repeated exposure to concentrations slightly higher than the exposure limit will cause blurring of vision, papilledema, numbness of the extremities, confusion, hallucinations, somnolence, fainting attacks, and bronchospasm. Methyl iodide is a potential carcinogen.

### *Laboratory findings*

(1)  Impairment of hepatic cell function may be indicated by appropriate laboratory tests.
(2)  Urine may contain casts, red blood cells, and protein.
(3)  Blood pH may be reduced.
(4)  Blood methanol level may reach toxic concentrations.

## Prevention

Gas masks are relatively ineffective because methyl bromide and methyl chloride penetrate the skin readily. Safety dispensers must always be used when applying methyl bromide as a fumigant.

## Treatment

### *Acute poisoning*

(1)  Remove from further exposure and observe carefully for the first 48 h. Restrain hyperactive patients.
(2)  General measures:
    (a)  Treat pulmonary edema (see p. 55).
    (b)  Control convulsions by the cautious use of diazepam.
(3)  Special problems:
    (a)  Bronchospasm complicating pulmonary edema or bronchial pneumonia is treated by aminophylline given intravenously; repeat as necessary.
    (b)  Treat renal failure.
    (c)  Treat acidosis.
    (d)  Treat methanol intoxication if necessary.
    (e)  Treat bacterial pneumonia with organism-specific chemotherapy.

### *Chronic poisoning*

Remove from further exposure.

**Prognosis**

Patients who survive 48–72 h usually recover completely, but neurotoxic effects may persist for months.

## TETRACHLOROETHANE

**Formula**: $CHCl_2CHCl_2$; bp: 146°C; vapor pressure at 20°C: 11 mmHg.

Tetrachloroethane is used as a solvent in industry and occurs as a contaminant in other chlorinated hydrocarbons. It is occasionally present in household cleaners.

Tetrachloroethane is the most poisonous of the chlorinated hydrocarbons. The exposure limit is 1 ppm. Tetrachloroethane causes a long-lasting narcosis with delayed onset and severe damage to the liver and kidneys. The pathologic findings include acute yellow atrophy of the liver. If death has been immediate, congestion of lungs, kidneys, brain, and gastrointestinal tract may be the only evidence of poisoning.

**Clinical findings**

The principal manifestations of tetrachloroethane poisoning are coma, jaundice, and oliguria.

*Acute poisoning* (from inhalation, ingestion, or skin absorption)

Initially tetrachloroethane causes irritation of the eyes and nose, followed by headache and nausea. Cyanosis and central nervous system depression progressing to coma appear after 1–4 h.

Liver and kidney damage, after apparent recovery or after repeated exposures to amounts less than that necessary to cause acute symptoms, is indicated by nausea and vomiting, abdominal pain, jaundice, and oliguria with uremia. The relative damage to the liver or kidneys varies.

*Chronic poisoning* (from inhalation or skin absorption)

Headache, tremor, dizziness, peripheral paresthesia, hypesthesia, or anesthesia.

### Laboratory findings

(1) An increase in the large mononuclear cells above 12% in the differential blood smear indicates exposure.
(2) Tests to evaluate possible liver damage are described on p. 75.
(3) The urine may contain protein, red blood cells, or casts.

### Prevention

Household products should not contain tetrachloroethane, and less toxic solvents should be substituted for tetrachloroethane in industrial processes whenever possible.

The exposure limit should never be exceeded. If a contaminated area must be entered, a gas mask with a canister approved for tetrachloroethane is safe for 30 min if the concentration does not go over 20 000 ppm (2%). For a concentration over 20 000 ppm, an airline hose mask or self-contained $O_2$ supply is necessary. Workers entering a high-concentration area must wear a rescue harness and lifeline attended by a responsible person outside the contaminated area.

If direct contact is unavoidable, aprons and gloves made of solvent-proof synthetics must be worn. Skin creams will not prevent penetration.

Alcohol ingestion increases the susceptibility to tetrachloroethane.

### Treatment

Treatment is as described for carbon tetrachloride poisoning (see p. 174).

### Prognosis

Rapid progression of jaundice indicates a poor outcome. In some instances mild symptoms will persist for up to 3 months and then progress to acute yellow atrophy and death. Anuria may persist for as long as 2 weeks and still be followed by complete recovery.

## TRICHLOROETHYLENE

**Formula**: $CHClCCl_2$; bp: 88°C; vapor pressure at 20°C; 60 mmHg. Tetrachloroethane (see p. 177) may be present as an impurity in technical products.

Trichloroethylene is used as an industrial solvent; in typewriter correction fluids; and in household cleaners for walls, clothing, and rugs. It has been used as an inhalation anesthetic or analgesic but is too dangerous for this use. The exposure limit is 50 ppm. The adult fatal dose by ingestion or inhalation is estimated to be 5 ml. Trichloroethylene reacts to form dichloroethylene, phosgene, and carbon monoxide on contact with alkalis such as soda lime.

The most striking effect of trichloroethylene is depression of the central nervous system. Other areas affected (in order of decreasing severity of involvement) include the myocardium, liver, and kidney. Trichloroethylene will induce acute ventricular arrhythmias, including ventricular fibrillation, or these may be precipitated by the administration of epinephrine while the heart rate is slowed. Trichloroethylene is suspected to be carcinogenic.

Findings in fatalities from exposure to commercial trichloroethylene include degenerative changes in the heart muscle, central nervous system, liver, and renal tubular epithelium. The presence of tetrachloroethane as a contaminant in commercial trichloroethylene may contribute to the cellular damage.

**Clinical findings**

The principal manifestation of acute trichloroethylene poisoning is unconsciousness.

*Acute poisoning* (from inhalation, skin absorption, or ingestion)

Depending on concentration, symptoms progress more or less rapidly through dizziness, headache, nausea and vomiting, and excitement to loss of consciousness. Irregular pulse may indicate ventricular arrhythmia, which may progress to ventricular fibrillation. Recovery of consciousness is rapid, but nausea and vomiting may persist for several hours. Pulmonary edema may occur.

*Chronic poisoning* (from inhalation or skin absorption)

Symptoms and signs include weight loss, nausea, anorexia, fatigue, visual impairment, painful joints, dermatitis, and wheezing. Jaundice is uncommon.

## *Laboratory findings*

(1) The ECG may reveal ventricular irregularities during acute poisoning.
(2) Trichloroethylene metabolites in urine can be used as an indicator of absorption. A level of more than 20 mg of metabolites per 24 h indicates improper control of exposure.
(3) Tests to evaluate liver damage are described on p. 75.

## Prevention

Cross-ventilation should be sufficient to prevent any noticeable odor when trichloroethylene is used as a cleaning agent in the home.

## Treatment

### *Acute poisoning*

Move the patient to fresh air and give artificial respiration. Remove contaminated clothing. Do not give epinephrine or other stimulants that may cause ventricular arrhythmias. If symptoms are severe, treat as for carbon tetrachloride poisoning (see p. 174). Treat pulmonary edema (see p. 55).

### *Chronic poisoning*

Remove the patient from further exposure. If liver function is impaired, give a high-carbohydrate diet.

## Prognosis

Survival for 4 hours is ordinarily followed by complete recovery.

## 1,1,1-TRICHLOROETHANE

**Formula:** $CCl_3CH_3$; bp: 74.1°C.

1,1,1-Trichloroethane (methylchloroform) is used as a solvent for cleaning and degreasing, in paint removers, in typewriter correction fluids, and in crafts. Potential carcinogens such as vinylidene chloride may be present in technical grades as contaminants. The exposure limit is 350 ppm. The adult fatal dose by ingestion or inhalation is estimated to be 5 ml.

The main effect of 1,1,1-trichloroethane is central nervous system depression. The myocardium is sensitized to catecholamine-induced arrhythmias. Kidney and liver damage are minimal in experimental animals and have not occurred after use of 1,1,1-trichloroethane as an anesthetic agent. Repeated exposure of guinea pigs to a state of anesthesia has produced reversible hepatitis.

Fatalities have occurred when workers have entered unventilated tanks or from use in restricted areas. In one fatality from exposure to an estimated 60 000-ppm concentration of 1,1,1-trichloroethane, the only significant pathologic findings related to the exposure were petechial hemorrhages in the lungs and brain.

### Clinical findings

*Acute poisoning* (from inhalation or ingestion)

Symptoms progress through headache, dizziness, nausea, fainting, unconsciousness, respiratory depression, arrhythmias, and fall in blood pressure. Kidney and liver damage may appear after severe exposure.

*Laboratory findings*

(1) Infrared spectroscopy or gas chromatography can be used to quantitate 1,1,1-trichloroethane in expired air.
(2) Elevation of urinary urobilinogen has occurred several days after exposure insufficient to alter SGOT or SGPT levels.

### Treatment

Treat as for acute trichloroethylene poisoning (see p. 181).

### Prognosis

Patients who survived the initial anesthetic effects have recovered completely.

## TETRACHLOROETHYLENE

**Formula**: $CCl_2CCl_2$; bp: 121°C: vapor pressure at 20°C: 15 mmHg.

Tetrachloroethylene (perchlorethylene) is used as a solvent in commercial dry cleaning and degreasing. About 300 million kilograms are used annually in the USA. The exposure limit is 50 ppm, and toxic effects occur at 230 ppm. The blood level in one fatality was 4.4 mg/dl, and the brain level was 36 mg/100 g. Pathologic findings include central fatty necrosis and fatty infiltration in the liver and moderate cloudy swelling of renal tubular epithelium.

## Clinical findings

The principal manifestation of acute tetrachloroethylene poisoning is unconsciousness.

*Acute poisoning* (from inhalation or ingestion)

Symptoms and signs include headache, dizziness, irresponsible behavior, loss of inhibitions, and ventricular premature beats. Physical activity and catecholamines exacerbate ventricular arrhythmias. Peripheral nerve damage is indicated by tingling, numbness, and muscle weakness.

*Laboratory findings*

(1) The ECG reveals ventricular arrhythmias during acute poisoning.
(2) Blood tetrachloroethylene levels above 0.4 mg/dl have been associated with cardiac effects.
(3) Evaluate liver damage with appropriate tests.

## Prevention

The exposure limit should not be exceeded.

## Treatment

Treat as for trichloroethylene poisoning (see p. 181).

## Prognosis

Patients who survived the initial effects have recovered completely.

## DICHLOROMETHANE

**Formula**: $CH_2Cl_2$; bp: 40°C; vapor pressure at 25°C: 440 mmHg.

Dichloromethane (methylene dichloride, methylene chloride) is used as an ingredient in paint removers and as an industrial solvent. It has been used as an anesthetic agent, but fatalities occurred. The exposure limit is 100 ppm. The adult fatal dose by ingestion or inhalation is estimated to be 25 ml.

The main effect of methylene chloride is central nervous system depression. Kidney and liver damage have not occurred after its use as an anesthetic agent or after toxic exposures. It is decomposed by heat to phosgene and is metabolized in the body to carbon monoxide, with release of chloride ion resulting in acidosis. In one experiment, the carboxyhemoglobin level increased 14% in 3 h in one subject exposed to 986 ppm of methylene chloride. In massive exposures, intravascular hemolysis can occur. Pathologic findings are not specific.

## Clinical findings

*Acute poisoning* (from inhalation or ingestion)

Symptoms progress rapidly to unconsciousness and lack of response to painful stimuli. Respiration is at first fast, then slowed. Liquid methylene chloride spilled on the skin can cause erythema and blistering. Pulmonary edema can occur. One individual died of acute coronary insufficiency during exposure, possibly as a result of the stress of increased carboxyhemoglobin. Toxic encephalopathy has occurred after repeated exposures to levels above 500 ppm. One individual had painful joints, swelling of the extremities, mental impairment, diabetes, and skin rash after exposure to a paint stripper containing dichloromethane. Some of the symptoms persisted up to 6 months.

Gross hematuria occurs as a result of intravascular hemolysis. The swallowing mechanism may be disturbed by pharyngeal erosions, with resulting aspiration pneumonia.

*Chronic poisoning*

Chronic poisoning with dichloromethane has not been reported.

*Laboratory findings*

(1) Hemoglobin products in the urine indicate intravascular hemolysis.

(2) The carboxyhemoglobin level may be increased and the blood pH reduced.
(3) Radiographic examination reveals the extent of ulceration of the duodenum and jejunum.
(4) Blood in the stools indicates gastrointestinal injury.

## Treatment

### Inhaled dichloromethane

Treat as for acute trichloroethylene poisoning (see p. 181).

### Ingested dichloromethane

(1) Emergency measures – Remove by gastric lavage or emesis using activated charcoal (see pp. 31–32).
(2) General measures:
    (a) Treat hemolytic reaction (see p. 80).
    (b) Give hydrocortisone, 200 mg every 4 h.
(3) Special problems:
    (a) Treat aspiration pneumonia with antibiotics.
    (b) Blood transfusions may be necessary if gastrointestinal bleeding is excessive.
    (c) Treat acidosis.
    (d) Treat pulmonary edema (see p. 55).

## Prognosis

Patients who have ingested dichloromethane may have narrowing of the intestinal lumen as a result of erosions.

## ETHYLENE DICHLORIDE

**Formula**: $CH_2ClCH_2Cl$; bp: 83.5°C; vapor pressure at 20°C: 61 mmHg.

Ethylene dichloride (1,2-dichloroethane) is used as a solvent in the rubber, plastics, and insecticide industries. It is sometimes used in rubber and plastic cement for hobby and household use. The fatal adult dose by ingestion is approximately 5 ml. The exposure limit in air is 10 ppm. Ethylene dichloride depresses and injures almost all cells, but especially those of the central nervous system, liver, kidneys, and heart.

Postmortem evidence of injury includes the following: edema of the brain with congestion of the intracranial vessels; edema, hemorrhage, and vascular congestion in the lungs, heart, and spleen; fatty degeneration in the liver; congestion, edema, and tubular injury in the kidneys.

### Clinical findings

The principal manifestations of poisoning with ethylene dichloride are coma, pulmonary edema, and renal injury.

*Acute poisoning* (from inhalation, skin absorption, or ingestion)

Initial symptoms are cyanosis, fall in blood pressure, vomiting, diarrhea, cardiovascular collapse, and coma. If exposure is severe, these progress rapidly to pulmonary edema and respiratory difficulty. If the effects are not immediately fatal, the patient may have a temporary symptom-free interval followed by jaundice and oliguria or anuria.

*Chronic poisoning* (from inhalation or skin absorption)

Weight loss, low blood pressure, jaundice, oliguria, or anemia may occur after repeated minimal exposure.

*Laboratory findings*

The urine may show red blood cells, protein, and casts. Liver function impairment may be revealed by appropriate tests (see p. 75). Nitrogen retention due to renal injury is indicated by an increase in non-protein nitrogen, urea, or creatinine.

### Prevention

Maintain the concentration of ethylene dichloride in air below 50 ppm at all times. Ethylene dichloride should not be used as a plastic cement unless atmospheric levels are controlled.

**Treatment**

Treat as for methyl bromide poisoning (see p. 177).

**Prognosis**

Survival for 48 hours usually implies that complete recovery will occur, although deaths have occurred up to 5 days after exposure.

## ETHYLENE CHLOROHYDRIN

**Formula**: $CH_2ClCH_2OH$; bp: 128°C; vapor pressure at 44°C: 20 mmHg.

Ethylene chlorohydrin is used to speed the germination of seeds and potatoes, as a cleaning solvent, and in chemical synthesis. Even in dangerous concentrations, it does not produce a warning odor or irritation of the nose or throat.

Deaths have occurred from exposure to liquid ethylene chlorohydrin in the open air, from skin absorption, or from exposure to vapors in warehouses. The exposure limit is 1 ppm. The fatal adult dose by ingestion or inhalation is 1–2 ml. Ethylene chlorohydrin presumably irritates and damages cells after it is hydrolyzed to an acid (perhaps hydrochloric acid), producing pulmonary edema, vascular damage, direct inhibition of the cardiac muscle, central nervous system depression, and impairment of liver and kidney function. Postmortem examination in fatal poisoning has revealed fatty infiltration of the liver, edema of the brain, congestion and edema of the lungs, dilatation of the heart with fatty degeneration of the myocardium, congestion of the spleen, and swelling and hyperemia of the kidneys with fat deposits and swollen epithelial cells in the tubules.

**Clinical findings**

The principal manifestations in acute poisoning with ethylene chlorohydrin are respiratory and circulatory failure. Chronic poisoning does not occur.

Symptoms begin 1–4 h after ingestion, inhalation, or skin absorption and include nausea and vomiting, headache, abdominal pain, excitability, dizziness, delirium, respiratory slowing, fall in blood pressure, twitching of muscles, cyanosis, and coma. Urine contains red cells, albumin, and casts. Death results from respiratory and circulatory failure.

**Prevention**

Ethylene chlorohydrin should never be used for cleaning in an open process. Exhaust ventilation in most open hoods is insufficient to prevent dangerous exposure.

Treatment of potatoes or seeds by ethylene chlorohydrin must be carried out in an entirely closed space which workers are not allowed to enter until the space has been force-ventilated for 24 hours. The liquid must be sprayed into the fumigating chamber from a totally closed system to prevent any skin contact or inhalation of vapor. Transfer of the liquid from drums to the spraying system must be by means of an enclosed system and not by pouring.

**Treatment of acute poisoning**

*Emergency measures*

Remove patient from further exposure to ethylene chlorohydrin vapor or liquid. Complete recovery must be ensured before the patient returns to work. Give artificial respiration if respiration is depressed. Give $O_2$ as soon as possible. Remove ingested ethylene chlorohydrin by thorough gastric lavage, using tap water. If gastric lavage cannot be accomplished immediately, use syrup of ipecac (see p. 90).

*General measures*

Treat shock (see p. 56) and pulmonary edema (see p. 55). Administration of ethanol to suppress metabolism of ethylene chlorohydrin to toxic intermediates has been suggested.

**Prognosis**

Survival for 18 hours after poisoning has always been followed by complete recovery.

# POLYCHLORINATED NAPHTHALENE AND POLYCHLORINATED AND POLYBROMINATED BIPHENYLS

Chloronaphthalenes, dichloronaphthalenes, polychlorinated naphthalene (Halowax), polybrominated biphenyl (PBB), and polychlorinated biphenyl

(PCB, Arochlor) are used as high-temperature dielectrics for electric wires, electric motors, transformers, and other electrical equipment. They are also used as heat-exchange fluids, plasticizers, coatings, fillers, adhesives, and in paints, inks, and duplicating papers. Depending on the amount of chlorination, the melting point for these compounds varies from 80 to 130°C.

The exposure limit for these compounds is as follows (in mg/m$^3$): chlorinated diphenyl oxide, 0.5; chlorodiphenyl (42% chlorine), 1; chlorodiphenyl (54% chlorine), 0.5; hexachloronaphthalene, 0.2; octachloronaphthalene, 0.1; tetrachloronaphthalene, 2; pentachloronaphthalene, 0.5; trichloronaphthalene, 5. At least seven fatalities have been reported in the USA. It has been estimated that 40% of the US population has body fat levels of PCBs greater than 1 ppm, but the long-term effects of such levels have yet to be determined.

These compounds produce skin irritation and acute degeneration of the liver after prolonged exposure. Pathologic findings include acute necrosis of the liver, edema of the kidneys and heart, and, in some cases, necrosis of the adrenals.

## Clinical findings

The principal manifestations in chronic poisoning with chlorinated naphthalene and chlorinated diphenyl are chloracne and jaundice. Acute poisoning from single exposures has not been reported.

After exposure to vapors the skin shows a pinhead to pea-sized papular, acne-like eruption consisting of straw-colored cysts formed by plugging of sebaceous glands. These progress to pustular eruptions. Symptoms and signs resulting from liver injury include drowsiness, indigestion, nausea, jaundice, liver enlargement, and weakness progressing to coma. Liver injury occurs at exposure levels of 1–2 mg/m$^3$. Genetic injury has been reported in animal experiments. An increased incidence of cancer has occurred in some workers exposed to PCBs. Laboratory tests may reveal hypobilirubinemia, hyperbilirubinemia, or triglyceridemia. Tests to evaluate the extent of liver damage are described on p. 75.

## Prevention

Occurrence of acne in workers indicates inadequate control of fumes.

**Treatment of chronic poisoning**

Remove from further exposure. Treat liver damage (see p. 76).

**Prognosis**

At least 50% of patients with liver damage from chlorinated naphthalenes or chlorinated biphenyls have died. If workers are removed from exposure at the onset of acne, recovery is likely. Because of the long-term stability of these compounds in human fat, there is increasing concern about their possible mutagenicity or carcinogenicity.

## PHOSGENE

Phosgene ($COCl_2$) is a gas that liquefies at 8°C. It is used in chemical synthesis and also results from the high-temperature decomposition of chlorinated hydrocarbons, especially carbon tetrachloride, chloroform, and methylene chloride. Thus solvents, paint removers, and non-flammable dry cleaning fluids containing these substances will decompose to phosgene in the presence of fire or heat; deaths have occurred from such decomposition. The exposure limit for phosgene in air is 0.1 ppm.

Phosgene is hydrolyzed to hydrochloric acid in the body and thus irritates and damages cells. Pathologic findings include extensive degenerative changes in the epithelium of the trachea, bronchi, and bronchioli and hemorrhagic edematous focal pneumonia.

**Clinical findings**

The principal manifestations in acute poisoning with phosgene are respiratory and circulatory failure. Chronic poisoning does not occur.

*Symptoms and signs*

After inhalation or skin absorption symptoms and signs may begin any time up to 24 hours after exposure. These include a burning sensation in the throat, tightness in the chest, feeling of oppression, dyspnea, and cyanosis, with rapid progression to severe pulmonary edema and death from respiratory and circulatory failure.

*Laboratory findings*

Radiologic examination of the chest shows diffuse opacities resulting from pulmonary edema.

## Prevention

Paint removers and non-flammable dry cleaners should never be used in an enclosed space in the presence of fire or heaters of any kind.

## Treatment

*Emergency measures*

Remove patient from further exposure to phosgene or thermodecomposition products of halogenated hydrocarbons. Give artificial respiration if respiration is depressed. Give $O_2$ as soon as possible.

*General measures*

(1) Give cortisone acetate, 1 mg/kg orally 1–3 times daily, or other steroid to reduce tissue response to injury.
(2) Treat pulmonary edema (see p. 55).

## Prognosis

Survival for 48 hours after exposure has always been followed by complete recovery.

## FLUOROCARBONS

The fluorocarbon (fluoroalkane) liquids and gases listed in Table 10.1 are used as refrigerants and aerosol propellants. They are either non-flammable or almost non-flammable, but at flame temperatures they decompose to fluorine, hydrofluoric acid, hydrochloric acid, and phosgene.

Laboratory experiments in animals have shown that, by usual exposure methods, these compounds are almost non-toxic. The only toxic effect from exposure is anesthesia, and this occurs at concentrations of 10% or more. Recent experimental studies indicate that, in combination with asphyxia, at least some of these agents sensitize mice, rats, and dogs to fatal cardiac arrhythmias. The arrhythmias in mice include bradycardia, atrioventricular block, and ventricular T wave depression. These effects are not reversed by atropine.

Many fatalities have occurred in the USA as a result of the intentional inhalation of fluorocarbons obtained from aerosol cans. It has also been suggested that the increase in mortality rates from asthma is a result of the use of fluorocarbon-propelled medications.

Pathologic findings have not been contributory.

**Table 10.1** Fluorocarbons

|  | Boiling point (°C) | Exposure limit (ppm) |
|---|---|---|
| Chlorodifluoromethane (Freon 22) | −40.8 | 1000 |
| Chloropentafluoroethane | −39.1 | 1000 |
| Chlorotrifluoromethane (Freon 13) | −81.1 | 1000 |
| Dichlorodifluoromethane (Freon 12) | −29.8 | 1000 |
| Dichlorofluoromethane (Freon 21) | −9.0 | 10 |
| 1,1-Dichloro-1,2,2,2-tetrafluoroethane (Freon 114) | −3.8 | 1000 |
| Difluorodibromomethane (Freon 12B2) | 24.5 | 100 |
| 1,1-Difluoroethylene | −70 | 1000 |
| Hexafluoroacetone | −26 | 0.1 |
| 1,1,1,2-Tetrachloro-2,2-difluoroethane (TCDFa) | 91.67 | 500 |
| 1,1,2,2-Tetrachloro-1,2-difluoroethane (TCDF) | 93 | 500 |
| Trichlorofluoromethane (Freon 11) | 23.7 | 1000 |
| 1,1,2-Trichloro-1,2,2 trifluoroethane (Freon 113) | 45.8 | 1000 |
| Trifluorobromomethane (Freon 13B1) | −58 | 1000 |

### Clinical findings

Intentional exposure is produced by spraying the propellant into a plastic or paper bag and then inhaling deeply from the bag. Individuals who die as a result of the inhalation frequently show extreme physical activity – running or shouting or both – immediately prior to death. Difluorobromomethane causes central nervous system depression at lower concentrations than other fluorinated hydrocarbons. TCDF and TCDFa are respiratory irritants and central nervous system depressants and irritants. Dichlorofluoromethane has chronic effects like those of chloroform (see p. 386). Fatal chemical pneumonia has occurred as a result of the delayed irritant effect of 1,1,2,3,3-pentafluoro-3-chloropropene.

**Treatment**

Death has been so rapid that no treatment has been possible.

## RIOT CONTROL AGENTS AND PERSONAL PROTECTION DEVICES

Tear gas is 2-chloroacetophenone (1-phenyl-2-chloroethanone) (bp: 244°C) in a hydrocarbon solvent with a fluorocarbon pressurizing agent for discharge as a fog from an aerosol container. Tear-gas guns contain 2-chloroaceto-phenone in a finely divided state with an explosive device to propel the charge several feet. Wadding of rubber, cardboard, or synthetic material is used to enclose the agent and increase the propelling force of the explosive.

Liquid riot control agents (Mace, Chemical Mace, Peacemaker, Streamer) contain 2-chloroacetophenone (1%) and one or more of a variety of solvents – including 1,1,1-trichloroethane (5%), a kerosene-like hydrocarbon (5%), or propylene glycol (50–90%) – to prolong and increase the effect on the skin and mucous membranes, plus a propellant fluorocarbon such as trichlorofluoromethane (see Table 10.1). Other forms of riot control agents may contain chloropicrin, bromobenzyl cyanide (BBC), and *o*-chlorobenzyl-idene malononitrile. The exposure limits for substances used for riot control are as follows: 2-chloroacetophenone (CN), 0.05 ppm; *o*-chlorobenzylidene malononitrile (CS), 0.05 ppm; and chloropicrin, 0.1 ppm.

### Clinical findings

The principal manifestation of acute poisoning by riot control agents is irrita-tion of the skin and mucous membranes. Tear gas produces burning and irrita-tion of the eyes with profuse tearing, irritation of the skin, laryngospasm, headache, and sometimes vomiting. If the duration of exposure is long, cor-neal burns, pigmentation, and second-degree burns of the skin may occur. Liquid riot control agents sprayed onto the eye can cause corneal perforation.

In addition to the effects of tear gas, tear-gas guns can cause direct injury from the wadding or from direct deposition of 2-chloroacetophenone in the eyes or under the skin. These guns sometimes explode, causing severe hand injuries. Severe eye injury, corneal scarring, glaucoma, cataract, and hemor-rhage have necessitated enucleation up to 15 years after the injury.

Liquid riot control agents (Mace, etc.) have caused second-degree burns and hyperpigmentation of the skin, blurred vision, corneal scarring, skin sensitization, and hypertension. Chloropicrin causes vomiting and choking, with the possibility of aspiration. Bromobenzyl cyanide is a nauseant and irritant. o-Chlorobenzylmalononitrile is a respiratory irritant that smells like pepper and causes uncontrollable sneezing.

## Treatment

Emergency care personnel may need to wear protective equipment. Remove the victim's contaminated clothing and wash exposed skin with soap and water. Irrigate eyes with water or normal saline solution (preferably sterile) for 15 minutes or longer. Injured eyes should be examined immediately by an ophthalmologist. Direct eye contact with riot control agents should be treated with 24-hour irrigation by means of a corneal contact irrigating device if the patient cannot be seen immediately by an ophthalmologist.

## References

Bond GR. Hepatitis, rash and eosinophilia following trichloroethylene exposure: a case report and speculation on mechanistic similarity to halothane induced hepatitis. *J Toxicol Clin Toxicol* 1996;34:461

Burg J, Gist G. Health effects of environmental contaminant exposure: an intrafile comparison of the trichloroethylene subregistry. *Arch Environ Health* 1999;54:231

Calvert GM, *et al*. Health effects associated with sulfuryl fluoride and methyl bromide exposure among structural fumigation workers. *Am J Public Health* 1998;88:1774

Chang Y-L, *et al*. Diverse manifestations of oral methylene chloride poisoning: report of a case. *J Toxicol Clin Toxicol* 1999;37:497

Cheng T-J, *et al*. Abnormal liver function in workers exposed to low levels of ethylene dichloride and vinyl chloride monomer. *J Occup Environ Med* 1999;41: 1128

De Haro L, *et al*. Central and peripheral neurotoxic effects of chronic methyl bromide intoxication. *J Toxicol Clin Toxicol* 1996;35:29

Garnier R, *et al*. Coin-operated dry cleaning machines may be responsible for acute tetrachloroethylene poisoning: report of 26 cases including one death. *J Toxicol Clin Toxicol* 1996;34:191

Giesy JP, Kannan K. Dioxin-like and non-dioxin-like toxic effects of polychlorinated biphenyls (PCBs): implications for risk assessment. *CRC Crit Reviews in Toxicol* 1998;28:511

Gobba F, *et al.* Two-year evolution of perchloroethylene-induced color-vision loss. *Arch Environ Health* 1999;53:196

Gustavsson P, Hogstedt C. A cohort study of Swedish capacitor manufacturing workers exposed to polychlorinated biphenyls (PCBs). *Am J Ind Med* 1997;32:234

Horowitz BZ, *et al.* An unusual exposure to methyl bromide leading to fatality. *J Toxicol Clin Toxicol* 1998;36:353

Ichihara G, *et al.* Occupational health survey on workers exposed to 2-bromopropane at low concentrations. *Am J Ind Med* 1999;35:523

Kuspis DA, Krenzelok EP. Oral frostbite injury from intentional abuse of a fluorinated hydrocarbon. *J Toxicol Clin Toxicol* 1999;37:873

Mehrotra P, *et al.* Two cases of ethylene dibromide poisoning. *Vet Human Toxicol* 2001;43:91

Onofrj M, *et al.* Optic neuritis with residual tunnel vision in perchloroethylene toxicity. *J Toxicol Clin Toxicol* 1998;36:603

Paulu C, *et al.* Tetrachloroethylene-contaminated drinking water in Massachusetts and the risk of colon-rectum, lung, and other cancers. *Environ Health Perspect* 1999;107:265

Plaa GL. Chlorinated methanes and liver injury: Highlights of the past 50 years. *Annu Rev Pharmacol Toxicol* 2000;40:43

Sala M, *et al.* Organochlorine in the serum of inhabitants living near an electrochemical factory. *Occup Environ Med* 1999;56:152

Szlateny CS, Wang RY. Encephalopathy and cranial nerve palsies caused by intentional trichloroethylene inhalation. *Am J Emerg Med* 1996;14:464

**Table 10.2** Halogenated hydrocarbons (for treatment, see p. 174)

| | Exposure limit (ppm) | Fatal dose (LD50 in mg/kg, LC in ppm) | Mucous membrane, skin, lung, cornea irritation | Liver, kidney damage | CNS effects | Carcinogen | Miscellaneous |
|---|---|---|---|---|---|---|---|
| Allyl bromide | | 30 | + | + | + | | |
| Allyl chloride | 1 | 2000 ppm | + | + | + | | |
| Benzoyl chloride | | | + | + | + | | |
| Benzyl chloride | 1 | 1230 | + | + | + | | |
| Bis(2-chloroethyl) sulfide | | 20 | + | + | | | |
| Bis(2-chloroethoxy) methane | 1? | 65 | + | + | | + | |
| Bis(2-chloroisopropyl) ether | 15 | 240 | + | + | | + | |
| Bis(chloromethyl) ether | 0.001 | 210 | + | + | | + | |
| Bromoacetone | | 600* | + | | + | | |
| Bromodichloromethane | | 450 | + | + | + | + | |
| Bromoform | 0.5 | 400 | | + | + | | |
| Butyl chloride | | 2670 | + | + | + | | |
| Carbon tetrabromide | 0.1 | 1000 | | + | + | | |
| Chloroacetaldehyde | 1 | 23 | + | | + | | |
| Chloroacetic acid | | 76 | + | | + | | |
| Chlorobenzene | 75 | 2900 | + | + | + | | |
| Chlorobromomethane | 200 | 4300 | + | | + | | |
| 2-Chloro-1,3-butadiene | 10 | 300 | + | + | + | + | Cardiac |
| Chlorobutane | | 2670 | + | | + | | |
| Chlorodibromomethane | | 800 | + | + | + | + | |
| 2-Chloroethylvinyl ether | | 250 | + | | | | |
| Chloromethylmethyl ether | 0 | 817 | + | + | | + | |
| 3-Chloro-1,2-propanediol | | 152 | + | + | + | | |
| o-Chlorostyrene | 50 | 5200 | + | + | | | |
| o-Chlorotoluene | 50 | 1600 | + | + | + | | |

*Continued*

Table 10.2 (continued)

| | Exposure limit (ppm) | Fatal dose (LD50 in mg/kg, LC in ppm) | Mucous membrane, skin, lung, cornea irritation | Liver, kidney damage | CNS effects | Carcinogen | Miscellaneous |
|---|---|---|---|---|---|---|---|
| Dibromochloropropane | 0.01 | 60 | + | + | + | | |
| Dibromoethane | 0 | 117 | + | + | + | + | |
| Dichloroacetic acid | | 2820 | + | | | | |
| Dichloroacetylene | 0.1 | 19 ppm | + | | | | |
| Dichlorobenzene (o- or p-) | 50 | 500 | + | + | + | | |
| 1,1-Dichloroethane | 200 | 725 | | | + | | |
| 1,1-Dichloroethylene | 10 | 5750 | + | + | + | + | |
| 1,2-Dichloroethylene | 200 | 770 | + | | + | | |
| 2,2′-Dichloroethyl ether | 5 | 75 | + | | + | | |
| 2,3-Dichloro-1,4-naphthoquinone | | 1300 | + | + | + | | |
| Dichloropropane | 75 | 860 | + | + | + | | Cardiac |
| Dichloropropanol | | 90 | + | + | + | | |
| Dichloropropene | 1 | 250 | + | + | | | |
| 1,1-Difluoroethylene | 1 | 2000* | | | + | | |
| Epichlorohydrin | 2 | 90 | + | + | + | + | |
| Ethyl bromide | 200 | 2200 ppm | + | + | + | | Cardiac |
| Ethyl chloride | 1000 | 13 000 ppm | + | + | + | | Cardiac |
| Hexachloroacetone | | 700 | + | + | | | |
| Hexachlorobutadiene | 0.02 | 87 | + | + | + | + | |
| Hexachlorocyclo-pentadiene | 0.1 | 1 ppm | + | + | + | + | |
| Hexachloroethane | 10 | 4000 | + | + | + | | |
| Hexafluoroacetone | 0.1 | 300 | | + | | | Testicular |
| Pentachlorobenzene | | 2000 | + | | | + | |
| Pentachloroethane | | 500 | + | + | + | | |
| Propylene chlorohydrin | | 220 | + | + | + | | Hemolysis |

*Continued*

*Table 10.2  (continued)*

| | Exposure limit (ppm) | Fatal dose (LD50 in mg/kg, LC in ppm) | Mucous membrane, skin, lung, cornea irritation | Liver, kidney damage | CNS effects | Carcinogen | Miscellaneous |
|---|---|---|---|---|---|---|---|
| Sodium trichloroacetate | | 3320 | | | + | | |
| sym-Tetrabromoethane | 1 | 400 | + | + | + | | |
| Tetrachloroethylene† | 50 | 4000 | + | + | + | | Cardiac |
| 1,2,4-Trichlorobenzene | 5 | 756 | + | + | + | | |
| Trichlorobenzoic acid | | 1600 | + | | | | |
| 1,1,2-Trichloroethane | 10 | 580 | + | + | + | | |
| 1,2,3-Trichloropropane | 50 | 320 | | | + | | |
| Vinyl bromide | 5 | 250 ppm | + | + | + | + | |
| Vinyl chloride† | 5 | 20 000 ppm | | + | + | + | |
| Vinyl fluoride | 1 | | | | + | | |

*mg/m³; †tetrachloroethylene causes peripheral neuropathy, and vinyl chloride causes Raynaud's phenomenon and acroosteolysis

# 11 Alcohols and glycols*

## METHANOL

**Formula**: $CH_3OH$; bp: 64.5°C; vapor pressure at 20°C: 94 mmHg.

Methanol (methyl or wood alcohol) is used as an antifreeze, a paint remover, a solvent in shellac and varnish, in chemical synthesis, and as a denaturant in denatured alcohol. Preparations containing ethanol denatured with methanol and other chemicals appear to have greater toxicity than can be explained by their content of methanol and ethanol. For example, Solox (which contains approximately 5% methanol, 1% gasoline, 1% ethyl acetate, and 1% methylisobutylketone in ethanol) has caused severe hypoglycemia in addition to the usual findings from ethanol and methanol intoxication.

The fatal internal dose is 60–250 ml. The exposure limit is 200 ppm. More than 100 deaths in a single year in the USA have resulted from ingestion or inhalation of methanol, often as a substitute for ethanol.

The high oral or inhalation toxicity of methanol in comparison with that of ethanol has not been satisfactorily explained. Toxicity is probably due to metabolism of methanol to formic acid or formaldehyde, and formaldehyde has been shown to have selective injurious effects on retinal cells. Methanol is distributed in the body according to the water content of tissues.

Methanol is metabolized and excreted at a rate approximately one-fifth that of ethanol. After a single dose, excretion from the lungs and kidneys may continue for at least 4 days. Severe acidosis is produced by the metabolic product formic acid. The pH of the urine may reach 5.0.

Administration of ethanol reduces the toxic effects of methanol by blocking the metabolism of methanol to formaldehyde and formic acid; this allows the kidneys to excrete unchanged methanol.

In fatal cases the liver, kidneys, and heart show parenchymatous degeneration. The lungs show desquamation of epithelium, emphysema, edema, congestion, and bronchial pneumonia. The brain may show edema, hyperemia, and petechiae. The eye shows degenerative changes in the retina and edema of

---

*See also Table 11.3

the optic disk, and there may be optic nerve atrophy. The corneal epithelium may show degenerative changes.

## Clinical findings

The principal manifestations of methanol poisoning are visual disturbances and acidosis.

*Acute poisoning* (from ingestion, inhalation, or skin absorption)

(1) Mild – Fatigue, headache, nausea, and, after a latent period, temporary blurring of vision.
(2) Moderate – Severe headache, dizziness, nausea and vomiting, and depression of the central nervous system. Vision may fail temporarily or permanently after 2–6 days.
(3) Severe – The above symptoms progress to rapid, shallow respiration from acidosis; cyanosis; coma; fall in blood pressure; dilatation of the pupils; and hyperemia of the optic disk, with blurring of the margin. About 25% of those with severe poisoning (blood bicarbonate level < 20 mEq/l) die of respiratory failure.

*Chronic poisoning* (from inhalation)

Visual impairment may be the first sign of poisoning; this begins with mild blurring of vision and progresses to contraction of visual fields and sometimes complete blindness.

*Laboratory findings*

Severe acidosis is indicated by a blood bicarbonate level below 15 mEq/l. A blood methanol level above 50 mg/dl is an indication for hemodialysis.

## Prevention

Poison labels should be placed on all methanol containers. Workers should be instructed in the dangers of methanol ingestion. Spirit duplicators should be used only with adequate exhaust ventilation.

**Treatment**

*Acute poisoning*

(1) Emergency measures – If ingestion of methanol is discovered within 2 hours, give syrup of ipecac (see p. 90). Lavage thoroughly with 2–4 liters of tap water with sodium bicarbonate (20 g/l) added.
(2) Antidotes – Use if blood methanol exceeds 20 mg/dl.
    (a) Give ethanol, 50% (100 proof), 1.5 ml/kg orally initially, diluted to not more than 5% solution, followed by 0.5–1 ml/kg every 2 h orally or intravenously for 4 days in order to reduce metabolism of methanol and to allow time for its excretion. The blood ethanol level should be in the range 1–1.5 mg/ml.
    (b) Give fomepizole (see p. 89).
(3) General measures:
    (a) Combat acidosis by administration of sodium bicarbonate (see p. 71).
    (b) Give up to 4 liters of fluids daily orally or intravenously to maintain adequate urine output.
    (c) Extracorporeal dialysis should be used when symptoms progress rapidly and do not respond to administration of ethanol, fomepizole or alkalinizing agents or if the blood methanol level is above 50 mg/dl. Extracorporeal dialysis is at least four times as effective as peritoneal dialysis in removing methanol.
    (d) Maintain adequate nutrition by giving small meals at regular 3- to 4-h intervals.
    (e) Maintain body warmth.
    (f) Treat coma (see p. 63).
(4) Special problems – Control delirium by use of pentobarbital sodium, 100 mg every 6–12 h, or give diazepam, 10 mg slowly intravenously. Avoid respiratory depression.

*Chronic poisoning*

Remove from exposure.

## Prognosis

In acute methanol poisoning, particularly when it is unrecognized, 25–50% of victims do not recover. Visual impairment is not likely to show much improvement after 1 week.

## References

Burns AB, *et al*. Use of pharmacokinetics to determine the duration of dialysis in management of methanol poisoning. *Am J Emerg Med* 1998;16:538

Burns MJ, *et al*. Treatment of methanol poisoning with intravenous 4-methyl-pyrazole. *Ann Emerg Med* 1997;30:829

Girault C, *et al*. Fomepizole (4-methyl pyrazole) in fatal methanol poisoning with early CT scan cerebral lesions. *J Toxicol Clin Toxicol* 1999;37:777

Hantson P, *et al*. Methanol poisoning during late pregnancy. *J Toxicol Clin Toxicol* 1996;35:187

Hantson P, *et al*. Neurotoxicity to the basal ganglia shown by magnetic resonance imaging (MRI) following poisoning by methanol and other substances. *J Toxicol Clin Toxicol* 1996;35:151

Hantson P, Mahieu P. Pancreatic injury following acute methanol poisoning. *J Toxicol Clin Toxicol* 2000;38:297

Jacobsen D, McMartin KE. Antidotes for methanol and ethylene glycol poisoning. *J Toxicol Clin Toxicol* 1996;35:127

Liu JJ, *et al*. Methanol-related deaths in Ontario. *J Toxicol Clin Toxicol* 1999;37:69

Liu JJ, *et al*. Prognostic factors in patients with methanol poisoning. *J Toxicol Clin Toxicol* 1998;36:175

Roberge RJ, *et al*. Putaminal infarct in methanol intoxication: case report and role of brain imaging studies. *Vet Human Toxicol* 1998;40:95

## ETHANOL

**Formula**: $C_2H_5OH$; bp: 78°C; vapor pressure: 44 mmHg at 20°C.

Ethanol (ethyl or grain alcohol) is used as a solvent, an antiseptic, a chemical intermediate, and a beverage. For many commercial uses ethanol is denatured. The following formulas are most common in pharmaceutical and household preparations: formulas 1 and 3A contain 5% methanol; formula 23A contains 10% acetone; formula 23H contains acetone and 1.5% methylisobutylketone; formula 39C contains 1% diethyl phthalate; formula

40 contains 1.25 ml of tertiary butyl alcohol and 0.25 g of brucine sulfate in each liter. The strength of alcoholic beverages is ordinarily given in vol%, indicating volumes of alcohol in 100 volumes of the beverage, or in proof spirits, in which the proof number is approximately twice the concentration in vol%. Thus, 100° proof is approximately 50 vol%. The usual concentration of ethanol in beverages is as follows: beer, 3–5%; wine, 10–12%; fortified wine, 20%; distilled spirits, 40%. Fermented beverages may contain more complex alcohols, which are more toxic.

The fatal dose for an average adult is 300–400 ml of pure ethanol (600–800 ml of 100° proof whiskey) if consumed in less than 1 h, while serious symptoms have been produced in children by 1 ml/kg of denatured alcohol containing 5% methanol. The exposure limit is 1000 ppm. Chronic users have a greater tolerance for ethanol.

Ethanol, being a small, hydrophilic molecule, is rapidly absorbed from the gastrointestinal tract or alveoli and is distributed according to the water content of tissues. It is oxidized by way of acetaldehyde to $CO_2$ and water at a rate of 100–110 mg/kg/h. The ethanol metabolizing system saturates at a plasma ethanol level of 1 mg/ml. The volume of distribution ($V_d$) for ethanol is 0.6 l/kg (see p. 99).

Ethanol depresses the central nervous system irregularly in descending order from cortex to medulla, depending on the amount ingested. The range between a dose that produces anesthesia and one that impairs vital functions is small. Thus, an amount that produces stupor is dangerously close to a fatal dose. Effects are potentiated by concomitant ingestion of barbiturates and other depressant drugs.

The pathologic findings in acute fatalities from ethanol include edema of the brain and hyperemia and edema of the gastrointestinal tract. Postmortem findings in patients dying after chronic ingestion of large amounts of ethanol include degenerative changes in the liver, kidneys, and brain; atrophic gastritis; and cirrhosis of the liver.

### Interactions

Ethanol enhances the effects of coumarin anticoagulants, antihistamines, hypnotics, sedatives, tranquilizers, insulin, monoamine oxidase inhibitors, and antidepressants. Disulfiram-like intolerance to ethanol may occur from sulfonylureas, thiocarbamates, metronidazole, tolazoline, furazolidone, chloramphenicol, and quinacrine.

## Clinical findings

The principal manifestation of ethanol poisoning is central nervous system depression.

### *Acute poisoning* (from ingestion)

(1) Mild (blood ethanol 0.05–0.15%; 0.5–1.5 mg/ml) – Decreased inhibitions, slight visual impairment, slight muscular uncoordination, and slowing of reaction time. Approximately 25% of individuals in this group are clinically intoxicated.

(2) Moderate (blood ethanol 0.15–0.3%; 1.5–3 mg/ml) – Definite visual impairment, sensory loss, muscular uncoordination, slowing of reaction time, and slurring of speech. From 50 to 95% of individuals in this group are clinically intoxicated.

(3) Severe (blood ethanol 0.3–0.5%; 3–5 mg/ml) – Marked muscular uncoordination, blurred or double vision, approaching stupor. Severe hypoglycemia sometimes occurs, with hypothermia, conjugate deviation of the eyes, extensor rigidity of the extremities, unilateral or bilateral Babinski's sign, convulsions, and trismus. Children are especially susceptible. Fatalities begin to occur in this range.

(4) Coma (blood ethanol above 0.5%; 5 mg/ml) – Unconsciousness, slowed respiration, decreased reflexes, and complete loss of sensations. Deaths are frequent in this range.

### *Chronic poisoning* (from ingestion) See Table 11.1.

(1) General – Weight loss.

(2) Gastrointestinal – Cirrhosis of the liver and gastroenteritis with anorexia and diarrhea.

(3) Nervous system
   (a) Polyneuritis with pain, and motor and sensory loss in the extremities.
   (b) Optic atrophy.
   (c) Mental deterioration with memory loss, tremor, impaired judgement, and loss or impairment of other abilities.

**Table 11.1** Chronic toxicity of ethanol

**Psychoneurologic syndromes**
    Acute alcoholism
    Intoxication, excitement, coma
    Withdrawal syndromes
    Hallucinosis, convulsions, delirium tremens
    Nutritional syndromes
    Wernicke–Korsakoff syndrome, pellagra (thiamine deficiency)
**Gastrointestinal syndromes**
Acute and chronic gastritis, malabsorption syndrome, fatty liver, cirrhosis, acute and
    chronic pancreatitis
**Hematologic syndromes**
Anemia due to acute or chronic blood loss
Cytoplasmic vacuolization of erythroid precursors
Megaloblastic marrow alterations (inhibition of folate metabolism) with anemia
Sideroblastic bone marrow abnormalities
Stomatocytic erythrocyte changes
Hemolytic anemia, thrombocytopenia
Defective granulocyte mobilization
**Neuromuscular syndromes**
Peripheral polyneuropathy
Acute and chronic alcoholic myopathy
**Cardiovascular syndromes**
Alcoholic cardiomyopathy
**Metabolic syndromes**
Lactic acidosis, hypoglycemia, hypomagnesemia, hypouricemia, hyperlipidemia
**Pulmonary syndromes**
Pulmonary aspiration, respiratory infections. Lung volumes, airway resistance, diffusion,
    gas exchange all adversely affected
**Conditions aggravated by alcohol**
Traumatic encephalopathy, epilepsy, Hodgkin's disease, porphyria, peptic ulcer
**Drugs that contraindicate concomitant use of alcohol**
Disulfiram, sedatives, hypnotics, tranquilizers, phenformin

(d) Ethanol withdrawal syndrome or acute alcoholic mania (delirium tremens) usually follows abstinence after a prolonged bout of steady drinking. Symptoms include uncontrollable fear; sleeplessness; tremors; restlessness progressing to visual, auditory, or gustatory hallucinations, and delirium. Exaggerated reflexes, tachycardia, and sometimes convulsions can occur. The most severe form of alcoholic withdrawal is delirium tremens.

(e) Acute alcoholic psychosis (Korsakoff's syndrome) is characterized by severe mental impairment, suggestibility, disorientation, and impairment of memory.

(f) In alcoholism of many years' duration, acute myopathy occasionally occurs after a period of unusually high alcohol intake. Symptoms are aching and tender muscles associated with muscular edema and degeneration of muscle fibers. The symptoms of pathologic change in the heart muscle are palpitation, extrasystoles, tachycardia, or other arrhythmias. The disease may progress to irreversible myocardial fibrosis and then to circulatory failure.

*Laboratory findings*

(1) Most laboratories report blood ethanol levels that are 10–20% lower than serum or plasma ethanol levels. Blood ethanol levels (Table 11.2) correlate well with clinical findings except in chronic ethanol abusers, in whom levels are higher (see Acute Poisoning, above). Blood levels above 0.05–0.15% (0.5–1.5 mg/ml) are legal evidence of intoxication in many jurisdictions. Ethanol concentration in expired air can also be used to indicate blood level.

**Table 11.2** Blood ethanol levels after intake of alcoholic beverages

| Beverage (% ethanol) | Amount ingested (ml) | Peak blood level in a 60-kg person (mg/ml)* |
|---|---|---|
| Beer (3%) | 500 | 0.46 |
| Wine (10%) | 250 | 0.77 |
| Distilled spirits (40%) | 50 | 0.62 |

*The blood ethanol level falls at a rate of approximately 0.185 mg/ml/h. To calculate the expected blood ethanol level at any other body weight, use the following formula:

$$\left[\frac{60\,\text{kg}}{\text{Subject's weight in kg}}\right] \times \begin{array}{c}\text{Expected level}\\\text{from table}\end{array} = \begin{array}{c}\text{Expected level}\\\text{in subject}\end{array}$$

(2) In chronic alcoholism liver function should be evaluated by appropriate tests (see p. 75).

(3) Urinalysis may be positive for reducing sugar, acetone, or diacetic acid. Urine ethanol levels correlate well with blood ethanol levels.

(4) Blood glucose levels should be determined after ingestion of ethanol-containing substances, especially in children.

(5) Cardiomyopathy is indicated by electrocardiographic changes, including arrhythmias, extrasystoles from diverse foci, and deformed T waves.

(6) Elevation of serum amylase indicates pancreatitis.

## Prevention

Alcoholics Anonymous (see listing in local phone book) may be able to assist those patients who genuinely desire help.

Disulfiram (Antabuse) administration induces sensitivity to ethanol and may be helpful in training the patient to avoid ethanol.

## Treatment

### *Acute poisoning*

(1) Emergency measure – Remove unabsorbed ethanol by gastric lavage with tap water or by emesis (see p. 29).

(2) General measures for treatment of coma:
    (a) Maintain adequate airway. Give artificial respiration if necessary.
    (b) Maintain normal body temperature.
    (c) Give 2 g of sodium bicarbonate in 250 ml of water every 2 h to maintain neutral or slightly alkaline urine.
    (d) Avoid administration of excessive fluids.
    (e) Avoid depressant drugs.
    (f) In the presence of hypoglycemia, administer 5–10% glucose intravenously plus thiamine, 100 mg intramuscularly.
    (g) Hemodialysis is indicated if the blood ethanol level is above 5 mg/ml.

### *Chronic poisoning*

(1) Emergency measures:
    (a) In acute alcoholic mania, give diazepam, 10 mg slowly intravenously initially, followed by 5 mg intravenously every 5–10 minutes until mania is controlled. Then give 5–10 mg orally every 1–8 h as necessary.

   (b) Avoid physical restraint; maintain calm, quiet, and uniform surroundings.

(2) General measures:

   (a) In patients with a history of seizures, give 500 mg of phenytoin and repeat in 4–6 h. Phenytoin, 300 mg daily, is then continued.

   (b) Give high-vitamin, high-protein diet plus thiamine, 100 mg 3 times daily; pyridoxine, 100 mg/d; folic acid, 5 mg 3 times daily; ascorbic acid, 500 mg twice daily.

   (c) Give oral fluids to 4 l/d. Give 1–2 liters of 5% dextrose in saline intravenously if patient is unable to take fluids orally.

   (d) Naltrexone is approved for use in treating addiction to alcohol. Give 50 mg daily.

## Prognosis

In acute, uncomplicated alcoholism, survival for 24 hours is ordinarily followed by recovery.

In alcoholic psychosis, survival is likely but complete recovery is rare. In the presence of mental deterioration, complete withdrawal from ethanol may be followed only by minimal improvement.

## References

Burge SK, Schneider FD. Alcohol-related problems: recognition and intervention. *Am Family Physician* 1999;59:361

Cydulka RK, *et al*. Injured intoxicated drivers: citation, conviction, referral, and recidivism rates. *Ann Emerg Med* 1998;32:349

Davidson P, *et al*. Intoxicated ED patients: a 5-year follow-up of morbidity and mortality. *Ann Emerg Med* 1997;30:593

Dufour M, Fuller RK. Alcohol in the elderly. *Annu Rev Med* 1995;46:123

Finsterer J, *et al*. Malnutrition-induced hypokalemic myopathy in chronic alcoholism. *J Toxicol Clin Toxicol* 1998;36:369

Floyd RL, *et al*. Alcohol use prior to pregnancy recognition. *Am J Prev Med* 1999;17:101

Garro AJ, Lieber CS. Alcohol and cancer. *Annu Rev Pharmacol Toxicol* 1990;30:219

Higgins JP, *et al*. Alcohol, the elderly, and motor vehicle crashes. *Am J Emerg Med* 1996;14:265

Khan F, *et al.* Overlooked sources of ethanol. *J Emerg Med* 1999; 17:985

Koeppel C, *et al.* Carbohydrate-deficient transferrin for identification of drug overdose patients at risk of an alcohol withdrawal syndrome. *J Toxicol Clin Toxicol* 1996;34:297

Maio RF, *et al.* Adolescent injury in the emergency department: opportunity for alcohol interventions? *Ann Emerg Med* 2000;35:252

Marinella MA. Alcoholic ketoacidosis presenting with extreme hypoglycemia. *Am J Emerg Med* 1997;15:280

Monti PM, *et al.* Toward bridging the gap between biological, psychobiological and psychosocial models of alcohol craving. *Addiction* 2000;95:S229. (Naltrexone)

Smith GS, *et al.* Fatal nontraffic injuries involving alcohol: a metanalysis. *Ann Emerg Med* 1999;34:659

Weinrieb RM, O'Brien CP. Naltrexone in the treatment of alcoholism. *Annu Rev Med* 1997;48:477

## ETHYLENE GLYCOL AND DIETHYLENE GLYCOL

These agents are dense liquids with sweetish, acrid tastes. Their vapor pressures at room temperature are negligible. **Formula** (ethylene glycol): $CH_2OHCH_2OH$; bp: 198°C. **Formula** (diethylene glycol): $HOCH_2CH_2O-CH_2CH_2OH$; bp: 245°C.

The fatal dose of ethylene glycol is approximately 100 g; of diethylene glycol, 15–100 g. Up to 60 deaths in a single year have been reported from ethylene glycol or diethylene glycol. The exposure limit for particulate ethylene glycol is $10 \, mg/m^3$; for vapor, it is 50 ppm.

Ethylene glycol and its esters are distributed with body water, and some are metabolized to oxalic acid, which is thought to play a role in some of the toxic effects. The ethers of ethylene glycol, as well as diethylene glycol and its esters and ethers (none of which appear to be metabolized to oxalic acid), produce brain and kidney damage by unknown mechanisms. Many of these glycols produce profound acidosis. The half-life of ethylene glycol in the presence of normal kidney function and without acidosis is 17 h.

The pathologic findings are congestion and edema of the brain, focal hemorrhagic necrosis of the renal cortex, and hydropic degeneration of the liver and kidneys. Calcium oxalate crystals may be found in the brain, spinal cord, and kidneys.

## Clinical findings

The principal manifestations of acute poisoning with these agents are anuria and narcosis.

### Acute poisoning (from ingestion)

The initial symptoms in massive dosage (>100 ml in a single dose) are those of alcohol intoxication. These symptoms soon progress to vomiting, cyanosis, headache, tachypnea, tachycardia, hypotension, pulmonary edema, muscle tenderness, stupor, anuria, prostration, and unconsciousness with convulsions. Hypoglycemia may occur. Death may occur within a few hours from respiratory failure or within the first 24 hours from pulmonary edema. Patients who have prolonged coma or convulsions may have irreversible brain damage. Hypocalcemic tetany as a result of calcium precipitation may follow ethylene glycol poisoning. Massive doses of these glycols may cause intravascular hemolysis.

If the ingestion of small amounts (15–30 ml) is repeated daily or if the patient recovers from acute poisoning, oliguria may begin in 24–72 h and progress rapidly to anuria and uremia.

### Chronic poisoning (from inhalation)

Continued exposure to the vapors from a process utilizing ethylene glycol is reported to induce unconsciousness, nystagmus, and lymphocytosis.

### Laboratory findings

The urine may contain calcium oxalate crystals, albumin, red blood cells, and casts. The blood pH or glucose level may be reduced. Methemoglobinemia may occur. Hypocalcemia and hyperkalemia may be present. A serum ethylene glycol level above 20 mg/dl indicates the necessity for treatment. Elevated serum creatinine (>1.4 mg/dl) and reduced creatinine clearance rate indicate the necessity for hemodialysis. Other useful tests: serum electrolytes including calcium and magnesium, osmolality (gap >10 mosm/l), blood ethanol, arterial pH (<7.3), serum bicarbonate (<20 mEq/l).

**Treatment**

*Acute poisoning*

(1) Emergency measures – Remove ingested glycols by gastric lavage or emesis (see pp. 29–32).
(2) Antidote
   (a) Give fomepizole (see p. 89). Continue administration until serum ethylene glycol falls below 20 mg/dl.
   (b) Give ethanol as in the treatment of methanol poisoning (see p. 201) to prevent metabolism of ingested ethylene glycol to oxalate.
   (c) Give calcium gluconate, 10 ml of 10% solution diluted in 1 liter of 5% glucose, intravenously as necessary to maintain normal serum calcium levels. Calcium administration may cause anuria owing to precipitation of calcium oxalate in the kidney.
(3) General measures:
   (a) Give artificial respiration with $O_2$ if respiration is depressed.
   (b) In the absence of renal impairment, force fluids to 4 liters or more daily to increase excretion of the glycol.
   (c) Use dialysis.
   (d) Avoid stimulants.
   (e) For hypoglycemia, give 5% dextrose intravenously.
   (e) Control convulsions with diazepam, 0.1 mg/kg slowly intravenously.
(4) Special problems – Treat pulmonary edema (see p. 55), uremia (see p. 67), shock (see p. 56), acidosis (see p. 71), and methemoglobinemia (see p. 78).

*Chronic poisoning*

Remove from exposure.

**Prognosis**

Complete recovery of renal function may follow 2 weeks of complete anuria. Cerebral damage may, however, be permanent.

## References

Barceloux DG, *et al*. American Academy of Clinical Toxicology practice guidelines on the treatment of ethylene glycol poisoning. *J Toxicol Clin Toxicol* 1999;37:537

Jobard E, *et al*. 4-Methylpyrazole and hemodialysis in ethylene glycol poisoning. *J Toxicol Clin Toxicol* 1996;34:373

Kowalczyk M, *et al*. Ethanol treatment in ethylene glycol poisoned patients. *Vet Human Toxicol* 1998;40:225

Moreau CL, *et al*. Glycolate kinetics and hemodialysis clearance in ethylene glycol poisoning. *J Toxicol Clin Toxicol* 1998;36:659

Morgan BW, *et al*. Ethylene glycol ingestion resulting in brainstem and midbrain dysfunction. *J Toxicol Clin Toxicol* 2000;38:445

Sivilotti MLA, *et al*. Toxicokinetics of ethylene glycol during fomepizole therapy: implications for management. *Ann Emerg Med* 2000;36:114

Wax PM. It's happening again – another diethylene glycol mass poisoning. *J Toxicol Clin Toxicol* 1996;34:517

**Table 11.3** Alcohols and glycols (for treatment, see p. 211)

| | Exposure limit (ppm) | Fatal dose (mg/kg) | Irritation | CNS effects | Bone marrow damage | Kidney, liver damage | Miscellaneous |
|---|---|---|---|---|---|---|---|
| Allyl alcohol | 0.5 | 64 | + | + | + | + | Skin burns |
| Amyl alcohol | 100 | 200 | + | + | + | | Headache |
| 2-Butoxy ethanol | 20 | 300 | + | + | + | + | Hemolysis |
| Butyl alcohol | 50 | 790 | + | + | | + | |
| Butyl carbitol | | 2400 | + | + | | + | |
| Carbitol | | 3620 | + | + | | + | |
| Cyclohexanol | 50 | 2060 | + | + | + | + | Tremor |
| Decanol | | 4720 | + | + | | + | |
| Diacetone alcohol | 50 | 4000 | + | + | | + | Anemia |
| Dipropylene glycol | | 14 000 | + | | | + | |
| Dipropylene glycol methyl ether | | 5660 | + | + | | + | |
| 2-Ethoxy ethanol | 5 | 500 | + | + | | + | Hemolysis |
| 2-Ethoxy ethyl acetate | 5 | 1950 | + | + | | + | |
| Furfuryl alcohol | 10 | 160 | + | + | | | |
| Glycerin | | 1428 | | | | | |
| Hexylene glycol | 25 | 3200 | + | + | | | |
| Isopropoxyethanol | 25 | 4900 | + | | + | | |
| 2-Methoxy ethanol | 5 | 100 | + | + | + | + | Hemolysis |
| 2-Methoxy ethyl acetate | 5 | 1250 | + | + | + | + | Hematuria |
| 1-Methoxy-2-propanol | 100 | 5660 | | + | | + | |
| Methylcyclohexanol | 50 | 1750 | + | + | | + | |
| Methylisobutylcarbinol | 25 | 1000 | + | + | | | |
| Octanol | | 18 g | + | + | | + | |
| Polypropylene glycol | | 2400 | | + | | | Cardiac |
| Propylene glycol | | 20 g | | + | | | Convulsions |
| Propynol | 1 | 20 | + | + | | | |
| Tetrahydrofurfuryl alcohol | | 2300 | + | + | | | |

## ISOPROPYL AND n-PROPYL ALCOHOL

**Formula** (isopropyl alcohol [isopropanol]): $(CH_3)_2CHOH$; bp: 82.5°C; vapor pressure at 23.8°C: 40 mmHg. **Formula** (n-propyl alcohol): $CH_3(CH_2)_2OH$; bp: 97–98°C.

Isopropyl alcohol is used as rubbing alcohol, after-shave lotion, and window cleaner. n-Propyl alcohol is used in industry. These alcohols are about twice as toxic as ethanol; the fatal dose by ingestion is 250 ml. The exposure limit is 200 ppm for n-propyl alcohol and 400 ppm for isopropyl alcohol. About 15% of an ingested dose of isopropyl alcohol is metabolized to acetone.

Pathologic findings after fatalities from isopropyl alcohol poisoning include hemorrhagic tracheobronchitis, bronchopneumonia, and hemorrhagic pulmonary edema. Pulmonary damage may occur as a result of pulmonary excretion of the alcohol.

### Clinical findings

The principal manifestation of acute isopropyl or n-propyl alcohol poisoning is central nervous system depression.

*Symptoms and signs* (from inhalation, ingestion, or skin absorption)

Symptoms are similar to those of ethanol intoxication, with more marked and more persistent nausea, vomiting, abdominal pain, hematemesis, refractory narcosis, areflexia, depressed respirations, and oliguria followed by diuresis. Deep coma has resulted from sponging with isopropyl alcohol. Generalized tenderness, induction, and edema of muscles may occur. Vapor exposure causes eye irritation. Prolonged contact with the skin can cause corrosion.

*Laboratory findings*

(1) Elevated blood urea nitrogen.
(2) Elevated SGOT.
(3) Melena.
(4) Fall in hemoglobin level as a result of hemolysis.
(5) Acetonuria, acetonemia, and hypoglycemia.

## Treatment of acute poisoning

### *Emergency measures*

(1) In respiratory depression, give $O_2$ by artificial respiration.
(2) Give activated charcoal (see pp. 31–32). Gastric lavage with protected airway (see p. 29) is useful even if delayed. Do not attempt emesis if respiration is depressed.
(3) Maintain blood pressure (see p. 57).
(4) Give glucose intravenously and correct electrolyte imbalance and dehydration (see p. 69).

### *Special measures*

(1) In severe poisoning with blood level above 500 mg/dl, hemodialysis can be lifesaving.
(2) Treat renal failure (see p. 67).

## Prognosis

Symptoms persist 2–4 times as long as after ethanol ingestion. Patients who survive 48–72 h ordinarily recover completely.

## Reference

Leeper SC, *et al*. Topical absorption of isopropyl alcohol induced cardiac and neurologic deficits in an adult female with intact skin. *Vet Human Toxicol* 2000;42:15

# 12  Esters, aldehydes, ketones, and ethers*

## TRIORTHOCRESYL PHOSPHATE

Tricresyl phosphate, $(CH_3C_6H_4)_3PO_4$, exists in three isomeric forms: $o$-, $m$-, and $p$-. Only the $o$-form (triorthocresyl phosphate, TOCP) is of toxicologic importance; it is a liquid that fumes appreciably at 100°C. Triorthocresyl phosphate is used in lubricants, in fireproofers, and as a plasticizer in plastic coatings. Fatty foods stored in plastics containing free triorthocresyl phosphate will become contaminated. Triphenyl phosphate has similar effects but is less hazardous.

The fatal dose of triorthocresyl phosphate by ingestion is estimated to be 1 g/kg, but the toxic dose is 6 mg/kg. Food contaminated to the extent of 0.4% has caused serious poisoning. The exposure limit is 0.1 mg/m³. The exposure limit for triphenyl phosphate is 3 mg/m³.

Demyelinization of nerves is the most prominent finding. Degenerative changes are also found in the muscles, anterior horn cells, and pyramidal tracts. As a result of these changes a flaccid paralysis develops that affects the more distal muscles of the legs and arms.

Triorthocresyl phosphate inhibits non-specific cholinesterase but not acetylcholinesterase. The relationship between this inhibition and the nerve demyelinization is unknown.

### Clinical findings

The principal manifestation of triorthocresyl phosphate poisoning is muscular paralysis.

*Acute poisoning* (From ingestion, inhalation, or skin absorption)

Symptoms begin 1–30 days after exposure and include weakness of the distal muscles progressing to foot drop, wrist drop, and loss of plantar reflex. Laryn-

---

*See also Table 12.1

geal, ocular, and respiratory muscles are affected in severe poisoning. Death is from respiratory paralysis.

### *Chronic poisoning*

The above symptoms may be produced by cumulative exposure over several months.

### Prevention

Foods should never be stored in plastic containers containing unreacted triorthocresyl phosphate. Containers sold for food purposes are safe.

Processes utilizing triorthocresyl phosphate at high temperatures must be totally enclosed to avoid contamination of workroom air.

### Treatment

### *Acute poisoning*

(1) Emergency measures – Remove ingested poison by gastric lavage or emesis (see pp. 29–32). Give artificial respiration as needed.
(2) General measures – If respiratory depression or weakness of respiratory muscles occurs, give artificial respiration with $O_2$. Assisted respiration may be necessary for several weeks.

### *Chronic poisoning*

Treat as for acute poisoning.

### Prognosis

In paralysis from triorthocresyl phosphate, recovery may be gradual over a period of 1 year. Complete recovery may never occur.

## FORMALDEHYDE

Formaldehyde (HCHO) is a gas that is ordinarily available as a 40% solution (formalin) for use as a disinfectant, an antiseptic, a deodorant, a tissue fixative, or an embalming fluid. The polymerized form, trioxymethylene (paraformaldehyde), can be decomposed by heat to formaldehyde for fumigating purposes. The fatal dose of formalin is 60–90 ml. The exposure limit for formaldehyde is 2 ppm (NIOSH). The American Society of Heating, Refrigeration and Air Conditioning Engineers has set a ceiling limit for formaldehyde of 0.12 mg/m³ for indoor air. Polymers of formaldehyde are used to give paper and cloth wet strength and as adhesives in particle board and plywood. These polymers sometimes contain free formaldehyde. They decompose slowly, with the liberation of formaldehyde over a period of years. Air concentrations of formaldehyde ranging up to 1.9 ppm have been found in mobile homes with extensive use of particle board, plywood, and urea-formaldehyde insulation.

Although formaldehyde is a normal metabolite in humans, in high concentrations it can react chemically with most substances in cells and thus depress all cellular functions and lead to death of the cells. At least part of the toxic effect appears to be the result of conversion of formaldehyde to formic acid. Formaldehyde in very high concentrations is a carcinogen in animals, probably as a result of its capacity to irritate.

Pathologic findings from the ingestion of formaldehyde are necrosis and shrinking of the mucous membranes. Degenerative changes may be found in the liver, kidneys, heart, and brain.

### Clinical findings

The principal manifestations of formaldehyde poisoning are collapse and anuria.

#### Acute poisoning

Ingestion causes immediate and severe abdominal pain followed by collapse, loss of consciousness, and anuria. There may be vomiting and diarrhea. Death is from circulatory failure. Exposure to formaldehyde in air causes respiratory tract and eye irritation. Such reactions can occur in some individuals at concentrations well below 1 ppm. Laryngeal edema and skin sensitivity reactions with urticarial swelling can also occur at these low concentrations.

#### Skin manifestations

Clothing and papers containing free formaldehyde cause sensitivity dermatitis in some individuals.

### Laboratory findings

The urine may contain protein, casts, or red blood cells.

## Treatment of acute poisoning

### Emergency measures

(1) Dilute, inactivate, or adsorb ingested formaldehyde by giving milk, activated charcoal (see pp. 31–32), or tap water. Do not use gastric lavage or emetics. Any organic material will inactivate formaldehyde.
(2) Treat shock (see p. 56).

### Special problems

Treat anuria (see p. 67). Esophageal stricture may occur.

## Prognosis

Patients who survive for 48 hours will probably recover.

## ACETALDEHYDE, METALDEHYDE, PARALDEHYDE

Metaldehyde – a tasteless, water-insoluble solid – and paraldehyde (bp: 124°C) – a water-soluble (1:8) liquid with a burning taste and smell – are polymers of acetaldehyde (bp: 20°C), a highly volatile, irritating, water-miscible liquid. In the presence of acids paraldehyde decomposes readily and metaldehyde slowly to acetaldehyde. In the presence of moisture paraldehyde slowly decomposes to acetaldehyde and acetic acid. Deaths have occurred from administration of decomposed paraldehyde; it should be stored in small, well-filled bottles in the dark at a temperature of 25°C or lower and tested for acidity before administration. It should not be administered if the container has been opened for more than 24 hours. Paraldehyde is used as a hypnotic, metaldehyde as snail bait, and acetaldehyde as a reagent in chemical synthesis. Deaths have occurred from ingestion of 3 g (100 mg/kg) of metaldehyde. Amounts over 400 mg/kg are rapidly fatal. The exposure limit for acetaldehyde is 100 ppm. Levels for paraldehyde and metaldehyde have not been established.

Paraldehyde and metaldehyde presumably are decomposed slowly to acetaldehyde in the body. In the case of paraldehyde, the rate apparently does not exceed the rate of acetaldehyde oxidation, so that acetaldehyde does not accumulate. With metaldehyde, however, the rate of decomposition to acetaldehyde may exceed the rate of oxidation of acetaldehyde, since persons who have died of metaldehyde poisoning have shown symptoms suggestive of acetaldehyde poisoning.

Acetaldehyde, a highly reactive chemical, is irritating and depressive to all cells. Metaldehyde apparently acts only after decomposition to acetaldehyde. Paraldehyde produces depression of the central nervous system without slowing of respiration.

Pathologic findings in deaths from acetaldehyde poisoning are pulmonary irritation and edema. After paraldehyde or metaldehyde poisoning findings are not characteristic.

## Clinical findings

The principal manifestations of poisoning with these agents are irritation and coma.

### *Acute poisoning*

(1) Acetaldehyde – Exposure to the vapors causes severe irritation of mucous membranes, reddening of the skin, coughing, pulmonary edema, and narcosis. Ingestion causes nausea and vomiting, diarrhea, narcosis, and respiratory failure.
(2) Paraldehyde – Ingestion ordinarily induces sleep without depression of respiration, although deaths occasionally occur from respiratory and circulatory failure after doses of 10 ml or more.
(3) Metaldehyde – Ingestion of less than 50 mg/kg causes nausea, retching, severe vomiting, abdominal pain, temperature elevation, muscular rigidity, and hyperventilation. Ingestion of more than 100 mg/kg causes hyperreflexia, convulsions, and coma. Death from respiratory failure can occur up to 48 hours after ingestion. Liver and kidney injury also occurs.

*Chronic poisoning*

(1) Acetaldehyde – Repeated exposure to the vapors causes dermatitis and conjunctivitis.
(2) Paraldehyde – Chronic medicinal use of paraldehyde produces mental deterioration and delirium tremens.
(3) Metaldehyde – Amounts less than that necessary to produce acute poisoning are without effect.

*Laboratory findings*

(1) The blood glucose level may be depressed.
(2) The blood methemoglobin level may be raised.
(3) Liver or kidney function impairment may be revealed by appropriate tests (see p. 75). The serum transaminase level may be elevated.
(4) Serum creatine kinase elevation indicates muscle damage from convulsions.
(5) Blood acetaldehyde levels above 0.5 mg/dl are toxic.

## Treatment (For aldehydes, ketones, ethers, and esters)

*Acute poisoning from exposure to fumes*

(1) Emergency measures:
    (a) Remove from exposure.
    (b) Maintain airway and respiration.
    (c) Give $O_2$ by inhalation.
(2) General measures – Treat pulmonary edema (see p. 55).

*Acute poisoning from ingestion*

(1) Emergency measures:
    (a) Remove poison by gastric lavage or emesis (see pp. 29–32). Activated charcoal is useful. For metaldehyde, gastric lavage with 2–5% sodium bicarbonate solution will reduce conversion to acetaldehyde. Follow with saline catharsis. Gastric lavage and catharsis are effective up to 12–24 h after poisoning, since metaldehyde is slowly absorbed and is also excreted into the gastrointestinal tract.
    (b) Maintain airway and respiration. Give $O_2$ if respiration is depressed.

(2) Antidote – In metaldehyde poisoning in which convulsions cannot be controlled, cautious trial of D-penicillamine, *N*-acetylcysteine, ascorbic acid, or thiamine has been suggested on the basis that they lower blood acetaldehyde levels. Cautious trial of naloxone has also been suggested, since naloxone blocks the effect of salsolinol, a condensation product of acetaldehyde and dopamine that may contribute to convulsions.

(3) General measures:

    (a) Treat coma (see p. 63).

    (b) Treat hypoxia (see p. 52).

    (c) Treat pulmonary edema (see p. 55).

    (d) Give glucose intravenously for hypoglycemia.

    (e) Treat methemoglobinemia (see p. 78).

    (f) Treat convulsions with diazepam, 0.1 mg/kg slowly intravenously. Do not use paraldehyde. Barbiturates and anticonvulsants such as phenytoin should not be given, since these inhibit acetaldehyde metabolism.

    (g) Treat renal failure (see p. 67) or hepatic failure (see p. 76).

    (h) In metaldehyde poisoning, maintain alkaline urine and treat acidosis by administering sodium bicarbonate or other alkalinizing agents (see p. 71).

### *Chronic poisoning from exposure to fumes*

Remove from further exposure.

### *Chronic poisoning from paraldehyde ingestion*

(1) Remove from further exposure.

(2) Treat mental symptoms.

### **Prognosis**

Patients who survive for 48 hours after acute poisoning are likely to recover. Complete recovery after chronic poisoning from paraldehyde is not likely. Mental deficiency after metaldehyde poisoning may persist for a year or more.

## References

Kim Y, *et al*. Evaluation of exposure to ethylene glycol monoethyl ether acetates and their possible haematological effects on shipyard painters. *Occup Environ Med* 1999;56:378

Pandey CK, *et al*. Toxicity of ingested formalin and its management. *Hum Exp Toxicol* 2000;19:360

Taskinen HK, *et al*. Reduced fertility among female wood workers exposed to formaldehyde. *Am J Ind Med* 1999;36:206

**Table 12.1** Aldehydes, ketones, ethers, and esters (for treatment, see p. 221)

| | Exposure limit (ppm) | LD50 (mg/kg) or LC (ppm) | Irritation | CNS effects | Liver and kidney damage | Carcinogen | Miscellaneous and remarks |
|---|---|---|---|---|---|---|---|
| **Aldehydes** | | | | | | | |
| Acetal | | 3500 | | + | | | |
| Acrolein | 0.1 | 40 | + | + | | | |
| Benzaldehyde | | 28 | | + | | | Convulsions |
| Crotonaldehyde | 0.3$^C$ | 104 | + | | | | Sensitizer |
| 2-Furaldehyde | 2 | 65 | + | | + | | Pulmonary edema |
| Glutaraldehyde | 0.2 | 100 | + | + | | | |
| Malonaldehyde | | 606 | + | | | | Mutagen |
| n-Valeraldehyde | 50 | 310 ppm | + | | | | |
| **Ketones** | | | | | | | |
| Acetone | 500 | 2857 | + | + | | | Hypoglycemia |
| Acetophenone | 10 | 740 | + | + | | | |
| Benzoquinone | 0.1 | 130 | + | + | + | + | |
| Butanone-2 | 200 | 2737 | + | + | | | Neuropathy |
| Cyclohexanone | 25 | 1400 | + | + | | | |
| Diethyl ketone | 200 | 2140 | + | + | | | Neuropathy? |
| Diisobutyl ketone | 25 | 1416 | + | + | | | |
| Dipropyl ketone | 50 | 3730 | + | + | | | |
| Ethyl amyl ketone | 25 | 2500 | + | + | | | |
| Ethyl butyl ketone | 50 | 2760 | + | + | | | |
| Hexanone-2 | 5 | 914 | + | + | | | Neuropathy |
| Isophorone | 5 | 1870 | + | + | + | | |
| Ketene | 0.5 | 53 ppm | + | | | | Like phosgene |

*Continued*

*Table 12.1 (continued)*

| | Exposure limit (ppm) | LD50 (mg/kg) or LC (ppm) | Irritation | CNS effects | Liver and kidney damage | Carcinogen | Miscellaneous and remarks |
|---|---|---|---|---|---|---|---|
| Mesityl oxide | 15 | 710 | + | + | | | |
| Methylamyl ketone | 50 | 730 | + | + | | | |
| Methylcyclohexanone | 50 | 1000 | | + | | | |
| Methylisobutylketone | 50 | 1600 | + | + | | | |
| 4-Methyl-pentanone-2 | 50 | 1600 | + | + | | | Neuropathy |
| Methylvinylketone | 0.2C | | + | | | | Sensitizer |
| 1,4-Naphthoquinone | | 190 | + | | | + | Sensitizer, anemia |
| Ninhydrin | | 250 | + | | | | |
| Pentanone-2 | 200 | 1600 | + | + | | | |
| **Ethers** | | | | | | | |
| Allyl glycidyl ether | 5 | 390 | + | + | | | |
| Benzoyl peroxide | 5* | 5700 | + | | + | + | Sensitizer |
| n-Butyl glycidyl ether | 25 | 1520 | + | + | | | |
| Diglycidyl ether | 0.1 | 170 | + | + | + | + | Anemia |
| Dioxane | 20 | 2000 | + | + | + | + | |
| Ethylene oxide | 1 | 72 | + | + | + | + | |
| Glycidol | 25 | 420 | + | + | | | |
| Isopropyl ether | 250 | 8470 | + | + | | | |
| Isopropyl glycidyl ether | 50 | 1300 | + | + | | | |
| Methylal | 1000 | 5708 | + | + | + | | |
| Phenyl ether | 1 | 3370 | + | | + | | Nausea |
| Phenyl glycidyl ether | 0.1 | 1400 | + | + | | | |
| β-Propiolactone | 0.5 | 25 ppm | + | | | + | |

*Continued*

Table 12.1 (continued)

| | Exposure limit (ppm) | LD50 (mg/kg) or LC (ppm) | Irritation | CNS effects | Liver and kidney damage | Carcinogen | Miscellaneous and remarks |
|---|---|---|---|---|---|---|---|
| Propylene oxide | 20 | 440 | + | + | | + | |
| Tetrahydrofuran | 200 | 1650 | + | + | + | | |
| Trimellitic anhydride | 0.005 | 1900 | + | + | | | Lung damage |
| Vinyl cyclohexene | 0.1 | 2563 | + | | | + | |
| Vinyl cyclohexene dioxide | 10 | 800 | + | | | + | |
| **Esters** | | | | | | | |
| Amyl acetate | 100 | 6500 | + | + | + | | Anesthetic effect |
| Butyl acetate | 150 | 3200 | + | + | | | |
| Butyl acrylate | 2 | 900 | + | | + | + | Sensitizer |
| Butyl lactate | 5 | 200 ip | + | | | | |
| Dibutylphosphate | | 3200 | + | | | | |
| Diethylphthallate | 5* | 1000 | + | | | | |
| Dioctylphthallate | | 6513 | + | | | | Teratogen |
| Ethyl acetate | 400 | 4100 | + | + | + | | Sensitizer |
| Ethyl acrylate | 5 | 800 | + | + | + | | Heart damage |
| Ethyl formate | 100 | 1100 | + | + | | | Like formic acid |
| Ethyl methacrylate | | 3630 | + | + | | | |
| Ethyl silicate | 10 | 6270 | + | + | | | Acid corrosive |
| Hexyl acetate | 50 | 2000 ppm | + | + | | | |
| Hydroxyethylacrylate | | 650 | + | | | | |
| Hydroxypropylacrylate | 0.5 | 250 | + | | | | Sensitizer |
| Isopropyl acetate | 100 | | + | | | | |
| Methyl acetate | 200 | 3700 | + | + | | | Like methanol |
| Methyl acrylate | 10 | 280 | + | + | | | |

*Continued*

Table 12.1  (continued)

| | Exposure limit (ppm) | LD50 (mg/kg) or LC (ppm) | Irritation | CNS effects | Liver and kidney damage | Carcinogen | Miscellaneous and remarks |
|---|---|---|---|---|---|---|---|
| Methyl formate | 100 | 1620 | + | + | | | Like formic acid |
| Methyl methacrylate monomer | 100 | 5000 | + | + | | | Burning Plexiglas is similar |
| Methylmethane sulfonate | | 225 | + | | | + | |
| Propyl acetate | 200 | 6640 | + | + | | | |
| Triallyl phosphate | | 71 | | | | + | |
| Tributylphosphate | 0.2 | 1189 | + | | | | |
| Triethylphosphate | | 1500 | + | | | | |
| Trimethylphosphate | | 840 | + | | | | |
| Trimethylphosphite | 2 | 1600 | + | + | | | Eye damage |
| Tris (2,3 dibromopropyl) phosphate | | 1010 | | | | + | Sensitizer |
| Vinyl acetate | 10 | 1613 | + | | | | |

*mg/m$^3$; $^C$ceiling.

# 13  Hydrocarbons*

## PETROLEUM DISTILLATES: KEROSENE, SOLVENT DISTILLATE, AND GASOLINE

Kerosene, mineral seal oil, diesel oil: bp: 150–300°C. Solvent distillate (Stoddard solvent): bp: 100–150°C. Gasoline, naphtha, petroleum ether, mineral spirits (benzine), paint thinner, petroleum spirit, ligroin: bp: 20–100°C. The vapor pressure of distillates whose boiling point is above 100°C is negligible at 25°C. Lubricating oils, mineral seal oil, and petrolatum are non-toxic by ingestion unless aspiration occurs.

All the petroleum distillates are liquids. They contain mostly branched-chain or straight-chain aliphatic hydrocarbons and are used as fuels and solvents.

Petroleum distillates have far greater toxic effects when they are aspirated into the tracheobronchial tree than when they are merely ingested: ingestion of 500–1000 ml may produce only minor symptoms, but aspiration of as little as 1 ml can result in overwhelming chemical pneumonitis. The exposure limit for non-aromatic petroleum distillates (petroleum naphtha) is 500 ppm; for gasoline, 300 ppm; for mineral oil mist, 5 mg/m$^3$; and for rubber solvent naphtha, 400 ppm. The presence of benzene increases the toxicity (see p. 231). The exposure limit for Stoddard solvent, which contains aromatic hydrocarbons (benzene and derivatives), is 100 ppm. The exposure limit for ligroin, which contains aromatic hydrocarbons other than benzene, is 300 ppm. Pesticides, camphor, metals, or halogenated compounds dissolved in petroleum distillates also increase their toxicity.

Petroleum distillates are fat solvents and alter the function of nerves to produce depression, coma, and sometimes convulsions. The effects on liver, kidneys, and bone marrow may be caused by contaminants such as benzene.

Petroleum distillates with boiling points above 150°C have little toxicity when they are absorbed after ingestion. Direct aspiration of these substances into the lungs during ingestion appears to be the principal cause of the pulmonary irritation. Because these petroleum hydrocarbons have a low surface

---

*See also Table 13.1

tension and low viscosity, small quantities will spread over a large surface area, such as the lung.

Pathologic findings in acute poisoning include pulmonary edema, bronchial pneumonia, and gastrointestinal irritation. Degenerative changes in the liver and kidneys and hypoplasia of the bone marrow occur after prolonged inhalation of high concentrations.

## Clinical findings

The principal manifestations of poisoning with these agents are pulmonary irritation and central nervous system depression.

### *Acute poisoning* (from inhalation or ingestion)

Nausea and vomiting; cough; and pulmonary irritation progressing to pulmonary edema, bloody sputum, and bronchial pneumonia with fever and cough. Pneumothorax and emphysema may complicate recovery. If a large amount (>1 ml/kg) is ingested and retained, symptoms of central nervous system depression and irritation occur and include weakness, dizziness, slow and shallow respiration, unconsciousness, and convulsions. Ventricular fibrillation can occur rarely after ingestion or inhalation. Petroleum distillates are irritating to skin.

### *Chronic poisoning* (from inhalation)

Dizziness, weakness, weight loss, anemia, nervousness, pains in the limbs, peripheral numbness, and paresthesias.

### *Laboratory findings*

(1)  The red blood cell count may be reduced.
(2)  The bone marrow may show hypoplasia.
(3)  The urine may contain protein and red cells.
(4)  In the presence of pulmonary symptoms, get chest X-ray.

## Treatment

### Acute poisoning

(1) Emergency measures – Only hydrocarbons that are solvents for a toxic agent or are themselves toxic need be evacuated; most hydrocarbons are not toxic *per se*. Extreme care must be used to prevent aspiration. Gastric lavage with a cuffed endotracheal tube in place to prevent further aspiration should be done within 15 minutes. In the absence of depression or convulsions or impaired gag reflex, emesis can also be induced using syrup of ipecac (see p. 90) without increasing the hazard of aspiration.

(2) General measures – Give artificial respiration with $O_2$ if respiration is depressed. Maintain airway.

(3) Special problems – Treat bacterial aspiration pneumonia with organism-specific chemotherapy. Treat pulmonary edema (see p. 55). Administration of high doses of corticosteroids appears to be useful in the late stages of pulmonary injury from petroleum hydrocarbons.

### Chronic poisoning

Treat as for acute poisoning.

## Prognosis

After the first 24 hours, the extent of pulmonary involvement indicates severity. Infiltration of more than 30% of the lungs requires 2–4 weeks for resolution. Long-term pulmonary effects are not seen.

## References

Chyka PA. Benefits of extracorporeal membrane oxygenation for hydrocarbon pneumonitis. *J Toxicol Clin Toxicol* 1996;34:357

Cox MJ, *et al*. Severe burn injury from recreational gasoline use. *Am J Emerg Med* 1996;14:39

Kamijo Y, *et al*. Pulse steroid therapy in adult respiratory distress syndrome following petroleum naphtha ingestion. *J Toxicol Clin Toxicol* 2000;38:59

Rush MD, *et al*. Skin necrosis and venous thrombosis from subcutaneous injection of charcoal lighter fluid (naphtha). *Am J Emerg Med* 1998;16:508

Shusterman EM, *et al.* Soft tissue injection of hydrocarbons: a case report and review of the literature. *J Emerg Med* 1999;17:63

Spiller HA, Krenzelok EP. Epidemiology of inhalant abuse reported to two regional poison centers. *J Toxicol Clin Toxicol* 1996;35:167

## AROMATIC HYDROCARBONS: BENZENE, XYLENE, TOLUENE

**Benzene:** liquid; bp: 80°C; vapor pressure at 26°C: 100 mmHg; exposure limit: 1 ppm. **Xylene:** commercial preparation a mixture of *o-*, *m-*, *p-* ;bp: 140°C; vapor pressure at 28°C: 10 mmHg; exposure limit: 100 ppm. **Toluene:** liquid; bp: 110°C; vapor pressure at 31°C: 40 mmHg; exposure limit: 100 ppm. Coal tar naphtha is a mixture of benzene, toluene, xylene, and other aromatic hydrocarbons.

These compounds are commonly used as solvents in rubber and plastic cement. Toluene is the usual ingredient in the cement used for glue sniffing. In experimental animals the toxicities of benzene, toluene, and the three xylenes are similar either by injection or by inhalation, and the lethal quantity ranges from 2 to 5 g/kg; benzene is the most toxic. The toxic level of benzene in humans is around 0.2 g/kg, and for toluene and xylene it is 0.5–1 g/kg. In practice, the low vapor pressure of xylene reduces the inhalation hazard from this substance. In large amounts these compounds depress the central nervous system; repeated exposure to small amounts of benzene or toluene depresses the bone marrow.

In acute fatalities, the postmortem findings include petechial hemorrhages, noncoagulated blood, and congestion of all organs. In fatalities from chronic exposure to benzene or toluene, the findings include severe bone marrow aplasia; anemia; necrosis or fatty degeneration of the heart, liver, and adrenals; and hemorrhages.

### Clinical findings

The principal manifestation of acute poisoning is coma. Anemia occurs after chronic exposure to benzene or toluene.

*Acute poisoning*

(1) Inhalation or ingestion – Symptoms from mild exposure are dizziness, weakness, euphoria, headache, nausea and vomiting, tightness in the chest, and staggering. If exposure is more severe symptoms progress to visual blurring, tremors, shallow and rapid respiration, and ventricular irregularities including fibrillation, paralysis, unconsciousness, and convulsions. Violent excitement or delirium may precede unconsciousness. Kidney or liver damage may occur.

(2) Skin contact – Irritation, scaling, and cracking.

*Chronic poisoning* (from inhalation)

Symptoms include headache, loss of appetite, drowsiness, nervousness, and pallor. Anemia, petechiae, and abnormal bleeding occur after exposure to benzene or toluene. The anemia may progress to complete aplasia of the bone marrow, especially after benzene poisoning. Continued repeated inhalation of toluene to the point of euphoria has caused irreversible encephalopathy with ataxia, tremulousness, emotional lability, and diffuse cerebral atrophy. The incidence of leukemia in workers chronically exposed to benzene is 5–10 times that in non-exposed populations.

*Laboratory findings in benzene exposure*

(1) The red blood cell count may be diminished to 20% of normal.
(2) The white blood cell count may be diminished to 5–10% of normal. The differential count shows that the greatest decrease is in polymorphonuclear leukocytes.
(3) The thrombocytes may be reduced to 10–50% of normal.
(4) The tourniquet test (Rumpel–Leede) is positive.
(5) The bone marrow may appear normal, hypoplastic, or hyperplastic.

**Prevention**

Adequate ventilation must always be supplied in workrooms where benzene is being used. The benzene concentration in air should be checked frequently. Where high vapor concentrations are unavoidable, forced air masks should be used. A lifeline attended by a responsible person outside the contaminated enclosure is essential. If skin contact is unavoidable, neoprene gloves must be worn.

## Treatment

### Emergency measures

Remove patient from contaminated air and give artificial respiration with $O_2$. Remove ingested hydrocarbon by gastric lavage, being careful to avoid aspiration (see p. 230).

### General measures

(1) Control excitement or convulsions with diazepam, 0.1 mg/kg slowly intravenously.
(2) Keep at complete bed rest until respiration is normal.
(3) *Do not give* epinephrine or ephedrine or related drugs. They may induce fatal ventricular fibrillation. Monitor ECG to detect ventricular abnormalities foreshadowing possible cardiac arrest.

### Special problems

Treat anemia by repeated blood transfusions. Treat respiratory or pulmonary problems as described on p. 230. Treat kidney or liver damage (see pp. 67 and 75).

## Prognosis

In acute poisoning death may occur up to 3 days after poisoning.

Rapid progression of symptoms and lack of response to removal of the hydrocarbon indicate a poor outcome. In chronic poisoning from benzene, a steady decrease in the cellular elements of the blood or bone marrow indicates a poor outcome. If the cellular elements remain at a constant low level or rise gradually, recovery is likely. Patients have recovered after as much as a year of almost complete absence of formation of new blood elements.

## References

Deleu D, Hanssens Y. Cerebellar dysfunction in chronic toluene abuse: beneficial response to amantadine hydrochloride. *J Toxicol Clin Toxicol* 2000;38:37

Einav S, *et al*. Bradycardia in toluene poisoning. *J Toxicol Clin Toxicol* 1996;35: 295

Finkelstein MM. Leukemia after exposure to benzene: temporal trends and implications for standards. *Am J Ind Med* 2000;38:1

Kamijo Y, *et al*. Fatal bilateral adrenal hemorrhage following acute toluene poisoning: a case report. *J Toxicol Clin Toxicol* 1998;36:365

Khuder SA, *et al*. Assessment of complete blood count variations among workers exposed to low levels of benzene. *J Occup Environ Med* 1999;41:821

Plenge-Boenig, Karmaus W. Exposure to toluene in the printing industry is associated with subfecundity in women but not in men. *Occup Environ Med* 1999;56:443

Wiebelt H, Becker N. Mortality in a cohort of toluene exposed employees (rotogravure printing plant workers). *J Occup Environ Med* 1999;41:1134

## NAPHTHALENE

Melting point: 80°C; bp: 218°C; vapor pressure at 80°C: 9.8 mmHg.

Naphthalene, obtained from coal tar, is used as a moth repellent and synthetic intermediate.

The fatal dose of ingested naphthalene is approximately 2 g. This chemical is most dangerous in children up to age 6, in whom absorption occurs rapidly. The exposure limit is 10 ppm. Naphthalene causes hemolysis with subsequent blocking of renal tubules by precipitated hemoglobin. Hepatic necrosis has been reported. Hemolysis only occurs in individuals with a hereditary deficiency of glucose-6-phosphate dehydrogenase in the red cells (primarily black males), which results in a low level of reduced glutathione and increased susceptibility to hemolysis by metabolites of naphthalene.

### Clinical findings

The principal manifestations from naphthalene poisoning are hemolysis, jaundice, oliguria, and convulsions.

*Acute poisoning* (from ingestion or inhalation)

(1) Ingestion – Nausea and vomiting, diarrhea, oliguria, hematuria, anemia, jaundice, and pain on urination progressing to oliguria or anuria. In more serious poisoning, excitement, coma, and convulsions may occur.

(2) Inhalation – Headache, mental confusion, and visual disturbances have been reported from exposure to boiling naphthalene.

## *Chronic poisoning*

(1) Repeated ingestion will cause the symptoms described for acute poisoning.
(2) Local effects – Continued handling of naphthalene may produce a dermatitis characterized by itching, redness, scaling, weeping, and crusting of the skin. Eye contact causes corneal irritation and injury. Workers exposed to high levels of naphthalene fumes have developed lens opacity.

## *Laboratory findings*

(1) The red blood cell count may be 20–40% of normal. The white blood cell count may be increased. Hemolysis may be present.
(2) Urine may contain hemoglobin, protein, and casts.

## Prevention

Store naphthalene safely. Exhaust ventilation is necessary during work with naphthalene. Naphthalene workers should have periodic eye, blood, and urine examinations.

## Treatment

### *Emergency measures*

Remove ingested naphthalene by gastric lavage or emesis (see pp. 29–32). Treat convulsions (see p. 60).

### *General measures*

(1) Alkalinize urine – Give sodium bicarbonate, 5 g orally every 4 h or as necessary to maintain alkaline urine. Give fluids, up to 15 ml/kg/h, with furosemide, 1 mg/kg, to produce maximum diuresis and reduce injury to the kidney from hemoglobin products.
(2) Give repeated small blood transfusions until hemoglobin is 60–80% of normal.
(3) Hemodialysis or exchange transfusions should be used in the presence of severe central nervous system symptoms.

*Special problems*

Treat anuria (see p. 66).

**Prognosis**

Rapid progression to coma and convulsions indicates poor prognosis. Anuria may persist for 1–2 weeks with eventual complete recovery.

Local effects disappear 1–6 months after discontinuing exposure.

**Reference**

Bieniek G. Urinary naphthols as an indicator of exposure to naphthalene. *Scan J Work Environ Health* 1997;23:414

## ATMOSPHERIC ORGANIC COMPOUNDS

Organic compounds are liberated into the air during combustion and by the evaporation of solvents. These substances range from methane ($CH_4$) through aldehydes such as formaldehyde (HCHO) and acrolein ($CH_2$=CHCHO) to branched-chain, unsaturated hydrocarbons or polycyclic aromatic hydrocarbons (PAH). Many of these substances take part in reactions involving nitrogen dioxide, ozone, and energy from sunlight. Some combine to form particles that contribute to reduced visibility.

The main source of organic compounds in the atmosphere is internal combustion engines. An automobile without crankcase or exhaust controls wastes 10% of the supplied fuel into the atmosphere, or 18 g (0.04 lb) per mile at a fuel consumption of 1 gallon each 15 miles. Of this total, 60% is in the exhaust, 24% in crankcase blowby, and 15% in carburetor and fuel tank evaporation. Exhaust emissions from cars with catalytic converters should not exceed 100 ppm of hydrocarbons.

Diesel vehicles emit 2% of the supplied fuel to the atmosphere, or 12 grams per mile for a vehicle using fuel at a rate of 5 miles per gallon. Evaporative losses from diesel vehicles are low, since they use low-volatility fuel.

The national maximum for hydrocarbons in community air is 0.24 ppm of compounds other than methane. The atmosphere of metropolitan regions without controls contains 2 ppm of hydrocarbons 90% of the time and 5 ppm

20% of the time. Large organic molecules contaminating the atmosphere as a result of human activities may contribute to the incidence of cancer.

## References

Fung F, Clark RF. Styrene-induced peripheral neuropathy. *J Toxicol Clin Toxicol* 1999;37:91

Himmelstein MW, *et al*. Toxicology and epidemiology of 1,3-butadiene. *CRC Crit Reviews Toxicol* 1998;27:1

Romunstad P, *et al*. Cancer incidence and cause specific mortality among workers in two Norwegian aluminum reduction plants. *Am J Ind Med* 2000;37:175

Rudell B, *et al*. Bronchoalveolar inflammation after exposure to diesel exhaust: comparison between unfiltered and particle trap filtered exhaust. *Occup Environ Med* 1999;56:527

Zmirou D, *et al*. Personal exposure to atmospheric polycyclic aromatic hydrocarbons in a general adult population and lung cancer risk asessment. *J Occup Environ Med* 2000;42:121

**Table 13.1** Hydrocarbons (for treatment, see p. 230)

| | Exposure limit (ppm) | LD50 (mg/kg) or LC (ppm) | Irritation | Kidney and liver damage | Bone marrow damage | CNS effects | Myocardial sensitizer | Carcinogen |
|---|---|---|---|---|---|---|---|---|
| Acetylene | 2500 | | | | | + | + | |
| Benzo(α)pyrene | 0.2* | 420 | | | | | | + |
| Biphenyl | 0.2 | 2400 | + | | | + | | |
| 1,3-Butadiene | 2 | 5480 | + | + | + | + | | |
| Butane | 800 | | | | | + | | |
| p-tert-Butyltoluene | 1 | 778 | + | | | + | | |
| Chrysene | 0.2* | | | | | | | + |
| Cumene | 50 | 1400 | + | + | | + | | |
| Cyclohexane† | 300 | 813 | + | + | | + | | |
| Cyclohexene† | 300 | | + | + | | + | | |
| Cyclopentadiene | 75 | | + | + | | + | | |
| Cyclopentane‡ | 600 | | + | | | + | | |
| Decahydronaphthalene | | 4200 | + | | | + | | |
| Dicyclopentadiene | 5 | 350 | + | + | | + | | |
| Divinyl benzene | 10 | 4644 | + | | | + | | |
| Ethane | | | | | | + | | |
| Ethylbenzene | 100 | 3500 | + | | | + | | |
| Ethylidene norbornene | 5 | 2527 | + | + | + | | | |
| Fluoranthrene | 0? | 2000 | | | | | | + |
| Heptane | 400 | | + | | | + | + | |
| n-Hexane‡ | 50 | 190 | + | | + | + | + | |
| Hexanes (branched) | 500 | | + | | | + | + | |
| Indene | 10 | 2300 | + | + | | | | |
| Mesityl oxide | 15 | 710 | | | | + | | |
| Methane | | | | | | + | | |
| Methylacetylene | 1000 | | | | | + | | |

*Continued*

*Table 13.1 (continued)*

| | Exposure limit (ppm) | LD50 (mg/kg) or LC (ppm) | Irritation | Kidney and liver damage | Bone marrow damage | CNS effects | Myocardial sensitizer | Carcinogen |
|---|---|---|---|---|---|---|---|---|
| Methylcyclohexane | 400 | 4000 | + | + | | + | | |
| Nonane | 200 | 3200 ppm | + | | | + | | |
| Octane | 300 | | + | | | + | | |
| Paraffin wax | 2* | | | | | | | + |
| Pentane | 600 | | + | | | + | | |
| Propane | 1000 | | | | | + | | |
| Styrene | 50 | 316 | + | | | + | | |
| Terphenyls | 5* | 500 | + | + | | | | |
| Tetrahydronaphthalene | | 2860 | + | | | + | | |
| Trimethylbenzene | 25 | 5000 | + | | + | | | |
| Vinyltoluene | 50 | 1072 | + | | | + | | |

*mg/m$^3$; †May contain benzene; ‡Peripheral neuropathy

# 14 Corrosives

## OXALIC ACID

**Formula**: COOH-COOH; soluble in water; fumes appreciably when heated to 100°C.

Oxalic acid and oxalates are used as bleaches and metal cleaners in industry and in household products. The leaves of garden rhubarb (*Rheum* species) contain a high concentration of oxalate.

The fatal dose by ingestion is estimated to be 5–15 g. The exposure limit for oxalic acid is 1 mg/m$^3$. Oxalic acid is a corrosive acid. Oxalates combine with serum calcium to form insoluble calcium oxalate. The reduction in available calcium leads to violent muscular stimulation with convulsions and collapse.

In deaths following oxalic acid poisoning, calcium oxalate crystals are found in the renal tubules and in other tissues. The kidneys show cloudy swelling, hyaline degeneration, and sclerosis of the tubules. Corrosive changes may be found in the mouth, esophagus, and stomach. Cerebral edema also is a frequent finding.

### Clinical findings

The principal manifestation of oxalic acid poisoning is anuria.

*Acute poisoning* (from ingestion of oxalic acid)

Symptoms begin with local irritation and corrosion of the mouth, esophagus, and stomach, with pain and vomiting. These symptoms are followed shortly by muscular tremors, convulsions, weak pulse, and collapse. Death may occur within minutes. After apparent recovery or if oxalate is ingested, acute renal failure may occur from blocking of the renal tubules by calcium oxalate.

*Chronic poisoning* (from skin contact or inhalation)

Prolonged skin contact may cause discoloration and gangrene by a local corrosive effect. Prolonged inhalation of fumes produced by boiling oxalic acid solutions leads to oxalic acid poisoning with renal impairment.

### *Laboratory findings*

(1) Calcium oxalate crystals, red blood cells, and protein are found in the urine.
(2) Other clinical laboratory tests are noncontributory.

### Prevention

Avoid prolonged skin contact. Avoid fumes from boiling oxalic acid.

### Treatment

### *Acute poisoning*

(1) Emergency measures – Precipitate oxalate by giving calcium in any form orally, such as milk, lime water, chalk, calcium gluconate, calcium chloride, or calcium lactate. Do not use gastric lavage or emesis if tissue corrosion has occurred. Dissolve 10 g (2 teaspoons) of calcium lactate in (or add milk to) lavage or emesis fluids.
(2) Antidote – Give 10% calcium gluconate or calcium chloride, 10 ml slowly intravenously, and repeat if symptoms persist.
(3) General measures:
    (a) If renal function remains normal, give fluids to 4 liters daily to prevent precipitation of calcium oxalate in the renal tubules.
    (b) Treat as for acid ingestion (see p. 245).

### *Chronic poisoning*

Remove from further exposure.

### Prognosis

If calcium antidotes can be given promptly, recovery is likely.

## MISCELLANEOUS ACIDS AND ACID-LIKE CORROSIVES

The acids and acid-like corrosives listed in Table 14.1 are used for cleaning metals and other products and in a variety of chemical reactions.

Ingestion of 1 ml of a corrosive acid has caused death. (Exposure limits are listed in Table 14.1.) Death may occur up to 1 month after exposure to corrosive fumes such as nitrogen oxide, as in silo gas poisoning. Corrosive acids destroy tissues by direct chemical action. The tissue protein is converted to acid proteinate, which dissolves in the concentrated acid. Hemoglobin is converted to dark acid hematin and is precipitated. The intense stimulation by acid causes reflex loss of vascular tone.

The pathologic findings are those of corrosion and irritation. After ingestion, corrosive penetration of the esophagus and stomach are commonly found. The area of contact is stained brown or black except in the case of nitric and picric acids, which produce a yellow stain. Precipitated blood ('coffee-grounds' material) is frequently found in the stomach. The epithelium of the esophagus may desquamate in portions or as a whole. The eye shows denudation of the corneal epithelium and, in severe cases, edema and necrosis of the deeper tissues.

### Clinical findings

The principal manifestation of acid poisoning is corrosion.

### *Acute poisoning*

(1) Ingestion – severe, burning pain in the mouth, pharynx, and abdomen followed by vomiting and diarrhea of dark precipitated blood. The blood pressure falls sharply. Brownish or yellowish stains may be found around or in the mouth. Asphyxia occurs from edema of the glottis.

   After initial recovery, onset of fever indicates mediastinitis or peritonitis from perforation of the esophagus or the stomach. However, the patient may have a rigid abdomen without perforation. If the patient recovers from the immediate damage, scar formation is more likely to produce stricture of the pylorus than stricture of the esophagus.

(2) Inhalation – Inhalation of acid fumes or irritating gases causes coughing, choking, and variable symptoms of headache, dizziness, and weakness followed after a 6- to 8-h latent period by pulmonary edema with tight-

**Table 14.1** Acids and acid-like corrosives (for treatment see p. 245)

|  | Exposure limit (ppm) | TC (ppm) LD (g/kg) |
|---|---|---|
| Acetic acid (glacial) | 10 | 816 ppm |
| Acetic anhydride | 5 | 1000 ppm |
| Acetyl chloride |  | 2 ppm |
| Acrylic acid | 2 | 4000 ppm |
| Benzalchloride |  | 80 ppm |
| Benzoyl chloride | 0.5 | 2 ppm |
| Benzoyl peroxide | 5* |  |
| Benzyl chloride | 1 |  |
| Benzyltrichloride | 0.1 | 1.6 ppm |
| Bromine | 0.1 | 140 ppm |
| Calcium chloride |  | 1 g/kg |
| Chlorine | 0.5 | 137 ppm |
| Chlorine dioxide | 0.1 | 500 ppm |
| Chlorine trifluoride | 0.1 |  |
| Chloroacetylchloride | 0.05 | 1000 ppm |
| Dibutylphosphate | 1 |  |
| 2,2-Dichloropropionic acid | 1 | 500 ppm |
| Ethyl chlorocarbonate |  | 145 ppm |
| Formic acid | 5 | 7.3* |
| Hydrazoic acid | 0.1 | 0.3 ppm |
| Hydrobromic acid | 3 | 814 ppm |
| Hydrochloric acid | 5 | 1300 ppm |
| Lactic acid |  | 210 ppm |
| Maleic anhydride | 0.1 | 9.8 ppm |
| Methacrylic acid | 20 | 221* |
| Methyl silicate | 1 | 250 ppm |
| Methyl trichlorosilane |  | 450 ppm |
| Osmic acid | 0.0002 | .133* |
| Peroxyacetic acid |  | 450 ppm |
| Perchloric acid |  | 0.4 g/kg |
| Phosphoric acid | 1* |  |
| Phosphorus pentachloride | 0.1 | 205* |
| Phosphorus trichloride | 0.2 | 50 ppm |
| Phthallic anhydride | 1 |  |
| Propionic acid | 10 |  |
| Silicon tetrahydride | 5 |  |
| Sodium metabisulfite | 5* |  |
| Sulfamic acid |  | 1 g/kg |
| Sulfosalicylic acid |  | 1.3 g/kg |
| Tartaric acid |  | 5 g/kg |
| Thioglycolic acid | 1 | 0.1 g/kg |
| Titanium tetrachloride |  | 100* |
| Trichloroacetic acid | 1 | 0.4 g/kg |

*mg/m³

ness in the chest, air hunger, dizziness, frothy sputum, and cyanosis. The accompanying physical findings are moist rales, low blood pressure, and high pulse pressure. Hemoptysis and shortness of breath may continue for several weeks after a single exposure to chlorine or other corrosive vapor.

(3) Skin contact – Symptoms are severe pain and brownish or yellowish stains. Burns usually penetrate the full thickness of the skin, have sharply defined edges, and heal slowly with scar formation.

(4) Eye contact – Conjunctival edema and corneal destruction occur from even dilute acids in the eyes. The symptoms are pain, tearing, and photophobia.

*Chronic poisoning* (from inhalation)

Long exposure to acid fumes may cause erosion of the teeth followed by jaw necrosis. Bronchial irritation with chronic cough and frequent attacks of bronchial pneumonia are common. Gastrointestinal disturbances are also noted.

*Laboratory findings*

In acute poisoning hemoconcentration may be indicated by a rise in red blood cell count and hematocrit.

*X-Ray findings*

After inhalation of corrosives, diffuse mottling of the lung fields may be seen on X-rays.

**Prevention**

The exposure limit must always be observed (see Table 14.1). Water bubbler eye fountains and showers must be available where skin or eye contact with acids is possible.

Tight-fitting goggles, rubber aprons, and rubber gloves *must* be worn when handling acids. Employees must be drilled in the constant use of safety equipment.

Enclosed spaces containing corrosive gases should be thoroughly ventilated before being entered. Use of proper gas masks is advisable.

### Treatment

*Ingestion*

(1) Emergency measures:
   (a) Do not use gastric lavage or emesis.
   (b) Dilute the acid – Ingested acid must be diluted within seconds by drinking quantities of water or milk. If vomiting is persistent, administer fluids repeatedly. Ingested acid must be diluted approximately 100-fold to render it harmless to tissues.
   (c) Relieve pain – Give morphine sulfate, 5–10 mg every 4 h as necessary. Avoid central nervous system depression.
(2) General measures:
   (a) Treat asphyxia from glottal edema by maintaining an adequate airway (see p. 54).
   (b) Treat shock – Maintain normal blood pressure by transfusion and by the administration of 5% dextrose in saline (see p. 57).
   (c) If symptoms are severe and perforation of the stomach or esophagus is suspected, give nothing by mouth until endoscopic examination has been done.
   (d) Maintain nutrition by giving carbohydrate or hyperalimentation fluid intravenously.
(3) Special problems – Esophageal stricture may require dilation.

*Eye contact*

(1) Emergency measures – Dilute the acid. Flood affected area with quantities of water in a shower or by means of a water bubbler eye fountain for at least 15 minutes (see p. 33). The eyelids must be held apart during the washing.
(2) Antidote – Do not use chemical antidotes. The heat liberated in the chemical reaction may actually increase injury.
(3) General measures – Eye burns require the immediate attention of an ophthalmologist. If an ophthalmologist is not immediately available, wash the eyes and apply sterile bandages without any medication. Allay pain by the systemic administration of analgesics. Then take the patient to an ophthalmologist.

*Skin contact*

(1) Emergency measures – Remove acid by flooding with water for at least 15 minutes. If the clothing is contaminated, a stream of water must be directed under the clothing while the clothes are being removed in order to remove the acid rapidly.
(2) Antidote – Do not use chemical antidotes (see above).
(3) General measures – Treat damaged areas as for thermal burns.

*Inhalation*

(1) Give artificial respiration.
(2) Treat shock (see p. 56).
(3) Treat pulmonary edema (see p. 55).
(4) Treat bacterial pneumonia with organism-specific chemotherapy.

*Chronic poisoning*

Remove from further exposure.

**Prognosis**

In one series 32 of 105 persons who ingested acid died. Damage to the esophagus and stomach after ingestion may progress for 2–3 weeks. Death from peritonitis may occur as late as 1 month after ingestion. Approximately 95% of those who ingest acid and recover from immediate effects have persistent esophageal stricture.

Skin burns from acid are followed by extensive scarring. Skin grafting is required if a good cosmetic effect is desired. Corneal damage almost always results in blindness.

After inhalation of corrosive atmospheres, convalescence may be prolonged and frequent relapses may occur. Death may occur 30 days or more after exposure to such corrosive atmospheres as silo gas.

**References**

Ho C-K, *et al.* Suspected nasopharyngeal carcinoma in three workers with long term exposure to sulphuric acid vapour. *Occup Environ Med* 1999;56:426

Meggs WJ, *et al.* Nasal pathology and ultrastructure in patients with chronic airway inflammation (RADS and RUDS) following an irritant exposure. *J Toxicol Clin Toxicol* 1996;34:383

Sexton JD, Pronchik DJ. Chlorine inhalation: the big picture. *J Toxicol Clin Toxicol* 1998;36:87

## NITROGEN OXIDES

The nitrogen oxides important in air contamination and in reactions that form atmospheric oxidants (see p. 252) include nitric oxide (NO, colorless), nitrogen dioxide ($NO_2$, brown color), nitrogen trioxide ($N_2O_3$, colorless), and nitrogen pentoxide ($N_2O_5$, colorless). Nitrous oxide ($N_2O$, laughing gas, colorless) and dinitrogen tetroxide ($N_2O_4$, colorless) do not occur in the atmosphere in significant amounts. Nitric acid ($HNO_3$) is produced in the atmosphere by reaction between oxides of nitrogen and water vapor.

The nitrogen oxides are emitted into the atmosphere as a result of combustion of any nitrogen-containing substances. Thus, missile fuels, explosives, cigarettes, and agricultural wastes liberate nitrogen oxides. Nitrogen dioxide is also liberated during the rapid decomposition of plant material, as happens in silos. In an enclosed silo the concentration of nitrogen dioxide may reach as high as 1500 ppm. In addition, combustion at high temperatures of nitrogen-free fuels in the presence of air oxidizes the nitrogen of the air to nitric oxide ($N_2 + O_2 = 2NO$). At 1800K, 1% of the reactants will be converted, and at 2675K, 5% of the reactants will be converted. Unmodified auto or diesel exhaust contains 1100 ppm of nitric oxide, producing an emission of 0.13 lb per gallon of fuel or 4 g per mile for a vehicle consuming 1 gallon of fuel each 15 miles. Since 1977 federal regulations in the USA have limited all new automobiles to an emission of 0.31 g of nitrogen oxides per mile. Cigarette smoke contains 200–650 ppm of nitrogen oxides, and pipe smoke contains 1100 ppm.

On reaching the air nitric oxide oxidizes spontaneously to nitrogen dioxide, which gives smog its brown color. This reaction is slow if the concentration of nitric oxide is below 1 ppm, but it is accelerated by the presence of other contaminants in the air, especially ozone. This color can be seen most clearly by looking into an air-polluted basin from above the temperature inversion boundary on any day with low wind velocity.

The exposure limit for industrial exposure to nitrogen dioxide is 3 ppm (NIOSH 1 ppm) and for submarines in the US Navy 0.5 ppm. The industrial exposure limit for nitric acid is 2 ppm. The exposure limit for nitric oxide is 25 ppm. The fatal dose of nitric acid is 1 ml. The national maximum annual average for nitrogen dioxide in community air has been set at 0.05 ppm in the USA. A concentration of 0.2 ppm was exceeded for a total of 487 hours in San Francisco in 1967 and for 2594 hours in the same year in Burbank, California.

Experimental studies in humans have used nitrogen dioxide, since it is reasonably stable and reproducible conditions can be established. The taste and odor of this compound can be detected at 1 ppm by experienced subjects. Chest discomfort occurs at a concentration of 15 ppm for 1 h, the sensation becoming unpleasant at 25 ppm. After 1 minute at 50 ppm, subjects feel substernal pain. Longer exposure at this concentration has caused inflammatory changes in the lungs that ordinarily are reversible. Higher concentrations have been fatal.

Pathologic findings show that the effects on the lungs from inhaled silo gas (nitrogen dioxide) are typical of bronchiolitis fibrosa cystica. These effects include hemorrhage; fibrous stroma replacing the terminal bronchi, alveolar ducts, and sacs; hyaline membrane formation; and hyalinization of the basement membrane.

Exposure of rats to 0.5 ppm for 4 h causes reversible degranulation of lung cells. Mice exposed continuously for 3 months to 0.5 ppm are more susceptible when exposed to pneumococci. Monkeys lose weight when exposed at this concentration, but other animals are not affected. Continuous exposure of rats to 2 ppm of nitrogen dioxide for 3 days caused epithelial hyperplasia in the terminal bronchioles, and exposure for more than 1 year caused thinning of the membrane lining the lungs. Intermittent exposure of rats to 4 ppm for a year caused no discernible permanent damage to the lungs.

### Clinical findings

The principal manifestation of nitrogen dioxide poisoning is dyspnea. For nitric acid, see p. 242.

*Acute poisoning* (from inhalation)

Progressive weakness, dyspnea, cough, and cyanosis begin 1–3 weeks after single or repeated exposure to concentrations of 50–300 ppm. Concentrations above 300 ppm cause fulminating pulmonary edema or bronchopneumonia with onset within hours or days. Exposure to pure nitric oxide causes methemoglobinemia.

*Laboratory findings*

Pulmonary function tests reveal reductions in inspiratory capacity and vital capacity and impaired diffusion capacity. These findings improve as the inflammatory process subsides, but some impairment of function may be permanent.

## Prevention

Silos and other enclosed spaces in which decomposition of organic material can liberate nitrogen dioxide should be ventilated thoroughly before being entered.

## Treatment

*General measures*

Give 35–50% $O_2$ for dyspnea and cyanosis.

*Special problems*

(1) Treat pulmonary edema (see p. 55).
(2) Treat bronchopneumonia with organism-specific chemotherapy.

## Prognosis

Recovery from the acute phase requires 1–6 months. Emphysematous change persists depending on the severity of the original damage.

**References**

Rosenlund M, Bluhm G. Health effect resulting from nitrogen dioxide exposure in an indoor ice arena. *Arch Environ Health* 1999;54:52

Tabacova S, *et al*. Exposure to oxidized nitrogen: lipid peroxidation and neonatal health risk. *Arch Environ Health* 1999;53:214

## DIMETHYL SULFATE AND DIETHYL SULFATE

**Formula** (dimethyl sulfate): $(CH_3)_2SO_4$; bp: 188°C; vapor pressure at 76°C: 15 mmHg. **Formula** (diethyl sulfate): $(C_2H_5)_2SO_4$; bp: 209°C; vapor pressure at 47°C: 1 mmHg.

Dimethyl sulfate is used in organic synthesis. The lethal dose is 1–5 g. The exposure limit is 0.1 ppm. Diethyl sulfate is also used in organic synthesis. The lethal dose is probably in excess of 10 g. No exposure limit has been established.

Dimethyl sulfate hydrolyzes in the presence of water to methanol and sulfuric acid. It is caustic to mucous membranes of the eyes, nose, throat, and lungs. Pulmonary edema is the usual cause of death. Diethyl sulfate hydrolyzes slowly in water to monoethyl sulfate and ethanol. Monoethyl sulfate is corrosive to mucous membranes.

Pathologic changes are those of extreme irritation. The eyes, nose, mouth, throat, lungs, liver, heart, and kidneys are affected.

### Clinical findings

The principal manifestation of acute dimethyl sulfate or diethyl sulfate poisoning is extreme irritation.

*Symptoms and signs* (from inhalation, skin absorption, or ingestion)

The immediate effects of vapor exposure are irritation and erythema of the eyes progressing to lacrimation, blepharospasm, and chemosis. Cough, hoarseness, and edema of the tongue, lips, larynx, and lungs occur later.

Ingestion or direct contact with mucous membranes causes corrosion equivalent to that from sulfuric acid. After absorption, pulmonary edema and injury to the liver and kidneys are the most prominent findings.

Diethyl sulfate is suspected of being a carcinogen after long exposure.

*Laboratory findings*

(1) Hematocrit determination may reveal hemoconcentration. Hypoglycemia also occurs.
(2) The urine may contain protein and red blood cells.

## Prevention

If dimethyl sulfate or diethyl sulfate is spilled the building must be evacuated and the agent decomposed by hosing with water or spraying with 5% sodium hydroxide (caustic soda).

Workers who enter contaminated areas must wear positive-pressure airline hose masks or self-contained breathing apparatus. Canister type gas masks are not safe.

## Treatment of acute poisoning

*Emergency measures*

Remove the patient to fresh air and wash skin or mucous membranes with copious amounts of water. Showers and bubbler eye fountains must be available where these agents are used. Washing should continue for at least 15 minutes. Treat skin corrosion the same as a burn. Observe exposed individuals for at least 24 hours for the development of symptoms.

*General measures*

(1) Maintain adequate arterial $O_2$ saturation – if necessary, by artificial ventilation with 60–100% $O_2$.
(2) Treat bronchospasm
   (a) Give isoproterenol, 1:200, 0.5 ml in 3 ml of saline, by intermittent positive-pressure nebulizer for 15-minute periods every 2–4 h. Cardiac arrhythmias may occur.
   (b) Give aminophylline, 250–500 mg in 50 ml of saline intravenously over 30 min every 6 h as necessary. Cardiac arrhythmias and tachycardia may occur.
(3) Administration of hydrocortisone, 300 mg in divided doses daily for 2 days, may be useful to limit pulmonary injury.

*Special problems*

Treat pulmonary edema (see p. 55).

**Prognosis**

The first 24 hours after poisoning constitute the most dangerous period. If pulmonary edema can be controlled, recovery is likely. Complete recovery from eye irritation may take up to 1 month.

## ATMOSPHERIC OXIDANTS

Atmospheric oxidants are defined as substances in the atmosphere with an oxidizing power sufficiently great to liberate iodine from a solution of potassium iodide. One oxidant, ozone ($O_3$), accelerates the cracking of rubber. Oxidants, which make up the eye irritants in photochemical smog, result from the action of sunlight on air containing nitrogen dioxide and certain organic compounds.

**Sources**

The reactions that initiate the formation of oxidants depend on the absorption of light energy. The amount of energy in a light quantum is given by the expression $h$ (Planck's constant, with a value of $6.62 \times 10^{-27}$ erg second) $\times \nu$ (frequency of the light). For this reason the light in the ultraviolet spectrum is more important, since it has greater energy. The following reactions are considered to be important in the absorption of light energy ($h\nu$) and the production of monatomic oxygen ($O\bullet$) and free organic radicals ($R\bullet$):

$$NO_2 + h\nu = NO + O\bullet \qquad\qquad RONO + h\nu = RO\bullet + NO$$
$$RCHO + h\nu = R\bullet + HC\bullet O \qquad RONO + h\nu = R\bullet + NO_2$$
$$RCO\bullet R' + h\nu = R'\bullet + RCO\bullet$$

Other reactions, including some or all of the following, occur in the dark:

$$O\bullet + O_2 = O_3 \qquad\qquad CH_3OO\bullet + O_2 = CH_3O\bullet + O_3$$
$$O_3 + NO = O_2 + NO_2 \qquad CH_3O\bullet + NO = CH_3ONO$$
$$O\bullet + C_4H_8 = \bullet CH_3 + C_3H_5O \qquad CH_3O\bullet + O_2 = H_2CO + HOO\bullet$$
$$\bullet CH_3 + O_2 = CH_3OO\bullet \qquad O_3 + 2NO_2 = N_2O_5 + O_2$$

The following reaction scheme from ethylene ($C_2H_4$) to peroxyacetylnitrate (PAN) has been suggested:

$$C_2H_4 + O_3 = C_2H_4O_3$$
$$2C_2H_4O_3 = HCHO + CH_3O + CH_3CO + O_3$$
$$CH_3CO + O_2 = CH_3CO_3$$
$$CH_3CO_3 + NO_2 = CH_3CO \cdot O \cdot ONO_2 \text{ (PAN)}$$

The concentration of ozone does not begin to rise until nitric oxide (NO) has been completely converted to nitrogen dioxide ($NO_2$). Although nitrogen dioxide alone contributes to the formation of a small amount of ozone, the levels found in urban atmospheres do not occur unless some of the carbon compounds indicated in the above schemes are present. These include aldehydes, ketones, and unsaturated hydrocarbons. The reactivity of these substances in atmospheres forms the basis for the restriction of their use in various solvents for paints, lacquers, and other finishes. Methane ($CH_4$), which makes up about half of the organic compounds in the atmosphere, does not react. Some of the reaction intermediates are possible contributors to eye irritation, but they are so unstable that analysis or experimental testing has not been possible. PAN has been tested in volunteers and found to be irritating to the eyes at concentrations of 0.5 ppm, a concentration higher than that likely to occur in the atmosphere. A mixture of chemicals may be more irritating than the individual substances.

At the peak of oxidant concentration in the atmosphere (shortly after midday), ozone makes up more than 90% of the total. By nightfall, ozone falls to a low level but oxidants may still be present. The chemical make-up of all the dark-reaction oxidants has not as yet been defined. One compound has been identified as PAN (see above); its concentration during air pollution episodes is not known.

Ozone is also produced by electrical discharges such as lightning and by the effect of intense ultraviolet light. At an altitude of 75 000 ft the concentration of ozone is raised to 16 ppm by the direct action of sunlight. Unless some means is used to decompose the ozone, the concentration inside pressurized aircraft flying at heights between 30 000 and 40 000 ft reaches 0.3–0.4 ppm. Some ozone found at ground level is brought down to this level by atmospheric mixing, but this amount does not exceed 0.01–0.03 ppm except during lightning storms.

In the USA the national maximum 1-hour average for ozone in community air has been set at 0.12 ppm. In 1967 the level in San Jose, California, exceeded 0.1 ppm for 272 h; in Burbank, California, for 1191 h; and in Pasadena, California, for 1245 h. In the same year a level of 0.05 ppm was exceeded for 1032 h in San Jose, 2198 h in Burbank, and 2243 h in Pasadena, while San Francisco had 129 h above 0.05 ppm and 25 h above 0.1 ppm. The industrial exposure limit for ozone is 0.1 ppm.

**Effects on humans and animals**

The odor threshold for ozone in the most sensitive individuals is 0.01 ppm, but it is only recognized by all persons at 0.05 ppm. At a concentration of 0.1 ppm of ozone or oxidants, more than 5% of individuals will have symptoms of eye irritation. Mice exposed for 3 h to this concentration plus a streptococcus had a statistically significant increase in the mortality rate as compared to mice exposed only to the streptococcus. Guinea pigs exposed to 0.1 ppm of ozone and tubercle bacilli continuously for 17 weeks also showed an increased mortality rate as compared to guinea pigs exposed only to tubercle bacilli.

Patients with obstructive lung diseases such as asthma or emphysema, when exposed to an ambient atmosphere containing 0.1–0.15 ppm of oxidants, showed increased breathing resistance, increased $O_2$ consumption, and decreased arterial $O_2$ concentration, as compared to the same patients exposed to charcoal-filtered air during episodes with outside air at 0.1–0.15 ppm of oxidants. Recovery from the effects of oxidant-containing ambient air required several days.

Experiments have shown that exposure to 0.2 ppm of ozone for 3 h reduces visual acuity, increases peripheral vision, decreases night vision, and alters the balance of the muscles controlling the position of the eye.

Asthmatic patients report more attacks when the daily peak of oxidants goes over 0.25 ppm. A level of 0.3 ppm of ozone causes cough and some respiratory tract irritation after 30 minutes of exposure. This same concentration of PAN raised $O_2$ consumption during voluntary exercise. Progressively higher concentrations are more irritating; lung function is distinctly impaired at ozone concentrations of 0.6 ppm.

## Mechanisms of ozone action

Ozone and other oxidants presumably produce their irritant action as a result of their chemical reactivity at the point of contact. These oxidants would be expected to react so rapidly on contact with any organic compounds that they could not be absorbed as such into the bloodstream. Thus, effects on tissues not directly exposed to ozone or oxidants are difficult to explain. Peroxidized fatty acids have been suggested as carriers of the energy. For example, subjects exposed to 1 ppm of ozone for 10 min showed a reduction in the ability of hemoglobin in the red blood cells to release $O_2$ in the tissues. The shape of red blood cells was altered by exposure of subjects to ozone at concentrations down to 0.2 ppm.

An effect of ozone similar to that of ionizing radiation has been suggested. Ionizing radiation appears to act on tissues by producing free radicals, and ozone could also have this effect. Substances that combine quickly with free radicals are effective as protective agents against both ionizing radiation and ozone. Both ozone and ionizing radiation cause chromosomal damage and age animals prematurely. However, in one series of experiments, exposure to ozone protected mice against simultaneous exposure to radiation.

## Treatment

The use of activated charcoal absorbers in rooms has been suggested as a means of lowering air contaminant concentrations.

## Reference

Sanderson WT, *et al*. Ozone-induced respiratory illness during the repair of a Portland cement kiln. *Scan J Work Environ Health* 1999;25:227

## SULFUR OXIDES

The following sulfur oxides occur as atmosphere contaminants: sulfur dioxide ($SO_2$) and sulfur trioxide ($SO_3$) along with the products of their reactions with water, sulfurous acid ($H_2SO_3$), and sulfuric acid ($H_2SO_4$), respectively. Sulfur monochloride ($S_2Cl_2$) and thionyl chloride ($SOCl_2$) are used in industrial processes. A number of salts of sulfur oxides are used as bleaches, oxidizers, reducing agents, and cleaning agents. Their estimated fatal doses and exposure limits (if established) are as follows: sodium hydrogensulfate (sodium bisulfate, $NaHSO_4$), 10 g; sodium sulfite ($Na_2SO_3$), 10 g; sodium hydrosulfite (sodium sulfoxylate, $Na_2S_2O_4$), 30 g; sodium hydrogensulfite (sodium bisulfite, $NaHSO_3$), 10 g, 5 mg/m³; sodium metabisulfite ($Na_2S_2O_5$), 10 g, 5 mg/m³; sodium, potassium, or ammonium persulfate ($Na_2S_2O_8$, $K_2S_2O_8$, $[NH_4]_2S_2O_8$), 10 g, 0.5 mg/m³; sodium thiosulfate ($Na_2S_2O_3$), 50 g. Sodium hydrosulfite releases sulfur dioxide on contact with acids. Persulfate salts release ozone and sulfuric acid on contact with water.

Sulfur dioxide reduces visibility by taking part in reactions between organic compounds and nitrogen oxides to form particulates. Oxidation to sulfur trioxide, which then combines with water to form small droplets of sulfuric acid, also reduces visibility.

Sulfur oxides arise from combustion of fuel oil and coal, from petroleum refining, and from the chemical and metallurgical industries.

In the USA the national maximum annual average for sulfur dioxide in community air is 0.03 ppm, and the maximum 24-h average is 0.14 ppm. For industrial exposures, the exposure limit for sulfur dioxide is 2 ppm; for sulfur trioxide, 2 ppm; for sulfuric acid, 1 mg/m³; for sulfurous acid, 10 ppm; for thionyl chloride, 1 ppm; and for sulfur monochloride, 1 ppm. The estimated fatal dose of sulfuric acid is 1 ml; of sulfurous acid, 10 ml.

Trained observers can recognize the presence of sulfur dioxide at a concentration of 0.3 ppm, but concentrations up to 1 ppm have little effect on lung function except for possible increase in respiratory rate. Increased resistance to breathing begins to occur at 1.6 ppm in normal individuals and possibly at 0.7 ppm in patients with respiratory disease. Concentrations in air pollution disasters such as occurred in Donora, Pennsylvania, and in London have ranged from 1 to 3 ppm. The eye irritation level is 10 ppm. Rats show decreased life span with accelerated aging and heart, lung, and kidney damage on uninterrupted exposure to 1 ppm.

Sulfites are potent sensitizers, and anaphylaxis can occur from exposure to residues in food or drugs.

### Clinical findings and treatment

See pp. 16 and 242–246.

**Prevention**

Persons sensitive to sulfites should be identified and warned to avoid foods that may contain residues. Physicians should not prescribe drugs containing sulfites for sensitive individuals.

## ALKALIS AND PHOSPHATES (potassium hydroxide, sodium hydroxide [lye], sodium phosphates, potassium carbonate, and sodium carbonate)

These agents (see Table 14.2) are used in the manufacture of soaps and cleansers and in chemical synthesis. Urine sugar test tablets contain sodium hydroxide. 'Button batteries' often contain sodium hydroxide or potassium hydroxide, which are released if batteries are ingested.

The fatal doses of alkalis are listed in Table 14.2.

The alkalis combine with protein to form proteinates and with fats to form soaps, thus producing soft, necrotic, deeply penetrating areas on contact with tissues. The solubility of these products allows further penetration that may continue for several days.

Sodium and potassium hexametaphosphates, polyphosphates, tripolyphosphates, pyrophosphates, and other phosphates used as water softeners form complexes with calcium and, after ingestion, are capable of seriously reducing the serum level of ionic calcium. They have less corrosive effects on mucous membranes than sodium or potassium hydroxide. Hydrolysis of the polymeric phosphates can also produce acidosis.

Pathologic findings include gelatinous necrotic areas at the sites of contact.

Intense stimulation by alkalis causes reflex loss of vascular tone and cardiac inhibition.

### Clinical findings

The principal manifestation of poisoning with alkalis is corrosion.

#### Acute poisoning

(1) Ingestion of strong alkalis – Ingestion of alkali is followed by severe pain, vomiting, diarrhea, and collapse. The vomitus contains blood and

**Table 14.2** Alkali corrosives

|  | Exposure limit (ppm) | TC (ppm) LD (g/kg) |
|---|---|---|
| 2-Aminobutane | 5 | 0.2 g/kg |
| 2-Aminopropane | 5 | 4000 ppm |
| Butylamine | 5 | 0.4 g/kg |
| Calcium hydroxide | 5* |  |
| Calcium oxide | 2* |  |
| Cement (Portland) | 5* |  |
| Cesium hydroxide | 2* | 0.5 g/kg |
| Cyclohexylamine | 10 | 7500 ppm |
| 2-N-Dibutylaminoethanol | 0.5 | 1 g/kg |
| Diethanolamine | 2* | 0.7 g/kg |
| Diethylamine | 5 | 4000 ppm |
| Diethylaminoethanol | 2 | 200 ppm |
| Diethylene triamine | 1 | 1 g/kg |
| Diisopropylamine | 5 | 2207 ppm |
| Dimethylamine | 5 | 4540 ppm |
| Ethanolamine | 3 | 0.5 g/kg |
| Ethylamine | 5 | 3000 ppm |
| 1,2-Ethanediamine | 10 | 4000 ppm |
| Isopropylamine | 5 |  |
| Lithium hydride | 0.025* | 10* |
| Lithium hydroxide |  | 960* |
| Methylamine | 5 | 2400* |
| Potassium carbonate |  | 1.2 g/kg |
| Potassium hydroxide | 2* |  |
| Potassium permanganate† |  | 0.1 g/kg |
| Sodium carbonate |  | 1200* |
| Sodium hydroxide | 2* |  |
| Sodium silicate |  | 0.25 g/kg |
| Tetrasodium pyrophosphate | 5* |  |
| Triethanolamine | 5* |  |
| Triethylamine | 1 |  |
| Trimethylamine | 5 |  |

*mg/m$^3$; †forms methemoglobin

desquamated mucosal lining. If death does not occur in the first 24 h, the patient may improve for 2–4 days and then have a sudden onset of severe abdominal pain, board-like abdominal rigidity, and rapid fall in blood pressure indicating delayed gastric or esophageal perforation. Button batteries can cause corrosive damage to the esophagus and upper gastro-intestinal tract.

Even though the patient recovers from the immediate damage, esophageal stricture can occur weeks, months, or even years later to make swallowing difficult. Carcinoma is a risk in later life.

(2) Ingestion of other alkalis – Ingestion of hexametaphosphate, tripolyphosphate, and other phosphates in the form of detergents or laxatives causes a shock-like state, fall in blood pressure, slow pulse, cyanosis, coma, and sometimes tetany as a result of reduction in ionic calcium.

(3) Eye contact – Eye contact with concentrated alkali causes conjunctival edema and corneal destruction. Dilute solutions of the amines shown in Table 14.2 can cause corneal damage.

(4) Skin contact – Alkalis penetrate skin slowly. The extent of damage therefore depends on duration of contact.

(5) Diethylaminoethanol and 2-*N*-dibutylaminoethanol inhibit cholinesterase (see pp. 128–129 for clinical findings).

*Chronic poisoning* (from skin contact)

A chronic dermatitis may follow repeated contact with alkalis.

*Laboratory findings*

The red blood cell count and hematocrit are increased. Button batteries lodged in the esophagus or a Meckel's diverticulum can be seen on X-ray.

**Prevention**

Store corrosive alkalis safely. The manufacturer's 'safety caps' on containers should not be replaced with regular caps. Water bubbler eye fountains and showers must be available where skin or eye contact with alkalis is possible. Tight-fitting goggles, rubber aprons, and rubber gloves must be worn when handling alkalis in concentrated solutions. Employees must be drilled in the constant use of safety equipment.

**Treatment**

*Ingestion*

(1) Emergency measures – Dilute the alkali by giving water or milk to drink immediately, and allow vomiting to occur. Avoid gastric lavage or

emetics, which increase the possibility of perforation. Esophagoscopy is the only way to exclude the possibility of corrosion in the upper gastrointestinal tract; if corrosion is suspected, esophagoscopy should usually be performed within 24 hours.

(2) Antidote – For hypocalcemia after phosphate ingestion, give calcium gluconate, 5 ml of 10% solution slowly intravenously, to restore ionic calcium to normal level.

(3) General measures – Give nothing by mouth until esophagoscopy has been done. Treat perforation with organism-specific chemotherapy. After the acute injury has subsided, esophageal dilation can be done.

(4) Specific measures – Button batteries lodged in the esophagus should be removed endoscopically or surgically. Batteries that have passed beyond the esophagus will ordinarily be expelled within 1–3 days; surgical intervention is unnecessary unless the battery lodges in a diverticulum. Catharsis may speed passage of the battery through the intestinal tract.

### Eye contact

(1) Emergency measures – Wash eye for 15 minutes with running water and then irrigate eye for 30–60 min with normal saline solution.

(2) General measures – Apply sterile bandages, allay pain by systemic administration of analgesics, and take the patient to an ophthalmologist for evaluation of the injury.

### Skin contact

Wash with running water until skin is free of alkali as indicated by disappearance of soapiness.

### Chronic poisoning

Remove from further contact and treat dermatitis (see p. 83).

### Prognosis

Approximately 25% of those who ingest strong alkali die from the immediate effects. Damage to the esophagus and stomach after ingestion may progress for 2–3 weeks. Death from peritonitis may occur as late as 1 month after ingestion. Approximately 95% of those who ingest strong alkali and recover from the immediate effects have persistent esophageal stricture.

Button batteries that pass the esophagus usually travel through the gastro-intestinal tract with little or no damage.

Corneal damage is almost always permanent; corneal transplant may be useful.

### Reference

Fizgibbons LJ, Snoey ER. Severe metabolic alkalosis due to baking soda inges-tion: case reports of two patients with unsuspected antacid overdose. *J Emerg Med* 1999;17:57

## AMMONIA AND AMMONIA SOLUTION

Ammonia ($NH_3$) is a gas at ordinary temperatures; vapor pressure at 27°C: 500 mmHg. 'Ammonium hydroxide' is the old term used to describe a solu-tion of ammonia in water, which actually comprises solvated ammonia mole-cules plus small amounts of $NH_4^+$ and $OH^-$ ions.

Ammonia is used in organic synthesis, as a refrigerant, and as a fertilizer. 'Ammonium hydroxide' is used in organic synthesis and as a cleaner.

The exposure limit of ammonia is 25 ppm. The fatal dose of ammonia solution by ingestion is about 30 ml (1 oz) of a 25% solution.

Ammonia and ammonium hydroxide injure cells directly by alkaline caus-tic action and cause extremely painful irritation of all mucous membranes.

The pathologic findings in inhalation poisoning are pulmonary edema, pulmonary irritation, and pneumonia. After ingestion the findings are the same as with alkalis (see p. 257), although usually less severe.

### Clinical findings

The principal manifestation of acute poisoning with these compounds is extreme irritation.

#### *Ingestion*

Ingested ammonia causes severe pain in the mouth, chest, and abdomen, with cough, vomiting, and shock-like collapse. Gastric or esophageal perforation may occur later, with exacerbation of abdominal pain, fever, and abdominal rigidity. Lung irritation and pulmonary edema may appear rapidly or after a delay of 12–24 h.

## Inhalation

Ammonia fumes (1000 ppm) cause irritation of the eyes and upper respiratory tract, with cough, vomiting, conjunctival injection, and redness of the mucous membranes of the lips, mouth, nose, and pharynx. Higher concentrations cause swelling of the lips and conjunctiva, temporary blindness, restlessness, tightness in the chest, frothy sputum indicating pulmonary edema, cyanosis, and rapid, weak pulse.

## Skin contact

If skin contact is prolonged more than a few minutes, it causes severe burning pain and corrosive damage.

## Eye contact

Eye contact with concentrated ammonia causes immediate and severe pain followed by conjunctival edema and corneal clouding. Cataract formation and atrophy of the retina and iris may occur later.

## Prevention

Employees working in areas where ammonia is used must be trained in escape methods and in the use of safety equipment, including goggles, gas masks, showers, eye fountains, water hoses, exits, lifelines, and first-aid equipment. Ammonia equipment must be constantly inspected to prevent accidents. All valves should be labeled to prevent accidental opening.

If a contaminated area must be entered, a full-face airline mask or self-contained oxygen mask must be worn. Protective clothing is also necessary if the concentration is above 10 000 ppm.

## Treatment

### *Emergency measures*

(1) Ingestion – Dilute ingested poison as described on p. 259.
(2) Eye contamination – Wash eyes in a water bubbler eye fountain for at least 15 minutes. Follow this by repeated irrigation with normal saline solution. The patient should be taken to an ophthalmologist for further treatment.
(3) Inhalation – Remove patient from contaminated area and keep at bed rest.
(4) Skin contamination – Wash skin for at least 15 minutes.

### *Antidote*

Milk may be given by mouth, or water can be used externally.

### *General measures*

Treat as described on p. 245.

### *Special problems*

(1) Treat pulmonary edema (see p. 55).
(2) Treat esophageal stricture (see p. 245).

## Prognosis

Patients who survive 48 hours are likely to recover. Eye contact is frequently followed by permanent blindness.

## FLUORINE, HYDROGEN FLUORIDE, AND DERIVATIVES

Fluorine, hydrogen fluoride, and many derivatives of fluorine are gases at ordinary temperatures. Sulfur pentafluoride is a liquid.

Fluorine is used in organic synthesis. Hydrogen fluoride (hydrofluoric acid) is used in the petroleum and semiconductor industries and in etching glass. Cryolite (sodium aluminum fluoride) is used in aluminum reduction and many other industrial processes. Fluoride salts are used in the prevention of dental caries and in rodenticides. A 90 g tube of fluoride toothpaste contains 67 mg of fluoride. Methyl sulfonyl fluoride is used as a fumigant.

The exposure limits for fluorine and derivatives are as follows: fluorine, 1 ppm; hydrogen fluoride, 3 ppm; fluoride salts, 2.5 mg/m³; boron trifluoride, 1 ppm; bromine pentafluoride, 0.1 ppm; carbonyl fluoride, 2 ppm; chlorine trifluoride, 0.1 ppm; nitrogen trifluoride, 10 ppm; oxygen difluoride, 0.05 ppm; perchloryl fluoride, 3 ppm; selenium hexafluoride, 0.05 ppm; sulfur hexafluoride, 1000 ppm; sulfur pentafluoride, 0.01 ppm; sulfur tetrafluoride, 0.1 ppm; sulfuryl fluoride, 5 ppm; tellurium hexafluoride, 0.02 ppm. The fatal dose of sodium fluoride is 5–10 mg of fluorine per kilogram, and toxic effects occur below 1 mg of fluorine per kilogram. The fatal plasma level of fluorine is 3 mg/l. Patients with osteoporosis tolerate up to 60 mg of sodium fluoride per day, but osteosclerosis may occur at a urinary excretion level of 10 mg of fluoride per day in workers exposed to fluoride. The fatal dose of fluorosilicates is about the same as for fluorides, but that of cryolite is much higher (above 10 g). The LD50 for methyl sulfonyl fluoride in experimental animals is 3.5 mg/kg.

Fluorine and fluorides act as direct cellular poisons by interfering with calcium metabolism and enzyme mechanisms. Fluorides form an insoluble precipitate with calcium and lower the plasma calcium level. Fluorine, hydrogen fluoride (hydrofluoric acid), and most fluorine derivatives are corrosive to tissues.

Skin or mucous membrane contact with hydrogen fluoride produces deeply penetrating, necrotic ulcerations.

Neutral fluorides in 1–2% concentrations will cause inflammation and necrosis of mucous membranes. After death rigor mortis sets in rapidly. Postmortem findings are cerebral hyperemia and edema, pulmonary edema, and degenerative changes in the liver and kidneys.

In fatalities caused by inhalation of hydrogen fluoride or fluorine, pulmonary edema and bronchial pneumonia are the most prominent findings.

In deaths following prolonged absorption of fluoride, the bone structure shows thickening with calcification in the ligamentous attachments. Bone marrow space is greatly reduced.

## Clinical findings

The principal manifestation of fluorine and fluoride poisoning is corrosion.

*Acute poisoning*

(1) Inhalation – Inhalation of hydrogen fluoride, fluorine, and most fluorine derivatives causes coughing, choking, and chills lasting 1–2 h after exposure. After an asymptomatic period of 1–2 days, fever, cough, tightness in the chest, rales, and cyanosis indicate pulmonary edema. These symptoms progress for 1–2 days and then regress slowly over a period of 10–30 days. Sulfuryl fluoride causes narcosis, convulsions, and pulmonary irritation. Nitrogen trifluoride causes methemoglobin formation. Bromine pentafluoride causes nephrosis and hepatitis. Sulfur hexafluoride (sulfur fluoride) is nearly non-toxic.

(2) Ingestion – Ingestion of neutral fluorides such as sodium fluoride or sodium silicofluoride causes salivation, nausea and vomiting, diarrhea, and abdominal pain. Later, weakness, tremors, shallow respiration, carpopedal spasm, and convulsions occur. Death is by respiratory paralysis. If death does not occur immediately, jaundice and oliguria may appear. Reduction in serum calcium may induce cardiac arrhythmias. Experience with oral fluoride supplements used to prevent tooth decay has been reassuring; no adverse effects occur unless enormous amounts are ingested.

(3) Contact – Skin or mucous membrane contact with hydrogen fluoride solution results in damage depending on the concentration. Concentrations above 60% result immediately in severe, extremely painful burns. Such burns are deep and heal slowly. Concentrations lower than 50% may cause slight immediate irritation of the skin or none at all. The acid penetrates readily, however, and a deep-seated ulceration results if contact continues for more than a few minutes. A fatality has occurred from systemic poisoning following exposure of 2.5% of the body surface to hydrofluoric acid.

*Chronic poisoning* (from inhalation or ingestion)

Intake of more than 6 mg of fluorine per day results in fluorosis. Symptoms are weight loss, brittle bones, anemia, weakness, general ill health, stiffness of joints, and discoloration of the teeth when exposure occurs during tooth formation.

### Laboratory findings

(1) In acute poisoning from fluoride salts or skin exposure to hydrofluoric acid, serum calcium and serum magnesium are reduced.

(2) ECG may show evidence of reduced serum calcium.

(3) In chronic exposure, X-ray evidence of osteosclerosis and calcification of ligaments is indicative of fluorosis.

(4) In severe fluorosis, both red and white blood cell counts may be diminished.

(5) Fluorine workers should have urine fluoride determinations at 6-month intervals.

## Prevention

Hydrogen fluoride workers must be carefully instructed in the dangers of skin contact with hydrogen fluoride and in the necessity for immediate removal of even dilute solutions by prolonged washing. Showers and water bubbler eye fountains must be available where hydrogen fluoride is being used. Processes utilizing hydrogen fluoride must be totally enclosed. Workers should wear long rubber gauntlets, long rubber aprons, high rubber boots, and wide plastic face shields while handling hydrogen fluoride. Full safety suits that are checked daily for leaks may be necessary. Forced-air face masks should be worn if the air concentration of hydrogen fluoride is sufficiently high to cause nasal irritation. Tools and benches must be decontaminated immediately by washing with ammonia or lye solutions after hydrogen fluoride is spilled.

## Treatment

### Skin or mucous membrane burns

Wash thoroughly under a stream of water for 15–60 min. Do not wait until symptoms appear before giving treatment. Coat the burn with a magnesium oxide–water paste containing 20% glycerin. Do not use oily ointments. Open all blisters; if hydrogen fluoride has penetrated under the fingernails, consider removing the nails using local anesthesia. Wash these areas for 15–30 min. The injection of 0.5 ml of 10% calcium gluconate with local anesthetic per square centimeter under the burn area is effective but painful and must be repeated; an alternative that is proving far more acceptable and effective is injection of 0.5–2 ml of 10% calcium gluconate or calcium chloride into the radial or ulnar artery. Treat systemic effects promptly (see below).

### *Eye burns*

Wash eyes with running water for 15 min (see p. 33) and then irrigate the eye with normal saline for 30–60 min. Cover the eyes with sterile bandages, allay pain by giving systemic analgesics, and take the patient to an ophthalmologist for evaluation of injury. Do not use chemical antidotes.

### *Inhalation*

Remove patient to fresh air. Keep at complete rest. Treat pulmonary edema (see p. 55).

### *Ingestion of hydrogen fluoride*

Treat as for acid ingestion (see p. 245).

### *Ingestion of neutral fluorides*

(1) Emergency measures – Give soluble calcium in any form: milk, calcium gluconate solution, or calcium lactate solution. For calcium salts, the concentration should be 10 g in 250 ml of water. Give calcium gluconate, 10 g, and magnesium sulfate, 30 g, in 200 ml of water orally to precipitate and remove fluoride from the intestine.

(2) Antidote – Give calcium gluconate, 10 ml of 10% solution intravenously slowly; repeat until symptoms disappear. If serum magnesium level is low, give milk of magnesia, 10 ml every hour.

(3) General measures:
   (a) Give milk and cream every 4 h to relieve irritation of the esophagus and stomach.
   (b) Treat shock (see p. 54).
   (c) Give maximum amounts of fluids either orally or intravenously.

### *Fluorosis*

Remove from further exposure.

## Prognosis

After ingestion of neutral fluoride, survival for 48 hours is followed by recovery. After inhalation, survival for 3–4 days is usually followed by recovery. Skin burns require 1–2 months to heal. In fluorosis from chronic exposure, removal from exposure for a year or more may be necessary before joint stiffness begins to reverse. The prognosis in burns of the esophagus or stomach from hydrofluoric acid is the same as in acid burns (see p. 246).

## References

Chan BSH, Duggin GG. Survival after a massive hydrofluoric acid ingestion. *J Toxicol Clin Toxicol* 1996;35:307

Gallerani M, *et al.* Systemic and topical effects of intradermal hydrofluoric acid. *Am J Emerg Med* 1998;16:521

Kao W-F, *et al.* Ingestion of low-concentration hydrofluoric acid: an insidious and potentially fatal poisoning. *Ann Emerg Med* 1999;34:35

Susheela AK, Jethanandani P. Circulating testosterone levels in skeletal fluorosis patients. *J Toxicol Clin Toxicol* 1996;34:183

Yamaura K, *et al.* Recurrent ventricular tachyarrhythmias associated with QT prolongation following hydrofluoric acid burns. *J Toxicol Clin Toxicol* 1996;35:311

# 15  Metallic poisons*

## ANTIMONY AND STIBINE

Antimony is used in alloys, type metal, foil, batteries, ceramics, textiles, safety matches, ant paste, and a number of chemicals, including tartar emetic (antimony potassium tartrate). Acid treatment of metals containing antimony releases the colorless gas stibine ($SbH_3$).

The exposure limit for antimony is $0.5 \, mg/m^3$. The exposure limit for stibine is 0.1 ppm. The fatal dose of antimony compounds by ingestion is 100–200 mg. Fatalities from antimony poisoning are rare. The mechanism of poisoning is similar to that of arsenic poisoning, presumably by inhibition of enzymes through combination with sulfhydryl (–SH) groups.

Antimony is strongly irritating to mucous membranes and to tissues. Stibine causes hemolysis and irritation of the central nervous system. Pathologic findings include fatty degeneration of the liver and parenchymatous degeneration in the liver and other organs. The gastrointestinal tract shows marked congestion and edema.

### Clinical findings

The principal manifestations of antimony poisoning are gastrointestinal disturbances. Stibine causes hemolysis.

#### Acute poisoning

(1) Ingestion – The symptoms are nausea, vomiting, and severe diarrhea with mucus and later with blood. Hemorrhagic nephritis and hepatitis may also occur.
(2) Inhalation (of stibine) – Headache, nausea and vomiting, weakness, jaundice, hemolysis, anemia, weak pulse.

---

*See also Table 15.2

*Chronic poisoning* (from fume and dust exposure)

Itching skin pustules, bleeding gums, conjunctivitis, laryngitis, headache, weight loss, and anemia. Antimony is suspected of being a carcinogen.

### *Laboratory findings*

(1) The red blood cell count is diminished. Eosinophils may reach 25% of total white cells.
(2) The urine contains hemoglobin and red cells.

### Prevention

Adequate fume and dust control is necessary to prevent the exposure limit from being exceeded.

### Treatment

### *Acute poisoning*

(1) Emergency measures
   (a) Remove ingested antimony compounds by gastric lavage or emesis (see pp. 29–32).
   (b) Remove patient from further exposure to stibine.
(2) Antidote – None.
(3) General measures – Treat hemolysis from stibine (see p. 80).

### *Chronic poisoning*

Remove from further exposure.

### Prognosis

If the patient survives for 48 hours recovery is probable.

### ARSENIC AND ARSINE

Arsenic is used in ant poisons, insecticides, weed killers, paint, wallpaper, ceramics, and glass. The action of acids on metals in the presence of arsenic forms arsine gas. Alloys such as ferrosilicon may release arsine upon contact with water, since the ferrosilicon may be contaminated with arsenic.

The fatal dose of arsenic trioxide is about 120 mg. In the USA, the allowable food residue is limited by federal law to 1.4 mg/kg. The exposure limit for arsine is 0.05 ppm (NIOSH 0.002 mg/m$^3$); for arsenic, arsenic acid, arsenates, arsenites, and other compounds of arsenic, it is 0.5 mg/m$^3$ (NIOSH 0.002 mg/m$^3$). Organic arsenicals, such as arsphenamine, acetarsone, methane arsonic acid, and dimethylarsinic (cacodylic) acid, release arsenic slowly and are therefore less likely to cause acute poisoning, although at least one fatality has occurred from the vaginal use of acetarsone suppositories. The fatal dose for these compounds is estimated at 0.1–0.5 g/kg.

Arsenic presumably causes toxicity by combining with sulfhydryl (–SH) enzymes and interfering with cellular metabolism.

If death occurs within a few hours, the stomach mucosa shows inflammation but other pathologic changes are absent. If death occurs more than a few hours after poisoning, pathologic examination shows inflammatory changes and partial desquamation of the intestinal mucosa. The capillaries of the gastrointestinal tract are distended, and ecchymoses may be found. In immediate deaths from arsine poisoning, intravascular hemolysis is found. If death is delayed for several days after poisoning with arsenic in any form, the liver and kidneys show degenerative changes.

## Clinical findings

The principal manifestations of arsenic poisoning are gastrointestinal disturbances. The principal manifestation of arsine poisoning is hemolysis.

### *Acute poisoning*

(1) Ingestion – After ingestion of overwhelming amounts of arsenic (10 times the MLD), initial symptoms are those of violent gastroenteritis: burning esophageal pain, vomiting, and copious watery or bloody diarrhea containing shreds of mucus. Later the skin becomes cold and clammy, the blood pressure falls, and weakness is marked. Death is from circulatory failure. Convulsions and coma are the terminal signs. If death is not immediate, jaundice and oliguria or anuria appear after 1–3 days.

Doses approaching the MLD cause restlessness, nausea and vomiting, headache, dizziness, chills, cramps, irritability, and variable paralysis that may progress over a period of several weeks. Ventricular arrhythmias may occur.

(2) Inhalation – Inhalation of arsenic dusts may cause acute pulmonary edema, restlessness, dyspnea, cyanosis, cough with foamy sputum, and rales.

(3) Arsine – Exposure to arsine causes burning and stinging of the face and, after 3–4 h, tightness of the chest, dysphagia, nausea and vomiting, diarrhea, and electrocardiographic abnormalities. Later, pulmonary edema, massive hemolysis, cyanosis, hemoglobinuria, renal failure, and liver damage can occur. The liver and spleen may be enlarged. At 10 ppm, arsine rapidly causes delirium, coma, and death.

*Chronic poisoning* (from ingestion or inhalation)

The following are affected variably:

(1) Central nervous system – Polyneuritis, optic neuritis, anesthesias, paresthesias such as burning pains in the hands and feet.

(2) Skin – Bronzing, alopecia, localized edema, dermatitis.

(3) Gastrointestinal tract – Cirrhosis of the liver, nausea and vomiting, abdominal cramps, salivation.

(4) General effects – Anemia and weight loss. Aplastic anemia, leukopenia, and anemia have occurred.

(5) Cardiovascular system and kidneys – Chronic nephritis, cardiac failure, dependent edema.

(6) Tryparsamide administration has caused visual impairment and optic atrophy.

(7) Melarsoprol has caused mild cardiac damage, hypertension, neuritis, colic, proteinuria, and rare fatalities.

(8) Glycobiarsol has caused sensitivity reactions and hepatitis after oral administration.

(9) Acetarsone (acetarsol) has caused sensitivity dermatitis, exfoliative dermatitis, jaundice, and angioneurotic edema.

(10) Arsenic and its compounds are carcinogenic for skin, lungs, and liver and possibly other organ systems.

*Laboratory findings*

(1) Acute poisoning
- (a) The urine may contain red blood cells, protein, and casts. Inorganic arsenic may exceed 1 mg/24 h.
- (b) Arsenic compounds may appear as barium-like radio-opaque material after ingestion.
- (c) In fatal arsenic poisoning the blood level has ranged from 1 to 15 µg/ml.
- (d) After arsine inhalation the urine contains hemoglobin and hemosiderin. The serum contains hemoglobin and methemalbumin.

(2) Chronic poisoning
- (a) Urinary excretion of inorganic arsenic at a rate above 100 µg/24 h or a blood inorganic arsenic level above 0.1 mg/l indicates exposure.
- (b) Renal or hepatic function may be impaired as shown by suitable tests (see pp. 67 and 75).
- (c) Blood counts reveal neutrophilic leukopenia as well as anemia.

## Prevention

Store arsenic safely. The exposure limit of arsine in air must be observed at all times. Acid treatment of metals or dilution of acid sludge must be done with adequate fume control.

## Treatment

### Acute poisoning from arsenic

(1) Emergency measures – Remove ingested arsenic by gastric lavage or emesis (see pp. 29–32). Follow with a saline cathartic.
(2) Antidote – Give dimercaprol (see p. 87) for 2 days, then penicillamine (see p. 94) or succimer (see p. 97). Discontinue antidote when the urine arsenic level falls below 500 µg/24 h.
(3) General measures:
- (a) Treat dehydration by giving 5% glucose in normal saline intravenously.
- (b) Treat shock (see p. 56).
- (c) Treat pulmonary edema (see p. 55).

(d) Treat anuria (see p. 66).

(e) Treat liver damage (see p. 76).

(f) In severe poisoning use hemodialysis after dimercaprol therapy to remove combined dimercaprol and arsenic.

### Acute poisoning from arsine

Treat hemolytic reaction (see p. 80). Exchange transfusions are useful to remove the hemoglobin–arsine complex. Dialysis is necessary during the period of hemoglobinuric renal failure. Antidotes appear to be useless.

### Chronic poisoning

Remove from further exposure and give dimercaprol (see p. 87) or penicillamine (see p. 94). Signs of arsenic intoxication disappear slowly.

### Prognosis

In acute arsenic poisoning, survival for more than 1 week is usually followed by complete recovery. Complete recovery from chronic arsenic poisoning may require 6 months to 1 year.

### References

Apostoli P, *et al.* Biological monitoring of occupational exposure to inorganic arsenic. *Occup Environ Med* 1999;56:825

Kamijo Y, *et al.* Survival after massive arsenic poisoning self-treated by high fluid intake. *J Toxicol Clin Toxicol* 1998;36:27

Lewis DR, *et al.* Drinking water arsenic in Utah: a cohort mortality study. *Environ Health Perspect* 1999;107:359

Romeo L, *et al.* Acute arsine intoxication as a consequence of metal burnishing operations. *Am J Ind Med* 1997;32:211

Tsai S, *et al.* Mortality for certain diseases in areas with high levels of arsenic in drinking water. *Arch Environ Health* 1999;54:186

# BERYLLIUM

Beryllium is used in alloys for electrical and other equipment. It is present in some fluorophors used in cathode ray tubes but is no longer used in fluorophors in fluorescent lamps.

The fatal dose of beryllium is not known. The exposure limit in air for beryllium is $0.002 \, mg/m^3$.

Between 1941 and 1966, 760 cases of berylliosis were recorded in a national registry in the USA (Massachusetts General Hospital, Boston). Between 1966 and 1973, 76 new cases were recorded. Beryllium appears to inhibit certain magnesium-activated enzymes. The relationship between this effect and the pathologic changes induced by beryllium is not understood.

Soluble beryllium salts are directly irritating to skin and mucous membranes and induce acute pneumonitis with pulmonary edema. At least some of the changes present in acute pneumonitis and chronic pulmonary granulomatosis develop as a result of hypersensitivity to the beryllium in the tissues.

At pathologic examination, granulomas consisting of monocytes, lymphocytes, and fibrous tissue are found at the site of beryllium localization. In deaths from acute pneumonitis, the lung alveoli are filled with mononuclear and plasma cells.

## Clinical findings

The principal manifestation of beryllium poisoning is dyspnea.

### Acute poisoning

(1) Inhalation – Acute pneumonitis, with chest pain, bronchial spasm, fever, dyspnea, cyanosis, cough, blood-tinged sputum, and nasal discharge. Right heart failure may occur as a result of increased pulmonary arterial resistance. Onset of symptoms occurs 2–5 weeks after an exposure of 1–20 days.

(2) Skin contact – Cuts from beryllium-contaminated objects form deep ulcerations that are slow to heal. Acute dermatitis from contact with dust simulates first- and second-degree burns.

(3) Eye contact – Dust contamination causes acute conjunctivitis with corneal maculae and diffuse erythema.

*Chronic poisoning*

(1) Inhalation – In chronic pulmonary granulomatosis (berylliosis), weight loss and marked dyspnea begin 3 months to 11 years after the first exposure. The disease may pursue a steady downhill course or may be marked by exacerbations and remissions. Right heart failure may occur as a result of increased pulmonary resistance. Fever is variable. The incidence of lung cancer is increased in workers exposed to beryllium.

(2) Skin contact – Eczematous dermatitis with a maculopapular, erythematous, vesicular rash appears in a large percentage of workers exposed to beryllium dusts. In such patients patch tests with dilute beryllium solutions show positive reactions.

*Laboratory findings*

These are noncontributory.

*X-Ray findings*

(1) Radiologic examination in acute pneumonitis reveals a diffuse increase in density of the lung fields.

(2) In chronic pulmonary granulomatosis, radiologic examination reveals a 'snowstorm' appearance of the lungs.

**Prevention**

Dusts and fumes from beryllium processes must be rigidly controlled. No beryllium is allowable in air. Chest X-rays are not useful in controlling exposure or in case-finding. Positive radiologic findings may be seen in the absence of symptoms or may occur only at the onset of symptoms. Workers may be asymptomatic and have normal chest X-rays during exposure to beryllium, and yet they may develop symptoms and positive chest X-ray findings many years after discontinuing exposure.

**Treatment**

*Acute pneumonitis*

(1) Emergency measures:

(a) Complete bed rest is necessary.

(b) If cyanosis is present, give 40–60% $O_2$ by mask or intratracheal tube as necessary to maintain arterial $pO_2$ above 60 mmHg. Ventilatory assistance may be necessary.

(2) Antidote – The administration of calcium edetate has been suggested (see p. 88).

(3) General measures:

(a) Relieve bronchial spasm – Give epinephrine, 0.2 mg (0.2 ml of 1:1000 solution) subcutaneously, or aminophylline, 0.25 g intravenously every 6 h.

(b) Treat bronchial pneumonia – Give organism-specific chemotherapy.

(c) For right heart failure – Digitalize.

(d) Give prednisone or equivalent corticosteroid, 25–50 mg/d orally, to decrease the hypersensitivity reaction to beryllium. These hormones relieve symptoms but are not curative.

### Chronic granuloma of lungs (berylliosis)

Moderate activity is allowable. Maintain arterial $pO_2$ above 60 mmHg by intermittent $O_2$ administration – if necessary, by mechanical ventilation. Adequate oxygenation delays the onset of pulmonary hypertension and cor pulmonale.

### Skin granuloma and ulcers

Excise beryllium-contaminated areas of skin surgically.

### Beryllium dermatitis or conjunctivitis

(1) Remove from further exposure. Wash skin and eyes thoroughly (see pp. 31–32).

(2) Apply local anesthetic ointment to control pain.

### Prognosis

Recovery from acute pneumonitis requires 2–6 months. Deaths have been rare. Approximately 2% of patients with chronic pulmonary granulomatosis from beryllium (berylliosis) die. Adrenocortical hormones appear to improve symptoms without appreciably affecting the outcome of the disease.

### Reference

Middleton DC. Chronic beryllium disease: uncommon disease, less common diagnosis. *Environ Health Perspect* 1998;106:765

## CADMIUM

Cadmium is used for plating metals and in the manufacture of bearing alloys and silver solders. Cadmium plating is soluble in acid foods such as fruit juices and vinegar. When products containing cadmium are heated above its melting point (321°C), cadmium fumes are released.

The fatal dose by ingestion is not known. Ingestion of as little as 10 mg will cause marked symptoms. At least 10 fatalities have occurred after exposure to cadmium fumes. The exposure limit for cadmium dusts or cadmium oxide fumes is 0.05 mg/m$^3$ (NIOSH 0.04 mg/m$^3$). Cadmium is damaging to all cells of the body.

The pathologic findings in cases of fatal cadmium ingestion are severe gastrointestinal inflammation and liver and kidney damage. In fatal acute poisoning from the inhalation of cadmium fumes, pathologic examination reveals inflammation of the pulmonary epithelium and pulmonary edema. Pathologic examination in fatalities following prolonged exposure to cadmium fumes reveals emphysema.

### Clinical findings

#### Acute poisoning

(1) Ingestion – Nausea and vomiting, diarrhea, headache, muscular aches, salivation, abdominal pain, shock, liver damage, and renal failure.

(2) Inhalation of cadmium fumes causes a metallic taste in the mouth, shortness of breath, pain in the chest, cough with foamy or bloody sputum, weakness, and pains in the legs. Chest examination reveals bubbling rales. Urine formation may be diminished later. Progression of the disease is indicated by onset of fever and by development of signs of lung consolidation.

*Chronic poisoning* (from inhalation)

Loss of sense of smell, cough, dyspnea, weight loss, anemia, irritability, and teeth stained yellow. The liver and kidneys may be damaged. The incidence of carcinoma of the prostate is increased in workers exposed to cadmium.

*Laboratory findings*

(1) Hematuria and proteinuria are present.
(2) The red and white blood cell counts are low. The erythrocyte sedimentation rate may be elevated.
(3) After ingestion or chronic inhalation, hepatic cell function may be impaired as shown by appropriate tests.

*X-Ray findings*

After inhalation, early chest X-rays show a diffuse increase in lung density; later findings are those of bronchial pneumonia.

## Prevention

The exposure limit for cadmium fumes must always be observed. Acid foods should never be stored or prepared in cadmium-plated cooking utensils.

## Treatment

*Inhalation*

(1) Remove patient from further exposure.
(2) Treat pulmonary edema (see p. 55).
(3) Calcium disodium edetate (see p. 88) given intravenously or intramuscularly appears to be effective. Give 25 mg/kg twice daily for 1 week and repeat if necessary after a 2-day interval. Do not give dimercaprol.

*Ingestion*

(1) Allay gastrointestinal irritation – Give milk or beaten eggs every 4 h.
(2) Catharsis – Remove unabsorbed cadmium by catharsis with Fleet's Phospho-Soda, 30–60 ml diluted 1:4 in water.

(3) Give calcium disodium edetate (see p. 88) if symptoms persist. Do not give dimercaprol.
(4) Treat liver damage (see p. 75).
(5) Treat renal failure (see p. 67).

**Prognosis**

Symptoms from cadmium ingestion usually last no more than 24 hours. In fume inhalation, the mortality rate has been approximately 15%. Survival for more than 4 days is followed by recovery, but complete recovery may take 6 months.

**References**

Mason HJ, *et al*. Follow up of workers previously exposed to silver solder containing cadmium. *Occup Environ Med* 1999;56:553

McDiarmid MA, *et al*. Follow-up of biologic monitoring results in cadmium workers removed from exposure. *Am J Ind Med* 1997;32:261

Ritz B, *et al*. Effect of cadmium body burden on immune response of school children. *Arch Environ Health* 1999;53:272

Viaene MK, *et al*. Neurobehavioural effects of occupational exposure to cadmium: a cross sectional epidemiological study. *Occup Environ Med* 2000;57:19

## CHROMIUM

Chromium is used in chemical synthesis, steel-making, electroplating, and leather tanning and as a radiator anti-rust.

The fatal dose of a soluble chromate such as potassium chromate, potassium bichromate, or 'chromic acid' – a solution of chromium (VI) oxide ($CrO_3$) in water – is approximately 5 g. The toxicity of chromium compounds depends on the valence state of the metal. The exposure limit for metal dust and chromium salts of valence 2 or 3 is 0.5 mg/m$^3$. Most soluble and insoluble compounds of valence 6, including chromic acid, chromates, bichromates, zinc chromate, lead chromate, and chromite ore, have an exposure limit of 0.05 mg/m$^3$. The exposure limit for tertiary butyl chromate is 0.1 mg/m$^3$, and that for chromyl chloride is 0.025 ppm or 0.15 mg/m$^3$. Up to 20% of chromium workers develop dermatitis.

Chromium and chromates are irritating and destructive to all cells of the body. 'Chromic acid' causes severe burns. In fatalities from acute poisoning, hemorrhagic nephritis is found.

## Clinical findings

The principal manifestation of chromium poisoning is irritation or corrosion.

*Acute poisoning* (from ingestion)

Dizziness, intense thirst, abdominal pain, vomiting, shock, and oliguria or anuria. Death is from uremia.

*Chronic poisoning* (from inhalation or skin contact)

Repeated skin contact leads to incapacitating eczematous dermatitis with edema, and ulceration that heals slowly. Breathing chromium fumes over long periods causes painless ulceration, bleeding, and perforation of the nasal septum accompanied by a foul nasal discharge. Conjunctivitis, lacrimation, and acute hepatitis with jaundice have also been observed. Findings in acute hepatitis include nausea and vomiting, loss of appetite, and an enlarged, tender liver.

The incidence of lung cancer is increased up to 15 times normal in workers exposed to dusty chromite, chromic oxide, and chromium ores. All chromium compounds in which the metal has a valence of 6 are considered to be carcinogens.

## Laboratory findings

(1) Proteinuria and hematuria are present.
(2) Hepatic cell function impairment may be revealed by appropriate tests (see p. 75).

## Prevention

The exposure limit must always be observed. Chromic mist, fumes, and dust must be controlled. Chromate solutions must not come into contact with the skin.

## Treatment

### Acute poisoning

(1) Emergency measures – Remove swallowed chromate by gastric lavage or emesis (see pp. 29–32).
(2) Antidote – Administration of ascorbic acid has been suggested as a way to convert hexavalent chromium to less toxic trivalent chromium.
(3) General measures – If oliguria or anuria is present, carefully maintain fluid and electrolyte balance (see p. 69).

### Chronic poisoning

(1) Treat weeping dermatitis with 1% aluminum acetate wet dressings. Avoid further exposure to chromate.
(2) Treat liver damage by giving high-carbohydrate, high-protein, high-vitamin diet.

## Prognosis

In acute poisoning, rapid progression to anuria indicates a poor outcome. Dermatitis and liver damage will respond when the patient is removed from further exposure.

## References

Barcelous DG. Chromium. *J Toxicol Clin Toxicol* 1999;37:173

Gibb HJ, *et al.* Lung cancer among workers in chromium chemical production. *Am J Ind Med* 2000;38:115

Kolacinski Z, *et al.* Acute potassium dichromate poisoning: a toxicokinetic case study. *J Toxicol Clin Toxicol* 1999;37:785

Loubieres Y, *et al.* Acute, fatal, oral chromic acid poisoning. *J Toxicol Clin Toxicol* 1999;37:333

Schaffer AW, *et al.* Increased blood cobalt and chromium after total hip replacement. *J Toxicol Clin Toxicol* 1999;37:839

## LEAD

Lead is used in type metal, storage batteries, industrial paint, solder, electric cable covering, pottery glaze, rubber, toys, gasoline (tetraethyl lead), and brass alloys. Other sources include plastic beads or jewelry coated with lead to give a pearl appearance; illicit whiskey; home-glazed pottery; leaded glass; the dust in shooting galleries; ashes and fumes from burning old painted wood, newspapers, magazines, and battery cases; and artists' paint pigments. The amount of lead in a sample of ash resulting from burning black-ink newsprint was less than 5 mg/kg, and that in a sample of ash from burned colored-ink newsprint (comics) was 57.7 mg/kg.

The amount of lead in economic circulation or that has been lost from use is enormous. From 1720 to 1997, 63 411 900 tons of lead were added to the supply in the USA. Most of the annual use of lead is in batteries, but in total, more than 7 million tons of lead have been used in gasoline additives in the USA. Another source of environmental lead contamination comes from the weights used to balance wheels on motor vehicles. An estimated 25 million kg of lead are in use for this purpose and possibly as much as 10% of the total is deposited on streets and highways annually. Much of the lead from gasoline additives, wheel weights, and paints is distributed on the earth's surface. Lead levels in the soil along busy highways may exceed 10 g/kg and house dust may have 7.5 g/kg, compared to an average of 15 mg/kg in the earth's crust. Undisturbed surface soils in urban areas usually contain more than 500 mg of lead per kilogram in the top cm.

The fatal dose of absorbed lead has been estimated to be 0.5 g. Accumulation and toxicity occur if more than 0.5 mg/d is absorbed. The half-life of lead in bone is 32 years, and the half-life of lead in the kidney is 7 years. The exposure limit for lead and lead arsenate in air is 0.15 mg/m$^3$. The average level of lead in community air should not exceed 1.5 µg/m$^3$ per calendar quarter. The exposure limit for lead in food is 2.56 mg/kg. The exposure limit for tetraethyl or tetramethyl lead is 0.07 mg of lead per cubic meter.

Since 1972, 3 350 000 children between ages 1 and 5 years have been screened for blood lead levels in the USA. Of these, 6.6% had a blood lead level in the toxic range. In the past, as many as 200 deaths per year were due to lead encephalopathy; most were in children who lived in homes built before 1940 and resulted from exposure to lead-based paints.

The most serious toxic effects result from effects of lead on the brain and peripheral nervous system. The brain and liver lead levels may be 5–10 times the blood level. The lead in these tissues is only slowly removable by deleading agents. Since only uncombined lead is removed effectively by deleading agents, the increased excretion of lead brought about by such agents is only temporary. The deleading agent only becomes effective again when further lead has been released from combination.

Erythrocyte δ-aminolevulinic acid dehydratase, an enzyme important in hemoglobin synthesis, is one of the most sensitive indicators of the effect of lead. The free erythrocyte protoporphyrin level is an even more sensitive indicator of lead toxicity. Free erythrocyte protoporphyrin levels above 25–50 μg/dl are considered abnormal; however, because free erythrocyte protoporphyrin levels are also high in iron deficiency states, they cannot be used alone to diagnose lead poisoning. The activity of erythrocyte δ-aminolevulinic acid dehydratase is partially inhibited at blood lead levels of 10 μg/dl. Half of all individuals had blood lead levels greater than this in 1980. In 1976, the mean blood lead level was 15.8 μg/dl.

In acute poisoning pathologic findings include inflammation of the gastrointestinal mucosa and renal tubular degeneration. In chronic lead poisoning, cerebral edema and degeneration of nerve and muscle cells occur. There may be cellular infiltration around capillaries and arterioles. The liver and kidneys show intranuclear inclusion bodies.

**Clinical findings** (see Table 15.1)

Any symptoms suggestive of incipient encephalopathy should be considered an emergency. A rapid presumptive diagnosis can be based on the presence of the following: blood lead level above 50–80 μg/dl; free erythrocyte protoporphyrin above 200–250 μg/dl; and the appearance of radio-opaque material on a plain film of the abdomen and radio-opaque lead lines in the wrists and knees. Any positive finding in addition to suggestive symptoms may be sufficient indication to start therapy. Any child who has minor symptoms of poisoning can develop acute encephalopathy suddenly if the blood lead level is above 80 μg/dl.

To determine abnormal lead exposure give calcium disodium edetate, 25 mg/kg as a single intramuscular injection or intravenously over 1.5 h as a 0.5% solution in 5% dextrose in water. Collect all urine for 24 h if kidney function is normal or for 3–4 days in renal insufficiency. Compare the urine lead level after calcium disodium edetate with prior urine lead levels.

The principal manifestations of lead poisoning are gastrointestinal or central nervous system disturbances and anemia.

*Acute poisoning* (from ingestion or injection of soluble or rapidly absorbed compounds of lead)

Metallic taste, abdominal pain, vomiting, diarrhea, black stools, oliguria, collapse, and coma.

*Chronic poisoning* (from ingestion, skin absorption, or inhalation of particulate or organic lead)

The diagnosis should be considered in any walking or crawling child with any of the symptoms given below who lives in or visits a house built before 1940.

(1)  Early – Loss of appetite, weight loss, constipation, apathy or irritability, occasional vomiting, fatigue, headache, weakness, metallic taste, lead line on gums, loss of recently developed skills, and anemia.

(2)  More advanced – Intermittent vomiting; irritability; nervousness; uncoordination; vague pains in arms, legs, joints, and abdomen; sensory disturbances of extremities; paralysis of extensor muscles of arms and legs with wrist and foot drop; disturbance of menstrual cycle; and abortion.

(3)  Severe – Persistent vomiting, ataxia, periods of stupor or lethargy, encephalopathy (with visual disturbances), elevated blood pressure, papilledema, cranial nerve paralysis, delirium, convulsions, and coma. Severe symptoms occur most frequently in lead poisoning in children or in adults exposed to tetraethyl lead.

(4)  Exposure to tetraethyl lead or tetramethyl lead causes insomnia, disturbing dreams, emotional instability, hyperactivity, convulsions, and even toxic psychosis. The organic compounds of lead localize in neural tissue.

*Laboratory findings*

The following findings are suggestive of lead poisoning (Table 15.1).

(1)  Blood – Hemoglobin below 13 g/dl of blood. A blood lead level above 5 µg/dl indicates exposure to lead, and one above 25 µg/dl suggests the need for a search for the source of lead and its elimination. The risk of encephalopathy is great at blood lead levels over 80 µg/dl; a level of 100 µg/dl should be considered an emergency, although much higher levels have been found in asymptomatic individuals.

**Table 15.1** Symptoms and signs in the diagnosis of lead poisoning

|  | *Suggestive* | *Incipient intoxication* | *More advanced or definite plumbism* |
|---|---|---|---|
| General appearance | Patient feels restive, moody, easily excited, 'flustered'. | Pallor, lead line, jaundice. | Lead line, jaundice, emaciation, 'premature aging', weight loss, lethargy. |
| Digestive system | Persistent metallic taste, slight loss of appetite, slight constipation. | Metallic taste, definite loss of appetite, slight abdominal colic, constipation. | Nausea and vomiting, marked abdominal pain, rigid abdomen, marked constipation, blood in stool. |
| Nervous system | Patient is irritable and unco-operative. | Slight headache, insomnia, slight dizziness, palpitation, increased irritability, increased reflexes. | Persistent headaches, ataxia, confusion. Marked reflex changes, tremor, fibrillary twitching, neuritis, visual disturbances, encephalitis (hallucinations, convulsions, coma), paralysis. |
| Miscellaneous changes | None. | Muscle soreness, easy fatigability, hypotension. | General weakness, joint pains, hypertension, bone density. |
| Urine examination | Urine excretion of lead greater than 0.08 mg/d. | Trace of protein, few granular casts. | Increase in protein and casts. Coproporphyrinuria, hematuria, glycosuria, aminoaciduria, oliguria. |
| Blood changes | Polycythemia or anemia, polychromatophilia, increased platelets, percentage of reticulocytes about doubled. | Increase in reticulocytes. From 50 to 100 stippled cells per 100 000 erythrocytes. Blood lead over 60 µg/dl. Decrease in hemoglobin. Decrease in total number of red blood cells below 4 million. Increase in all forms of basophilic cells. Increase in percentage of mononuclears. Anisocytosis and poikilocytosis. Nucleated red cells present in peripheral circulation. Decreased platelets. | |

Free erythrocyte protoporphyrin is a sensitive test of lead toxicity (as well as of iron deficiency), and erythrocyte porphyrin fluorescence can be measured directly on diluted whole blood as a screening test.

(2) Urine

   (a) Urinary lead excretion greater than 0.08 mg/d or urine copro-porphyrin above 0.15 mg/24 h. A urine coproporphyrin level above 0.8 mg/l occurs only in symptomatic poisoning in adults. A urine δ-aminolevulinic acid level above 6 mg/l indicates that some lead effects have occurred. A level above 19 mg/l is associated with symptoms of lead poisoning. Glycosuria, hematuria, and proteinuria also occur.

   (b) Urinary excretion of more than 1 μg of lead per milligram of calcium edetate after intramuscular administration of calcium edetate at 25 mg/kg but not exceeding 1 g total.

(3) Spinal fluid – Lumbar puncture should be avoided unless necessary for diagnosis. Spinal fluid examination reveals elevated protein, pleocytosis, and increased spinal fluid pressure in approximately one third of children with lead poisoning.

### X-Ray findings

X-ray evidence of transverse bands of increased density at the ends of grow-ing bones is present in chronic poisoning in children and is most likely at ages 2–5 years. Multiple bands represent repeated episodes of poisoning. A film of the abdomen reveals opaque particles, especially in the rectosigmoid area, if paint or other lead products have been ingested recently. Cerebral edema is evident on CT scans.

### Prevention

Lead-containing paint should not be used indoors. Painters and lead workers must change clothing and bathe before eating. Effective dust-control filter masks should be worn when sanding or wire-brushing lead-containing paint. Lead-containing paint should only be burned with adequate fume control, since lead-containing fumes are emitted. Precautions must be taken to keep lead in air below the exposure limit. Children must not be allowed to play with lead toys. Cheap jewelry often contains lead.

## Treatment

It may be necessary to start treatment as soon as blood and urine samples are obtained for lead analysis.

### Emergency measures

Remove ingested soluble lead compounds by gastric lavage with dilute magnesium sulfate or sodium sulfate solution or by emesis (see pp. 29–32). Treat cerebral edema with mannitol and prednisolone or other corticosteroid (see below).

### Antidotes

Dimercaprol and calcium disodium edetate, and later succimer, should be given to all patients with clinical symptoms of lead poisoning and should be considered for asymptomatic patients with blood lead levels over 80–100 µg/dl or free erythrocyte protoporphyrin levels over 250–300 µg/dl of whole blood.

(1) Urine flow – Initiate urine flow first. Give 10% dextrose in water intravenously, 10–20 ml/kg body weight over a period of 1–2 h. If urine flow does not start, give mannitol, 20% solution, 5–10 ml/kg body weight intravenously over 20 minutes. Fluid must be limited to requirements, and catheterization may be necessary in coma. Daily urine output should be 350–500 ml/m$^2$/24 h. Excessive fluids further increase cerebral edema.

(2) For children – Give dimercaprol, 4 mg/kg intramuscularly every 4 h for 30 doses. Beginning 4 h later, give calcium disodium edetate at a separate injection site, 12.5 mg/kg intramuscularly every 4 h as 20% solution, with 0.5% procaine added, for a total of 30 doses. If significant improvement has not occurred by the fourth day, increase the number of injections by 10 for each drug. In patients without encephalopathy who respond well, dimercaprol can be discontinued after the third or fourth day and edetate reduced to 50 mg/kg/24 h for the remainder of the 5-day course of injections. Two to 3 weeks after the first course, if the blood lead level is still above 80 µg/dl, give a second course of 30 injections each of both drugs. Courses of calcium disodium edetate should not exceed 500 mg/kg, with at least 1 week between courses.

For follow-up care, place the child in a protected environment to make certain that further ingestion of lead does not occur; give penicillamine or succimer orally. Penicillamine dosage: 30 mg/kg daily in 3–4 doses, for 3–6 months or until blood lead level falls below 60 μg/dl. The maximum dose is 500 mg/d. Give penicillamine on an empty stomach 90 minutes before meals. Succimer dosage: 10 mg/kg every 8 h for 5 days then twice daily for 14 days. Repeat course after 14 day interval until blood lead is below 25 μg/dl.

(3) For adults – Adults with acute encephalopathy should be given dimercaprol and calcium disodium edetate in the same way as for children. For other symptomatic adults, the course of dimercaprol and calcium disodium edetate can be shortened or calcium disodium edetate only can be given in a dosage of 50 mg/kg intravenously as 0.5% solution in 5% dextrose in water or normal saline by infusion over not less than 8 h for not more than 5 days. Follow with oral penicillamine 500–750 mg/d orally for 1–2 months or until urine lead level drops below 0.3 mg/24 h.

### General measures in acute encephalopathy

(1) For cerebral edema, give mannitol, 20% solution, 5 ml/kg by intravenous injection at a rate not to exceed 1 ml/min. Give prednisolone, 1–2 mg/kg intravenously or intramuscularly, or other corticosteroid in equivalent doses, every 4 h.

(2) Do not use catharsis or enemas in the presence of severe symptoms.

(3) Control convulsions with cautious administration of phenobarbital, hydantoin anticonvulsants, or diazepam. Associated depression of respiration may increase cerebral edema and can be hazardous in the acute stage.

(4) Reduce fever with cooling blanket.

(5) Maintain urine output at 350–500 ml/m$^2$/24 h by giving 10% dextrose in water parenterally. Avoid administration of sodium-containing fluids.

(6) Withhold oral fluid, food, and medication for at least 3 days.

### Special problems

(1) In the presence of impaired renal function, dialysis is mandatory.

(2) Wrist drop and foot drop may be corrected by splinting and passive exercise until function returns.

(3) Toxicity from tetraethyl lead and tetramethyl lead does not respond to chelation therapy. Give barbiturates or diazepam to control hyperactivity.

**Prognosis**

Until recently the mortality rate in patients with lead encephalopathy was about 25%. About half of those who survived had permanent mental deterioration. The effect of calcium disodium edetate on the prognosis in lead encephalopathy has not been determined as yet.

**References**

Angle CR. Childhood lead poisoning and its treatment. *Annu Rev Pharmacol Toxicol* 1993;33:409.

Apostoli P, *et al.*, eds. International conference on lead. *Am J Ind Med* 2000;38: 229

Araki S, *et al.* Subclinical neurophysiolgical effects of lead: a review on peripheral, central, and autonomic nervous system effects in lead workers. *Am J Ind Med* 2000;37:193

Bruening K, *et al.* Dietary calcium intakes of urban children at risk of lead poisoning. *Environ Health Perspect* 1999;107:431

Chisolm JJ Jr. Safety and efficacy of meso-2,3-dimercaptosuccinic acid (DMSA) in children with elevated blood lead concentrations. *J Toxicol Clin Toxicol* 2000;38:365

Chuang H-Y, *et al.* Relationship of blood lead levels to personal hygiene habits in lead battery workers: Taiwan, 1991–1997. *Am J Ind Med* 1999;35:595

Dona A, *et al.* Flour contamination as a source of lead intoxication. *J Toxicol Clin Toxicol* 1999;37:109.

Esernio-Jenssen D, *et al.* Severe lead poisoning from an imported clothing accessory: 'watch' out for lead. *J Toxicol Clin Toxicol* 1996;34:329 (simulated pocket watch)

Kakosy T, *et al.* Lead intoxication epidemic caused by ingestion of contaminated ground paprika. *J Toxicol Clin Toxicol* 1996;34:507

Kessel I, O'Connor JT. *Getting the Lead out: The Complete Resource on How to Prevent and Cope with Lead Poisoning*. Plenum Publishing, 1997

Korrick SA, *et al*. Lead and hypertension in a sample of middle-aged women. *Am J Public Health* 1998;89:330

Kulshrestha MK. Lead poisoning diagnosed by abdominal x-rays. *J Toxicol Clin Toxicol* 1996;34:107

Landrigan PJ, *et al*. The reproductive toxicity and carcinogenicity of lead: a critical review. *Am J Ind Med* 2000;38:231

Levin SM, Goldberg M. Clinical evaluation and management of lead-exposed construction workers. *Am J Ind Med* 2000;37:23

Markowitz M. Lead poisoning: a disease for the next millennium. *Curr Probl Pediatr* 2000;30:62

McKinney PE. Acute elevation of blood lead levels within hours of ingestion of large quantities of lead shot. *J Toxicol Clin Toxicol* 2000;38:435

Murgueytio AM, *et al*. Relationship between lead mining and blood lead levels in children. *Arch Environ Health* 1999;53:414

Needleman HL, Bellinger D. The health effects of low level exposure to lead. *Annu Rev Public Health* 1991;12:111

Norton RL, *et al*. Blood lead of intravenous drug users. *J Toxicol Clin Toxicol* 1996;34:425

O'Connor ME, Rich D. Children with moderately elevated lead levels: is chelation with DMSA helpful? *Clin Pediatr* 1999;38:325

Osterode W, *et al*. Dose dependent reduction of erythroid progenitor cells and inappropriate erythropoietin response in exposure to lead: aspects of anaemia induced by lead. *Occup Environ Med* 1999;56:106

Panariti E, Berxholi K. Lead toxicity in humans from contaminated flour in Albania. *Vet Human Toxicol* 1998;40:91

Prpic-Majic D, *et al*. Lead poisoning associated with the use of ayurvedic metal-mineral tonics. *J Toxicol Clin Toxicol* 1996;34:417

Ratzon N, *et al*. Effect of exposure to lead on postural control in workers. *Occup Environ Med* 2000;57:201

Reynolds SJ, *et al*. Prevalence of elevated blood leads and exposure to lead in construction trades in Iowa and Illinois. *Am J Ind Med* 1999;36:307

Root RA. Lead loading of urban streets by motor vehicle wheel weights. *Environ Health Perspectives* 2000;108:937

Roscoe RJ, *et al*. Blood lead levels among children of lead-exposed workers: a meta-analysis. *Am J Ind Med* 1999;36:475

Rothenburg S, *et al*. Maternal blood lead level during pregnancy in south central Los Angeles. *Arch Environ Health* 1999;54:151

Scelfo GM, Flegal AR. Lead in calcium supplements. *Environ Health Perspect* 2000;108:309

Scharman EJ, Krenzelok EP. A sodium rodizonate lead testing kit for home use – valid for paint and soil samples? *J Toxicol Clin Toxicol* 1996;34:699

Shannon M, Graef JW. Lead intoxication in children with pervasive developmental disorders. *J Toxicol Clin Toxicol* 1996;34:177

Silbergeld EK. Preventing lead poisoning in children. *Annu Rev Public Health* 1997;18:187

Soong W, *et al*. Long-term effect of increased lead absorption on intelligence of children. *Arch Environ Health* 1999;54:297

Spriewald BM, *et al*. Lead induced anaemia due to traditional Indian medicine: a case report. *Occup Environ Med* 1999;56:282

Viskum S, *et al*. Improvement in semen quality associated with decreasing occupational lead exposure. *Am J Ind Med* 1999;35:257

## MANGANESE

Manganese is used in the manufacture of steel and dry cell batteries. Manganese dietary supplements are available. Their toxicity is unknown.

The exposure limits for manganese and manganese compounds are as follows: dust, $5\,mg/m^3$; fumes, $1\,mg/m^3$; tetroxide, $1\,mg/m^3$; manganese cyclopentadienyl tricarbonyl, $0.1\,mg/m^3$; methyl manganese cyclopentadienyl tricarbonyl, $0.2\,mg/m^3$. Manganese cyclopentadienyl tricarbonyl and methyl manganese cyclopentadienyl tricarbonyl are used as anti-knock additives in gasoline. These substances are readily absorbed through the skin. The toxic amount from inhalation is not known. Fatalities are rare.

The mechanism of manganese poisoning is not known. Inhalation of manganese fumes or dusts produces progressive deterioration in the central nervous system. Large oral doses of manganese compounds are without systemic effect in experimental animals.

The findings in one death suspected to be from ingesting manganese-contaminated drinking water were atrophy and disappearance of cells of the globus pallidus. Experimental animals show inflammatory changes in both grey and white matter.

### Clinical findings

The principal manifestations of poisoning with these compounds are central nervous system disturbances.

*Acute poisoning* (from ingestion, inhalation, or skin absorption)

Single exposure to the manganese cyclopentadienyl tricarbonyls causes edema, bleeding, hypotension, nerve atrophy, renal damage, hyperactivity, convulsions, and coma.

*Chronic poisoning* (from ingestion or inhalation)

(1) Ingestion – Drinking manganese-contaminated well water caused lethargy, edema, and symptoms of extrapyramidal tract lesions in one outbreak. Chronic poisoning from ingesting manganese in other forms has not been reported.

(2) Inhalation – Inhalation of manganese dusts causes acute bronchitis, nasopharyngitis, pneumonia, headache, itching, numbness of the extremities, impairment of libido, sleep disturbances, dermatitis, and liver enlargement. Later, there are gradually progressive signs that simulate Parkinsonism. These include weakness in the legs, increased muscle tone, hand tremor, slurred speech, muscle cramps, spastic gait, fixed facial expression, and mental deterioration.

(3) Chronic exposure to the manganese cyclopentadienyl tricarbonyls causes effects like those of tetraethyl lead (see p. 284).

*Laboratory findings*

(1) Hepatic cell function may be impaired as shown by appropriate tests (see p. 75).

(2) Increased hemoglobin and red blood cell count; decrease in monocytes.

(3) Cerebrospinal fluid may contain traces of globulin.

**Prevention**

Workers should change clothing and bathe on leaving work. Quarterly physical examinations of all exposed workers will aid in the discovery of early changes.

Batteries must not be buried near water supplies.

## Treatment of chronic poisoning

### Immediate measures

Remove from further exposure.

### Antidote

Calcium edetate is effective in removing manganese but has no permanent effect on symptomatic patients in the late stages of manganism.

### General measures

Oral levodopa, beginning with 0.1 g 3–5 times a day and gradually increasing to a total daily dose of 8 g/d, or DL-5-hydroxytryptophan, up to 3 g daily, is reported to be effective against some central nervous system symptoms.

## Prognosis

While liver damage and respiratory system damage from manganese are reported to improve with administration of calcium disodium edetate, this antidote has no effect on the symptoms of central nervous system deterioration. If exposure is discontinued when central nervous system symptoms first appear, recovery is possible.

## Reference

Barceloux DG. Manganese. *J Toxicol Clin Toxicol* 1999;37:293

## MERCURY

Mercury is the only metal that is a liquid at room temperature. Air saturated with mercury at 20°C contains about 15 mg/m$^3$. At 40°C saturated air contains 68 mg/m$^3$.

Mercury and its salts are used in the manufacture of thermometers, felt, paints, explosives, lamps, electrical apparatus, and batteries. The diethyl and dimethyl mercury compounds are used in treating seeds. Mercurous chloride (calomel) and organic mercurials were formerly used medicinally.

The fatal dose of mercuric salts such as mercuric chloride (corrosive sublimate) is 1 g. Ingested metallic mercury is ordinarily not toxic, since it is not absorbed. However, metallic mercury retained in the lung or injected intravenously can produce toxicity, although often it does not. Mercury vapor is in the monatomic state and is lipophilic. It is transferred to brain cells, where it is oxidized to $Hg^{2+}$ to produce toxic effects. Inhaled mercury vapor causes acute pneumonitis. Mercurous chloride, ammoniated mercury, mercury proto-iodide, and organic antiseptic mercurials such as acetomeroctol, merbromin, mercocresol, nitromersol, phenylmercuric salts and esters, and thimerosal (Merthiolate) are not likely to cause acute poisoning because they are poorly absorbed. The single fatal dose of these compounds is 2–4 times the fatal dose of soluble inorganic mercury salts. The mercurial diuretics (mersalyl, meralluride, mercurophylline, mercumatilin, mercaptomerin, chlormerodrin, and merethoxylline) are almost as toxic as mercuric chloride in experimental animals when mercury content is compared. The exposure limit for mercury or mercury compounds is 0.05 mg/m$^3$ as mercury. Alkyl mercury compounds such as methyl mercury chloride, methyl mercury cyanide, methyl mercury hydroxide, methyl mercury pentachlorophenate, methyl mercury toluene sulfonate, ethyl mercury chloride (Ceresan), ethyl mercury phosphate, and ethyl mercury toluene sulfonate are more toxic than mercuric chloride, and the exposure limit is 0.01 mg of mercury per cubic meter. Other organic mercury compounds, such as hydroxymercuriphenol and cyanomethyl-mercuri-guanidine, are as toxic as an equivalent amount of mercury in mercuric chloride.

Environmental contamination from industrial discharge of organic mercury compounds has resulted in organic mercurial poisoning from eating fish from the discharge area (Minamata disease) and in teratogenesis. Seed grains treated with organic mercury fungicides have caused poisoning when used as food. The concentration of alkyl mercury compounds (methyl mercury) in food should not exceed 0.5 mg/kg; for foods at this level, intake should be limited to not more than 0.5 kg per week.

Mercury depresses cellular enzymatic mechanisms by combining with sulfhydryl (–SH) groups; for this reason soluble mercuric salts are toxic to all cells. The high concentrations attained during renal excretion lead to specific damage to renal glomeruli and tubules.

In fatalities from mercury poisoning the pathologic findings are acute tubular and glomerular degeneration or hemorrhagic glomerular nephritis.

The mucosa of the gastrointestinal tract shows inflammation, congestion, coagulation, and corrosion.

## Clinical findings

The principal manifestations of mercury salt poisoning are gastrointestinal, hepatic, and renal damage.

### Acute poisoning

(1) Ingestion – Ingestion of mercuric salts causes metallic taste, thirst, severe abdominal pain, vomiting, and bloody diarrhea. Diarrhea of mucus shreds and blood may continue for several weeks. One day to 2 weeks after ingestion, urine output diminishes or stops. Death is from uremia. Esophageal, gastric, or intestinal stenosis may occur after mercuric chloride ingestion.

(2) Inhalation – Inhalation of a high concentration of mercury vapor can cause almost immediate dyspnea, cough, fever, nausea and vomiting, diarrhea, stomatitis, salivation, and metallic taste. The symptoms may resolve or may progress to necrotizing bronchiolitis, pneumonitis, pulmonary edema, and pneumothorax. This syndrome is often fatal in children. Acidosis and renal damage with renal failure may occur. Inhaling volatile organic mercurials in high concentrations causes metallic taste, dizziness, clumsiness, slurred speech, diarrhea, and sometimes fatal convulsions.

(3) Alkyl mercury compounds are concentrated in the central nervous system, with ataxia, chorea, athetosis, tremors, and convulsions. Damage tends to be permanent.

### Chronic poisoning

(1) Injection or ingestion – Injection of organic mercurial compounds or ingestion of insoluble or poorly dissociated mercuric salts – including mercurous chloride and organic mercurial compounds – over a prolonged period causes urticaria progressing to weeping dermatitis, stomatitis, salivation, diarrhea, anemia, leukopenia, liver damage, and renal damage progressing to acute renal failure with anuria. Injection of organic mercurial diuretics has caused depression or irregularities of

cardiac function and anaphylaxis. In children, repeated administration of calomel in 'teething powders' caused a syndrome known as erythredema polyneuropathy (acrodynia, or 'pink disease'). Symptoms are photophobia, anorexia, restlessness, stomatitis, pains in the arms and legs, pink palms, oliguria, and severe diarrhea. The symptoms may persist for weeks or months.

(2) Inhalation or skin contact – Inhalation of mercury vapor, dusts, or organic vapors or skin absorption of mercury or mercury compounds over a long period causes mercurialism. Findings are extremely variable and include tremors, salivation, stomatitis, loosening of the teeth, blue line on the gums, pain and numbness in the extremities, nephritis, diarrhea, anxiety, headache, weight loss, anorexia, mental depression, insomnia, irritability, instability, hallucinations, and evidence of mental deterioration.

## *Laboratory findings*

(1) The lowest blood concentration of methyl mercury associated with identifiable symptoms is 0.2 μg/ml. A tentative blood standard for methyl mercury or other organic mercury derivatives has been set: these should not exceed 0.1 μg/ml. Neuromuscular toxicity occurs at blood levels of inorganic mercury below 0.1 μg/ml.

(2) Urinary excretion of more than 0.3 mg of mercury per 24 h indicates the possibility of mercury poisoning. An average urinary mercury excretion rate above 0.1 mg/24 h in a group of mercury workers indicates the need for corrective measures for the work situation. An individual who shows over 0.2 mg/24 h in urine should be removed from further exposure if the urinary excretion of mercury goes above 0.05 mg/24 h. In the USA the county or state health department will make arrangements for mercury analyses.

(3) Proteinuria and hematuria (may be absent in chronic poisoning).

## Prevention

The exposure limit must be observed at all times; frequent air sampling is necessary. Floors in rooms where mercury is used must be impervious and free from cracks. Spilled mercury should be picked up immediately by water pump suction or by a wet sweeping compound. After handling mercury or mercury compounds the skin must be thoroughly cleaned. The administration of mercury in any form to children should be avoided. Ammoniated mercury should be replaced by less hazardous agents.

## Treatment

### Acute poisoning

(1) Emergency measures – Remove ingested poison by gastric lavage with tap water or by emesis and catharsis (see pp. 29–32).
(2) Antidote – Give dimercaprol (see p. 87). Penicillamine and succimer are also effective (see pp. 94, 97). Neither penicillamine nor dimercaprol is effective against the neurologic effects of alkyl mercury compounds but succimer can increase the elimination of methyl mercury from the brain. A chelating agent should be continued until the urine mercury level falls below 50 µg/24 h.
(3) General measures:
   (a) Treat anuria (see p. 66) and shock (see p. 56).
   (b) Treat stenotic lesions of the gastrointestinal tract after appropriate endoscopy.

### Chronic poisoning

Remove from further exposure. Give dimercaprol (see p. 87). Treat oliguria (see p. 67). Maintain nutrition by intravenous or oral feeding.

## Prognosis

In acute and chronic poisoning, recovery is likely if dimercaprol treatment is given for at least 1 week. Recovery from mental deterioration caused by chronic mercury poisoning may never be complete. Brain damage from alkyl mercury compounds is more likely to be permanent. Improvement requires 1–2 years.

## References

Bauer EP, Fuortes LJ. An assessment of exposure to mercury and mercuric chloride from handling treated herbarium plants. *Vet Human Toxicol* 1999;41:154

Bradberry SM, *et al*. Elemental mercury-induced skin granuloma: a case report and review of the literature. *J Toxicol Clin Toxicol* 1996;34:209

Crinnion WJ. Long-term effects of chronic low-dose mercury exposure. *Altern Med Rev* 2000;5:209

Deleu D, *et al*. Peripheral polyneuropathy due to chronic use of topical ammoniated mercury. *J Toxicol Clin Toxicol* 1998;36:233

Engqvist A, *et al*. Speciation of mercury excreted in feces from individuals with amalgam fillings. *Arch Environ Health* 1999;53:205

Fiedler N, *et al*. Neuropsychological and stress evaluation of a residential mercury exposure. *Environ Health Perspect* 1999;107:343

Forman J, *et al*. A cluster of pediatric metallic mercury exposure cases treated with *meso*-2,3-dimercaptosuccinic acid (DMSA). *Environ Health Perspect* 2000;108:575

Garza-Ocanas L, *et al*. Urinary mercury in twelve cases of cutaneous mercurous chloride (calomel) exposure: effect of sodium 2,3-dimercaptopropane-1-sulfonate (DMPS) therapy. *J Toxicol Clin Toxicol* 1996;35:653

Mathieson T, *et al*. Neuropsychological effects associated with exposure to mercury vapor among former chloralkali workers. *Scan J Work Environ Health* 1999;25:342

McKinney PE. Elemental mercury in the appendix: an unusual complication of a Mexican-American folk remedy. *J Toxicol Clin Toxicol* 1999;37:103

Ozuah PH. Mercury poisoning. *Curr Probl Pediatr* 2000;30:91

Pfab R, *et al*. Clinical course of severe poisoning with thiomersol. *J Toxicol Clin Toxicol* 1996;34:453

Ruha A-M, *et al*. Combined ingestion and subcutaneous injection of elemental mercury. *J Emerg Med* 2001;20:39

Souza EM, *et al*. Subcutaneous injection of elemental mercury with distant skin lesions. *J Toxicol Clin Toxicol* 2000;38:441

Torres-Alanis O, *et al*. Intravenous self-administration of metallic mercury: report of a case with a 5-year follow-up. *J Toxicol Clin Toxicol* 1996;35:83

## NICKEL CARBONYL

Nickel carbonyl – formed by passing carbon monoxide over finely divided metallic nickel – is a liquid that boils at 43°C. It is important in the Mond process for refining nickel. It is also used in petroleum refining.

The exposure limit for nickel carbonyl is 0.05 ppm. Inhaled nickel carbonyl decomposes to metallic nickel, which deposits on the epithelium of the lung. This finely divided nickel is rapidly absorbed and damages the lung and brain. Postmortem examination in deaths caused by nickel carbonyl inhalation reveals edema and hyperemia of the lungs and brain. Areas of necrosis and hemorrhage are found in the brain and lungs.

## Clinical findings

The principal manifestation of nickel carbonyl poisoning is dyspnea.

### *Acute poisoning*

Inhalation of nickel carbonyl immediately causes cough, dizziness, headache, and malaise, which ordinarily can be relieved by removal to fresh air. Progressive dyspnea, cough, cyanosis, fever, rapid pulse, and nausea and vomiting may follow in 12–36 h, and death from respiratory failure within 4–12 days.

### *Chronic poisoning*

Workers exposed to nickel carbonyl have a high incidence of lung cancer. Some workers develop dermatitis.

## Prevention

The exposure limit for nickel carbonyl must always be observed. No person with chronic pulmonary disease should work where nickel carbonyl exposure can occur. Contaminated atmospheres can only be entered by using an air-line face mask.

## Treatment

### *Acute poisoning*

(1) Emergency measures – Treat cyanosis and dyspnea by giving 100% $O_2$ by mask. If pulmonary edema is present treat as described on p. 55.
(2) Antidote – Give sodium diethyldithiocarbamate (dithiocarb), 10 mg/kg every 4 h. Until dithiocarb is available give disulfiram, 10 mg/kg every 8 h for the first day, then 5 mg/kg every 8 h. Check availability of dithiocarb at the local Poison Control Center.
(3) General measures – After any exposure, keep the patient at absolute bed rest for the first 4 days after poisoning, even if asymptomatic. Thereafter,

keep at bed rest until cyanosis is relieved. Corticosteroid administration may be helpful. Maintain arterial oxygen saturation with positive pressure 60% oxygen at 12 cm of water pressure.

### Chronic poisoning

Remove from further exposure.

### Prognosis

Survival for more than 14 days is followed by recovery. Cyanosis and dyspnea are indices of the severity of poisoning.

### References

Barceloux DG. Nickel. *J Toxicol Clin Toxicol* 1999;37:239

Bradberry SM, Vale JA. Therapeutic review: Do diethyldithiocarbamate and disulfiram have a role in acute nickel carbonyl poisoning? *J Toxicol Clin Toxicol* 1999;37:259

Kurta DL, *et al.* Acute nickel carbonyl poisoning. *Am J Emerg Med* 1993;11:64

## PHOSPHORUS, PHOSPHINE, AND PHOSPHIDES

Phosphorus exists in several allotropic forms, the most important of which are red phosphorus, a granular, nonabsorbed, and nonpoisonous form; and white phosphorus, a yellow, waxy, water-insoluble and fat-soluble, highly poisonous form that will burn on contact with air. Red phosphorus is sometimes contaminated with white phosphorus. The striking surface of a safety match contains 50% red phosphorus. White phosphorus is used in rodent and insect poisons, fireworks, and fertilizer manufacture. The action of water or acids on metals will liberate phosphine (hydrogen phosphide, $PH_3$) if phosphorus is present as a contaminant. Phosphine may also be present in acetylene. Phosphides, which are used as rat poisons, release phosphine on contact with water. Phosphorus sesquisulfide (tetraphosphorus trisulfide) has low toxicity. The heads of 20 large wooden matches contain 220 mg phosphorus sesquisulfide.

The fatal dose of white phosphorus or phosphides is approximately 1 mg/kg. The exposure limit for white phosphorus is $0.1 \, mg/m^3$; for phosphine, 0.3 ppm; and for phenyl phosphine, 0.05 ppm.

Phosphorus causes tissue destruction, with disturbances in carbohydrate, fat, and protein metabolism in the liver. Deposition of glycogen in the liver is inhibited; deposition of fat is increased.

Chronic absorption of phosphorus increases bone formation under the epiphyseal cartilage and impairs blood circulation in bone by bone formation in haversian and marrow canals. These changes lead to necrosis and sequestration of bone; they occur most frequently in the mandible.

The pathologic findings in white phosphorus poisoning are jaundice, fatty degeneration and necrosis of the liver and kidneys, and hemorrhages, congestion, and erosion of the gastrointestinal tract. Pathologic findings from phosphine inhalation are pulmonary hyperemia and edema and focal myocardial necrosis. Zinc phosphide ingestion causes both fatty degeneration and necrosis of the liver and pulmonary hyperemia and edema.

## Clinical findings

The principal manifestations of poisoning with these compounds are jaundice and collapse.

### Acute poisoning

(1) Ingestion – Ingestion of white phosphorus is followed within 1–2 h by nausea and vomiting, diarrhea, cardiac arrhythmias, and a garlic odor of breath and excreta. The breath and excreta may appear to smoke. Death in coma or cardiac arrest may occur in the first 24–48 h, or symptoms may improve for 1 or 2 days and then return, with nausea and vomiting, diarrhea, liver tenderness and enlargement, jaundice, prostration, fall in blood pressure, oliguria, hypocalcemic tetany, hypoglycemia, and multiple petechial hemorrhages. Onset of Cheyne–Stokes respiration followed by convulsions, coma, and death may occur up to 3 weeks after poisoning. Phosphide ingestion causes jaundice, liver tenderness and enlargement, and pulmonary edema with dyspnea and cyanosis. Death may occur up to a week after poisoning.

(2) Skin contact – White phosphorus allowed to dry on the skin will ignite and cause second- to third-degree burns surrounded by blisters. These burns heal slowly.

(3) Inhalation – Inhalation of phosphorus is followed after 1–3 days by the symptoms of acute phosphorus poisoning. Phosphine or phosphide inhalation causes nausea and vomiting, fatigue, cough, jaundice, paresthesias, ataxia, intention tremor, diplopia, fall in blood pressure, dyspnea, pulmonary edema, collapse, cardiac arrhythmias, convulsions, and coma. Death usually occurs within 4 days; it may be delayed 1–2 weeks. Renal damage and leukopenia may appear after several days. Exposure to phenyl phosphine at 0.6 ppm causes hypersensitivity to sound and touch and hyperemia of the skin. Exposure at levels above 2 ppm causes hematologic effects, with decrease in red blood cell count, dermatitis, and nerve and testicular degeneration.

*Chronic poisoning* (from ingestion or inhalation of white phosphorus, phosphine, or phosphides)

The first symptom is toothache, followed by swelling of the jaw and then necrosis of the mandible ('phossy jaw'). Other findings are weakness, weight loss, loss of appetite, anemia, and spontaneous fractures.

*Laboratory findings*

(1) Impairment of liver function is shown by appropriate tests (see p. 75).
(2) Blood urea nitrogen and bilirubin are increased. Acidosis may occur.
(3) Hematuria and proteinuria may be present.

**Prevention**

The exposure limits for phosphorus, phosphine, and phosphides in the air must be observed at all times. Special clothing, to be changed daily, should be provided for phosphorus workers. Workers must bathe on leaving work and must be educated in the hazards of phosphorus exposure. Safety showers and eye fountains must be provided where white phosphorus is being used. Dental examination should be made frequently, depending on exposure.

## Treatment

### Acute poisoning

(1) Emergency measures – Remove poison by gastric lavage with 5–10 liters of tap water. If a gastric tube is not immediately available, induce emesis. Remove phosphorus contamination from the skin or eyes by copious irrigation with tap water for at least 15 minutes.

(2) General measures – Treat pulmonary edema (see p. 55). Treat shock (see p. 56). Give 10% calcium gluconate, 10 ml intravenously, to maintain serum calcium. Give 1–4 liters of 5% glucose in water or 10% invert sugar (Travert) in water intravenously daily until a high-carbohydrate diet can be given by mouth. Treat hepatic failure (see p. 75).

### Chronic poisoning

Remove from further exposure. Treat jaw necrosis by surgical excision of sequestered bone.

## Prognosis

In poisoning from ingestion of phosphorus, the mortality rate is about 50%. In phosphine inhalation, survival for 4 days is ordinarily followed by recovery.

## References

Abder-Rahman H. Effect of aluminum phosphide on blood glucose level. *Vet Human Toxicol* 1999;41:31

Abder-Rahman HA, *et al*. Aluminum phosphide fatalities, new local experience. *Med Sci Law* 2000;40:164

Singh S, *et al*. Aluminum phosphide ingestion – a clinico-pathologic study. *J Toxicol Clin Toxicol* 1996;34:703

## ZINC FUMES AND METAL FUME FEVER

Zinc fumes are produced in welding, metal cutting, and smelting zinc alloys or galvanized iron. Zinc fumes are most often responsible for metal fume fever, but other metal fumes, including magnesium oxide fumes, will also cause the disease. Soluble zinc salts such as zinc chloride are used in smoke generators.

The exposure limit for zinc oxide fumes is 5 mg/m³; for zinc chloride fumes, 1 mg/m³; and for magnesium oxide fumes, 10 mg/m³. No fatalities from breathing zinc oxide or zinc chloride fumes have been reported in recent years.

Fumes from zinc or soluble zinc salts irritate the lungs. Other physiologic changes are not known. The pathologic findings in fatalities from zinc chloride or zinc fume inhalation are pulmonary edema and damage to the respiratory tract.

## Clinical findings

The principal manifestations of acute zinc fume or other metal fume poisoning are muscular aches and fever. Chronic poisoning does not occur. Inhalation of zinc oxide or other metal oxide fumes causes fever, chills, nausea and vomiting, muscular aches, and weakness. Inhaling fumes of soluble zinc salts such as zinc chloride may cause pulmonary edema with cyanosis and dyspnea.

## Prevention

Zinc chloride smoke generators should not be operated in such a way that workers will be exposed. Fumes from smelting zinc must be controlled by proper air exhaust.

## Treatment of acute poisoning

### Specific measures

Treat pulmonary edema (see p. 55). Give prednisone, 25–50 mg orally daily, or other corticosteroid, to reduce tissue response to inhaled metal fumes. Decrease dosage as the patient improves.

### Other measures

Treat metal fume fever by bed rest and give aspirin for fever and pain.

## Prognosis

In zinc fume fever recovery occurs in 24–48 h. In pulmonary edema from zinc chloride fumes the mortality rate has been 10–40%.

## References

Barcelous DG. Cobalt. *J Toxicol Clin Toxicol* 1999;37:201

Barceloux DG. Copper. *J Toxicol Clin Toxicol* 1999;37:217

Barceloux DG. Molybdenum. *J Toxicol Clin Toxicol* 1999;37:231

Barceloux DG. Selenium. *J Toxicol Clin Toxicol* 1999;37:145

Barceloux DG. Vanadium. *J Toxicol Clin Toxicol* 1999;37:265

Barceloux DG. Zinc. *J Toxicol Clin Toxicol* 1999;37:279

Fuortes L, Schenck D. Marked elevation of urinary zinc levels and pleural-friction rub in metal fume fever. *Vet Human Toxicol* 2000;42:164

Hantson P, *et al*. Accidental ingestion of a zinc and copper sulfate preparation. *J Toxicol Clin Toxicol* 1996;34:725

Irsigler GB, *et al*. Asthma and chemical bronchitis in vanadium plant workers. *Am J Ind Med* 1999;35:366

Quadrani DA, *et al*. A fatal case of gun blue ingestion in a toddler. *Vet Human Toxicol* 2000;42:96 (Selenium)

**Table 15.2** Uncommon poisons

| | Exposure limit (ppm) | Effects | Treatment |
|---|---|---|---|
| *Bacillus subtilis* enzymes | 0.00006* | Irritant, sensitizer | Remove from exposure |
| Bismuth telluride | 10* | Pulmorary lesions; irritant | Remove from exposure |
| Bismuth telluride with selenium | 5* | Granulomatous pulmonary lesions | Remove from exposure |
| Carbon dioxide gas | 5000 | 3% – dyspnea and headache; 10% – visual disturbances, tinnitus, tremor, and loss of consciousness | Give artificial respiration |
| Cerium fumes | | Pulmonary fibrosis, emphysema | Remove from exposure |
| Cobalt dust and fumes | 0.02* | Inhalation causes shortness of breath, lung densities, dermatitis with hyperemia and vesiculation. Ingestion causes hypotension, pericardial effusion, polycythemia, congestive failure, pain, vomiting, nerve deafness, convulsions, enlargement of the thyroid | Give calcium disodium edetate (see p. 88) |
| Copper fumes or copper powder | 0.2* 1* | Metal fume fever, sneezing, nausea; renal damage may occur | Give calcium disodium edetate (see p. 88) |
| Epoxy hardeners (catalyst) | | Consist of amines, organic acids or acid anhydrides, or polyamines. These cause irritation, sensitivity reactions, and corrosion of skin or mucous membranes after prolonged contact. Vapor hazard possible | Remove ingested hardener by gastric lavage or emesis. Remove skin contamination by gentle scrubbing with soap and water. Avoid use of organic solvents, which may increase absorption |
| Epoxy monomer (unpolymerized resin) | | Skin irritant and sensitizer | Remove by scrubbing gently with soap and water |
| Epoxy resin (polymerized) | | Inert, but may decompose at high temperature with release of irritating products, causing pulmonary edema | Treat pulmonary edema |

*Continued*

*Table 15.2 (continued)*

| | Exposure limit (ppm) | Effects | Treatment |
|---|---|---|---|
| Ferrovanadium | 1* | Irritation of the eyes and respiratory tract, bronchitis, pneumonitis | Remove from exposure |
| Fluorocarbon polymer fumes (Teflon) | | Malaise; weakness; numbness and tingling in arms, fingers; pain in throat; and some difficulty in breathing. (From high-temperature decomposition of solid or aerosol Teflon or other fluorinated hydrocarbons.) | Remove from exposure |
| Germanium compounds | | Bronchitis; pneumonitis; liver, kidney damage; hemolysis | Remove from exposure |
| Germanium tetrahydride | 0.2 | Like arsine | See p. 274 |
| Hafnium | 0.5* | Salts are irritants and can cause liver damage | Remove from exposure |
| Indium | 0.1* | Pulmonary damage | Remove from exposure |
| Iron, dicyclopentadienyl | 10* | No effect? | |
| Iron oxide fumes | 5* | Pneumoconiosis; irritant | Remove from exposure |
| Iron salt fumes | 1* | | |
| Iron pentacarbonyl | 0.1 | Dizziness, headache, vomiting, coma | |
| Magnesium metal | | Skin implants cause necrosis, gangrene, subcutaneous emphysema | Remove from exposure |
| Magnesium oxide fumes | 10* | Fever | Remove from exposure |
| Molybdenum, insol | 10* | Possible irritation, CNS effects, liver and kidney damage | Remove from exposure |
| Molybdenum salts | 5* | Irritation, weight loss, ataxia in animals | Remove from exposure |
| Nickel | 1.5* | Skin sensitization with itching dermatitis, asthma. Lung cancer | Remove from exposure |
| Nickel compounds | 0.1* | | |
| Platinum metal, platinum salts | 1* 0.002* | Irritant, sensitizer, dermatitis, asthma | Remove from exposure |

*Continued*

Table 15.2 (continued)

| | Exposure limit (ppm) | Effects | Treatment |
|---|---|---|---|
| Polyurethane polymer | | High temperature decomposition releases CN⁻, NO | See p. 324 |
| Polyvinyl chloride polymers | | High-temperature decomposition releases HCl, phosgene, CO | See p. 245 |
| Rhodium salts | 0.01* | Irritant and possible sensitizer | Remove from |
| Rhodium fumes | 1* | | exposure |
| Selenate and selenium compounds orally | | Damages liver, kidneys, gastrointestinal tract, heart, lungs. Death has occurred from therapeutic use | Treat symptomatically. Both calcium edetate and dimercaprol have been shown to increase toxicity in experimental animals |
| Selenium fumes | 0.2* | Garlic breath, gastrointestinal upset, nervousness | |
| Selenium hexafluoride, hydrogen selenide | 0.05 | Pneumonitis, pulmonary edema, bronchial pneumonia | |
| Selenium oxide | 0.2* | Severe irritation, broncho-spasm, difficulty in breathing, chills, fever, headaches, pneumonitis with consolidation clearing after 1–4 weeks | |
| Silane | 5 | Irritant | Remove from exposure |
| Solder, rosin core pyrolysis products | | Eye, bronchial, and pulmonary irritation. Sensitizer | Remove from exposure |
| Tantalum | 5* | Irritant, lung damage | Remove from exposure |
| Tellurium fumes | 0.1* | Garlic odor of breath, metallic taste, nausea, loss of appetite, liver injury | Treat symptomatically |
| Tributyl tin | 0.1* | Severe irritation to necrosis | Remove from exposure and treat symptomatically |
| Triethyl tin | 0.1* | Brain damage that may be permanent | |
| Triphenyl tin | 0.1* | Liver damage | |

*Continued*

*Table 15.2 (continued)*

| | Exposure limit (ppm) | Effects | Treatment |
|---|---|---|---|
| Tungsten, insoluble salts and metal | 5* | Pulmonary fibrosis? | Remove from exposure |
| Tungsten, soluble salts | 1* | CNS effects | |
| Uranium salts | 0.2* | Pulmonary irritation, severe kidney degeneration, and cancers from radiation effects | Give calcium disodium edetate (see p. 88) |
| Vanadium fumes | 0.05* | Rhinorrhea, sneezing, sore chest, wheezing, dyspnea, weakness, bronchitis, pneumonitis | Give ascorbic acid, 1 g/d. Calcium edetate may be useful (see p. 88) |
| Vanadium dust | 0.05* | | |
| Welding fumes | 5* | Irritation, pulmonary damage, fever | Remove from exposure |
| Yttrium salts | 1* | Pulmonary irritation, fibrosis | Remove from exposure |
| Zirconium oxide and salts | 5* | Granulomas from skin application. Possible pneumonitis | Remove from exposure |

*$mg/m^3$

# 16 Cyanides, sulfides, and carbon monoxide

**HYDROGEN CYANIDE AND DERIVATIVES: ACRYLONITRILE, CYANAMIDE, CYANOGEN CHLORIDE, CYANIDES, NITROPRUSSIDES, AND CYANOGENETIC GLYCOSIDES (see Table 16.1)**

Hydrogen cyanide (HCN) is used as a fumigant and in chemical synthesis. Acrylonitrile is used in the production of synthetic rubber. Cyanamide is used as a fertilizer and as a source of hydrogen cyanide. Cyanogen chloride is used in chemical synthesis. Cyanide salts are used in metal cleaning, hardening, and refining and in the recovery of gold from ores. Nitroprussides are used in chemical synthesis and as hypotensive agents. The seeds of apple, cherry, peach, apricot, plum, jetberry bush, and toyon contain cyanogenetic glycosides such as amygdalin that release cyanide on digestion. The fatal dose of these seeds varies from 5 to 25 seeds for a small child. They are only dangerous if the seed capsule is broken.

Natural oil of bitter almonds contains 4% hydrogen cyanide, and artificial oil of bitter almonds contains mandelonitrile. Some species of the lima bean (*Phaseolus lunatus*) contain 300 mg of HCN per 100 g of bean. American white lima beans contain 10 mg of HCN per 100 g of bean. The dried root of cassava (*Manihot utilissima*, tapioca) may contain 245 mg of HCN per 100 g of root. Hydrolysis and leaching can reduce the amount of HCN to 1 mg per 100 g. When raw plant material containing cyanogenetic glycoside is ingested, enzymes in the plant material release HCN. In the absence of enzymes in ingested material, bacterial enzymes in the intestine release HCN. One man was poisoned after eating about 48 apricot kernels that had been roasted at 300°F (*c.* 150°C) for 10 min. Laetrile, claimed to be a cancer cure, is reported to be made from apricot kernels and contains a cyanide-releasing substance. It has caused fatal cyanide poisoning.

Cyanide apparently poisons by inhibiting the cytochrome oxidase system for $O_2$ utilization in cells. Other enzyme systems are also inhibited, but to a lesser degree.

**Table 16.1** Hydrogen cyanide and derivatives

| | Boiling point (°C) | Exposure limit (ppm) | LD50 (mg/kg) or LC (ppm) | Cyanide-releasing | Remarks |
|---|---|---|---|---|---|
| Acetone cyanohydrin | 82 | 4.7 | 4 | + | Irritant |
| Acetonitrile | 81.6 | 40 | 269 | + | Irritant |
| Acrylonitrile | 78.5 | 2 | 78 | + | Bullae, carcinogen |
| Benzonitrile | 190.7 | | 720 | 0 | |
| Benzylcyanide | 234 | | 45 | + | Irritant |
| Bromobenzylcyanide | Solid | | 100 | + | Irritant |
| n-Butyronitrile | 118 | 22* | 27 | + | |
| Cyanamide | Solid | 2* | 125 | 0 | |
| Cyanide salts | Solid | 5* | 2 | + | |
| Cyanoacetic acid | 108 | | 1500 | 0 | |
| Cyanogen | Gas | 10 | 350 ppm | + | |
| Cyanogen chloride | 61 | 0.3 | 6 | + | |
| Ferrocyanide | Solid | | | + | |
| Fumaronitrile | 186 | | 132 | + | |
| Hydrogen cyanide | 25.7 | 4.7 | 4 | + | |
| Malononitrile | Solid | 8* | 19 | + | Irritant |
| Mandelonitrile | Liquid | | 6 | + | Irritant |
| Methyl acrylonitrile | 90 | 1 | 15 | + | Carcinogen |
| Methyl 2-cyanoacrylate | Liquid | 2 | 1600 | | Irritant |
| Methyl isocyanate | 39 | 0.02 | 2 ppm | | Irritant, sensitizer |
| Nitroprusside (see p. 480) | Solid | | 20 | + (?) | Like nitrite |
| m-Phthalodinitrile | Solid | 5* | 250 | 0 | Irritant |
| Propionitrile | 97 | 14* | 40 | + | |
| Thiocyanate, Na or K | Solid | | 200 | + | |
| o-Tolunitrile | 204 | | 3200 | + | |
| Trichloroacetonitrile | 84.6 | | 250 | + | Extreme irritation |

*mg/m³

Cyanide first causes a marked increase in respiration by affecting chemoreceptors in the carotid body and respiratory center and then paralyzes all cells. Pathologic findings in fatal cases are not characteristic. The odor of bitter almonds may be noticeable at autopsy; however, the ability to perceive this odor is genetically determined, and some humans do not possess it. Ingestion of potassium cyanide or sodium cyanide causes congestion and corrosion of the gastric mucosa.

## Clinical findings

The principal manifestations of poisoning with these compounds are rapid respiration, fall in blood pressure, convulsions, and coma.

### Acute poisoning

(1) Cyanide, cyanogen chloride, acetonitrile, and other cyanide releasing substances – Ingestion or inhalation of large amounts of these compounds (10 times the MLD) causes immediate unconsciousness, convulsions, and death within 1–15 min. Ingestion, inhalation, or absorption through the skin of an amount near the MLD causes dizziness, rapid respiration, vomiting, flushing, headache, drowsiness, fall in blood pressure, rapid pulse, and unconsciousness. Death in convulsions occurs within 4 hours with all cyanide derivatives except sodium nitroprusside, which may cause death as late as 12 hours after ingestion.

(2) Acrylonitrile – Inhalation of acrylonitrile causes nausea and vomiting, diarrhea, weakness, headache, and jaundice. Skin contact with acrylonitrile has caused epidermal necrolysis.

(3) Calcium cyanamide – Ingestion causes flushing of skin and mucous membranes, headache, dizziness, and fall in blood pressure. These symptoms are greatly accentuated by the concomitant ingestion of ethanol. At least one fatality has occurred from ethanol ingestion after calcium cyanamide (calcium carbimide) ingestion.

### Chronic poisoning

Repeated inhalation of small amounts of cyanogen chloride causes dizziness, weakness, congestion of lungs, hoarseness, conjunctivitis, loss of appetite, weight loss, and mental deterioration. Similar symptoms have also been reported from inhaling cyanide in low concentrations for 1 year or more. Chronic ingestion of cyanide in the form of cassava is suspected of causing tropical ataxic neuropathy. Thyroid insufficiency also occurs as a result of conversion of cyanide to thiocyanate. A trimer of methylene amino-acetonitrile caused conjunctivitis and respiratory tract inflammation in rubber workers. Workers exposed to acrylonitrile show an increased incidence of cancer. Laetrile has caused agranulocytosis.

*Laboratory findings*

A severe metabolic acidosis occurs in acute cyanide poisoning.

**Prevention**

Many individuals cannot detect the odor of cyanide. The exposure limit of cyanide in work rooms must not be exceeded at any time. Emergency treatment kits containing 0.2-ml ampules of amyl nitrite, 10-ml ampules of 3% sodium nitrite, and 25-ml ampules of 25% sodium thiosulfate, with suitable syringes and needles, should be immediately available where cyanide is being used. Rescue personnel should wear protective clothing and rescue breathing apparatus.

**Treatment**

*Inhaled cyanide*

(1) Emergency measures:
  (a) Remove to uncontaminated atmosphere.
  (b) Give amyl nitrite inhalation, 1 ampule (0.2 ml) every 5 min. Stop administration if the systolic blood pressure goes below 80 mmHg.
  (c) Give artificial respiration with 100% $O_2$ in order to maintain high blood $O_2$ tension.
(2) Antidote – All cyanide antidotes are toxic, and unnecessary therapy is dangerous, especially in children.
  (a) Sodium nitrite – As soon as possible give 3% sodium nitrite solution intravenously at a rate of 2.5–5 ml/min. Stop administration if the systolic blood pressure goes below 80 mmHg. The administered nitrite forms methemoglobin, which combines with cyanide to form cyanmethemoglobin. The amount of nitrite administered must be based on the hemoglobin level and on the weight of the individual. Table 16.2 gives the amount of sodium nitrite necessary to convert 26% of hemoglobin to methemoglobin. Further administration of nitrite should be based on methemoglobin determinations, and the total methemoglobin should not exceed 40%.
  (b) Sodium thiosulfate – Follow sodium nitrite with 25% sodium thiosulfate solution intravenously at a rate of 2.5–5 ml/min.

**Table 16.2** Variation of sodium nitrite and sodium thiosulfate dose with hemoglobin concentration*

| Hemoglobin (g/dl) | Initial dose sodium nitrite (mg/kg) | Initial dose sodium nitrite 3% (ml/kg) | Initial dose sodium thiosulfate 25% (ml/kg) |
|---|---|---|---|
| 7 | 5.8 | 0.19 | 0.95 |
| 8 | 6.6 | 0.22 | 1.10 |
| 9 | 7.5 | 0.25 | 1.25 |
| 10 | 8.3 | 0.27 | 1.35 |
| 11 | 9.1 | 0.30 | 1.50 |
| 12 | 10.0 | 0.33 | 1.65 |
| 13 | 10.8 | 0.36 | 1.80 |
| 14 | 11.6 | 0.39 | 1.95 |

*Reproduced with permission from Berlin DM Jr. The treatment of cyanide poisoning in children. *Pediatrics* 1970;46:793

Thiosulfate converts cyanide to thiocyanate. The dose of thiosulfate should be based on hemoglobin determination as with nitrite (see Table 16.2).

(c) Hydroxocobalamin, which converts to non-toxic cyanocobalamin in the presence of cyanide, is available in some countries. The suggested initial dose is 4 g (50 mg/kg).

### Ingested cyanide

(1) Emergency measures:
  (a) Give amyl nitrite inhalation, 1 ampule (0.2 ml) every 5 min.
  (b) Gastric lavage (see p. 31) should be delayed until nitrite and thiosulfate antidotes have been given.
  (c) Give artificial respiration with 100% $O_2$ in order to maintain high blood $O_2$ tension (see above).
(2) Antidote – Treat as for inhaled cyanide (see above).

### Ingested calcium cyanamide

There is no known antidote.

After gastric lavage (see p. 31) treat symptomatically.

## Prognosis

In acute cyanide poisoning, survival for 4 h is usually followed by recovery.

## References

Chin RG, Calderon Y. Acute cyanide poisoning: a case report. *J Emerg Med* 2000;18:441

Houeto P, *et al.* Pharmacokinetics of hydroxocobalamin in smoke inhalation victims. *J Toxicol Clin Toxicol* 1996;34:397

Laforge M, *et al.* Ferrocyanide ingestion may cause false positives in cyanide determination. *J Toxicol Clin Toxicol* 1999;37:337

Lam KK, Lau FL. An incident of hydrogen cyanide poisoning. *Am J Emerg Med* 2000;18:172

Legras A, *et al.* Herbicide: Fatal ammonium thiocyanate and aminotriazole poisoning. *J Toxicol Clin Toxicol* 1996;34:441

Suchard JR, *et al.* Acute cyanide toxicity caused by apricot kernel ingestion. *Ann Emerg Med* 1998;32:742

## HYDROGEN SULFIDE, OTHER SULFIDES, MERCAPTANS, CARBON DISULFIDE, AND PROPANE SULTONE

Hydrogen sulfide is released spontaneously by the decomposition of sulfur compounds and is found in petroleum refineries, tanneries, mines, and rayon factories. It is produced by bacterial action on sewage effluents containing sulfur compounds when dissolved $O_2$ has been consumed owing to excessive organic loading of surface water. Such compounds are used by the canning industry as antioxidants during certain seasons and in many instances are discharged to surface waters, where they drastically reduce dissolved $O_2$. Carbon disulfide is used as a solvent, especially in the rayon industry. Mercaptans are released in petroleum refining and are used as warning odors in liquefied propane, butane, and natural gas. Phenylmercaptan and *p*-chlorophenyl mercaptan are used as pesticides. Calcium polysulfide (Vleminckx's solution), sodium sulfide, ammonium sulfide, and thioacetamide release hydrogen sulfide in contact with water or acids. Propane sultone is used as a chemical intermediate.

Hydrogen sulfide ($H_2S$) is a gas. Carbon disulfide ($CS_2$) is a liquid that boils at 46°C. It ignites at the temperature of boiling water (100°C).

Ethylmercaptan ($C_2H_5SH$) and methylmercaptan (methanethiol, $CH_3SH$) are gases.

The exposure limit for hydrogen sulfide is 10 ppm; carbon disulfide, 10 ppm; methylmercaptan, butylmercaptan, ethylmercaptan, and phenyl-mercaptan, 0.5 ppm; perchloromethylmercaptan, 0.1 ppm; phosphorus pentasulfide, 1 mg/m$^3$; and allylpropyl disulfide, 2 ppm. No exposure limit for propane sultone has been established. Hydrogen sulfide in community air should not exceed 0.03 ppm. The approximate fatal dose of carbon disulfide by ingestion is 1 g; of soluble sulfides, 10 g. The lethal dose of 2-mercapto-ethanol in rats is 300 mg/kg. Ingested sulfur is converted to sulfides in the gastrointestinal tract, and ingestion of 10–20 g has caused irritation of the gastrointestinal tract and renal injury.

Hydrogen sulfide causes both anoxic effects and damage to the cells of the central nervous system by direct action. Carbon disulfide damages chiefly the central nervous system, the peripheral nerves, and the hemopoietic system. The mercaptans are severe irritants.

There are no characteristic pathologic findings in sudden fatalities from hydrogen sulfide poisoning; if death is delayed 24–48 h, pulmonary edema and congestion of the lungs are found. Ingestion of carbon disulfide causes congestion and edema of the gastrointestinal tract. The characteristic unpleasant (rotten egg) odor is noticeable at autopsy. In deaths from carbon disulfide, degenerative changes may be found in the brain and spinal cord. Prolonged exposure to small concentrations of carbon disulfide has caused cerebro-vascular changes.

## Clinical findings

The principal manifestation of poisoning with these compounds is irritation.

### *Acute poisoning*

(1) Hydrogen sulfide is detectable by odor at 0.05 ppm, and 0.1 ppm causes irritation and sensory loss. Fifty ppm creates an unpleasant odor, but shortly the smell diminishes. After exposure to concentrations above 50 ppm symptoms are gradually progressive, with painful conjunctivitis, appearance of a halo around lights, headache, insomnia, nausea, rawness in the throat, cough, dizziness, drowsiness, and pulmonary edema.

Concentrations above 500 ppm cause immediate loss of consciousness, depressed respiration, and death in 30–60 min.

(2) Exposure to carbon disulfide at concentrations from 100 to 1000 ppm causes symptoms progressing from restlessness, irritation of the mucous membranes, blurred vision, nausea and vomiting, and headache to unconsciousness and paralysis of respiration. If consciousness returns, irritability, muscle spasms, visual disturbances, and even psychotic behavior are observed during recovery.

(3) Skin contact with carbon disulfide causes reddening and burning and, later, cracking and peeling. If the liquid remains in contact with the skin for several minutes, a second-degree burn may result.

(4) Ingestion of carbon disulfide or soluble sulfides causes vomiting, headache, cyanosis, respiratory depression, fall in blood pressure, loss of consciousness, tremors, convulsions, and death.

(5) Ethylmercaptan, methylmercaptan, and other mercaptans in high concentrations cause cyanosis, convulsions, hemolytic anemia, fever, coma, and irreversible depression of cerebral function. Perchloromethylmercaptan is a severe pulmonary irritant. Allyl propyl disulfide (onion oil) is a mild pulmonary and mucous membrane irritant.

(6) Phosphorus pentasulfide is an eye and skin irritant. It liberates hydrogen sulfide on contact with water.

*Chronic poisoning*

(1) Hydrogen sulfide – Prolonged exposure causes persistent low blood pressure, nausea, loss of appetite, weight loss, impaired gait and balance, conjunctivitis, and chronic cough.

(2) Carbon disulfide – Continued exposure by inhalation or skin absorption first causes bizarre sensations in the extremities and then sensory loss and muscular weakness. Later symptoms are irritability, memory loss, blurred vision, loss of appetite, insomnia, mental depression, partial blindness, dizziness, weakness, and Parkinsonian tremor. Examination may reveal vascularization of the retina, dilatation of retinal arterioles, and blanching of the optic disk. The corneal and papillary reflexes may be diminished or lost. The mortality rate from coronary heart disease is increased in workers exposed to carbon disulfide. The incidence of abortions, sterility, and amenorrhea is increased in exposed women.

(3) Propane sultone – Single exposures have been carcinogenic in several animal species.

*Laboratory findings*

(1) The differential count may reveal a decrease in polymorphonuclear leukocytes and an increase in lymphocytes.
(2) Hematuria and proteinuria may be present.
(3) Hepatic cell function may be impaired as shown by appropriate tests (see p. 75).

**Prevention**

The exposure limit must be observed at all times. The odor of carbon disulfide or hydrogen sulfide should not be relied upon to give adequate warning. Loss of the sense of smell occurs rapidly. Workers should alternate between jobs requiring exposure to carbon disulfide and jobs in uncontaminated air. Airline face masks must be worn when entering highly contaminated areas. A safety harness and lifeline attended by a responsible person are necessary.

**Treatment**

*Acute poisoning*

(1) Emergency measures:
    (a) Remove from exposure.
    (b) Give artificial respiration with $O_2$ if respiration is affected.
    (c) Remove swallowed poison by gastric lavage or emesis (see pp. 29–32), using a saturated sodium bicarbonate solution to reduce gastric acidity and to prevent the formation of hydrogen sulfide, which is more rapidly absorbed.
    (d) Stimulants may induce ventricular arrhythmias.
(2) Antidote – Amyl nitrite or sodium nitrite (see p. 315) can be used to aid in the formation of sulfmethemoglobin, thus removing sulfide from combination in tissues. Pyridoxine, 25 mg/kg intravenously, or 10% urea, 1 g/kg intravenously, have been suggested as sulfide acceptors.
(3) General measures:
    (a) Treat pulmonary edema (see p. 55).

(b) Keep patient at bed rest for 3–4 days. Reduce sensory input in instances of delirium or excitement.

***Chronic poisoning***

Remove from further exposure.

**Prognosis**

In hydrogen sulfide poisoning, if the patient survives for the first 4 hours, recovery is assured. In carbon disulfide poisoning, gradual improvement takes place over several months, but complete recovery may never occur.

**References**

Buick JB, *et al*. Is a reduction in residual volume a sub-clinical manifestation of hydrogen sulfide intoxication? *Am J Ind Med* 2000;37:296

Horowitz BZ, *et al*. Calcium polysulfide overdose: a report of two cases. *J Toxicol Clin Toxicol* 1996;35:299

Milby TH, Baselt RC. Hydrogen sulfide poisoning: clarification of some controversial issues. *Am J Ind Med* 1999;35:192

Reiffenstein RJ, *et al*. Toxicology of hydrogen sulfide. *Annu Rev Pharmacol Toxicol* 1992;32:109

# CARBON MONOXIDE

Carbon monoxide is produced by the incomplete combustion of carbon or carbonaceous materials. All flame or combustion devices, including catalytic radiant heaters, are likely to emit carbon monoxide. The worldwide emission of carbon monoxide is approximately 232 million tons each year, of which the USA contributes 88 million tons. The total amount emitted each year would be sufficient to raise the concentration in the lower atmosphere about 0.03 ppm, but a biologic scavenging process prevents the lowest oceanic levels from rising above 0.03–0.10 ppm.

The exhaust from incomplete combustion of natural gas or petroleum fuels may contain as much as 5% carbon monoxide. An unvented natural gas heater may emit as much as 1 cu ft/min, which is enough to make the air in a small room dangerous within minutes. The exhaust from gasoline internal combustion engines contains 3–7% carbon monoxide. A gasoline vehicle with no

CYANIDES, SULFIDES, AND CARBON MONOXIDE

emission control device emits 2.7 lb of carbon monoxide per gallon of fuel, or 80 g per mile at 15 miles per gallon. Present standards for new cars require limitation of carbon monoxide emission to 0.5%. A diesel vehicle emits 0.074 lb of carbon monoxide per gallon of fuel, or 7 g per mile at 5 miles per gallon. Smoke from cigarettes, pipes, and cigars is also a potent source of carbon monoxide, containing 4%.

The industrial exposure limit for carbon monoxide is 35 ppm. In the USA an adverse level of carbon monoxide for community air has been set at 9 ppm for a continuous period of 8 h. As examples of community air pollution levels, Burbank, California, exceeded 20 ppm for 583 h and 10 ppm for 6044 h in 1967, whereas San Francisco exceeded 20 ppm for 20 h and 10 ppm for 264 h in the same year.

Carbon monoxide combines with hemoglobin to form carboxyhemoglobin, which is incapable of carrying $O_2$, and tissue anoxia results. One part of carbon monoxide in 200 parts of $O_2$ or 1000 parts of air will cause approximately 50% saturation of hemoglobin with carboxyhemoglobin. A human who breathes air with the lowest possible values of carbon monoxide will still have about 1% of red blood cell hemoglobin combined with carbon monoxide. An individual's exhaled air will contain about 3 ppm of carbon monoxide, which comes from the breakdown of hemoglobin liberated when red blood cells die at the end of their life span of about 120 days. A person who inhales smoke from 20 cigarettes during 1 day will have at least 6% of their hemoglobin saturated with carbon monoxide. Garage employees working in an atmosphere containing 7–240 ppm carbon monoxide were found to have 3–15% of their hemoglobin combined with carbon monoxide. In laboratory experiments subjects exposed to 50 ppm for 30 min had 3% saturation of hemoglobin with carbon monoxide. The relationship is such that a concentration in air of 6 ppm carbon monoxide will increase the amount of hemoglobin in combination with carbon monoxide by 1%. The time required for this equilibrium to occur is thought to be about 8 hours, although direct measurement has not been made at these low concentrations.

Hemoglobin has an affinity for carbon monoxide 210 times greater than for $O_2$. In addition, the presence of carbon monoxide increases the stability of the hemoglobin combination. Thus, the presence of carbon monoxide reduces the availability of $O_2$ to the tissues in 2 ways: (1) by direct combination with hemoglobin to reduce the amount of hemoglobin available to carry $O_2$ and (2) by preventing the release of some of the $O_2$ at the low $O_2$ pressure present in body tissues. As an example, a patient with anemia having a hemoglobin level of 50% of normal and with no carbon monoxide will have about twice as much $O_2$ available to tissues as will the patient with normal hemoglobin who has 50% of hemoglobin combined with carbon monoxide. The patient with anemia may have only slight symptoms, whereas the patient with carbon monoxide poisoning is likely to die. Inhaling the smoke from one cigarette reduces the amount of $O_2$ available to the tissues by about 8%, the equivalent of going from sea level to an altitude of 4000 ft. This effect could play a role in coronary insufficiency.

In addition to its strong affinity for hemoglobin, carbon monoxide also combines with the myoglobin of muscles and with certain enzymes. Interference with the operation of the cytochrome oxidase system is postulated to be the major toxic effect of carbon monoxide; consequently, hyperbaric $O_2$ administration is recommended for management of serious carbon monoxide poisoning – even after the carboxyhemoglobin level returns toward normal. Mice are able to survive with all of their red blood cell hemoglobin combined with carbon monoxide if the $O_2$ pressure is sufficiently high.

The visual ability of subjects watching a faint background to distinguish differences in light intensity is impaired when only 4% of the hemoglobin is combined with carbon monoxide. This same level of saturation is also able to interfere with certain psychologic tests (e.g. choosing the correct letter, choosing the correct color, crossing 't's). Errors in arithmetic and in the ability to underline plural words did not occur until 8–10% saturation of hemoglobin. The ability to discriminate time duration was reduced after exposure to carbon monoxide at 50 ppm for 90 min. The pulse rate during exercise at sea level was not affected when 6% of the hemoglobin was combined with carbon monoxide, but it was increased when 13% was combined. On the other hand, 4% saturation of hemoglobin significantly increased the $O_2$ debt incurred during severe exercise.

Pathologic examination in fatal cases of carbon monoxide poisoning reveals microscopic hemorrhages and necrotic areas throughout the body. Intense congestion and edema of the brain, liver, kidneys, and spleen also occur. The tissues may be bright red. Microscopic examination reveals damage to nerve cells, especially in the cerebral cortex and medulla. Myocardial damage may occur at carboxyhemoglobin levels of 25–50%.

## Clinical findings

The principal manifestation of carbon monoxide poisoning is dyspnea.

### *Acute poisoning* (from inhalation)

The absorption of carbon monoxide and the resulting symptoms are closely dependent on the concentration of carbon monoxide in the inspired air, the time of exposure, and the state of activity of the person exposed.

(1)  A concentration of 100 ppm (0.01%) will not produce symptoms during an 8-hour exposure. Cardiovascular changes can be detected in some individuals at carboxyhemoglobin levels above 5%.

(2)  Exposure to 500 ppm (0.05%) for 1 h during light work may cause no symptoms or only slight headache and shortness of breath. The blood will contain approximately 20% carboxyhemoglobin. A longer exposure to the same concentration, or greater activity, will raise the blood saturation to 40–50%, with symptoms of headache, nausea, irritability, increased respiration, chest pain, confusion, impaired judgment, and fainting on increased exertion. Cyanosis and pallor occur.

(3)  Concentrations over 1000 ppm (0.1%) cause unconsciousness, respiratory failure, and death if exposure is continued for more than 1 h. The blood will contain 50–90% carboxyhemoglobin. Hyperactivity, bizarre behavior, and convulsions can occur during the recovery period. Myonecrosis, neuropathy, renal failure, thrombotic thrombocytopenic purpura, and retrobulbar neuritis with neuroretinal edema have occurred after severe poisoning. In 7% of fatal carbon monoxide poisonings the carboxyhemoglobin level is below 40%.

### *Chronic poisoning*

Chronic poisoning in the sense of accumulation of carbon monoxide in the body does not occur. After the blood carboxyhemoglobin level has returned to normal, susceptibility to carbon monoxide is not increased unless cerebral damage was incurred. However, repeated anoxia from carbon monoxide absorption will cause gradually increasing central nervous system damage, with loss of sensation in the fingers, poor memory, positive Romberg's sign, and mental deterioration. Deaths due to cardiovascular disease are slightly increased in those exposed to low levels of carbon monoxide.

*Laboratory findings*

(1) The white blood cell count may be normal or may be elevated to 18 000 or higher.
(2) The blood level of carboxyhemoglobin should be measured spectrophotometrically.
(3) Proteinuria may be present.
(4) An ECG is useful to indicate possible myocardial damage.
(5) Radiologic evidence of perihilar and intra-alveolar edema indicates a poor prognosis.

## Prevention

The air concentration of carbon monoxide must be kept below the exposure limit at all times by proper ventilation. All combustion devices must be vented to the outside air. These devices include flame water heaters, stoves, gas refrigerators, and internal combustion engines.

## Treatment

*Emergency measures*

(1) Remove from exposure.
(2) Give 100% $O_2$ by mask until the blood carboxyhemoglobin is reduced below the dangerous level. The carboxyhemoglobin level should fall 50% in 1–2 h. After 2 h reduce $O_2$ concentration to 60%. Hyperbaric administration of oxygen is not justified.
(3) If respiration is depressed, give artificial respiration with 100% $O_2$ until respiration is normal.

*Antidote*

Give $O_2$ as under Emergency measures.

*General measures*

(1) Maintain normal body temperature.
(2) Maintain blood pressure (see p. 57).

(3) Give 20% mannitol, 1 g/kg intravenously over 20 min, to reduce cerebral edema.

(4) Give prednisolone, 1 mg/kg intravenously or intramuscularly every 4 h, or other corticosteroid, for cerebral edema.

(5) If hyperthermia is present, reduce body temperature by application of cooling blankets.

(6) Treat bacterial aspiration pneumonia with organism-specific chemotherapy.

(7) Bed rest for 2–4 weeks is useful in order to minimize late neurologic complications.

(8) Control convulsions or hyperactivity with diazepam, 0.1 mg/kg slowly intravenously. Later, phenytoin may be used.

**Prognosis**

If the victim recovers, symptoms regress gradually. If a high blood saturation persists for several hours, tremors, mental deterioration, and abnormal behavior may persist or reappear after a symptom-free interval of 1–2 weeks. These symptoms of central nervous system damage may be permanent. Complete recovery is not likely if symptoms of mental deterioration persist for 2 weeks.

**References**

Abdul-Ghaffar NUA, *et al*. Acute renal failure, compartment syndrome, and systemic capillary leak syndrome complicating carbon monoxide poisoning. *J Toxicol Clin Toxicol* 1996;34:713

Bozeman WP, *et al*. Confirmation of the pulse oximetry gap in carbon monoxide poisoning. *Ann Emerg Med* 1997;30:608

Daley WR, *et al*. An outbreak of carbon monoxide poisoning following a major ice storm in Maine. *J Emerg Med* 2000;18:87

Deitchman S, *et al*. A novel source of carbon monoxide poisoning: explosives used in construction. *Ann Emerg Med* 1998;32:381

Krenzelok EP, *et al*. Carbon monoxide: The silent killer with an audible solution. *Am J Emerg Med* 1996;14:484

Rao R, *et al*. Epidemic of accidental carbon monoxide poisonings caused by snow-obstructed exhaust. *Ann Emerg Med* 1997;29:290

Scheinkestel CD, *et al.* Hyperbaric or normobaric oxygen for acute carbon monoxide poisoning: a randomised controlled clinical trial. *Med J Austral* 1999;170:203

Varon J, *et al.* Carbon monoxide poisoning: a review for clinicians. *J Emerg Med* 1999;17:87

Wilson RC, *et al.* An epidemiological study of acute carbon monoxide poisoning in the West Midlands. *Occup Environ Med* 1999;55:723

# 17 Atmospheric particulates*

In the USA the federal maxima for suspended particulates in the atmosphere are 75 µg/m³ for the annual mean and 260 µg/m³ for the 24-hour average. Certain regions have established 60 µg/m³ as the annual mean maximum and 150 µg/m³ as the maximum 24-hour average.

Particles small enough to remain suspended in the air (aerosols) are formed by grinding, crushing, or burning or by condensation or coalescence. Methods of measurement of the amount of airborne particulate matter consist of the following:

(1) Dust fall is measured in tons per square mile.

(2) Sulfate deposition is measured in mg/100 cm².

(3) Coefficient of haze (COH) is determined by drawing 1000 linear feet of air through filter paper; the percentage of light transmission of the resulting spot is read and converted to a number ranging from zero at 100% transmission to 70 at 20% transmission. (The filter will not trap particles smaller than 0.3 µm.)

(4) A high-volume air filter draws air through a 9 x 12 inch sheet of filter paper for 24 hours; the amount of collected material is weighed and reported in µg/m³ of air passed through the filter. (The filter will not trap particles smaller than 0.3 µm.)

(5) Visibility or visual range is an indication of light scattering or light absorption in the atmosphere; for a given weight of material, particles in the range of 0.1–1 µm have the greatest effect on visibility.

(6) Size analysis: In addition to the quantity of particulate matter suspended in the air, the size of the particles is of utmost importance for their effect on humans. Only those particles ranging from 0.1 to 10 µm are effectively trapped in the lungs. Larger particles are removed by the upper respiratory tract, and smaller particles are not trapped to a significant extent.

---

*See also Table 17.1

The constituents of air-suspended particulates include lead, vanadium, chromium, beryllium, other metals, silica (see below), carbon particles, organic compounds, motor oil, soil, asbestos, sulfates, sulfuric acid droplets, metal sulfates, glass particles, pollen, micro-organisms, and plant and animal products.

Organic particulates can be divided into benzene-soluble substances (mostly organic compounds with high molecular weights) and non-benzene-soluble substances (plant pollens, micro-organisms, and other plant and animal products). The plant and animal products are important in allergic reactions, while the benzene-soluble substances include those with carcinogenic potential such as benzo(a)pyrene and other polycyclic hydrocarbons. These are emitted during incomplete combustion and are also present in the dust from asphalt roads.

Experimental studies have shown that extracts of airborne particulate matter are more likely to induce cancer if injected under the skin of experimental animals than if instilled into the lungs. Part of the reason for such a lack of activity in the lung may be the short time the particulate extracts remain in the lung. If hematite or carbon particles are added to the material instilled into the lung, the carcinogenic potency is increased. This action may result from adsorption and retention of the material in the lung. The carcinogenic effect in animals is characterized by a latent period of 12–24 months, or 50–80% of the animal's lifetime.

When the carcinogenic potency of airborne particulate matter from different regions was compared, that from Alabama was found to be more carcinogenic than that from Los Angeles. The lung cancer death rate was higher in Alabama than in Los Angeles in a study made on mortality rates for 1949–1951. These data do not reflect the great increase in air pollution in Los Angeles since 1950, the effect of which may require 40–50 years to become manifest, since the peak of deaths from lung cancer does not occur until age 55.

## SILICA

Dust containing silica is produced during rock cutting, drilling, crushing, grinding, mining, abrasive manufacture, pottery making, processing of diatomaceous earth, and volcanic eruptions. Talcum powder contains magnesium silicate. Many substances containing silica are capable of causing silicosis; particles less than 5 μm in diameter appear to be the most important in causing silicosis. The exposure limit for dusts containing crystalline quartz, such as tripoli, is 0.1 mg of respirable particles of quartz per cubic meter of air. Cristobalite and tridymite have an exposure limit of 0.05 mg/m$^3$. For diatomaceous earth and silica gel, the total respirable mass should not exceed 10 mg/m$^3$ of air; for precipitated silica, the respirable mass should not exceed 5 mg/m$^3$.

Silica particles smaller than 5 μm in diameter are taken up from alveoli by phagocytic cells that then travel along the lymph channels toward the lymph nodes. Some of these phagocytes do not reach the lymph nodes but collect in nodules along the lymph channels. These nodules then gradually increase in size through proliferation of fibrous tissue to form the silicotic nodule. Pathologic examination reveals nodular fibrosis of the lungs.

Progression of tuberculosis is greatly increased in silicosis, but susceptibility is apparently not increased.

## Clinical findings

The principal manifestation of silicosis is dyspnea.

### Acute pneumoconiosis

Acute pneumoconiosis from overwhelming exposure to silica dust has occurred.

### Chronic pneumoconiosis

Breathing silica dust in concentrations greater than the exposure limit for 6 months to 25 years causes progressive dry cough, shortness of breath on exertion, and decreased chest expansion. As the disease progresses the cough becomes productive of stringy mucus, vital capacity decreases further, and shortness of breath becomes more severe. If the patient gets tuberculosis the course is rapidly downhill, with increased cough, dyspnea, and weight loss, if the disease is not treated.

### X-Ray findings

Radiologic examination of the chest reveals first a diffuse granular appearance. As the disease progresses, the fibrosis becomes linear and later definitely nodular, especially in the inner midlung fields. If tuberculosis is superimposed on the original disease, large nodules, cavities, and pneumonic changes are found. X-rays alone should not be relied upon to make the diagnosis of silicosis, since other pneumoconioses may give a similar radiologic appearance.

### Laboratory findings

The vital capacity is gradually reduced as the disease progresses.

## Prevention

Frequent quantitative dust counts and analyses must be made in work requiring exposure to dust. Particle counts must be kept within safe limits. Workers exposed to dust should have yearly chest examinations.

Air-line face masks and protective suits must be worn in situations where dust cannot be controlled (e.g. sandblasting). Wetting processes to control dusts must be used wherever feasible. Dust-producing operations should be segregated.

Accidental spilling of baby powder on infants' faces during diaper changing has resulted in death; care must be taken to avoid such spills.

## Treatment

### Specific measures

Exposure to silica dust must be reduced to a safe amount. Complete change of occupation is not advisable (see Prognosis).

### General measures

(1) Activity should be restricted to an amount that does not produce dyspnea. However, exercise to tolerance is important for rehabilitation.

(2)  Administration of bronchodilators, such as epinephrine, 1:1000; isoproterenol, 1:100; terbutaline, 1:1000; or phenylephrine, 1:100, by aerosol
may improve effectiveness of positive-pressure breathing therapy.

**Prognosis**

A worker who develops silicosis need not in every case be removed from
occupational exposure, which might involve intolerable family upheavals and
economic hardship. However, exposure to silica must be reduced to a safe
amount as described above.

A radiologic appearance identical with that seen in silicosis may be produced by dusts which do not cause progressive disease. Workers should not
be frightened with the diagnosis of silicosis unless their histories indicate sufficient exposure to silica.

Silicosis may appear and progress more than 5 years after exposure is discontinued. Removal from exposure does not stop progression of the disease.
Individuals with minimal silicosis who avoid tuberculosis, acute pulmonary
infections, and excessive exertion will live approximately normal life spans if
further silica exposure is avoided. Tuberculosis may progress in patients with
silicosis in spite of therapy. Severe attacks of purulent bronchial pneumonia
are frequent in persons with silicosis, and emphysema is likely to progress
gradually.

## ASBESTOS

The word asbestos is used for any mineral that breaks down into fibers. The
most commonly used form, chrysotile, is fibrous serpentine, a magnesium silicate containing 40% silica. Its fibers are tubular in section and range down to
0.015 μm in diameter, which is invisible in the ordinary microscope. Another
form, crocidolite, is fibrous riebeckite, a sodium ferro-ferrisilicate containing
51% silica. Its fibers range down to 0.08 μm in diameter. Amosite is fibrous
grunerite, a magnesium ferrosilicate containing 49% silica. Fibers of this
form range down to 0.1 μm in diameter. Other forms include anthophyllite
and tremolite-actinolite. Uses of the various forms of asbestos in cloth, brake
linings, cement products, paper, flooring, gaskets, and paint amount to 3 million tons per year in the USA.

Although diffuse fibrosis of the lungs was first reported in 1907 in asbestos workers and bronchogenic cancer was reported to be associated with asbestosis in 1935, only since 1960 has disease associated with asbestos been recognized in the general population. At that time pleural calcification was found in farm families in Finland who lived near an asbestos mine. Another disease, mesothelioma of the pleura, has been found in the general population in an area of South Africa where crocidolite asbestos is an important mining product. In a study in London the history of exposure of patients with mesothelioma was investigated. Of the 45 patients who had not worked with asbestos, 9 had lived in a household with asbestos workers and 11 had lived within half a mile of an asbestos plant as much as 20 years previously. In New York City 24 out of 28 lungs examined carefully were found to contain significant numbers of chrysotile fibers. Again in London, a similar study found that almost 80% of lungs contained chrysotile fibers, and in these lungs it was the most abundant of all fibers detected. The relationship between asbestos found in some metropolitan water supplies and human disease is unknown.

Corrective measures to limit asbestos exposure in mines and mills in the USA and Canada have been in force for many years. The exposure limits for particles longer than $5\,\mu m$ (given in particles per milliliter of air) are as follows: amosite, 0.5; chrysotile, 2; crocidolite, 0.2; other forms, 2. Atmospheric sampling for asbestos and examination of material is difficult, since the fibers are extremely small. Electron microscopy, with magnification of at least 20 000 times (and preferably 40 000 times), is necessary to recognize the fibers of chrysotile. If samples are collected by filtration the pore size for most filters is $0.3\,\mu m$ or larger, and the efficiency of collection must be carefully determined. The following levels have been found in urban air: In New York City, Manhattan had asbestos levels of $25–60\,ng/m^3$ of air; the Bronx had $25–28\,ng/m^3$; and Staten Island had $11–21\,ng/m^3$. One nanogram of chrysotile asbestos could represent 1 million fibrils. In Manhattan, asbestos fireproofing has been commonly sprayed in buildings, resulting in widespread dissemination of asbestos over much of the region. Rural areas of Pennsylvania had levels of $10–30\,ng/m^3$ of air.

Pathologic findings include linear fibrosis of the lungs, pleural adhesions, and tumors and calcification of the pleura.

## Clinical findings

The principal manifestation of asbestosis is dyspnea.

### *Pulmonary fibrosis*

The most common disability, fibrosis of the lung, ordinarily has its onset 20–40 years after the beginning of exposure. Symptoms include difficulty in breathing, clubbing of the fingers, and reduction of vital capacity. The disease can develop with as little as 13 years of exposure, and one group exposed to concentrations in the atmosphere above the recommended limit had an incidence of fibrosis of 38%.

The incidence of pulmonary fibrosis after exposure to asbestos is increased by smoking. Non-smokers who had been exposed to asbestos for 20 years did not have pulmonary fibrosis, whereas 29 out of 45 smokers who had been exposed for the same length of time demonstrated pulmonary fibrosis on radiologic examination.

### *Pleural effusion*

Sudden spontaneous pleural effusion sometimes occurs in workers exposed to asbestos years before the diagnosis of asbestosis can be made. Onset of pleural effusion can be as soon as 3–4 years after the beginning of exposure to asbestos.

### *Cancer*

Cancers of the mesothelial lining of the pleural cavity are rare except as a result of occupational exposure to asbestos. In addition to cases associated with crocidolite mining in South Africa, many more have occurred in Great Britain in cities where there are factories for processing asbestos or ports at which asbestos was unloaded. Prior to 1962, only four cases of mesothelioma had been found in Great Britain; by 1965 the number reached 160, and by 1969 a total of 622 cases had been reported. At present about 60 new cases are detected yearly.

In a group of men who applied asbestos insulation for 15 years or more, the mortality rate from cancer of the lung and pleura was 9 times that of a comparable age group in the male population as a whole. The study group consisted of 152 asbestos workers who had 15 or more years of exposure. In this group there were 46 deaths, of which 12 resulted from cancer of the lung and pleura and 7 from cancer of the gastrointestinal tract or peritoneum. The mortality rate from gastrointestinal tract cancer was not considered to be increased over the incidence in the non-exposed population. The mean duration of exposure to asbestos was 26 years for the total group and 32 years for those who died. In another study the number of deaths in 21 755 white male workers in three asbestos products industries was compared with that in 6281 white males in a non-asbestos industry. Cancer of the respiratory system was significantly increased in workers in all of the asbestos industries – asbestos cement products, asbestos friction materials, and asbestos textiles – as compared to those in the non-asbestos industry. The mortality rate from respiratory diseases in workers in the asbestos building products industry and the asbestos friction products industry was twice that of those in the non-asbestos industry. Workers in the asbestos textile industry had a respiratory disease mortality rate more than four times that of those in the non-asbestos industry. Most of this increase could be accounted for by the incidence of asbestosis.

Asbestos as a contaminant of rice has been suggested as the cause of the high incidence of stomach cancer in Japan. The Japanese prefer rice that has been treated with talc after milling. This talc has been found to contain asbestos. Preliminary reports from Australia indicate that asbestos is also responsible for cancer of the large bowel.

### X-Ray findings

Radiologic examination of the chest reveals a diffuse increase in density of the lungs and pleural calcification.

### Prevention

Frequent quantitative dust counts and analyses must be made in work requiring exposure to asbestos. Particle counts must be kept within safe limits. Workers should have chest roentgenograms taken yearly. Non-smokers are much less susceptible to asbestos disease.

## Treatment

Exposure to asbestos must be reduced below the exposure limit. Activity should be restricted to an amount that does not produce dyspnea. Daily exercise to tolerance is important for rehabilitation.

## Prognosis

After onset of symptoms, asbestosis progresses more rapidly than silicosis (see p. 330).

## References

### *General references*

Dockery DW, Pope CA III. Acute respiratory effects of particulate air pollution. *Annu Rev Public Health* 1994;15:107

### *Asbestos*

Bianchi C, *et al*. Asbestos exposure in lung carcinoma: a necropsy-based study of 414 cases. *Am J Ind Med* 1999;36:360

Chang H, *et al*. Risk assessment of lung cancer and mesothelioma in people living near asbestos-related factories in Taiwan. *Arch Environ Health* 1999;54:194

Cocco P, Dosemeci M. Peritoneal cancer and occupational exposure to asbestos. *Am J Ind Med* 1999;35:9

Finkelstein MM. Maintenance work and asbestos-related cancers in the refinery and petrochemical sector. *Am J Ind Med* 1999;35:201

Gennaro V, *et al*. Mesothelioma and lung tumors attributable to asbestos among petroleum workers. *Am J Ind Med* 2000;37:275

Germani D, *et al*. Cohort mortality study of women compensated for asbestosis in Italy. *Am J Ind Med* 1999;36:129

Hillerdal G. Mesothelioma: cases associated with non-occupational and low dose exposures. *Occup Environ Med* 1999;56:505

Jaervholm B, *et al*. Pleural mesothelioma in Sweden: an analysis of the incidence according to the use of asbestos. *Occup Environ Med* 1999;56:110

Levin JL, *et al*. Asbestosis and small cell lung cancer in a clutch refabricator. *Occup Environ Med* 1999;56:602

Levin SM, *et al*. Medical examination for asbestos-related disease. *Am J Ind Med* 2000;37:6

Rees D, *et al*. Case-control study of mesothelioma in South Africa. *Am J Ind Med* 1999;35:213

Rosenthal GJ, *et al*. Asbestos toxicity: an immunologic perspective. *Rev Environ Health* 1999;14:11

Soulat JM, *et al*. High-resolution computed tomography abnormalities in ex-insulators annually exposed to asbestos dust. *Am J Ind Med* 1999;36:593

Wang X-R, *et al*. Pulmonary function of nonsmoking female asbestos workers without radiographic signs of asbestosis. *Arch Environ Health* 1999;53:292

### Organic particulates

Burkhart J, *et al*. Hazardous occupational exposure and lung disease among nylon flock workers. *Am J Ind Med* 1999;Suppl 1:145

Christiani DC, *et al*. Cotton dust and endotoxin exposure and long-term decline in lung function: results of a longitudinal study. *Am J Ind Med* 1999;35:321

Luce D, *et al*. Sinonasal cancer and occupational exposure to textile dust. *Am J Ind Med* 1997;32:205

Mandryk J, *et al*. Work-related symptoms and dose-response relationships for personal exposures and pulmonary function among woodworkers. *Am J Ind Med* 1999;35:481

Raza SN, *et al*. Respiratory symptoms in Lancashire textile weavers. *Occup Environ Med* 1999;56:514

### Silica

Checkoway H, Franzblau A. Is silicosis required for silica-associated lung cancer? *Am J Ind Med* 2000;37:252

Fillmore CM, *et al*. Cancer mortality in women with probable exposure to silica: a death certificate study in 24 states of the U.S. *Am J Ind Med* 1999;36:122

Finkelstein MM. Silica, silicosis, and lung cancer: a risk assessment. *Am J Ind Med* 2000;38:8

Marek K, Lebecki K. Occurrence and prevention of coal miners' pneumoconiosis in Poland. *Am J Ind Med* 1999;36:610

Pan G, *et al*. Nested case-control study of esophageal cancer in relation to occupational exposure to silica and other dusts. *Am J Ind Med* 1999;35:272

Rapiti E, *et al*. End stage renal disease among ceramic workers exposed to silica. *Occup Environ Med* 1999;56:559

Rosenman KD, *et al*. Connective tissue disease and silicosis. *Am J Ind Med* 1999;35:375

Wang X, Yano E. Pulmonary dysfunction in silica-exposed workers: a relationship to radiographic signs of silicosis and emphysema. *Am J Ind Med* 1999;36: 299

## Other particulates

Akila R, *et al.* Decrements in cognitive performance in metal inert gas welders exposed to aluminium. *Occup Environ Med* 1999;56:632

Enterline PE. Carcinogenic effects of man-made vitreous fibers. *Annu Rev Public Health* 1991;12:459

Henneberger PK, Attfield MD. Respiratory symptoms and spirometry in experienced coal miners: effects of both distant and recent coal mine dust exposures. *Am J Ind Med* 1997;32:268

Wang M-L, *et al.* Clinically important $FEV_1$ declines among coal miners: an exploration of previously unrecognised determinants. *Occup Environ Med* 1999;56:837

Wang X, *et al.* Respiratory symptoms and pulmonary function of coal miners; looking into the effects of simple pneumoconiosis. *Am J Ind Med* 1999;35:124

**Table 17.1** Effects of particulates*

| | Exposure limit (mg/m³ respirable) | Clinical findings | X-Ray | Prognosis† |
|---|---|---|---|---|
| Aluminum alkyls | 2 | Irritation | | |
| Aluminum oxide (Al₂O₃), emery, bauxite | 10 | Mild irritation to skin and mucous membranes | | |
| Aluminum powder | 10 | Interstitial emphysema, non-nodular fibrosis. | Fibrosis | Progressive |
| Aluminum pyro powder | 5 | As above | Fibrosis | Progressive |
| Aluminum welding fumes | 5 | Irritation | | |
| Asphalt (petroleum fumes) | 5 | None | No change | No disease |
| Barytes (barium sulfate) | 10 | None | Nodulation of lungs | Non-progressive |
| Carbon black | 3.5 | Possible lung cancer | | |
| Coal dust Bituminous Anthracite | 0.9 0.4 | Gradual progression of respiratory impairment | Nodulation or 'reticulation' | Non-progressive in early stages |
| Coal tar | 0.2 | Photosensitivity and irritant, lung cancer, acne | | |
| Coke oven emissions | 0.15 | Lung and kidney cancer | | |
| Cotton dust | 0.2 | Progressive dyspnea, emphysema, weakness (byssinosis) | Emphysema | Non-progressive in early stages |
| Dusts, nuisance | 10 | Irritation | No change | No change |
| Flour | 0.5 | Asthma, bronchitis, lung function | | No change |

*Continued*

*Table 17.1 (continued)*

| | Exposure limit (mg/m³ respirable) | Clinical findings | X-Ray | Prognosis† |
|---|---|---|---|---|
| Glass, rock fiber | 5, 15 fibers/cc | Skin irritation, no lung involvement | No change | No disease |
| Grain dust | 4 | Sensitizer, asthma | Pneumonia | Non-progressive |
| Graphite | 2 | Dyspnea, cough, ventricular hypertrophy | Nodulation | Progressive |
| Iron oxide | 5 | Asymptomatic | Stippling to numerous small round shadows | Non-progressive |
| Mica, soapstone | 3, 20‡ | Similar to silicosis (see p. 329) | Fibrosis, pleural calcification | Progressive |
| Mineral oil mist, petroleum mist | 5 | Pneumonitis, possible carcinogen | Pneumonia | Non-progressive |
| Paraffin wax fume | 2 | Pneumonitis, possible carcinogen | Pneumonia | Non-progressive |
| Perlite | 10 | None | No change | No change |
| Silicon | 10 | Deposits in eyes, ears, skin, nose, with possible injury | No change | No change |
| Silicon carbide Silicon tetrahydride | 10 5 | Pulmonary fibrosis | Fibrosis | Non-progressive |
| Sugar cane dust | | Cough, dyspnea, hemoptysis, chills and fever, weakness, weight loss | Miliary mottling | Non-progressive after acute stage; cortisone is helpful in severe involvement |

*Continued*

*Table 17.1 (continued)*

| | Exposure limit (mg/m$^3$ respirable) | Clinical findings | X-Ray | Prognosis[†] |
|---|---|---|---|---|
| Talc | 2 | Similar to silicosis (see p. 329). Massive inhalation in children may cause acute bronchitis and bronchiolitis with plugging of small bronchi and cardiopulmonary failure | Fine fibrosis, calcification of pericardium | Progressive |
| Titanium dioxide | 10 | Pulmonary irritation | Slight fibrosis? | Non-progressive |
| Wood dust Hard | 1 | Conjunctivitis, lacrimation, keratitis, irritation of the upper respiratory passages, cancer | No change | Non-progressive |
| Soft Red cedar | 5 0.5 | As above Sensitizer | No change | Non-progressive |
| Soapstone | 3 | | Fibrosis similar to silicosis | Progressive |
| Starch | 10 | Dermatitis | Lung deposits | Non-progressive |
| Stearates, Na, K | 10 | Irritant | No change | Non-progressive |
| Zinc stearate | 10 | Irritant | Lung deposits | Progressive |

*None of these dusts is toxic when ingested; [†]after withdrawal from exposure; [‡]million particles per cubic foot

# IV. Household hazards

# 18 Cosmetics*

## BROMATES

Bromates are used as neutralizers in cold waves. On contact with acids such as gastric hydrochloric acid, potassium bromate releases hydrogen bromate, which is an irritating acid.

The fatal dose of bromate is estimated to be 4 g, or 100 ml of a 3% solution. Ingestion of 0.5 g by a 6-year-old boy caused deafness and renal failure. The usual neutralizer contains 15 g of bromate, which is diluted in 500 ml of water to make a 3% solution. About 10 fatalities from bromate poisoning have been reported. Bromates are extremely irritating and injurious to tissues, especially those of the central nervous system and kidneys. The pathologic findings include kidney damage and hemolysis.

### Clinical findings

The principal manifestations of acute bromate poisoning are vomiting and collapse. Chronic poisoning has not been reported.

### Symptoms and signs (from ingestion)

Vomiting, diarrhea, abdominal pain, oliguria or anuria, lethargy, deafness, coma, convulsions, low blood pressure, and fast pulse. Cyanosis due to methemoglobinemia and hematuria due to hemolysis may occur as late reactions.

### Laboratory findings

Hematuria and proteinuria; elevated non-protein nitrogen during oliguria or anuria; methemoglobinemia.

---

*See also Table 18.1

## Prevention

Non-poisonous cold wave neutralizers are available and should be used. If poisonous neutralizers are used they must be stored and used safely.

## Treatment

### Emergency measures

Remove poison by gastric lavage or emesis (see pp. 29–32). The gastric lavage or emetic should contain 30–50 g of sodium bicarbonate and 50 g of sodium thiosulfate for each liter of water. At the end of gastric lavage give 15 ml of Fleet's Phospho-Soda or 10 g of sodium sulfate in 200 ml of the sodium bicarbonate–sodium thiosulfate solution. The prompt use of peritoneal dialysis or of hemodialysis has also been suggested.

### Antidote

Give sodium thiosulfate, 0.1–1 ml/kg intravenously as a 10% solution.

### General measures

(1) Relieve gastric irritation by giving milk or cream every hour.
(2) In the presence of cyanosis and respiratory difficulty, give $O_2$. If methemoglobin level is above 30% give methylene blue cautiously, beginning with half the usual amount (see p. 78).
(3) Treat dehydration by giving 5% dextrose in water. Use caution in the administration of electrolytes, depending on the state of kidney function.

### Special problems

Treat anuria (see p. 66).

## Prognosis

Deafness and renal impairment may be permanent. About 10% of those severely poisoned will die.

**Table 18.1** Miscellaneous cosmetics

| Cosmetic substance | Active chemical | Remarks | Treatment |
|---|---|---|---|
| Cold wave lotion (for cold wave neutralizer, see potassium bromate, p. 343, and perborate, p. 442) | Thioglycolates, thioglycerol | Gastrointestinal irritation occurs after ingestion. May cause sensitivity dermatitis with edema, burning of skin, itching, and papular rash; hypoglycemia, CNS depression, convulsions, and dyspnea are possible | Sensitivity dermatitis will disappear on discontinuing the use of cold wave preparations |
| Cuticle remover | Potassium hydroxide, 5% | See p. 257 | See p. 259 |
| Depilatories | Barium sulfide (see p. 133), thioglycolates (see above), alkalis | Gastrointestinal irritation occurs after ingestion | Treat as for alkalis (see p. 259) |
| Eyelash dye | Naphthylamine, phenylenediamines, toluenediamines, and other aromatic amino compounds | Sensitivity dermatitis or irritation of eyes may occur (see p. 167). Not likely to cause serious poisoning after ingestion of usual household preparations | Discontinue use |
| Face powder | Pigments, talc | Sensitivity dermatitis, pneumoconiosis (see p. 340) | Discontinue use |
| Hair dyes, permanent | Naphthylamines, phenylenediamines, toluenediamines, and other aromatic amino compounds | Excessive use may cause liver damage and skin sensitization (see p. 167). Serious acute poisoning is rare after ingestion of usual household preparations | See p. 169 |

*Continued*

*Table 18.1 (continued)*

| Cosmetic substance | Active chemical | Remarks | Treatment |
|---|---|---|---|
| Hair dyes, temporary | Silver, 0.1%; mercury, 0.1%: lead, 0.1%; arsenic, 0.1%; bismuth, 0.1%; pyrogallol, 1%; denatured alcohol, 50% | The small quantity of toxic ingredients present in hair dyes makes acute poisoning unlikely | Remove poison (see p. 29). Give dimercaprol if symptoms occur (see p. 87) |
| Hair lighteners | Ethanol, 25%; hydrogen peroxide, 6%; potassium persulfate, 10% | Mucous membrane and gastrointestinal irritation with nausea and vomiting and diarrhea | Discontinue further exposure |
| Hair spray lacquer (wave set) | Vegetable gums, synthetic gum, polyvinylpyrrolidone, carboxymethyl-cellulose, polyvinyl alcohol, denatured alcohol (50%) | Sensitivity dermatitis may occur. Inhalation causes pulmonary granulomatosis with increase in size of hilar lymph nodes and infiltration in the lung that sometimes resembles sarcoidosis | Discontinue further exposure |
| Hair straighteners | Sodium hydroxide (up to 15%) | See p. 257 | See p. 259 |
| Hair tonic | Capsicum, 0.5% | See p. 539 | See p. 539 |
|  | Ethanol, 75% | See p. 202 | See p. 207 |
| Lip dye, lipstick | Eosin, other pigments | Cheilitis, facial dermatitis, or stomatitis | Discontinue use |
| Perfume | Alcohol (to 90%) | See p. 202 | See p. 207 |
| Tanning agents | Dihydroxyacetone, dyes | Sensitivity dermatitis may occur | Discontinue use |

## DEMULCENTS AND PROTECTIVES

Many non-toxic compounds are used as skin protectives, as skin softeners, and as ingredients in cosmetics. The following compounds are not irritating, and toxic doses by ingestion would have to be in excess of 2 g/kg. Skin sensitization is unusual. Aspiration or inhalation of any of these products could cause a chemical pneumonitis. Implantation of any of these substances will cause foreign body reaction.

| | | |
|---|---|---|
| Algin | Kaolin | Sesame oil |
| Allantoin | Lanolin | Silicone |
| Aluminum hydroxide | Make-up, liquid | Sorbic acid |
| Calcium carbonate | Methylcellulose | Spermaceti |
| Calcium phosphate | Monoacetin | Starch |
| Caprylates | Neatsfoot oil | Stearic acid |
| Carbowax | Paraffin | Titanium oxide |
| Chlorophyll | Polysorbate | Triacetin |
| Cleansing cream | Polyvinyl acetate | Umbelliferone |
| Hair dye, vegetable | Polyvinylpyrrolidone | Zinc oxide |
| Hair oil, cream | Red oil | |
| Hand lotion, cream | Rosi | |
| Hydroxyethyl cellulose | Rouge | |

### Reference

Babl FE, *et al*. Oral and airway sequelae after hair relaxer ingestion. *Pediatr Emerg Care* 2001;17:36

# 19  Food poisoning

## BOTULISM

Botulinus toxin is a heat-labile protein that can be destroyed by boiling at 100°C for 1 min or heating in water at 80°C for 10 min.

Botulism is caused by the exotoxin produced by the anaerobic growth of *Clostridium botulinum* at pH >4.6 and temperatures >3°C. Growth frequently occurs in underprocessed, non-acid canned foods. Seven antigenic types of toxin occur – A, B, C, D, E, F, and G; types A, B, and E are the most important. Foods most often responsible are meats, fish, and vegetables; olives and fruits are occasionally responsible. Botulism can occur in infants fed honey, fresh fruit or vegetables, or other foods containing the spores. Exotoxin production then occurs in the gut. Wound botulism can occur. The fatal dose of a contaminated food may be 0.1 ml.

Botulinus toxin causes muscle paralysis by blocking the transfer of nerve impulses at the motor end plate. Pathologic findings are congestion and hemorrhage in all organs, especially in the central nervous system.

### Clinical findings

The principal manifestations of acute botulism are vomiting, double vision, and muscular paralysis.

In adult poisoning the symptoms begin 8 hours to 8 days after ingestion, with nausea, vomiting, and sometimes diarrhea and abdominal distress. Progression to muscular weakness with marked fatigability, ptosis, dysarthria, blurred or double vision, dilated pupils, difficulty in swallowing, weakness paralysis of the respiratory muscles, and quadriplegia. Gastrointestinal symptoms may be absent. Deep tendon reflexes are not abolished. Pupillary response to light may be diminished or lost. The toxin can be identified in food, blood, feces, stomach contents, or tissues. In infants there is progressive paralysis that may result in respiratory compromise. The paralysis gradually disappears after 3–4 weeks.

## Prevention

A temperature of 115°C is required to destroy *C. botulinum* spores; this temperature can only be reached by pressure cooking. Process canned foods according to the methods approved by the Department of Agriculture as described in *Home Canning of Fruits and Vegetables*, Catalog No. Al. 77:8; and *Home Canning of Meat*, Catalog No. Al. 77:6. The pamphlets are obtainable from the Superintendent of Documents, US Government Printing Office, Washington, DC 20402.

Boil or pressure cook suspect canned foods for 15 min before serving.

If poisoning occurs in any member of a family or a group, treat every person who may have eaten the suspect food. Do not wait for symptoms to develop.

## Treatment

### *Emergency measures*

(1) Immediately upon suspecting food poisoning, and if the patient is asymptomatic, remove the toxin by emesis. Otherwise, use airway-protected gastric lavage (see pp. 29–32). Follow by catharsis with Fleet's Phospho-Soda, 30–60 ml diluted 1:4, unless the patient has diarrhea.
(2) Draw blood for toxin determination in serum.
(3) Notify the local health department.

### *Antidote*

Give type ABE botulus antitoxin unless type A or type B has been identified and type AB antitoxin can be used. Dosage is 1 vial intravenously every 4 h until the symptoms no longer progress or until the toxin can no longer be demonstrated in the patient's serum. Serum sensitivity must be tested by injecting 0.1 ml of a 1:10 dilution of antitoxin in saline intradermally; wait 15 min before giving dose. Centers for Disease Control in Atlanta can advise on the use of antitoxin; telephone (404) 239-3670.

### *General measures*

Treat respiratory depression. Artificial respiration or assissted ventilation may be necessary to oxygenate the patient during the period of weakness. Prevent pulmonary aspiration by aseptic tracheal cleansing. If pneumonia develops treat with organism-specific chemotherapy.

**Prognosis**

Approximately 50% of those with severe poisoning die. Those who survive recover completely, but residual weakness may persist for more than a year. The mortality rate in infants is less than 5%.

**References**

Adler M, *et al*. Promising new approaches for treatment of botulinum intoxication. *J Appl Toxicol* 1999;19(Suppl):S3

Shapiro RL, *et al*. Botulism in the United States: a clinical and epidemiologic review. *Ann Intern Med* 1998;129:221

# BACTERIAL FOOD POISONING

Bacterial food poisoning is caused by toxins elaborated during the growth of staphylococci or other organisms (Table 19.1) in foods kept warm. Food poisoning typically occurs when food is allowed to stand at room temperature after it is cooked, either because spores that survive heating regrow or because the standing food is allowed to be contaminated. Reheating the food will not destroy staphylococcal toxins and may or may not destroy *Clostridium perfringens* toxins. Toxins from *Vibrio parahaemolyticus* and *Bacillus cereus* are destroyed by heating at 80°C. The foods most often responsible for this type of poisoning are ham, tongue, sausage, dried meat, fish products, milk and milk products (including cream and cream-filled bakery goods), and eggs.

Bacterial food poisoning is ordinarily self-limited since the bacteria do not continue to grow in the presence of normal bacterial flora. Symptoms presumably arise from the local effects of toxins. The mortality rate is approximately 1%.

**Clinical findings**

The principal manifestations of acute bacterial food poisoning are vomiting and diarrhea. Chronic poisoning has not been reported.

*Symptoms and signs*

Nausea and vomiting, diarrhea, abdominal cramps or pain, and weakness occur; the incubation period varies depending on the organisms (Table 19.1).

**Table 19.1** Bacterial food poisoning

| Source | Incubation period (hours) | Duration (days) | Occurrence |
|---|---|---|---|
| Staphylococcus | 1–6 | 1–2 | Carrier contamination |
| Clostridium perfringens | 8–22 | 1–2 | Spore growth |
| Bacillus cereus | 1–16 | 1 | Spore growth |
| Vibrio parahaemolyticus | 4–96 | 1–7 | Sea water contamination |

The symptoms ordinarily progress for 12–24 h and then regress. Abdominal pain and tenesmus may be severe. Prostration, mild fever, dehydration, and shock sometimes occur.

### Laboratory findings

The blood count may reveal hemoconcentration. Urinalysis may reveal a trace of protein. Diagnosis is based on recovery of organisms from food, stomach contents, or feces.

## Prevention

If foods containing meats, milk or milk products, fish, or eggs are not eaten immediately after being cooked, they should be chilled quickly and stored under refrigeration. Raw seafoods should not be eaten after storage. Seafoods should be protected from seawater contamination after cooking. Food handlers with skin or eye infections should not work until after recovery.

## Treatment

### Emergency measures

Control severe vomiting by administration of chlorpromazine (Thorazine), 25–100 mg rectally or intramuscularly, or other anti-emetic. Repeat every 4 h as necessary.

### General measures

Place the patient at bed rest and give nothing by mouth until vomiting has subsided for 4 hours. Then give oral fluids as tolerated for 12–24 h before beginning regular diet. If vomiting and diarrhea are severe, maintain fluid balance by giving 5% dextrose in saline intravenously. Diarrhea is self-limited and should not be suppressed.

**Prognosis**

If the patient lives for 48 hours, recovery is likely.

## SEAFOOD POISONING (see also Chapter 35)

### Ciguatera

One of the most common toxin-associated food poisoning in the USA.

Sources: barracuda, grouper, jack, moray eel, mullet, parrotfish, porgy, snapper, surgeonfish, triggerfish, wrasse.

Neurotoxin produced by dinoflagellates, which are also responsible for red tides

*Gambierdiscus toxicus* has been identified as the dinoflagellate responsible for ciguatera, but other species may play a role.

The toxin becomes more concentrated as it moves up the food chain, so the larger, carnivorous fish such as barracuda, groupers, snappers, and jacks pose more threat.

### Prevention

Avoid consuming fish caught during red tides. Since toxin is more concentrated in the liver, avoid eating fish liver.

Ciguatera
* Is not destroyed by cooking or freezing
* The flavor of fish is not affected
* Has both anticolinesterase and cholinergic properties
* However, its toxicity is thought to be due to its inhibition of calcium regulation through the passive cell membrane sodium channels.

Another contributing factor may be another toxin contained in ciguatera fish, maitotoxin, which is a polycyclic ether.

**Symptoms**

- Appear within 6 h and not every person will necessarily be similarly affected
- Gastrointestinal: vomiting,watery diarrhea, abdominal cramps are usually not serious and self-limited

Odd neurologic symptoms can appear early or after the gastrointestinal effects resolve.

- Sensory tingling in lips and extremities that do not follow a dermatomal pattern
- Perception of loose teeth or dental pain
- Distortion of temperature perception (cold objects perceived as hot or painful)

A minority of patients may develop bradycardia or hypotension or rash.

The presentation of a patient is similar to type E botulism, organophosphate insecticide and tetrodotoxin poisoning.

**Treatment**

If presents within 3 h after ingestion, gastric lavage followed by activated charcoal.

If presents later, supportive.

For 3–6 months after the acute illness, patients should avoid fish, nuts, nut oils and alcohol, as these agents are thought to exacerbate the ciguatera syndrome. (expert opinion)

Subsequent reactions to ciguatera tend to be more severe than the original.

**Scombroid poisoning**

Accounts for approximately 5% of food poisoning reported to CDC in the USA.

Sources: inadequte refrigeration of fish after it has been caught, which allows bacteria on the fish surface to grow (*Proteus, Klebsiella*). Fish with dark meat have higher levels of histamine and are more likely associated with scombroid: tuna, mackerel bonita, swordfish, jacks; other fish associated include mahimahi, bluefish, herring, anchovy, sardine.

### Prevention

Refrigerate the fish adequately from the time it is caught to the time it is prepared. The toxicity is not prevented by cooking. Usually the "sharp" taste change is subtle and not detected when consumed.

### Symptoms

- Usually causes a histamine-like reaction (flushing, headache, burning sensation, dizziness, sunburn appearance to skin) and can be mistaken for an allergy. Usually does not cause urticaria.
- May cause gastrointestinal symptoms, such as nausea, vomiting, diarrhea.
- May occur within minutes to hours after consuming.
- Normally resolves on its own, but treatment with anti-histamines, $H_2$ blockers such as cimetidine are helpful.

### Paralytic shellfish poisoning

Serious illness causes by toxins produced by dinoflagellates: *Protogonyaulax catanella* and *P. tamarensis*.

Sources: bivalve mollusks such as mussels, clams, oysters, scallops

### Symptoms

- Usually occur within 30 min after ingestion.
- Are primarily neurologic with paresthesias, headache, ataxia, vertigo, cranial nerve dysfunction, muscle weakness.
- Occasionally gastrointestinal symptoms occur.
- Mortality 8–9% due to respiratory failure.
- If a patient survives the first 12–18 h after ingestion, relatively good chance for recovery.

### Treatment

Early recognition of the poisoning. Gastric lavage, activated charcoal, respiratory support and mechanical ventilation. Protect form aspiration pneumonia.

# CHEMICAL FOOD POISONING

Storage of foods such as fruit juice or sauerkraut in containers lined with cadmium, copper, zinc, or antimony (enameled metal pans) will lead to acute gastric irritation manifested by nausea and vomiting and diarrhea. The disease usually lasts 24–48 hours. If necessary atropine, 0.5 mg, and bismuth subcarbonate, 5 g, may be given orally to relieve abdominal distress. If symptoms are persistent and indicate metal poisoning, specific treatment may be necessary. (See cadmium, p. 279; antimony, p. 270; copper, p. 535; zinc, p. 535.) Food poisoning may also occur when meat preservatives that contain sodium nitrite are used excessively or erroneously in place of salt (see p. 468).

## References

Bhat RV, *et al.* A foodborne disease outbreak due to the consumption of moldy sorghum and maize containing fumonisin mycotoxins. *J Toxicol Clin Toxicol* 1996;35:249

Roberts JA. Economic aspects of food-borne outbreaks and their control. *Br Med Bull* 2000;56:133

Pitt JI. Toxigenic fungi and mycotoxins. *Br Med Bull* 2000;56:184

Wittman RJ, Flick GJ. Microbial contamination of shellfish: prevalence, risk to human health, and control strategies. *Annu Rev Public Health* 1995;16:123

# 20 Miscellaneous chemicals*

## BLEACHING PRODUCTS (Clorox, Purex, Sani-Clor)

Bleaching solutions are 3–6% solutions of sodium hypochlorite in water. The solution used for chlorinating swimming pools is 20% sodium hypochlorite. These solutions are about as corrosive as similar concentrations of sodium hydroxide. Upon contact with acid gastric juice or acid solutions, they release hypochlorous acid, which is extremely irritating to skin and mucous membranes but apparently is rapidly inactivated by blood serum and has low systemic toxicity. Buffering the acid by the administration of antacids offers a rapid means of reducing the irritating effect. Do not use acid antidotes in the treatment of sodium hypochlorite poisoning. Sodium thiosulfate immediately reduces hypochlorite to non-toxic products but may produce hydrogen sulfide in contact with acid. Mixing sodium hypochlorite with ammonia produces gaseous chloramines, which release HCl and ammonia on contact with moisture. Chloramine-T is a water-soluble solid containing about 12% available chlorine, which is released slowly on contact with water.

The fatal dose of 3–6% sodium hypochorite for children is estimated to be about 30 ml if emesis does not occur. The fatal dose of chloramine -T may be as low as 0.5 g.

### Clinical findings

The principal manifestation of acute poisoning with bleaching solutions is severe irritation with vomiting. Chronic poisoning does not occur.

Inhalation of hypochlorous acid fumes causes severe pulmonary irritation with coughing and choking followed by pulmonary edema. Ingestion causes irritation and corrosion of mucous membranes with pain and vomiting. Systemic effects include fall in blood pressure, delirium, and coma. Edema of the pharynx and larynx may be severe. Aspiration causes severe tracheobronchial irritation and exudation. Esophageal stenosis may occur later. Perforation of the esophagus or stomach has occurred but is rare. Prolonged skin contact

---

*See also Table 20.1

with bleaching solution causes irritation. Chloramine-T causes cyanosis and respiratory failure.

**Treatment**

*Emergency measures*

(1) Remove bleaching solution from the skin by flooding with water.
(2) Dilute and decompose swallowed bleaching solution by giving milk, melted ice cream, or beaten eggs. Antacids such as milk of magnesia or aluminum hydroxide gel are also useful. Do not use emesis, lavage, or acid antidotes.
(3) Treat chloramine-T poisoning with nitrite and thiososulfate administration as for cyanide (p. 314)

*General measures*

Treat as for esophageal lesions due to sodium hydroxide poisoning (see p. 259).

**Prognosis**

Recovery is likely if treatment is started early.

**References**

Babl FE, *et al*. Airway edema following household bleach ingestion. *Am J Emerg Med* 1998;16:514

Ross MP, Spiller HA. Fatal ingestion of sodium hypochlorite bleach with associated hypernatremia and hyperchloremic metabolic acidosis. *Vet Human Toxicol* 1999;41:82

# SOAPS AND DETERGENTS

Soaps and detergents can be grouped into three general classes that differ in toxic effects: anionic detergents, non-ionic detergents, and cationic detergents.

### Anionic detergents

The anionic household detergents (hand dishwashing liquids, hair shampoo) are sulfonated hydrocarbons or phosphorylated hydrocarbons. Powdered, flake, or bar soaps are made of sodium, potassium, or ammonium salts of fatty acids. Laundry compounds (All, Tide, Cheer, etc.) have added water softeners such as sodium phosphate, sodium carbonate, or sodium silicate (see p. 257).

The anionic detergents irritate the skin by removing natural oils, causing redness, soreness, and papular dermatitis. In sensitive persons they also cause thickening of the skin with weeping, cracking, scaling, and blistering. Ingestion causes oropharyngeal irritation, abdominal discomfort, diarrhea, intestinal distension, and occasionally vomiting. Fatalities from ingestion have not been reported. Animal experiments on anionic detergents without additives indicate that the LD50 ranges from 1 to 5 g/kg. The maximum safe amount for children may be estimated at 0.1–1 g/kg. The following are typical compounds: alkyl sodium sulfate, sodium lauryl sulfate, sodium alkyl phosphate, sodium aryl alkyl sulfonate, dioctyl sodium sulfosuccinate (docusate), and sodium oleate. The presence of enzymes does not increase the toxicity, but the enzymes are potent sensitizers. In pregnant women concentrated soap enema at term has caused colitis and possible fetal injury.

Skin eruptions are treated by removal from further exposure. For ingestion of detergents or soap, give fluids and allow vomiting to occur. Flush skin or eyes with water. For laundry compounds containing sodium phosphate or sodium carbonate, see p. 259.

Additives in soaps or detergents, including deodorants, may be skin sensitizers. Enzyme additives cause asthma.

### Non-ionic detergents

These compounds are only slightly irritating to the skin and are apparently harmless by ingestion. Single doses of 20 g by mouth produce no symptoms. The following are typical examples: alkyl aryl polyether sulfates, alcohols, or sulfonates; alkyl phenol polyglycol ethers; polyethylene glycol alkyl aryl ethers; and sorbitan monostearate.

No treatment is necessary.

### Cationic detergents (see p. 452)

**Table 20.1** Miscellaneous chemicals

| Common name | Poisonous ingredient | Remarks | Treatment |
|---|---|---|---|
| Aquarium products | Sodium chloride<br>Copper sulfate<br>Sodium hydroxide | See p. 568<br>See p. 533<br>See p. 257 | See p. 568<br>See p. 535<br>See p. 259 |
| Baking powder | Tartaric acid (50%) | Renal injury is possible from more than 1 g/kg orally. Tetany from reduction of ionic calcium | Give 10 ml of 10% calcium gluconate IV |
| Baking soda | Sodium bicarbonate | Causes alkalosis in doses over 5 g/kg. Alkalosis can also occur from skin application | Treat alkalosis by giving fluids (see p. 69) |
| Bleach, powdered | N-Chlorosuccinimide; 1,3-dichloro-5,5-dimethylhydantoin (exposure limit 0.2 mg/m$^3$); dichloroisocyanurate; sodium perborate (see p. 442); trichloroisocyanate. These products also contain 10–20% sodium carbonate (see p. 257) | Bronchospasms; mild inflammation and edema of eyes and upper respiratory tract; irritation or corrosion of stomach. Large ingested doses (0.5–1 g/kg) may cause weakness, lethargy, tremors, salivation, lacrimation, dyspnea, and coma | Remove by gastric lavage or emesis |
| Carpet backing | Latex (rubber) emulsion | Intestinal obstruction is possible | Gastric lavage and catharsis |
| Chlorinated lime | Calcium hypochlorite (10–70% available chlorine) | Irritating in lower strengths; 70% preparation may cause corrosion and severe local injury | Emesis; treat as for bleaching solution (see p. 357) |
| Cleaners, abrasive | Sodium phosphates | See p. 257 | See p. 259 |

*Continued*

*Table 20.1 (continued)*

| Common name | Poisonous ingredient | Remarks | Treatment |
|---|---|---|---|
| Cleaners, liquid | Sodium phosphates<br>Kerosene<br>Pine oil<br>Glycerol ethers | See p. 257<br>See p. 228<br>See p. 536<br>See p. 209 | See p. 259<br>See p. 230<br>See p. 539<br>See p. 211 |
| Cleaning solvents (inflammable) | Petroleum hydrocarbons | Also called Stoddard solvent or French dry cleaner. See Kerosene (p. 228) | See p. 230 |
| Cleaning solvents (non-inflammable, 'safe') | Carbon tetrachloride<br>Trichloroethylene | 'Safe' only because it is non-inflammable. | See p. 174<br>See p. 181 |
| Cloth-marking ink | Aniline | Produces methemoglobinemia by skin absorption or ingestion | See p. 169 |
| Crayons, industrial | Lead chromate | See p. 280 | See p. 282 |
| Dishwashing compounds (machine) | Sodium polyphosphates, sodium carbonate, sodium silicates | Irritating and corrosive to mucous membranes (see p. 257). Cause hypocalcemia with shock, cyanosis, slow pulse, tetany | Give 5 ml of 10% calcium gluconate IV and repeat as necessary |
| Drain cleaners (e.g. Drano) | Sodium hydroxide (90%)<br>Sulfuric acid (100%) | See p. 257<br><br>See p. 242 | See p. 259<br><br>See p. 245 |
| Dyes, cloth | Synthetic dyes, salt | May produce gastric irritation or skin sensitization | Remove |
| Dyes, fish bait | Chrysoidin | Urinary bladder irritant and carcinogen | Avoid |
| Dye remover | Sodium hydrosulfite (80%)<br>Sodium carbonate (20%) | See p. 256<br><br>See p. 257 | See p. 256<br><br>See p. 259 |

*Continued*

Table 20.1 (continued)

| Common name | Poisonous ingredient | Remarks | Treatment |
|---|---|---|---|
| Fertilizer | Ammonium nitrate, phosphate, and metal salt | Produce mild gastric irritation and possibly methemoglobinemia (see p. 78) | Dilute with milk or water |
| Fireworks | Arsenic<br>Mercury<br>Antimony<br>Lead<br>Phosphorus | See p. 270<br>See p. 294<br>See p. 269<br>See p. 282<br>See p. 301 | See p. 273<br>See p. 298<br>See p. 270<br>See p. 288<br>See p. 304 |
| Fluorescent lamps | Beryllium salts<br>Mercury | See p. 275<br>See p. 294 | See p. 276<br>See p. 298 |
| Fuel tablets | Metaldehyde<br>Methenamine | See p. 219<br>See p. 501 | See p. 221<br>See p. 501 |
| Furniture polish | Turpentine<br>Petroleum hydrocarbons | See p. 536<br>See p. 228 | See p. 537<br>See p. 230 |
| Indelible pencils | Triphenylmethane dyes | Injurious to tissues. Puncture wound or eye contamination causes pain, edema, and necrosis. Treat eye contamination by washing with water for at least 15 minutes. Repeated instillation of 1% fluorescein solution (*must be sterile*) will remove the dye by forming a soluble salt (see p. 33). Treat puncture wounds by surgical debridement | |
| Ink eradicator | Sodium hypochlorite (5%) | See p. 356 | See p. 357 |
| Ink, writing | Synthetic dyes, ferrous sulfate, tannic acid | May produce gastric irritation | Give demulcents |
| Matches<br>Safety<br>Striking surface, safety<br>Strike-anywhere | <br>Potassium chlorate<br>Red phosphorus<br><br>Phosphorus sesqui-sulfide (p. 301), potassium chlorate (p. 453) | <br>See p. 453<br>See p. 301<br><br>May cause nausea and vomiting | <br>See p. 454<br>See p. 304<br><br>Remove by gastric lavage or emesis |

*Continued*

*Table 20.1 (continued)*

| Common name | Poisonous ingredient | Remarks | Treatment |
|---|---|---|---|
| Moth repellent | p-Dichlorobenzene | See p. 197 | See p. 174 |
| | Naphthalene | See p. 234 | See p. 235 |
| Paints | Potentially toxic metallic compounds as pigments | See pp. 279 and 288 | |
| Oil type | Ill effects from single ingestion caused by the vehicle (see Petroleum distillates, Xylene) | | See pp. 230 and 233 |
| | After multiple ingestions of dry paint lead poisoning is possible | | See p. 288 |
| Emulsion type (latex base) | These contain water as a vehicle and a variety of pigments and suspending agents, none of which are seriously toxic. The single acute toxic dose is more than 5 ml/kg. Large doses might cause gastrointestinal irritation without systemic toxicity | | Remove by gastric lavage |
| Paint, lacquer, and varnish removers. | Benzene | See p. 231 | See p. 233 |
| | Petroleum hydrocarbons | See p. 228 | See p. 230 |
| | Methylene chloride | See p. 183 | See p. 184 |
| | Methanol | See p. 199 | See p. 201 |
| Photographic developers | Metol, hydroquinone, p-phenylenediamine, and other amino compounds | Any of these compounds may sensitize the skin. The resulting dermatitis is characterized by weeping, crusting, and itching | Avoid further contact with the particular developer or compound responsible for the dermatitis |
| Photographic fixer | Sodium thiosulfate | Possible release of hydrogen sulfide on contact with acid (see p. 316) | |
| Plastic casting resin | Polyester monomer (65%), styrene monomer (34%) | Irritating to skin and mucous membranes | Remove by washing |

*Continued*

Table 20.1 (continued)

| Common name | Poisonous ingredient | Remarks | Treatment |
|---|---|---|---|
| Plastic resin hardener | Methyl ethyl ketone peroxide (60%), dimethyl phthalate (40%) | Corrosive to skin, mucous membranes, and eyes. See p. 151 | Remove by washing or cautious gastric lavage. Avoid emesis |
| Stamp pad inks | Aniline dyes | May produce gastric irritation, skin sensitization, methemoglobinemia | Remove. See p. 78 |
| Steam iron cleaner | Tetrasodium edetate (20%), sodium carbonate (20%) | Doses over 1 ml/kg cause tetany by reduction of ionic calcium. | Give 10 ml of 10% calcium gluconate IV |
| Water colors | Gum cambogia (gamboge) | See p. 543 | See p. 544 |

## References

Okumura T, *et al*. Intravenous detergent poisoning. *J Toxicol Clin Toxicol* 2000;38:347

Okumura T, *et al*. Severe respiratory distress following sodium oleate ingestion. *J Toxicol Clin Toxicol* 1998;36:587

# V. Medicinal poisons

# 21 Analgesics, antipyretics, and anti-inflammatory agents

## SALICYLATES

Aspirin (acetylsalicylic acid) is present in many analgesic tablets. Salicylic acid is used in corn applications and in dermatologic ointments or as sodium salicylate for internal use. Methyl salicylate (oil of wintergreen) is the active ingredient in many skin liniments and ointments used for analgesic purposes. Salicylamide, salsalate (Disalcid), and sodium thiosalicylate are less toxic than aspirin and are used as weak analgesics given orally.

The fatal dose of any salicylate is estimated to be 0.2–0.5 g/kg. In children the number of deaths caused by salicylates has declined precipitously over recent years; this is largely attributed to the use of child-proof containers. Toxic effects appear at varying plasma levels depending on the duration of poisoning (Figure 21.1) but are uncommon below 30 mg/dl. Ingestion of 1 teaspoon of methyl salicylate (4 g of salicylate) has been fatal to a 2½-year-old child. The exposure limit for salicylates in work atmospheres is 5 mg/m$^3$.

An association is now thought to exist between salicylate administration during certain viral infections (e.g. varicella, influenza) and the occurrence of Reye's syndrome; however, the exact nature of the relationship is not clear.

Salicylates in toxic doses stimulate the central nervous system directly to cause hyperpnea and also produce a metabolic derangement with accumulation of organic acids. During hyperpnea loss of $CO_2$ compensates for the metabolic increase in organic acids to maintain the blood pH at nearly 7.4, although in some instances arterial pH may rise. The pH of the urine remains continuously below 7. Renal losses of sodium and potassium accompanying organic acid excretion, accumulation of organic acid metabolites from the salicylate-induced metabolic derangement, and ketosis from starvation and dehydration bring on metabolic acidosis, especially in children under 4 years of age. Acidemia increases the fraction of un-ionized salicylic acid, facilitating its entry into the brain. Blood $pCO_2$, bicarbonate, and pH fall progressively, indicating inadequate buffering capacity in the blood. In severe poisoning in small children or adults with renal failure, hyperkalemia may become a problem.

At therapeutic doses salicylates interfere with platelet aggregation, causing a prolongation of bleeding time. At toxic doses salicylates lower plasma prothrombin levels by interfering with the utilization of vitamin K in the liver. In the presence of gastric acid aspirin produces direct mucosal injury and consequent bleeding. The presence of alcohol increases mucosal injury. Salicylates are absorbed readily from the gastrointestinal tract, more rapidly in the presence of an alkalinizing agent such as sodium bicarbonate. Elimination of salicylates by the body is almost entirely by means of renal excretion; thus, renal function must be adequate. In the presence of normal renal function approximately 50% of a toxic dose will be excreted within the first 24 h. Excretion is 3–10 times as rapid if the urine is alkaline. If renal function is adequate and urine is alkaline, serum salicylate will fall to half the initial level in about 6 h.

The pathologic findings in deaths from salicylate poisoning are erosion and congestion of the gastrointestinal tract and edema, hemorrhages, and degenerative changes in the kidneys, brain, lungs, and liver.

### Clinical findings

The principal manifestations of salicylate poisoning are hyperpnea and disturbed acid–base balance.

*Acute poisoning* (from ingestion or skin absorption)

(1) Mild – Burning pain in the mouth, throat, or abdomen; slight to moderate hyperpnea; lethargy; vomiting; tinnitus; hearing loss; and dizziness.

(2) Moderate – Severe hyperpnea, marked lethargy, excitability, delirium, fever, sweating, dehydration, lack of coordination, restlessness, and ecchymoses.

(3) Severe – Severe hyperpnea, coma, convulsions, cyanosis, oliguria, uremia, pulmonary edema, and respiratory failure. Some of the symptoms may result from hypoglycemia.

Anaphylactic reactions after doses of 0.3–1 g can occur in those allergic to salicylates; people with asthma are more likely to react to salicylates and should avoid them.

*Chronic poisoning* (from ingestion or skin absorption)

Tinnitus, abnormal bleeding (gastric or retinal), gastric ulcer, weight loss, mental deterioration, skin eruptions. Liver damage can occur in normal patients but is more likely in patients with systemic lupus erythematosus, juvenile rheumatoid arthritis, rheumatic fever, alcoholism, and possibly rheumatoid arthritis.

*Laboratory findings*

(1)  Determination of the blood salicylate level (Figure 21.1) when urine spot test for salicylates is positive (see (5)). (*Note:* Figure 21.1 does not apply to chronic poisoning.) The relationship between serum salicylate levels (in mg/dl) in the first 6 h after poisoning is as follows: less than 45, not intoxicated; 45–65, mild intoxication; 65–90, moderate intoxication; 90–120, severe intoxication; above 120, usually lethal. The serum salicylate level may continue to rise for 6–10 h after ingestion as a result of intestinal absorption. The ferric nitrate method of determining serum salicylate levels does not indicate the presence of salicylamide.

(2)  Blood bicarbonate below 8 mEq/l indicates significant acidosis and disturbances in carbohydrate metabolism.

(3)  Other blood chemistry values that must be known for adequate treatment of severe salicylate poisoning include arterial pH; serum chloride, potassium, and sodium; and blood glucose.

(4)  Hematuria and proteinuria may be present.

(5)  To test for salicylates in urine, add a few drops of tincture of ferric chloride or Trinder reagent to an aliquot of urine. A violet color indicates a phenolic compound (salicylate). Since this test is sensitive, it only indicates that the patient has taken salicylates; it does not indicate the quantity. If positive, obtain a serum salicylate level. Both reagents were found 100% sensitive. False positive results occur with non-steroidal anti-inflammatory drugs, selective serotonin re-uptake inhibitors, phenothiazines and acetaminophen, and with ketosis.

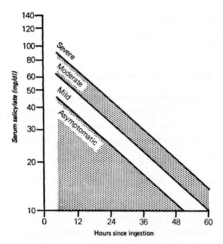

**Figure 21.1** Nomogram relating serum salicylate concentration and expected severity of intoxication at varying intervals following ingestion of a single dose of salicylate. Redrawn and reproduced, with permission, from Done AK. Salicylate intoxication. *Pediatrics* 1960;26:800

(6) Phenistix can be used to give semiquantitative indications of serum salicylate levels above 20 mg/dl. A Phenistix dipped into separated plasma or serum gives a tan color with levels below 40 mg/dl; a deeper brown color at 40–90 mg/dl; and a purple color above 90 mg/dl.

(7) Prothrombin levels may drop below 20% of normal.

(8) Long-term aspirin administration may result in abnormal liver function tests, including elevated alkaline phosphatase, AST, and ALT levels.

(9) Chronic salicylate administration increases urine cellular content, increases creatinine excretion, and reduces glomerular filtration rate.

(10) Blood loss in stools may vary from 1 to 3 g/d during chronic aspirin administration.

**Prevention**

Salicylates should not be given to children with varicella, influenza, or certain other viral infections. Make certain that parents understand the proper dosage of salicylates for children. Do not apply salicylic acid ointment repeatedly over a large part of the body surface. If salicylates are prescribed, parents should be advised against giving additional salicylates.

## Treatment

### Emergency measures

Remove salicylates by emesis with syrup of ipecac (see p. 90) unless respiration is depressed. Do not use apomorphine. Delay absorption of the remaining poison by giving activated charcoal (see pp. 31–32). If respiration is depressed, use airway-protected gastric lavage. Enteric-coated tablets can be removed by lavage with 1% sodium bicarbonate. Gastric lavage and catharsis will remove significant amounts of salicylates up to 12 h after ingestion.

### General measures

Intravenous alkaline fluids are used to treat hypotension and to alkalinize the urine rather than to reverse the acidosis *per se*.

(1) Draw blood for initial measurement of bicarbonate, chloride, potassium, sodium, glucose, and arterial pH levels.

(2) In mild poisoning with adequate urine output and no vomiting, give milk and fruit juice orally every hour up to a total of 100 ml/kg in the first 24 h.

(3) In severe poisoning begin hydration in the first hour with intravenous 5% dextrose or normal saline with 75 mEq/l sodium bicarbonate. After urine flow is established, treat potassium deficit. Monitor urine output; fluid retention can lead to cerebral edema with blurring of the optic disk, periorbital edema, and central nervous system depression. In the presence of fluid retention give furosemide, 0.25–1 mg/kg intravenously.

(4) Maintenance of alkaline urine enhances salicylate excretion, but is difficult in chronically poisoned infants. Further adjustment of sodium and potassium in fluids should be based on serum sodium and potassium determinations.

(5) Coma persisting after the salicylate level has returned to normal indicates the possibility of cerebral edema.

*Special problems*

(1) In the presence of abnormal bleeding or hypoprothrombinemia, give phytonadione, 10 mg intramuscularly. Fresh blood or platelet transfusion may be necessary.

(2) Do not give barbiturates, paraldehyde, morphine, or other central nervous system depressants.

(3) If renal function is impaired dialysis must be used to remove salicylates and control electrolyte imbalance.

(4) Reduce hyperpyrexia by tepid sponging. Do not use alcohol for sponging. Elevated body temperature must not be allowed to persist.

## Prognosis

If the blood bicarbonate level can be maintained above 15 mEq/l, recovery is likely. Chronic poisoning responds very slowly to treatment.

## References

Brubacher JR, Hoffman RS. Salicylism from topical salicylates: review of the literature. *J Toxicol Clin Toxicol* 1996;34:431

Chan TYK. Medicated oils and severe salicylate poisoning: quantifying the risk based on methyl salicylate content and bottle size. *Vet Human Toxicol* 1996;38:133

Chan TYK. Potential dangers from topical preparations containing methyl salicylate. *Human and Exp Toxicol* 1996;15:747

Lanas A, *et al*. Nitrovasodilators, low-dose aspirin, other nonsteroidal anti-inflammatory drugs, and the risk of upper gastrointestinal bleeding. *N Engl J Med* 2000;343:834

Schiavino D, *et al*. The aspirin disease. *Thorax* 2000;55(S2):S66

Sørensen HT, *et al*. Risk of upper gastrointestinal bleeding associated with use of low-dose aspirin. *Am J Gastroenterol* 2000;95:2218

Sporer KA, Khayam-Bashi H. Acetaminophen and salicylate serum levels in patients with suicidal ingestion or altered mental status. *Am J Emerg Med* 1996;14:443

Szczeklik A, Nizankowska E. Clinical features and diagnosis of aspirin induced asthma. *Thorax* 2000;55(S2):S42

## ACETAMINOPHEN, PHENACETIN

Acetaminophen (paracetamol) is used alone or in combination with other drugs in a number of proprietary analgesic compounds. Phenacetin is not available in the USA.

The popularity of acetaminophen has increased dramatically. Most fatalities from acetaminophen have occurred in adults who have intentionally taken 10 g or more (140 mg/kg).

Toxic doses of acetaminophen can injure the liver, kidneys, heart, and central nervous system. Liver damage from acetaminophen develops within hours as a result of oxidation of acetaminophen to toxic metabolites (epoxides); these damage the liver after the detoxifying agent glutathione has been depleted. N-Acetylcysteine, cysteamine, and methionine can act as glutathione precursors and are thought to block the formation of toxic oxidation products of acetaminophen. Acetaminophen is rapidly absorbed. Thirty minutes after ingestion of 1 g of acetaminophen, 10 g of activated charcoal (see pp. 31–32) reduces total absorption by only 30%.

### Clinical findings

The principal manifestation of poisoning with acetaminophen is hepatic failure. It does not cause acid–base disturbances such as those that occur with the salicylates.

### Acute poisoning (from ingestion)

Ingestion of 150 mg/kg or more causes nausea and vomiting, drowsiness, confusion, liver tenderness, low blood pressure, cardiac arrhythmias, jaundice, and acute hepatic and renal failure. Deaths have resulted from liver necrosis up to 2 weeks after ingestion.

### Chronic poisoning

Hepatic damage has been reported after daily ingestion of acetaminophen for a year or more, but this is rare. Chronic phenacetin ingestion is associated with renal failure.

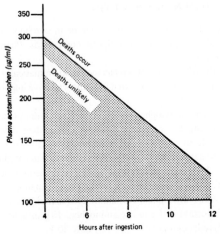

**Figure 21.2** Nomogram relating plasma acetaminophen concentration with time. Adapted from Prescott LF, *et al.* Cysteamine, methionine, and penicillamine in the treatment of paracetamol poisoning. *Lancet* 1976;2:109

### Laboratory findings

(1) Plasma acetaminophen levels peak 2½–4 or more hours after ingestion of the drug. In acute acetaminophen poisoning, unless the amount ingested is known to be less than 100–150 mg/kg body weight, the plasma acetaminophen level should be determined 3–4 or more hours after ingestion in order to determine treatment (Figure 21.2). The initial level and levels determined at intervals thereafter should be plotted on semilogarithmic paper to determine the relative potential for toxicity and the disappearance half-time (half-life) of the drug (see p. 100). A half-life greater than 4 h indicates liver damage. Fatalities are unlikely unless the 4-h plasma acetaminophen level is above 300 μg/ml. Liver damage is likely in all patients with 4-h plasma acetaminophen levels above 300 μg/ml, in 40% of those with 250–300 μg/ml, in 25% of those with 150–250 μg/ml, and in 5% of those with 120–150 μg/ml. Levels below

$120\,\mu g/ml$ are non-toxic. About 25% of patients with 4-h plasma acetaminophen levels above $300\,\mu g/ml$ will develop acute renal failure.

(2) Liver damage is indicated by serum aspartate aminotransferase (AST) or alanine aminotransferase (ALT) levels above $40\,IU/l$, a prothrombin time ratio above 1.3 compared to normal, or a plasma bilirubin level above 1 mg/dl. Liver damage is severe if aspartate or alanine aminotransferase levels exceed $1000\,IU/l$.

(3) Urine may contain protein, casts, hemoglobin, or red blood cells.

## Treatment

### *Emergency measures*

Remove ingested drug by emesis with syrup of ipecac (see p. 90) unless respiration is depressed. Do not use apomorphine. Activated charcoal interferes with absorption of *N*-acetylcysteine, but opinion is divided as to the clinical significance of this. Give a saline cathartic. If respiration is depressed use airway-protected gastric lavage (see pp. 29–32). Efforts to remove acetaminophen are useless after 4 h.

### *Antidote* (best given within 10 h after ingestion)

(1) If the 4-h plasma acetaminophen level (Figure 21.2) exceeds $150\,\mu g/ml$, administration of *N*-acetylcysteine (available as Mucomyst) is suggested. *N*-Acetylcysteine is given orally, 140 mg of 20% solution per kilogram as a loading dose, followed by 70 mg/kg every 4 h for 3 days. Some physicians use a shorter course of treatment. It may be necessary to administer the drug via a nasogastric tube. Adverse effects include nausea and vomiting.

(2) Cysteamine hydrochloride and methionine have also been suggested, but these may be less effective and are more toxic. They are not available for use in the USA.

### *General measures*

(1) If the prothrombin time ratio exceeds 3.0 give phytonadione, 1–10 mg intramuscularly. Fresh plasma or clotting factor concentrates may be necessary.

(2) Forced diuresis may be harmful; peritoneal dialysis, hemodialysis, and hemoperfusion are ineffective.

**Prognosis**

In acute poisoning patients who survive will probably recover.

**References**

Buckley NA, *et al.* Activated charcoal reduces the need for *N*-acetylcysteine treatment after acetaminophen overdose. *J Toxicol Clin Toxicol* 1999;37:753

Buckley NA, *et al.* Oral or intravenous *N*-acetylcysteine: which is the treatment of choice for acetaminophen poisoning? *J Toxicol Clin Toxicol* 1999;37:759

Caravati EM. Unintentional acetaminophen ingestion in children and the potential for hepatotoxicity. *J Toxicol Clin Toxicol* 2000;38:291 (over 200mg/kg)

Cetaruk EW, *et al.* Tylenol extended relief overdose. *Ann Emerg Med* 1997;30: 105

Clark RF, *et al.* The use of ondansetron in the treatment of nausea and vomiting associated with acetaminophen poisoning. *J Toxicol Clin Toxicol* 1996;34:163

Horowitz RK, *et al.* Placental transfer of *N*-acetylcysteine following human maternal acetaminophen toxicity. *J Toxicol Clin Toxicol* 1996;35:447

Jones AL. Mechanism of action and value of *N*-acetylcysteine in the treatment of early and late acetaminophen poisoning: a critical review. *J Toxicol Clin Toxicol* 1998;36:277

Langford JS, Sheikh S. An adolescent case of sulfhemoglobinemia associated with high-dose metoclopramide and *N*-acetylcysteine. *Ann Emerg Med* 1999;34:538

Perrone J, *et al.* Predictive properties of a qualitative urine acetaminophen screen in patients with self-poisoning. *J Toxicol Clin Toxicol* 1999;37:769

Scharman EJ. Use of ondansetron and other antiemetics in the management of toxic acetaminophen ingestions. *J Toxicol Clin Toxicol* 1998;36:19

Weiner AL, *et al.* A comparison of two bedside tests for the detection of salicylates in urine. *Acad Emerg Med* 2000;7:834

Woo OF, *et al.* Shorter duration of oral *N*-acetyl cysteine therapy for acute acetaminophen overdose. *Ann Emerg Med* 2000;35:363

Wright RO, *et al.* Hemolysis after acetaminophen overdose in a patient with glucose-6-phosphate dehydrogenase deficiency. *J Toxicol Clin Toxicol* 1996;34: 731

**Table 21.1** Miscellaneous drugs used in painful conditions

| Drug | Clinical findings and treatment |
| --- | --- |
| Gold compounds: aurothioglucose (Solganal), gold sodium thiosulfate, gold sodium thiomalate (Myochrysine) | Skin rash, stomatitis, pruritus, herpes, papular eruptions, nausea and vomiting, diarrhea, metallic taste, proteinuria, hematuria, uremia, nephrosis, hepatitis, fever, exfoliative dermatitis, photosensitivity, granulocytopenia, thrombocytopenic purpura, hypersensitivity pneumonitis, and aplastic anemia. **Remarks:** Patients should avoid exposure to sunlight, X-rays, and ultraviolet radiation while under treatment with gold compounds. **Treatment:** Give dimercaprol (see p. 87) or penicillamine (see p. 94) |
| Pyrazolones: phenylbutazone, antipyrine, aminopyrine, dipyrone | Convulsions, hepatic damage, leukopenia, agranulocytosis, rash, renal damage |
| Cincophen, neocincophen | Hepatic damage, acidosis. Do not use |
| Nonsteroidal anti-inflammatory agents: celecoxib (Celebrex), diclofenac (Voltaren), diflunisal (Dolobid), etodolac (Lodine), fenoprofen (Nalfon), flurbiprofen (Ansaid), ibuprofen (Motrin), indomethacin (Indocin), ketoprofen (Orudis), ketorolac (Toradol), meclofenamate (Meclomen), mefenamic acid (Ponstel), nabumetone (Relafen), naproxen (Naprosyn), oxaprozin (Daypro), piroxicam (Feldene), rofecoxib (Vioxx), sulindac (Clinoril), suprofen (Profenal), tolmetin (Tolectin) | Gastrointestinal irritation with erosion and hemorrhage or perforation, kidney damage, liver damage, heart damage, hemolytic anemia, agranulocytosis, thrombocytopenia, aplastic anemia, and meningitis can possibly occur with any of these drugs. Other symptoms include headache, dizziness, tinnitus, confusion, blurred vision, mental disturbances, skin rash, stomatitis, edema, reduced retinal sensitivity, corneal deposits, and hyperkalemia. Naproxen has caused cough, eosinophilia, and pulmonary infiltration. Sudden death has occurred after indomethacin in children. **Prevention:** Indomethacin and mefenamic acid are contraindicated and the others possibly hazardous in children. **Treatment:** Discontinue use. Remove oral overdoses by emesis if patient is alert, by gastric lavage if patient is depressed. Activated charcoal is useful (p. 31). Treat symptomatically (see p. 371) |

# INTERACTIONS (see p. 20)

If corticosteroids are withdrawn during continuing salicylate therapy salicylate toxicity can occur. Phenylbutazone decreases excretion of hydroxyhexamide, the active metabolite of acetohexamide. Phenylbutazone and congeners and indomethacin potentiate the effects of warfarin, tolbutamide, chlorpropamide, and phenytoin by displacement from binding sites.

Salicylate, phenylbutazone and congeners, and indomethacin enhance the effects of cortisone by displacement.

Salicylates enhance the effects of coumarin anticoagulants and hypoglycemic drugs. Salicylates potentiate the effects of methotrexate by protein displacement.

Probenecid raises the blood level of indomethacin by blocking its excretion. If indomethacin and furosemide are given together or if beta-blocking agents and indomethacin are given together, the response to the drugs is altered.

Salicylamide may greatly potentiate hepatic toxicity of acetaminophen.

### References

Guenthner T, *et al*. Goldschlager allergy in a gold allergic patient. *Vet Human Toxicol* 1999;41:246

Seifert SA, *et al*. Massive ibuprofen ingestion with survival. *J Toxicol Clin Toxicol* 2000;38:55

Spiller HA, *et al*. Prospective multicenter evaluation of tramadol exposure. *J Toxicol Clin Toxicol* 1996;35:361

## PHARMACOKINETICS AND TOXIC CONCENTRATIONS (see p. 100)

| | $pK_a$ | $T_{1/2}$ (h) | $V_d$ (l/kg) | % Binding | Toxic concentration (μg/ml) |
|---|---|---|---|---|---|
| Acetaminophen | 9.5 | 2–7 | 0.7–1 | 25 | 30, 50[†] |
| Aminopyrine | 5.0 | 2–7 | | 15 | |
| Aspirin | 3.5 | 2–24 | 0.1, 0.3* | 50–75 | 500 |
| Fenoprofen | 4.5 | 1.5–3 | 0.1 | 99 | 710[†] |
| Ibuprofen | 4.4 | 2 | 0.14 | 99 | |
| Indomethacin | 4.5 | 4–12 | 0.34–1.57 | 92–99 | 5 |
| Naproxen | 5 | 10–17 | 0.09 | 98–99 | 400 |
| Oxyphenbutazone | 4.7 | 27–64 | | 90–99 | |
| Phenacetin | | 0.7–1.25 | 1–2.1 | 30 | |
| Phenazone | | | | | 20, 25[†] |
| Phenylbutazone | 4.5 | 29–175 | 0.02, 0.25* | 98 | 120 |
| Procaine | | | | | 15, 20[†] |
| Salicylamide | | | | | 40[†] |
| Salicylic acid | | | | | 150, 300[†] |
| Sulfinpyrazone | 2.8 | 2–3 | | 98–99 | |
| Sulindac | | 7 | | 93 | |
| Tolmetin | 3.5 | 5.3 | 0.04 | 90 | |

*For children; [†]fatal

# 22 Anesthetics

## COCAINE

Cocaine is used as a local anesthetic on mucous membranes.

The fatal dose after application to mucous membranes may be as low as 30 mg. While ingested cocaine is much less toxic than cocaine taken or administered by other routes, including application to mucous membranes, it is still a serious problem. Fatalities have also occurred when ingested rubber balloons or plastic bags containing large quantities of cocaine have broken.

In toxic doses cocaine first stimulates and then depresses the central nervous system in descending order from the cortex to the medulla. The pathologic findings in fatal cases of cocaine poisoning are congestion of the gastrointestinal tract, brain, and other organs.

### Clinical findings

The principal manifestations of cocaine poisoning are convulsions and circulatory failure.

*Acute poisoning* (from ingestion, injection, or absorption through mucous membranes or skin abrasions)

The initial symptoms are restlessness, excitability, hallucinations, tachycardia, dilated pupils, chills or fever, sensory aberrations, abdominal pain, vomiting, numbness, and muscular spasms. These are followed by irregular respirations, convulsions, coma, and circulatory failure. Death may occur almost immediately after the use of cocaine or may be delayed for 1–3 h. Fatal pulmonary edema has occurred after intravenous administration of the free cocaine base.

*Chronic poisoning* (from ingestion, injection, or absorption through mucous membranes or skin abrasions)

Hallucinations, mental deterioration, weight loss, and change of character. The use of cocaine as snuff can cause perforation of the nasal septum.

### Laboratory findings

These are noncontributory.

### Prevention

Avoid using more than 50 mg (1 ml of 5% solution) of cocaine on mucous membranes. Less should be used for patients under 20 years of age. Cocaine should never be injected.

### Treatment

### Acute poisoning

(1) Emergency measures:
  (a) Maintain airway and respiration. Delay absorption of ingested drug by giving activated charcoal and then remove from the stomach by gastric lavage or emesis (see pp. 29–32). Limit absorption from an injection site by ice pack. Efforts to remove the drug after 30 min are probably useless.
  (b) Control convulsions by giving diazepam, 0.1 mg/kg slowly intravenously. Be prepared to give artificial respiration. Treat tachycardia and other cardiac arrhythmias.
(2) General measures:
  (a) Succinylcholine may be necessary if convulsions interfere with respiration.
  (b) Maintain blood pressure with fluids. Vasopressors are hazardous.
  (c) For hypertensive reactions give phentolamine, 5 mg slowly intravenously.
  (d) Evaluate for the possible presence of other recreational substances.
  (e) Treat hyperthermia (see p. 73).

## *Chronic poisoning*

Discontinue use of the drug. There are usually no withdrawal symptoms following cocaine withdrawal such as those that occur after morphine withdrawal.

## Prognosis

If the patient survives the first 3 h after acute poisoning recovery is likely.

## References

Baumann BM, *et al*. Cardiac and hemodynamic assessment of patients with cocaine-associated chest pain syndromes. *J Toxicol Clin Toxicol* 2000;38:283

Cornish JW, O'Brien CP. Crack cocaine abuse: an epidemic with many public health consequences. *Annu Rev Public Health* 1996;17:259

Counselman FL, *et al*. Creatine phosphokinase elevation in patients presenting to the emergency department with cocaine-related complaints. *Am J Emerg Med* 1997;15:221

Daisley H, *et al*. Fatal cardiac toxicity temporally related to poly-drug abuse. *Vet Human Toxicol* 1998;40:21 (Cocaine)

Erickson TB, *et al*. Analysis of cocaine chronotoxicology in an urban ED. *Am J Emerg Med* 1998;16:568

Fines RE, *et al*. Cocaine-associated dystonic reaction. *Am J Emerg Med* 1997;15:513

Jawahar D, *et al*. Cocaine-associated intestinal gangrene in a pregnant woman. *Am J Emerg Med* 1997;15:510

June R, *et al*. Medical outcome of cocaine bodystuffers. *J Emerg Med* 2000;18:221

Kontos MC, *et al*. Myocardial perfusion imaging with technetium-99m sestamibi in patients with cocaine-associated chest pain. *Ann Emerg Med* 1999;33:639

Perron AD, Gibbs M. Thoracic aortic dissection secondary to crack cocaine ingestion. *Am J Emerg Med* 1997;15:507

Sporer KA, Firestone J. Clinical course of crack cocaine body stuffers. *Ann Emerg Med* 1997;29:596

Wang RY. pH-Dependent cocaine-induced cardiotoxicity. *Am J Emerg Med* 1999;17:364

Winbery S, *et al*. Multiple cocaine-induced seizures and corresponding cocaine and metabolite concentrations. *Am J Emerg Med* 1998;16:529

## PROCAINE AND OTHER LOCAL ANESTHETICS (Tables 22.1 and 22.2)

A large number of local anesthetics are used by injection or on skin or mucous membranes. Procaine, lidocaine, and other local anesthetic agents are used for antiarrhythmic effects. They are rapidly absorbed from mucous membranes.

For maximum safe doses see Tables 22.1 and 22.2. Local anesthetics ordinarily have no systemic effects when ingested, since they are rapidly hydrolysed. Excessive doses may cause methemoglobinemia, since even the hydrolytic products are still capable of forming methemoglobin.

**Table 22.1** Local anesthetics for injection (for clinical findings and treatment see p. 383–4)

| | Maximum adult dose by injection or topical application | |
|---|---|---|
| Drug | (mg) | (ml) |
| Bupivacaine (Marcaine, Sensorcaine) | 250 | 25 of 1% |
| Chloroprocaine (Nesacaine) | 750 | 75 of 1% |
| Etidocaine (Duranest) | 750 | 75 of 1% |
| Lidocaine (Xylocaine) | 500 | 50 of 1% |
| Mepivacaine (Carbocaine) | 400 | 40 of 1% |
| Prilocaine (Citanest) | 600 | 60 of 1% |
| Procaine (Novocaine) | 1000 | 100 of 1% |
| Ropivacaine (Naropine) | 250 | 25 of 1% |
| Tetracaine (Pontocaine) | 50 | 10 of 0.5% |

**Table 22.2** Local anesthetics for topical use (For treatment, see p. 384)

| | Maximum adult dose for surface use | | Additional clinical findings |
|---|---|---|---|
| Drug | (mg) | (ml) | |
| Benoxinate | 10 | 2.5 of 0.4% | |
| Benzyl alcohol | 5000 | 100 of 5% | Irritation, tissue injury |
| Butyl aminobenzoate (Cetacaine) | 1000 | 7 of 14% | Sensitivity dermatitis |
| Dibucaine (Corticaine) | 50 | 1 of 5% | |
| Dyclonine (Dyclone) | 300 | 30 of 1% | |
| Ethyl aminobenzoate (benzocaine) | 1000 | 7 of 14% | Cyanosis from methemoglobinemia |
| Pramoxine | 200 | 20 of 1% | |
| Proparacaine (Ophthaine) | 5 | 1 of 0.5% | |

After injection or surface application large doses induce severe circulatory collapse by direct depression of blood vessel tone or by an effect on the central nervous system. Blood pressure lowering effects are more pronounced after intravenous injection in patients with heart or liver disease. In large doses local anesthetics first stimulate and then depress the central nervous system. In pregnant patients these agents cross the placenta and are not readily metabolized by the liver of the fetus. The pathologic findings in fatal cases of poisoning are not characteristic.

## Clinical findings

The principal manifestations of poisoning with these agents are hypotension and convulsions.

*Acute poisoning* (from injection, ingestion, or application to mucous membranes)

Dizziness, cyanosis due to methemoglobinemia, fall in blood pressure, muscular tremors, convulsions, coma, irregular and weak breathing, cardiac standstill, and bronchial spasm. Ingestion of 300–600 mg of lidocaine has caused convulsions and respiratory failure in a 17-month-old child, and rapid intravenous injection of 2 g has caused cardiac arrest in an adult. Mepivacaine has been injected into an unborn baby's head during administration of caudal anesthesia; this caused asphyxia, cyanosis, bradycardia, and convulsions and resulted in death.

*Hypersensitivity*

Hypersensitivity reactions sometimes occur after repeated applications of local anesthetics to skin or mucous membranes. The findings are itching, erythema, excoriation, edema, and vesiculation.

*Laboratory findings*

The ECG may show atrioventricular block.

## Prevention

Do not use doses larger than the suggested maximum doses (Tables 22.1 and 22.2) either topically or by injection. Hypersensitivity can be tested by applying the local anesthetic to the nasal mucosa on a cotton pledget for at least 5 min prior to injection. Signs of discomfort such as irritation, burning, or swelling indicate hypersensitivity. However, tests of hypersensitivity may be unreliable. If procaine or lidocaine is administered parenterally for the treatment of cardiac irregularities, give only by slow intravenous infusion with electrocardiographic monitoring and stop at the first untoward sign.

## Treatment

### Acute poisoning

(1) Emergency measures – Remove ingested drug by induced emesis followed by activated charcoal (see pp. 31–32). Limit absorption from injection site by ice pack. Maintain airway and give artificial respiration with $O_2$ until convulsions are controlled and blood pressure and pulse return to normal. Efforts to remove the drug are probably useless after 30 min.

(2) Special problems:
   (a) Control convulsions with diazepam, 0.1 mg/kg intravenously, or give succinylcholine chloride (see p. 62). Perform artificial respiration with $O_2$ until convulsions are controlled (see p. 61), and continue giving $O_2$ until blood pressure and pulse return to normal. Adequate arterial $O_2$ saturation must be maintained. If convulsions are not continuous, the administration of $O_2$ may be sufficient to maintain the patient until the blood level of local anesthetic falls.
   (b) Treat methemoglobinemia with methylene blue, 1%, 0.1 ml/kg intravenously over 10 min.

(3) General measures:
   (a) Treat hypoxia (see p. 52).
   (b) Do not give stimulants.
   (c) Treat fall in blood pressure by placing the patient in a head-down position; give intravenous saline (see p. 57).
   (d) Exchange transfusions may be necessary in newborns with local anesthetic toxicity.

### Hypersensitivity reactions

(1) Remove from further exposure.
(2) Treat dermatitis (see p. 83).

### Prognosis

Survival for 1 hour indicates that the patient will recover.

### Reference

Spiller HA, *et al*. Multi-center retrospective evaluation of oral benzocaine exposure in children. *Vet Human Toxicol* 2000;42:228

## VOLATILE AND GASEOUS ANESTHETICS

Chloroform, desflurane (Suprane), divinyl ether, enflurane (Ethrane), ether (diethyl ether, ethyl ether), ethyl chloride, halothane (Fluothane), isoflurane (Forane), methoxyflurane (Penthrane), sevoflurane (Ultane), and trifluoro-ethylvinyl ether (fluroxene, Fluoromar) are volatile liquid anesthetic agents. Ethylene, cyclopropane, and nitrous oxide are gases. Volatile and gaseous anesthetics are used to produce general anesthesia.

Fatal doses of liquid anesthetic agents by ingestion or inhalation are approximately as follows: ether, 30 ml; chloroform, 10 ml; divinyl ether, 30 ml; halothane, 10 ml; methoxyflurane, 10 ml; fluroxene, 10 ml; enflurane, 10 ml. The exposure limit for chloroform is 2 ppm; for diethyl ether, 400 ppm; for enflurane, 75 ppm; for halothane, 50 ppm.

Approximately 500 fatalities that are at least partly due to the administration of anesthetic agents occur each year in the USA. The overall fatality rate following administration of anesthetic agents is approximately 0.5–1 per 10 000. The incidence of hepatic necrosis following halothane administration is 1 per 10 000 after a single administration, which is not significantly different from that found with other anesthetic agents. The incidence of hepatic necrosis after halothane administration rises to 7 per 10 000 after multiple exposures. Hepatic necrosis after halothane administration is assumed to be an autoimmune response.

The gaseous and volatile anesthetics depress all functions of the central nervous system in descending order from the cortex to the medulla. Excessive amounts stop respiration. If $O_2$ is diminished and the percentage of inspired $CO_2$ is increased, ventricular arrhythmias, and damage to internal organs are likely to occur. Patients who die several days following administration of chloroform, ethyl chloride, halothane, or divinyl ether may show fatty degeneration and other degenerative changes in the liver, heart, and kidneys. The pathologic findings in deaths from cyclopropane, ether, or ethylene are not characteristic. Chloroform is a carcinogen in animals.

### Clinical findings

The principal manifestations of poisoning with these agents are unconsciousness and respiratory failure.

*Acute poisoning* (from inhalation or ingestion)

Excitement followed by unconsciousness and paralysis of respiration. Cardiac irregularities occur with cyclopropane, chloroform, and halothane if $CO_2$ in the inspired air is increased. Cardiac arrest also occurs. Convulsions are caused by increased $CO_2$ in alveolar air. Hypotension is greatest with halothane, chloroform, methoxyflurane, and cyclopropane. Cyanosis and respiratory depression are greatest with halothane and cyclopropane. Uncontrollable hyperthermia occurs rarely during or after anesthesia; this is a genetically determined response. Severe to fatal liver necrosis has been associated with single or repeated administration of halothane and fluroxene. High-output renal failure with polyuria, increased blood urea nitrogen, and hypernatremia has followed administration of methoxyflurane. Fatalities have occurred; these result from fluoride released by metabolic degradation of methoxyflurane. Nitrous oxide without adequate $O_2$ can cause fatal cardiac arrhythmias and anoxic brain damage with headache, cerebral edema, and permanent neurologic damage.

*Chronic poisoning* (from inhalation)

Repeated anesthesia with chloroform, methoxyflurane, halothane, or divinyl ether increases the likelihood of liver or kidney damage. Repeated industrial exposure to chloroform at levels above 10 ppm has caused liver damage. Chloroform is a carcinogen in animals.

*Laboratory findings*

In patients with jaundice following the use of liver-damaging anesthetic agents appropriate tests show impairment of liver function (see p. 74).

## Prevention

Avoid prolonged or repeated use of organ-damaging anesthetics. Maintain adequate oxygenation and $CO_2$ removal during the administration of volatile anesthetics. Monitor rectal temperature every hour during the recovery period.

## Treatment

### Emergency measures

Establish airway and maintain respiration. Remove volatile anesthetic by forced ventilation.

### General measures

(1) Maintain blood pressure by intravenous saline (see p. 57).
(2) Maintain body warmth.
(3) Maintain adequate airway by removing secretions from trachea by catheter suction.
(4) Prevent hypoxia (see p. 52).
(5) If hyperthermia occurs lower body temperature by application of wet towels. For malignant hyperthermia, give dantrolene sodium, 1 mg/kg every 15 min intravenously to a total of 10 mg/kg, and procainamide, 15 mg/kg intravenously over 10 min. Give normal saline intravenously at a rate of 1 liter every 10 min for 30 min. Lavage stomach, urinary bladder, rectum, and peritoneum with cool saline. Treat acidosis with intravenous sodium bicarbonate. Monitor serum total base, serum potassium, and arterial pH and treat appropriately. Maintain urine output at 1–2 liters daily with furosemide and mannitol. After the first day give dantrolene, 1 mg/kg orally daily for 3 days.

## *Special problems*

If liver damage occurs, change patient's diet to high-carbohydrate, low-protein, low-fat.

## Prognosis

Liver damage caused by chloroform may progress to cirrhosis and death.

## References

Berry PD, *et al*. Severe carbon monoxide poisoning during desflurane anesthesia. *Anesthesiology* 1999;90:613

Hoerauf K, *et al*. Genetic damage in operating room personnel exposed to isoflurane and nitrous oxide. *Occup Environ Med* 1999;56:433

O'Keeffe NJ, Healy TEJ. The role of new anesthetic agents. *Pharmacol Therap* 1999;84:233

Reeves M. Acute hepatitis following enflurane anaesthesia. *Anaesth Intensive Care* 1997;25:80

## INTERACTIONS (see p. 20)

Enflurane and halothane sensitize the myocardium to catecholamines. Diethyl ether increases the risk of heart failure and hypotension from propranolol. Procaine enhances the effect of muscle relaxants. Enzyme induction (see p. 20) enhances metabolism of anesthetic agents containing fluorine and increases their toxicity. Quinidine, procainamide, lidocaine, propranolol, and phenytoin reduce cardiac contraction and thus increase the possibility of heart failure during anesthesia.

# PHARMACOKINETICS AND TOXIC CONCENTRATIONS (see p. 100)

| | $pK_a$ | $T_{\frac{1}{2}}$ (h) | $V_d$ (l/kg) | % Binding | Toxic concentration (µg/ml) |
|---|---|---|---|---|---|
| Bupivacaine | 8.1 | 2.7 | 1 | 95 | |
| Cocaine | | 2.5 | | | 0.5, 1[†] |
| Etidocaine | 7.7 | 2.7 | 1.9 | 94 | |
| Lidocaine | 7.9 | 1.3–2.3 | 1.3–1.7* | 65 | 6, 10[†] |
| Mepivacaine | 7.5 | 1.9 | 1.2 | 75 | |
| Prilocaine | 7.9 | | | 50 | |

*For children.

# 23 Depressants

## SEDATIVES, HYPNOTICS, AND ANTICONVULSANTS

A large number of drugs cause sedation or hypnosis by depression of the central nervous system. Overdosage with these or with some anticonvulsant drugs leads to coma and respiratory failure. Fatal doses for most non-barbiturate depressants and anti-epileptics except chloral hydrate are in the range of 0.1–0.5 g/kg. For chloral hydrate the fatal dose may be as small as 30 mg/kg. For barbiturates see Table 23.2.

The hypnotics and sedatives cause progressive depression of the central nervous system in descending order from cortex to medulla. After toxic doses, the respiratory center is depressed and respiratory exchange is diminished, resulting in tissue anoxia. Pathologic findings in fatalities from central nervous system depressants include pulmonary edema, pneumonia, and cerebral edema.

### Clinical findings

The principal manifestations of poisoning with most of these agents are coma and respiratory depression.

### *Acute poisoning* (from ingestion or injection)

Early symptoms are sleepiness, mental confusion, and unsteadiness; these are followed rapidly by coma with slow, shallow respiration; flaccid muscles; hypotension; cyanosis; hypothermia or hyperthermia; and absent reflexes. Duration of coma is dependent on dose as well as on the specific medication taken (Table 23.2). In prolonged coma, moist rales are heard in the lower lung fields and can be an indication of pulmonary edema. Atelectasis or aspiration pneumonia with signs of lung consolidation and fever can also occur. Carbon dioxide retention under these conditions causes acidosis and, via effects on the carotid body, can lead to hypotension. Death occurs most often from pneumonia, pulmonary edema, or refractory hypotension. Cerebral edema contributes to the persistence of coma. Bullous lesions occurring over pressure points indicate usually that coma has lasted 12 h or more. Intravenous injection of any barbiturate may cause severe respiratory depression, laryngospasm, excitement, and severe fall in blood pressure. Combination with ethanol causes effects that appear to be more than additive.

### *Chronic poisoning* (from ingestion)

Symptoms of chronic intoxication are skin rash, mental confusion, ataxia, dizziness, drowsiness, hangover, emotional lability or depression, irritability, poor judgement, neglect of personal appearance, and other behavior disturbances. Prolonged use of any of these drugs will cause the above mental changes; many are habit-forming. In addition, reactions peculiar to each type of drug may occur (Tables 23.1, 23.2, 23.3). Sudden withdrawal from prolonged use of large amounts of barbiturates, methyprylon, glutethimide, and other sedatives causes anxiety, insomnia, dizziness, weakness, nausea and vomiting, muscular twitchings, tremors, and convulsions. The risk of teratogenicity is reported to be increased 2- to 3-fold with administration of antiepileptic drugs. Serious ocular effects, including microphthalmos, prominent iris vessels, and coloboma, are reported to occur in 11% of infants *in utero* when the mother has been taking hydantoins.

**Table 23.1** Non-barbiturate depressants

| Drug | Clinical findings (In addition to those on p. 390) |
| --- | --- |
| Carisoprodol (Soma) | Paralysis, visual disturbances, excitement, skin rash, asthma, fever, hypotension |
| Chloral hydrate | Acute: Gastric irritation, rapid circulatory collapse, cardiac arrhythmias. Chronic: Kidney, liver, and heart damage; psychosis; leukopenia |
| Ethchlorvynol (Placidyl) | Fatigue, headache, confusion, nausea, vomiting, hemolysis, pulmonary edema, acidosis, liver damage, pancytopenia |
| Glutethimide (Doriden) | Nausea, pancytopenia, thrombocytopenia, leukopenia, peripheral neuritis, osteomalacia, paresthesia, toxic psychosis, laryngospasm, nystagmus, double vision, pupillary dilatation, dry mouth, ileus, cerebellar ataxia, cerebral edema, convulsions |
| Meprobamate (Equanil, Miltown) | Chills, fever, peripheral edema, vascular collapse, cardiac arrest, aplastic anemia, nonthrombocytopenic purpura with petechiae and ecchymoses. Convulsions on withdrawal |

**Table 23.2** Depressants: barbiturates (for treatment of overdoses, see below)

| Drug | Estimated fatal dose (g) | Duration of coma (see p. 390) (days) |
| --- | --- | --- |
| Amobarbital (Amytal) | 1.5 | 5 |
| Barbital* | 2 | 5 |
| Butabarbital | 2 | 3 |
| Mephobarbital (Mebaral)[†] | 2 | 5 |
| Methohexital (Brevital) | 1 | 3 |
| Pentobarbital (Nembutal) | 1 | 3 |
| Phenobarbital (Luminal) | 1.5 | 7 |
| Secobarbital (Seconal) | 2 | 3 |
| Thiopental (Pentothal)[‡] | 1 | 1 |

*Not metabolized, excreted by kidney; [†]liver damage and agranulocytosis reported; [‡]stored in fat

## *Laboratory findings*

(1) The serum potassium level may be low in prolonged coma.

(2) Blood $pCO_2$ may be elevated.

(3) Drug blood levels associated with severe coma are related to the duration of action of the barbiturate. For barbiturates with which the coma lasts 1–3 days, the blood drug level associated with severe poisoning is 1–3 mg/dl. For those with which coma may last up to 5 days, the blood level is above 3 mg/dl. Blood levels of glutethimide over 3 mg/dl are also associated with serious poisoning. For phenobarbital and barbital, the blood level associated with severe poisoning is 5–8 mg/dl or higher. The severity of symptoms does not necessarily correlate well with the blood drug level.

## Prevention

Depressant drugs should be stored safely. Prescription containers should have a warning label and a child-proof cap. They should not be left where repeat doses can be taken inadvertently while the patient is falling asleep.

## Treatment

The following therapeutic recommendations apply to severe depression from any of the compounds listed in Tables 23.1, 23.2, and 23.3.

**Table 23.3** Depressants: anti-epileptics*†

| Drug | Clinical findings (in addition to those on p. 390) |
|---|---|
| Carbamazepine (Tegretol) | Aplastic anemia, agranulocytosis, abnormalities in liver function tests, jaundice, fatal hepatitis, urinary retention, skin rash, gastrointestinal upset, heart failure, hypertension, lens opacities. |
| Ethotoin (Peganone) | Nausea, vomiting, rash, diarrhea, lymphadenopathy |
| Felbamate (Felbatol) | Nausea, vomiting, rash, headache |
| Fosphenytoin (Cerebyx) | Hypotension, rash. Look for hemopoietic changes, liver effects |
| Gabapentin (Neurontin) | Ataxia, leukopenia, nystagmus |
| Lamotrigine (Lamictal) | Epidermal necrolysis, ataxia, nausea |
| Levetiracetam (Keppra) | Coordination difficulties, psychosis |
| Methsuximide (Celontin) and ethosuximide (Zarontin) | Periorbital edema, proteinuria, hepatic dysfunction, fatal bone marrow aplasia, delayed onset of coma |
| Mephenytoin (Mesantoin) | Hemolytic anemia, aplastic anemia, visual disturbances, lymph gland enlargement, fever |
| Oxcarbazepine (Trileptal) | Hyponatremia, ataxia, nystagmus, abdominal pain |
| Phenacemide (Phenurone) | Liver damage, aplastic anemia, leukopenia, behavioral effects, renal impairment, skin rash, suicidal tendencies |
| Phensuximide (Milontin) | Nausea, vomiting, muscular weakness, hematuria, casts, nephrosis |
| Phenytoin (diphenylhydantoin, Dilantin) | Swelling of gums, fever, liver and kidney damage, agranulocytosis, adenopathy, aplastic anemia, pulmonary changes, lupus erythematosus, lymph gland enlargement, epidermal necrolysis, cardiac irregularities, peripheral nerve damage, tremor, drug psychosis, rigidity |
| Primidone (Mysoline) | Painful gums, excessive fatigue |
| Tiagabine (Gabitril) | Nausea, dizziness, abdominal pain, diarrhea |
| Topiramate (Topamax) | Confusion, speech impairment, weight gain, hemiparesis |
| Trimethadione (Tridione) and paramethadione (Paradione) | Neutropenia, hematuria, agranulocytosis, nephrosis, photophobia, lupus, myasthenia, blurred vision |
| Valproic acid (Depakene), sodium valproate, divalproex (Depakote) | Gastrointestinal disturbances, hair loss, psychosis, altered bleeding time, altered liver enzymes, fatal hepatic failure |
| Vigabatrin (Sabril) | Abdominal pain, ataxia, headache |
| Zonisamide (Zonegran) | Urinary lithiasis, toxic epidermal necrolysis, aplastic anemia, oligohidrosis |

*For treatment of overdoses, see p. 394; †precautions: perform white count and urinalysis at least monthly or immediately on occurrence of upper respiratory infection, sore throat, or other change in status

*Emergency measures*

(1) Maintain adequate airway. Remove mucous secretions from the trachea by suction with a soft rubber catheter. If respiratory difficulty is present use an oropharyngeal airway. Intubate if comatose.

(2) Maintain adequate $O_2$ intake and $CO_2$ removal. Arterial $pO_2$ should be 70–100 mmHg, and $pCO_2$ should be below 40 mmHg. If respiration is depressed give $O_2$ as necessary to maintain adequate arterial oxygenation and ventilate the patient.

(3) In conscious patients delay absorption of the drug by giving activated charcoal. Follow by gastric lavage and catharsis (see pp. 29–32). Avoid induction of emesis. If respiration is depressed place a cuffed endotracheal tube before doing gastric lavage. For catharsis, 30–60 ml of 50% sodium sulfate or Fleet's Phospho-Soda diluted in 200 ml of water can be given. The chances of removing a significant amount of drug are better if treatment is started within 2 h after ingestion. Since the remaining drug in the gastrointestinal tract can contribute to relapse after initial improvement, repeated gastric lavage and catharsis combined with charcoal administration are useful, especially in ethchlorvynol and glutethimide poisoning. Glutethimide and meprobamate are fat-soluble and markedly slow gastric emptying; thus, gastric lavage is useful whenever the patient is seen. In comatose patients any of these procedures increases the hazard of aspiration pneumonia or cardiac arrest.

(4) Maintain blood pressure (see below).

*Antidote*

No specific antidote is known for the sedative and hypnotic drugs. All stimulant analeptic drugs are absolutely contraindicated. In the presence of severe respiratory depression these drugs are not effective; they do not shorten the duration of depression but only stimulate the medullary centers for short periods of time, and the initial stimulation will be followed by greater depression. Complications of stimulant therapy are cardiac failure, cardiac arrhythmias, hyperthermia, convulsions, delayed psychosis, and kidney damage with anuria.

### General measures

Procedures are to be carried out under 24-hour supervision by a physician who has had training in resuscitation techniques. Check and record the following every hour: rate and quality of the pulse, blood pressure, reaction of the pupils, respiration rate, temperature, color of the skin (cyanosis), reflexes (corneal, papillary, tendon), and response to painful stimuli (pinching or pinprick).

(1) Elevate the patient's head (15 degrees) to reduce cerebral venous pressure and the possibility of cerebral edema. Maintain pharyngeal suction if necessary. Give intermittent positive-pressure respiration to help prevent pneumonia.

(2) Every 2 h turn the patient and massage skin. Use an oscillating bed, if available.

(3) Endotracheal suction should be done hourly, or more often if necessary. Prior to suction ventilate with $O_2$ for 3 min. Introduce catheter without suction, apply suction, and remove catheter slowly while rotating gently. The procedure should be completed in not more than 15 seconds. Do not use endotracheal suction in the presence of pulmonary edema.

(4) If renal function is adequate give fluids up to 40 ml/kg daily at a rate not exceeding 3 ml/kg/h (e.g. 0.2% sodium chloride in 5% dextrose with 20 mEq of potassium chloride added per liter) to maintain a daily urine output of 15–30 ml/kg. Measure serum potassium, chloride, and sodium levels daily and adjust intravenous fluid as necessary. Forced alkaline diuresis to 10–15 l/d is only marginally useful in phenobarbital poisoning, and associated pulmonary edema is a significant hazard.

(5) Urine output exceeding 0.5 ml/kg/h in the absence of diuretics indicates adequate tissue perfusion. Maintain blood pressure by administering fluids. Excessive administration of fluids may lead to pulmonary edema. In hypotension that does not respond to fluid administration give dopamine hydrochloride. The rate of infusion must be titrated carefully to maintain blood pressure at the lowest level that will give adequate renal perfusion. A peristaltic infusion pump or pediatric microdrip may be necessary to adjust the infusion rate accurately. Vasopressor-induced arrhythmias are most common after barbiturates, hydantoins, or chloral hydrate.

(6) The role of hemodialysis, peritoneal dialysis, and extracorporeal resin or charcoal hemoperfusion in the treatment of depressant poisoning is not

yet clearly established. The recovery rate is better than 99% in patients treated with intensive supportive care. The hazards from dialysis are significant. For short-acting drugs dialysis can only increase the removal rate by 10–20%. For longer-acting drugs dialysis is more likely to be helpful; blood drug levels can be used as an indication. The following blood levels are indications for the use of dialysis therapy: for aprobarbital, amobarbital, talbutal, and allobarbital, 10 mg/dl; for barbital and phenobarbital, 15 mg/dl. Dialysis has not reduced the mortality rate in poisoning due to ethchlorvynol, glutethimide, or methaqualone. Conditions that increase the hazard of dialysis therapy include hypotension that has not responded to therapy, pulmonary edema, and reduced renal function.

### Special problems

(1) Treat hypothermia by application of blankets. Avoid rapid warming or burning of the patient by hot pads or hot-water bottles. Administer intravenous fluids at 37°C and gases at 40°C. Administration of 40% moistened $O_2$ at 40°C improves cardiac function and reduces the risk of hypothermic ventricular fibrillation.
(2) Treat hyperthermia by applying wet towels or cooling blanket until the patient's rectal temperature is down to 38°C.
(3) Treat pulmonary edema (see p. 55).
(4) Monitor urine output and prevent bladder distension by placing an indwelling catheter. Maintain accurate fluid input/output chart to facilitate monitoring electrolyte and fluid balance.
(5) Treat aspiration pneumonia with organism-specific chemotherapy.

### Prognosis

Determine prognosis by the severity of the clinical findings.

### Mild

Patient can be aroused. No treatment is necessary.

*Moderate*

Patient cannot be aroused. Respiration is full and regular. No cyanosis or pulmonary edema is present. Blood pressure is normal. Recovery occurs in 24–48 h with good nursing care and adequate fluid balance.

*Severe*

Coma with slow, shallow, irregular respiration; cyanosis; absence of all reflexes; low blood pressure; hypothermia of 0.5–2°C; dilated pupils; and absence of response to painful stimuli. The mortality rate should be less than 5%. Recovery of consciousness may require 3–5 days.

## NARCOTIC ANALGESICS (Table 23.4)

Narcotic analgesics control severe pain by their depressant effect on the brain.

Fatalities have occurred from overdose during therapeutic use, accidental ingestion, or intentional misuse. Overdoses of heroin in addicts caused more than 1200 deaths in narcotic addicts in New York City in 1970, and the number of deaths in the USA may exceed 10 000 per year. Accidental ingestion of methadone has led to the death of many children. Naloxone appears to be a pure antagonist, and doses of naloxone above 5 g have not caused death.

The narcotic analgesics produce variable effects on the central nervous system depending on the drug, the susceptibility of the patient, and the dosage. For example morphine and most of the other opium derivatives except codeine depress the cortex and medullary centers and stimulate the spinal cord. Codeine, on the other hand, is somewhat less depressing to the cortex and medullary centers but more stimulating to the spinal cord. Methadone and alphaprodine are similar to morphine in their depressant effects on the cortex and medullary centers in toxic doses.

The pathologic findings in death from narcotic analgesics are not characteristic.

### Clinical findings

The principal manifestations of poisoning with these drugs are slowing of respiration and coma.

**Table 23.4** Narcotic depressants and antagonists*

| Drug | Fatal dose[†] (g) | Clinical findings (In addition to those on p. 397) |
|---|---|---|
| Alfentanil (Alfenta) | 0.01 | Rigidity |
| Apomorphine | 0.1 | Violent emesis, cardiac depression |
| Buprenorphine (Buprenex) | 0.05 | |
| Butorphanol (Stadol) | 0.1 | |
| Codeine | 0.8 | Convulsions |
| Dextromethorphan (dormethan, Romilar) | 0.5 | Dizziness |
| Dezocin (Dalgan) | 0.5 | Nausea, dizziness, hypotension |
| Dihydrocodeine | 0.5 | |
| Diphenoxylate (Lomotil) | 0.2 | Constipation |
| Ethylmorphine (Dionin) | 0.5 | Irritation |
| Fentanyl (Sublimaze) | 0.002 | Muscle rigidity |
| Heroin | 0.2 | |
| Hydrocodone (Dicodid) | 0.2 | Tremors |
| Hydromorphone (Dilaudid) | 0.2 | |
| Levomethadyl (Laam) | 0.1 | Arrythmias |
| Levorphanol (Levo-Dromoran) | 0.1 | |
| Loperamide (Imodium) | 0.5 | Nausea, vomiting |
| Meperidine (pethidine, Demerol) | 1 | Fainting, edema |
| Methadone (Dolophine, Adanon) | 0.1 | |
| Morphine | 0.2 | |
| Nalbuphine (Nubain) | 0.3 | |
| Nalmefene[‡] | | Pain |
| Naloxone (Narcan)[‡] | | Hypertension |
| Naltrexone (Trexan)[‡] | | Liver damage |
| Omnopon (Pantopon) | 0.3 | |
| Opium (*Papaver somniferum*) | 0.3 | |
| Oxycodone (Percodan) | 0.5 | |
| Oxymorphone (Numorphan) | 0.05 | Restlessness |
| Paregoric (camphorated tincture of opium) | 60 | |
| Pentazocine (Talwin) | 0.3 | Nausea |
| Propoxyphene (Darvon) | 0.5 | Nausea, vomiting, skin, rash, ptosis, convulsions |
| Remifentanil (Ultiva) | 0.0002 | Rigidity |
| Sufentanil (Sufenta) | 0.002 | Rigidity |
| Tramadol (Ultram) | 0.5 | Convulsions |

[†]Estimated for an adult; may be much higher (up to 10 times) in narcotic addicts and much lower (1/20) in infants. [‡]Narcotic antagonist; naloxone is a pure antagonist, doses up to 5 g have not caused death.

*Acute poisoning* (from ingestion or injection)

Toxic doses of the narcotic analgesics cause unconsciousness; pinpoint pupils (dilated with anoxia); slow, shallow respiration; cyanosis; weak pulse; hypotension; spasm of gastrointestinal and biliary tracts; and in some cases pulmonary edema, spasticity, and twitching of the muscles. Death from respiratory failure may occur within 2–4 h after oral or subcutaneous administration or immediately after intravenous overdose. Convulsions may accompany codeine, meperidine, apomorphine, propoxyphene, or oxymorphone poisoning. The metabolite of meperidine, normeperidine, has significantly greater excitatory effect than meperidine. Metabolites of other drugs may also be more convulsant than the parent drugs. Convulsions are more likely with high doses, renal impairment, alkaline urine, the presence of enzyme-inducing drugs, or the presence of phenothiazines.

*Chronic poisoning* (from ingestion or injection)

The findings in chronic use or addiction are not marked. Pinpoint pupils and rapid changes in mood may occasionally be observed. All opiates if ingested chronically will cause physiologic dependence, however this must be differentiated from addiction which is a separate phenomenon.

*Withdrawal symptoms*

All the narcotic analgesics have strong addicting potential. The addict's craving is partly psychologic and partly due to fear of the severe symptoms of withdrawal. Sudden withdrawal from morphine or other narcotic analgesics causes yawning; lacrimation; pilomotor reactions; severe gastrointestinal disturbance with cramps, vomiting, diarrhea, or constipation; sweating; fever; chills; increase in respiratory rate; insomnia; tremor; and mydriasis. Death is rare. The narcotic antagonist naltrexone can precipitate withdrawal symptoms.

*Laboratory findings*

The abrupt production of withdrawal symptoms after the administration of nalorphine will indicate dependence. Analysis of urine or blood can also be used to determine drug use.

## Prevention

Narcotic analgesics should be used with caution in children under 12 years of age.

Repeated doses of narcotic analgesics must be avoided in the treatment of chronic painful conditions unless the benefit to be derived, such as improved functional status or comfort measures in terminal illness, outweighs the side-effects of and consequences of dependence.

The combination of monoamine oxidase inhibitor drugs (see p. 508) with any narcotic analgesic may cause coma with hyperthermia, respiratory failure, convulsions, cerebral edema, and unstable blood pressure. The combined use of LSD (see p. 529) and narcotic analgesics is also dangerous to life.

## Treatment

### Acute poisoning

(1) Emergency measures:
   (a) Maintain respiration with artificial respiration and then give antidote as prescribed below.
   (b) In fully conscious patients remove swallowed poison by thorough gastric lavage or emesis (see pp. 29–32). The chances of removing a significant amount of the drug are better if treatment is started within the first 2 h. If the patient is unconscious or respiration is depressed, emesis is contraindicated and the dangers of unprotected gastric lavage are not justified. If a massive dose has been ingested, catharsis is possibly useful after the patient is awake.
   (c) Treat coma (see p. 63) and shock (see p. 56).

(2) Antidote – For overdoses of any of the narcotic analgesics, give naloxone hydrochloride (Narcan), 0.01 mg/kg intravenously. Naloxone does not depress respiration. Repeat injection of the antagonist only as necessary to maintain response to stimuli. If an effective increase in pulmonary ventilation is not achieved with the first dose, the dose may be repeated every 2–3 min until respiration returns to normal and the patient responds to stimuli. The dose of naloxone may need to be 0.1–0.2 mg/kg in massive overdoses of narcotic analgesics. Observe the patient closely for the first 24–48 h in the case of methadone overdose. Naloxone is safe to use as a test in coma of unknown origin in which a narcotic is suspected. In

addicts or newborns of addicted mothers, injection of naloxone can precipitate acute, severe withdrawal. Naloxone does not antagonize
convulsant effects of narcotics and may enhance meperidine seizures.

(3) General measures – Maintain body warmth and adequate fluid vol-
ume/blood pressure. Treat shock.

(4) Other measures – Dialysis is obviated by the availability of antagonists.
Stimulants are contraindicated.

### Chronic poisoning or addiction

(1) The treatment of addiction is best undertaken under the direction of physicians who specialize in these problems.

(2) Clonidine, 17 μg/kg/d in divided doses for 10 days, has been used to
block the symptoms of rapid withdrawal from narcotic dependence.

(3) Because of inadequate treatment of chronic pain, recommendations have
been developed in the USA to guide physician's appropriate manage-
ment of these patients. Specific information is available at the following
web sites:
JCAHO standards at http://www.jcaho.org/standard/pm.html
American Pain Society at http://www.ampainsoc.org
American Pain Foundation at http://www.painfoundation.org
National Guideline Clearinghouse at http://www.guideline.gov
Americal Alliance of Cancer Pain Initiatives at http://www.aacpi.org

(4) Since regulation of narcotics is so strict, the physician who prescribes
narcotics should be familiar with the Controlled Substances Act of 1970.
The Bureau of Narcotics, US Department of Justice, has a pamphlet that
describes the Act for physicians.

### Prognosis

In acute poisoning, if naloxone can be given, recovery will usually occur
within 1–4 h.

### ANTIHISTAMINES (Table 23.5)

Many antihistamines are sold both over the counter and by prescription for the
treatment of allergies and colds and as sedatives. Some are also used as
motion sickness remedies.

At least 20 fatalities have been reported from accidental ingestion in children. Significant drug interactions between some antihistamines (terfenidine) and other drugs (erythromycin, ketoconazole, etc.) have resulted in fatal cardiac arrhythmias.

Antihistaminic drugs in toxic doses produce a complex of central nervous system excitatory and depressant effects, partly from atropine-like anticholinergic effects. The pathologic findings are not characteristic. Cerebral damage and kidney damage have been observed at autopsy.

### Clinical findings

The principal manifestations of poisoning with these drugs are convulsions and coma.

*Acute poisoning* (from ingestion)

Therapeutic doses of antihistaminic drugs cause a high incidence of adverse symptoms and signs, including drowsiness, dryness of the mouth, headache, nausea, tachycardia, urinary retention, and nervousness. Larger doses cause

**Table 23.5**  Antihistamines and similar drugs

| Name | Fatal doses |
|---|---|
| Astemizole (Hismanal)[§] | 25–250 mg/kg* |
| Azelastine (Astelin) | 25–250 mg/kg* |
| Brompheniramine (Dimetane) | 25–250 mg/kg* |
| Cetirazine (Zyrtec) | 25–250 mg/kg* |
| Chlorpheniramine (Chlor-Trimeton) | 25–250 mg/kg* |
| Clemastine (Tavist) | 10–100mg/kg* |
| Cyclizine (Marezine)[†] | 25–250 mg/kg* |
| Cyproheptadine (Periactin) | 25–250 mg/kg* |
| Dimenhydrinate (Dramamine) | 25–250 mg/kg* |
| Diphenhydramine (Benadryl) | 400 mg, 40 mg/kg[‡] |
| Fexofenidin (Allegra) | 25–250 mg/kg* |
| Hydroxyzine (Atarax) | 25–250 mg/kg* |
| Loratidine (Claritin) | 25–250 mg/kg* |
| Meclizine (Bonine)[†] | 25–250 mg/kg* |
| Orphenadrine (Disipal) | 25–250 mg/kg* |
| Terfenidine (Seldane)[§] | 25–250 mg/kg* |
| Trimethobenzamide (Tigan) | 25–250 mg/kg* |
| Triprolidine (Actidil) | 25–250 mg/kg* |

*Estimated acute fatal dose; [†]shown to cause birth defects in animals, hence contraindicated in pregnancy; [‡]reported acute fatal dose. [§]Off USA market due to cardiotoxicity.

two different types of effects – either drowsiness, disorientation, staggering gait, hallucinations, stupor, and coma; or hyperreflexia, tremors, excitement, nystagmus, hyperthermia, and convulsions. Symptoms may vary from patient to patient with the same drug, or a mixture of the above symptoms may be seen in the same patient.

### *Chronic poisoning*

Tripelennamine, methapyrilene, and pyrilamine have caused agranulocytosis or aplastic anemia.

### Prevention

Antihistamines should be sold with a poison label and stored safely. Patients should be warned to discontinue medication at the first symptoms.

### Treatment

### *Acute poisoning*

(1) Emergency measures:
   (a) If coma and respiratory depression are present, use resuscitative measures. *Do not use stimulants.*
   (b) Delay absorption of ingested drug by giving activated charcoal and then remove by airway-protected gastric lavage followed by catharsis (see pp. 29–32). Emetics may not work successfully.
   (c) Maintain blood pressure (see p. 57).
(2) General measures – Control convulsions by giving diazepam, 0.1 mg/kg slowly intravenously. Forced diuresis is not helpful.
(3) Special problems – Treat agranulocytosis (see p. 79). Treat arrhythmias (see pp. 59, 461). Treat hyperthermia by cooling applications.

### *Chronic poisoning*

Discontinue the drug at the onset of symptoms. For further treatment, see Acute poisoning, above.

**Prognosis**

Fewer than 10% of those seriously poisoned have died. Patients who live more than 24 h will probably survive.

## PHENOTHIAZINE DRUGS (Table 23.6)

Chlorpromazine and related drugs are synthetic chemicals derived in most instances from phenothiazine. They are used as anti-emetics, as antipsychotics, and as potentiators of analgesic and hypnotic drugs.

The acute fatal dose for these compounds appears to be in the range of 15–150 mg/kg, although severe symptoms have occurred with doses less than 1 mg/kg. Reported fatal doses are as follows: chlorpromazine, 350 mg in a 4-year-old and 2 g in an adult female; promazine, 1 g in a 2-year-old. Because these compounds enhance the effects of other drugs, administration during acute toxicity from antihistamines, alcohol, barbiturates, or morphine must be done cautiously. At least 25 deaths due to agranulocytosis and several deaths due to liver damage have been reported as due to poisoning with chlorpromazine or related drugs. The incidence of toxic reactions may be as high as 1–5% of patients receiving these drugs for more than 1 month.

The principal pathologic finding in patients who have died with liver damage is cirrhosis. In patients dying with agranulocytosis the pathologic findings have been acellular bone marrow and, sometimes, regurgitation of bile into

**Table 23.6** Phenothiazines and related drugs

| | Reported toxic effects | | |
| Name | Blood dyscrasias | CNS effects, convulsions | Liver damage |
| --- | --- | --- | --- |
| Chlorpromazine (Thorazine) | * | * | * |
| Fluphenazine (Permitil) | + | + | + |
| Mesoridazine (Serentil) | | + | |
| Perphenazine (Trilafon) | | * | + |
| Prochlorperazine (Compazine) | + | * | * |
| Promethazine (Phenergan) | | + | |
| Thiethylperazine (Torecan) | | + | |
| Thioridazine (Mellaril) | + | + | + |
| Thiothixene (Navane) | + | + | + |
| Trifluoperazine (Stelazine) | | * | |

*Deaths from toxic reaction reported.

the bile canaliculi with pigment deposition in the parenchymal cells of the liver. Damage to liver cells was not present.

## Clinical findings

The principal manifestations of poisoning with phenothiazines are drowsiness, hypotension, jaundice and leukopenia, and acute dystonic reactions.

### *Acute poisoning*

Acute toxic ingestion first manifests as agitation, delirium and seizures. After this initial hyperactivity, sedation, hypotension, hypothermia and coma occur. Antipsychotic overdosages are rarely fatal unless ingestion is combined with alcohol, other sedatives or tricyclic antidepressants.

Usual doses induce drowsiness and mild hypotension in as many as 50% of patients. Larger doses cause drowsiness, severe postural hypotension, hypothermia, tachycardia, dryness of the mouth, nausea, ataxia, anorexia, nasal congestion, fever, constipation, tremor, blurring of vision, stiffness of muscles, urinary retention, and coma. Therapeutic dosages of thioridazine have been associated with torsades de pointes. Intravenous injection of solutions containing more than 25 mg/ml of these drugs causes thrombophlebitis and cellulitis in a small number of patients. Hypotension and ventricular arrhythmias are the most common causes of death. Neuroleptic malignant syndrome (muscular rigidity, hyperthermia, elevated CPK, and mental status changes) can occur within an hour of ingestion or after 2 months from initiation of chronic antipsychotic use.

### *Chronic poisoning* (from ingestion)

Prolonged administration of chlorpromazine or related drugs may produce the following reactions:
(1) Leukopenia or agranulocytosis has appeared 4–8 weeks after therapy with doses over 50 mg/d. Findings include ulcerations of the gums, tongue, or pharynx; fever; weakness; disorientation; and anorexia.
(2) Jaundice, characteristically obstructive and without evidence of liver cell damage (at least in the early stages), may appear shortly after treatment or may be delayed 2–6 weeks.

(3) Generalized maculopapular eruptions with edema, scaling, and pruritus may appear after administration of chlorpromazine but are more likely to appear as sensitivity reactions in medical personnel who handle the preparation or after exposure to sunlight in persons taking the drug.

(4) A syndrome similar to Parkinson's disease occurs as a result of extrapyramidal and other central nervous system effects. In addition, tardive dyskinesia (syndrome of hyperkinetic involuntary movements) can occur.

(5) Prolonged administration of phenothiazines in high doses has caused skin pigmentation and corneal and lens opacities. The exposed areas of the face, neck, and hands show a purplish pigmentation that has the histologic appearance of melanin. Corneal and lens pigmentation or other changes are accompanied by reduction in visual acuity. Chorioretinopathy has been reported after thioridazine.

(6) Electrocardiographic abnormalities and sudden death thought to result from ventricular fibrillation have occurred.

(7) Endocrine effects include amenorrhea, galactorrhea, gynecomastia, and water dysregulation.

### *Laboratory findings*

(1) Liver function tests in the presence of jaundice reveal elevated serum bilirubin, elevated serum alkaline phosphatase, and the presence of bile in the urine.

(2) Serum cholesterol and blood sugar are sometimes elevated.

(3) In agranulocytosis the blood examination reveals white blood cell count decreased below 2000, polymorphonuclear neutrophils diminished or absent from the blood smear, and acellular and aplastic bone marrow.

(4) Phenothiazine compounds in urine can be detected by the addition of a few drops of tincture of ferric chloride to urine acidified with dilute nitric acid. A violet color results if phenothiazine compounds are present.

(5) An ECG may show a prolonged QT interval and a widened QRS complex.

### Prevention

Patients must be warned to discontinue the drug and report for examination immediately upon the appearance of sore throat, fever, jaundice, or other signs of reaction.

**Treatment**

*Acute poisoning*

(1) Emergency measures:
   (a) Establish airway and maintain respiration.
   (b) Discontinue related drugs at the first sign until the severity of the reaction can be evaluated. Remove overdoses by gastric lavage (see pp. 29–32). Emetics are not likely to be effective.
   (c) Treat severe hypotension by giving fluids (see p. 57). The use of sympathomimetic amines (norepinephrine, etc.) is contraindicated.
   (d) Monitor ECG and treat arrhythmias. Phenytoin or lidocaine are used because other antiarrhymics such as quinidine, procainamide and disopyramide cause similar conduction effects as phenothiazines.
(2) Antidote:
   (a) Diphenhydramine, 1–5 mg/kg intravenously, will reverse extra-pyramidal signs.
   (b) For ventricular arrhythmias give phenytoin, 0.5 mg/kg/min slowly intravenously. The injection rate should not exceed 50 mg in 3 min. Phenytoin can be repeated every 5 min up to a total dose of 10 mg/kg. Torsades is treated with magnesium.
(3) General measures – Control convulsions or hyperactivity with pento-barbital (see p. 60). Avoid other depressant drugs. Hemodialysis is not effective.

*Chronic poisoning*

(1) Immediate measures – Discontinue treatment at the first sign of jaundice, fever, sore throat, pigmentation, or ocular change.
(2) Treat hypotension with fluid volume.
(3) Neuroleptic malignant syndrome is treated with a cooling blanket aand either dantrolene sodium 1 mg/kg orally every 12 h or bromocriptine 5 mg orally every 8 h.

**Prognosis**

In agranulocytosis from phenothiazines recovery is likely if the patient survives for 2 weeks.

In liver damage from phenothiazines complete recovery usually occurs within 4–8 weeks after discontinuing the drug.

## BROMIDES

Sodium bromide (NaBr), potassium bromide (KBr), and ammonium bromide ($NH_4Br$) are water-soluble salts.

Some non-prescription medications (e.g. Bromo-Seltzer, Dr. Miles' Nervine) formerly contained bromides, but none currently available in the USA contain bromides. However, patients may still have access to the older preparations. Some prescription drugs contain bromides. Other preparations that release bromide, such as bromisovalum (Bromural) and carbromal, can lead to chronic bromide toxicity. Well water containing as little as 20 mg of bromide per liter has caused toxicity. Toxic signs from bromides occur in 1–10% of users, but fatalities from bromides alone are rare. Bromide displaces chloride from the plasma and cells; this produces depression of the central nervous system. Pathologic findings are pneumonia and pulmonary edema.

### Clinical findings

The principal manifestations of bromide poisoning are neuropsychologic, gastrointestinal and dermatologic.

#### Acute poisoning

Large doses of bromide cause nausea and vomiting, abdominal pain, coma, and paralysis.

#### Chronic poisoning

Symptoms from overdose are confusion, irritability, tremor, memory loss, anorexia, emaciation, headache, slurred speech, delusions, psychotic behavior, ataxia, stupor, and coma. Between 1 and 5% of bromide users will have an acneiform papular eruption of the face and hands.

#### Laboratory findings

Blood bromide levels should be determined in undiagnosed patients who are stuporous or show psychotic or irrational behavior. Toxicity can occur at blood bromide levels above 20 mg/dl. Serum chloride levels are falsely elevated as bromide interferes with the test.

## Prevention

Blood bromide levels should be determined monthly during bromide therapy to avoid levels above 50 mg/dl.

## Treatment

### Acute poisoning

(1) Emergency measures – Induce emesis if patient is alert. Protect airway and provide supportive treatment.
(2) Enhance bromide excretion with fluids and chloride. Give 5% dextrose/ 0.5 normal saline IV to maintain urine output of 4–6 ml/kg/h. Furosemide can be used to increase urine output.

### Chronic poisoning

Discontinue use.

## Prognosis

Patients with bromide poisoning recover completely in 1–6 months.

## SELECTIVE DEPRESSANTS (Table 23.7)

A large number of drugs are used as depressants to relieve anxiety, relax muscle spasm, or inhibit cough. The single dose of any of these compounds that would be fatal in an adult is 0.05–0.5 g/kg. Smaller doses might be dangerous in children or in elderly persons.

## Clinical findings

### Acute poisoning

Drowsiness, weakness, nystagmus, diplopia, decreased coordination, and lassitude, progressing to coma with cyanosis and respiratory depression. Aspiration pneumonia is a frequent complication of coma with respiratory depression. Newborn infants of mothers given any of these drugs may have prolonged effects as a result of slow detoxification.

### Chronic poisoning

Drowsiness, depression, weakness, anxiety, ataxia, headaches, blurred vision, gastric upset, and pruritic skin rashes characterized by urticaria or erythematous macular eruptions.

Drug dependence has been reported to result from abuse of many of the selective depressants. Convulsions can occur from abrupt withdrawal.

### Laboratory findings

Any of the formed elements of the blood may be decreased in number.

### Prevention

The patient should be warned to discontinue medication with these agents at the onset of any unusual symptoms. Severe hypotension may occur when any of these drugs are used. These agents should not be used in pregnancy.

### Treatment

### Acute poisoning

(1) Emergency measures:
   (a) Remove drug by ipecac emesis followed by administration of activated charcoal. Airway-protected gastric lavage is necessary in patients with depressed respiration (see pp. 29–32).
   (b) If coma and respiratory depression are present treat as for depressants (see p. 391). Alkaline diuresis has been suggested, but the hazard of pulmonary edema probably outweighs the benefits.
   (c) Maintain blood pressure.
(2) General measures – Avoid concurrent administration of other depressant drugs.

**Table 23.7** Selective depressants*

| Drug | Clinical findings (in addition to those on p. 409) |
|---|---|
| Alprazolam (Xanax) | Hypotension, skin rash |
| Baclofen (Lioresal) | Cholinergic effects, nausea, constipation, anorexia, urinary retention, impotence, confusion |
| Benzonatate (Tessalon) | Gastrointestinal upset, convulsions |
| Buspirone (BuSpar) | Nausea, headache, dizziness, sedation |
| Chlordiazepoxide (Librium) | Stimulation, rage reaction, severe generalized dermatitis, syncope without warning, mental confusion, jaundice from liver damage, agranulocytosis, convulsions |
| Chlorzoxazone (Paraflex) | Constipation or diarrhea, gastrointestinal disturbances with bleeding, liver damage, sensitivity reactions |
| Clonazepam (Klonopin) | Hair loss, hirsutism, gastrointestinal disturbances, hepatomegaly, sore gums, dysuria, lymphadenopathy, leukopenia, thrombocytopenia |
| Clorazepate (Tranxene) | Abnormal liver and kidney function tests, hypotension, skin rash |
| Clozapine (Clozaril) | Agranulocytosis, convulsions, hypotension, respiratory arrest |
| Dantrolene (Dantrium) | Liver damage, gastrointestinal upset or bleeding, speech and vision disorders, tachycardia |
| Diazepam (Valium) | Tinnitus, excitability, rage reaction, hallucinations. Synergism with other depressants. Lactic mitosis from prolonged use, phlebitis |
| Dolasetron (Anzemet) | ECG alterations, slow pulse, headache, diarrhea |
| Droperidol (Inapsine) | Hypotension, hallucinations, extrapyramidal symptoms, tachycardia, respiratory depression when used with narcotics |
| Estazolam (ProSom) | Diarrhea |
| Etomidate (Amidate) | Pain at injection site, apnea, muscle clonus, nausea, vomiting, hypotension |
| Flurazepam (Dalmane) | Hypotension, excitement, skin rash, leukopenia, elevated liver enzymes, jaundice |
| Gamma hydroxybutyric acid (GHB, Blue Nitro, many other brand names) Gamma butyrolactone (GBL) | Stupor, hypotonia, sudden coma |

*Continued*

*Table 23.7 (continued)*

| Drug | Clinical findings (in addition to those on p. 409) |
|---|---|
| Granisetron (Kytril) | Altered liver enzymes, headache |
| Haloperidol (Haldol) | Extrapyramidal reactions, persistent tardive dyskinesia, depression, headache, confusion, vertigo, grand mal seizures, exacerbation of psychosis, hypotension, leukopenia, endocrine malfunction, skin rash |
| Ketamine (Ketalar) | Rise in blood pressure and pulse rate, apnea in the presence of increased intracerebral pressure, laryngospasm and respiratory arrest, profuse salivation with respiratory obstruction, EEG changes similar to those of epilepsy. Contraindicated in patients with convulsions. Delirium, hallucinations, excitement, and irrational behavior occasionally occur during recovery. Tonic and clonic movements sometimes resemble seizures |
| Lorazepam (Ativan) | Nausea, change of appetite, headache, sleep disturbance |
| Loxapine (Daxolin), olanzapine (Zyprexa), pimozide (Orap) | Extrapyramidal effects, tardive dyskinesia, hypotension, hypertension, anticholinergic effects, gastrointestinal disturbances, convulsions, CNS depression, hypothermia, rhabdomyolysis, acute renal failure |
| Metaxolone (Skelaxin) | Nausea, sedation, irritability, rash |
| Methocarbamol (Robaxin) | Skin rash, conjunctivitis, blurred vision, fever |
| Midazolam (Versed) | Apnea, pain at injection site, ECG changes, confusion, rash |
| Molindone (Moban) | Hypotension, extrapyramidal effects, tardive dyskinesia |
| Oxazepam (Serax) | Syncope, liver or bone marrow damage, sensitivity reactions |
| Papaverine | Constipation, increased reflex excitability, liver damage |
| Pramipexole, ropinirole | Dizziness, fainting, nausea, hypotension, hallucinations |
| Propofol (Diprivan) | Slow pulse, hypotension, apnea, pain at injection site |
| Quazepam (Doral) | Incontinence, jaundice, anticholinergic effects |
| Quetiapine (Seroquel) | Hyperpyrexia, rigidity, hypotension, tardive dyskinesia |
| Riluzole (Rilutek) | Leukopenia, nausea, pain, possible liver or kidney damage |
| Risperidone (Risperidal) | Hypotension, prolactinemia, thrombocytopenia, sedation |
| Selegiline (Eldepryl) | Nausea, hallucinations, contraindicated with meperidine, tyramine foods |
| Temazepam (Restoril) | Anorexia, diarrhea |
| Triazolam (Halcion) | Nausea, vomiting, fatigue, tachycardia |
| Zolpidem (Ambien) | Diarrhea |

*Chronic poisoning*

Discontinue the drug at onset of any abnormal hematologic findings. Reduce dosage if drowsiness occurs.

**Prognosis**

Recovery is likely except in patients with aplastic anemia.

## NEUROMUSCULAR BLOCKING AGENTS (Table 23.8)

Agents that block neuromuscular transmission are used to promote relaxation during surgical anesthesia and occasionally to control convulsions. Dosages sufficient to relax peripheral muscles will also dangerously depress respiration. Thus an effective dose of any of these compounds is potentially a fatal dose if respiration is not maintained by artificial means. The incidence of fatalities during the use of general anesthetic agents is greatly increased by the concomitant use of skeletal neuromuscular blocking agents.

These compounds appear to block neuromuscular transmission by either of two methods. The curare derivatives and gallamine triethiodide paralyze muscles by increasing the resistance of the muscle to depolarization by the acetylcholine released by nerve stimulation. By giving neostigmine or edrophonium the resistance to depolarization can be partially overcome and the paralysis relieved. Atropine is ordinarily given along with neostigmine to block the effects of neostigmine on other systems. On the other hand, decamethonium bromide and succinylcholine chloride act by depolarizing the muscles, and no drugs are available that will overcome the paralysis thus induced. All of the skeletal neuromuscular blocking agents also depress autonomic ganglia to some extent, leading to fall in blood pressure.

The pathologic findings in deaths from skeletal neuromuscular blockade are not characteristic.

**Clinical findings**

Chronic poisoning does not occur. The principal manifestations of acute poisoning (from injection) are respiratory failure and circulatory collapse. Symptoms are heaviness of the eyelids, diplopia, and difficulty in swallowing and talking, followed rapidly by paralysis of the extremities, neck, intercostal

**Table 23.8** Skeletal neuromuscular blocking agents

| Drug | Initial dose* (mg/kg) | Maximum duration (min) | Antidote |
|---|---|---|---|
| **Prevents depolarization** | | | |
| Atracurium (Tracrium) | 0.5 | 45 | Edrophonium or neostigmine |
| Cisatracurium (Nimbex) | 0.1 | 90 | Edrophonium or neostigmine |
| Doxacurium (Nuromax) | 0.025 | 55 | Edrophonium or neostigmine |
| Metocurine iodide (Metubine) | 0.1 | 120 | Edrophonium or neostigmine |
| Mivacurium (Mivacron) | 0.1 | 30 | Edrophonium or neostigmine |
| Pancuronium (Pavulon) | 0.04 | 120 | Edrophonium or neostigmine |
| Pipecuronium (Arduan) | 0.05 | 90 | Neostigmine |
| Rocuronium (Zemuron) | 0.6 | 30 | Edrophonium or neostigmine |
| Vecuronium (Norcuron) | 0.1 | 30 | Edrophonium or neostigmine |
| **Depolarizes** | | | |
| Succinylcholine chloride (Anectine, etc.) | 0.1 | 30 | None |

*Dose that causes respiratory paralysis

muscles, and, lastly, the diaphragm. Venous pooling and vascular dilatation, with severe fall in blood pressure, also occur. Cardiac arrest during succinylcholine administration has occurred after head injury. Symptoms ordinarily progress for 1–10 min after the injection is discontinued. The time required for complete recovery is variable, but it may be several hours. Malignant hyperthermia has been reported after the use of succinylcholine. Pancuronium may cause tachycardia.

## Prevention

Skeletal neuromuscular blocking agents should be used only when facilities for giving artificial respiration and for controlling circulatory collapse are available. Local anesthetics, general anesthetics, and other drugs may prolong the effect of skeletal neuromuscular blocking agents. Atypical plasma cholinesterase is present in 1 out of 2000 patients, and in these individuals succinylcholine is hydrolyzed slowly and the effect is prolonged.

**Treatment**

*Emergency measures*

Intubate. Give artificial respiration and maintain blood pressure (see p. 57).

*Antidote*

For curare derivatives or gallamine triethiodide give either of the following: (1) Edrophonium (Tensilon) chloride, 10 mg (1 ml of 1% solution) intravenously; this may be repeated to a maximum of 30 mg. (2) Neostigmine (Prostigmin) methylsulfate, 1–2 ml of 1:2000 solution intravenously, with atropine, 1 mg. *Caution:* These antidotes may aggravate the circulatory collapse that occurs during muscular paralysis due to skeletal neuromuscular blocking agents.

**Prognosis**

If spontaneous respiration occurs, recovery is usually permanent.

## INTERACTIONS (See p. 20)

In the presence of tranquilizers or depressants, the action of ketamine may be prolonged. Hypertension and ventricular tachycardia from ketamine may occur if thyroid drugs are being used.

All central nervous system depressants, including ethanol, enhance the central nervous system depressant effects of other central nervous system depressants, anesthetics, tranquilizers, antihistamines, antidepressants, narcotic analgesics, and monoamine oxidase inhibitor antidepressants. Tolerance to one indicates tolerance to the others.

The effect of succinylcholine is enhanced by propanidid, procaine, echothiophate, hexafluorenium, polymyxins, and aminoglycosides.

Allyl barbiturates reduce the cytochrome P-450 enzyme necessary for metabolism of some drugs and chemicals. Excessive response to these drugs may occur.

Hypnotics, antihistamines, and narcotic analgesics slow intestinal absorption.

Phenytoin toxicity can occur in slow acetylators given disulfiram or isoniazid. Phenytoin levels rise and toxicity is possible when diazoxide is withdrawn. Diazepam, coumarins, phenylbutazone, thioridazine, and methylphenidate may increase blood levels of phenytoin, with possible toxicity.

Neuromuscular blockade from tubocurarine type agents is increased by propranolol, procainamide, quinidine, clindamycin, polymyxins, and aminoglycosides and by potassium loss induced by diuretics, carbenoxolone, amphotericin B, corticosteroids, or laxative abuse.

Long-term phenothiazine administration increases and short-term phenothiazine administration decreases anesthetic requirements. Phenothiazines are alpha sympathomimetic blocking agents and cause hypotension. They also alter catecholamine levels in the brain and interact dangerously with monoamine oxidase inhibitors. Vasopressors can be more or less effective in the presence of phenothiazines.

## References

### *Barbiturate and non-barbiturate depressants*

Ludwigs U, *et al.* Suicidal chloral hydrate poisoning. *J Toxicol Clin Toxicol* 1996;34:97

Roth BA, *et al.* Carisoprodol-induced myoclonic encephalopathy. *J Toxicol Clin Toxicol* 1998;36:609

Roberge RJ, *et al.* Flumazenil reversal of carisoprodol (Soma) intoxication. *J Emerg Med* 2000;18:61

Sing K, *et al.* Chloral hydrate toxicity from oral and intravenous administration. *J Toxicol Clin Toxicol* 1996;34:101

### *Anticonvulsants*

Chua HC, *et al.* Elimination of phenytoin in toxic overdose. *Clin Neurol Neurosurg* 2000;102:6

Faisy C, *et al.* Carbamazepine-associated severe left ventricular dysfunction. *J Toxicol Clin Toxicol* 2000;38:339

Kawasaki C, *et al.* Charcoal hemoperfusion in the treatment of phenytoin overdose. *Am J Kidney Dis* 2000;35:323

Kraus de Camargo OA, Bode H. Agranulocytosis associated with lamotrigine. *BMJ* 1999;318:1179

Mamiya K, *et al.* Phenytoin intoxication induced by fluvoxamine. *Therap Drug Monitoring* 2001;23:75

Manto M, *et al.* Hypoglycemia associated with phenytoin intoxication. *J Toxicol Clin Toxicol* 1996;34:205

Moss DM, *et al.* Cross-sensitivity and the anticonvulsant hypersensitivity syndrome. *J Emerg Med* 1999;17:503

Okumura A, *et al*. Predictive value of acetylcholine stimulation testing for oligohidrosis caused by zonisamide. *Pediatr Neurol* 2000;23:59

Pinkston R, Walker LA. Multiorgan system failure caused by valproic acid toxicity. *Am J Emerg Med* 1997;15:504

Schuerer DJE, *et al*. High-efficiency dialysis for carbamazepine overdose. *J Toxicol Clin Toxicol* 2000;38:321

Stephen LJ, *et al*. Transient hemiparesis with topiramate. *BMJ* 1999;318:845

Wong ICK, Lhatoo SD. Adverse reactions to new anticonvulsant drugs. *Drug Safety* 2000;23:35

### Narcotic analgesics

Brooks DE, *et al*. Clinical nuances of pediatric methadone intoxication. *Vet Human Toxicol* 1999;41:388

Kaplan JL, *et al*. Double-blind, randomized study of nalmefene and naloxone in Emergency Department patients with suspected narcotic overdose. *Ann Emerg Med* 1999;34:42

Litovitz T, *et al*. Surveillance of loperamide ingestions: an analysis of 216 Poison Center reports. *J Toxicol Clin Toxicol* 1996;35:11

Melandri R, *et al*. Myocardial damage and rhabdomyolysis associated with prolonged hypoxic coma following opiate overdose. *J Toxicol Clin Toxicol* 1996;34:199

Osterwalder JJ. Naloxone—for intoxications with intravenous heroin and heroin mixtures – harmless or hazardous? A prospective clinical study. *J Toxicol Clin Toxicol* 1996;34:409

Schneider RK, *et al*. Update in addiction medicine. *Ann Intern Med* 2001;134:387

Sporer KA. Acute heroin overdose. *Ann Intern Med* 1999;130:584

Stork CM, *et al*. Propoxyphene-induced wide QRS complex dysrhythmia responsive to sodium bicarbonate – a case report. *J Toxicol Clin Toxicol* 1995;33:179

Watson WA, *et al*. Opioid toxicity recurrence after an initial response to naloxone. *J Toxicol Clin Toxicol* 1998;36:11

### Bromides

Horowitz BZ. Bromism from excessive cola consumption. *J Toxicol Clin Toxicol* 1996;35:315

### Antihistamines and phenothiazines

Arnold SM, *et al*. Two siblings poisoned with diphenhydramine: a case of factitious disorder by proxy. *Ann Emerg Med* 1998;32:256

Bassett KE, *et al*. Cyclizine abuse by teenagers in Utah. *Am J Emerg Med* 1996;14: 472

Drotts DL, Vinson DR. Prochlorperazine induces akathisia in emergency patients. *Ann Emerg Med* 1999;34:469

Emadian SM, *et al*. Rhabdomyolysis: a rare adverse effect of diphenhydramine overdose. *Am J Emerg Med* 1996;14:574

Hasan MY, *et al*. Management of neuroleptic malignant syndrome with anticholinergic medication. *Vet Human Toxicol* 1999;41:79

Hwanitz E, *et al*. The efficacy and safety of clozapine versus chlorpromazine in geriatric schizophrenia. *J Clin Psychiatry* 1999;60:41

June RA, Nasr I. Torsades de Pointes with terfenadine ingestion. *Am J Emerg Med* 1997;15:542

Leung ATS, *et al*. Chlorpromazine-induced refractile corneal deposits and cataract. *Arch Ophthalmol* 1999;117:1662

Lewin NA, Wang RY. Neuroleptic agents. In Goldfrank LR, Flumenbaum NE, Lewin NA, *et al*. eds, *Goldfrank's Toxicologic Emergencies*. Norwalk, CT: Appleton & Lange, 1994:739–47

Russell SA, *et al*. Upper airway compromise in acute chlorpromazine ingestion. *Am J Emerg Med* 1996;14:467

Schmidt W, Lang K. Life-threatening dysrhythmias in severe thioridazine poisoning treated with physostigmine and transient atrial pacing. *Crit Care Med* 1997;25:1925

### *Selective depressants*

Acri AA, Henretig FM. Effects of risperidone in overdose. *Am J Emerg Med* 1998;16:498

Bedry R, *et al*. Non-fatal clozapine (Leponex) intoxication with toxicokinetic evaluation. *Vet Human Toxicol* 1999;41:20

Brubacher JR, *et al*. Delayed toxicity following ingestion of enteric-coated divalproex sodium (Epival*). J Emerg Med* 1999;17:463

Chapple D, *et al*. Baclofen overdose in two siblings. *Pediatr Emerg Care* 2001;17: 110

Chern C-H, *et al*. Continuous flumazenil infusion in preventing complications from severe benzodiazepine intoxication. *Am J Emerg Med* 1998;16:238

Elko CJ, *et al*. Zolpidem-associated hallucinations and serotonin reuptake inhibition: a possible interaction. *J Toxicol Clin Toxicol* 1998;36:195

Fernandez MC, *et al*. Gabapentin, valproic acid, and ethanol intoxication: elevated blood levels with mild clinical effects. *J Toxicol Clin Toxicol* 1996;34:437

Graudins A, Aaron CK. Delayed peak serum valproic acid in massive divalproex overdose – treatment with charcoal hemoperfusion. *J Toxicol Clin Toxicol* 1996;34:335

Green SM, *et al*. Inadvertent ketamine overdose in children: clinical manifestations and outcome. *Ann Emerg Med* 1999;34:492

Harmon TJ, *et al*. Loss of consciousness from acute quetiapine overdosage. *J Toxicol Clin Toxicol* 1998;36:599

Hustey FM. Acute quetiapine poisoning. *J Emerg Med* 1999;17:995

Insley Crouch B, *et al*. Benzonatate overdose associated with seizures and arrhythmias. *J Toxicol Clin Toxicol* 1998;36:713

Ishii A, *et al*. Nonfatal suicidal intoxication by clozapine. *J Toxicol Clin Toxicol* 1996;35:195

Karsenti D, *et al*. Hepatotoxicity associated with zolpidem treatment. *BMJ* 1999;318:1179

Kurta DL, *et al*. Zolpidem (Ambien): a pediatric case series. *J Toxicol Clin Toxicol* 1996;35:453

Lee W-L, *et al*. A case of severe hyperammonemia and unconsciousness following sodium valproate intoxication. *Vet Human Toxicol* 1998;40:346

Li J, *et al*. A tale of novel intoxication: a review of the effects of gamma-hydroxybutyric acid with recommendations for management. *Ann Emerg Med* 1998;31:729

Mady S, *et al*. Pediatric clozapine intoxication. *Am J Emerg Med* 1996;14:462

Mitchell RK, *et al*. Respiratory arrest after intramuscular ketamine in a 2-year-old child. *Am J Emerg Med* 1996;14:580

Okun MS, *et al*. GHB toxicity: what you need to know. *Emerg Med* 2000;32:10

Peng C-T, *et al*. Prolonged severe withdrawal symptoms after acute-on chronic baclofen overdose. *J Toxicol Clin Toxicol* 1998;36:359

Renwick AC, *et al*. Monitoring of clozapine and norclozapine plasma concentration-time curves in acute overdose. *J Toxicol Clin Toxicol* 2000;38:325

Roberge RJ, *et al*. Two chlorzoxazone (Parafon Forte) overdoses and coma in one patient: reversal with flumazenil. *Am J Emerg Med* 1998;16:393

Sleeper R, *et al*. Psychotropic drugs and falls: New evidence pertaining to serotonin reuptake inhibitors. *Pharmacotherapy* 2000;20:308

VanDierendonk DR, Dire DJ. Baclofen and ethanol ingestion: a case report. *J Emerg Med* 1999;17:989

Wiley CC, *et al*. Pediatric benzodiazepine ingestion resulting in hospitalization. *J Toxicol Clin Toxicol* 1998;36:227

## PHARMACOKINETICS AND TOXIC CONCENTRATIONS (see p. 100)

| | $pK_a$ | $T_{1/2}$ (h) | $V_d$ (l/kg) | % Bound | Toxic concentration (mg/ml) |
|---|---|---|---|---|---|
| Alfentanil | | | | | 0.1 |
| Alprazolam | | | 1.1 | 80 | 0.075, 0.1[†] |
| Amobarbital | 7.7 | 12–27 | 2.5–4 1 | 61 | 30 |
| Baclofen | 3.9, 9.6 | 3–4 | | 30 | |
| Barbital | | | | | 100 |
| Bromide | | 168 | | | 200, 2000[†] |
| Brompheniramine | | | | | 0.05, 0.2[†] |
| Buprenorphine | | | | | 0.02 (urine) |
| Butabarbital | 7.9 | 37.5 | 0.8 | 26 | 28, 73[†] |
| Butalbital | | | | | 10, 25[†] |
| Carbamazepine | | 18–55 | 1 | 72 | 10 |
| Chloral hydrate | 10.04 | 8–35 | 0.6 | 70–80 | |
| Chlorazepate | | | | 80–95 | 2 |
| Chlordiazepoxide | 4.6 | 8–28 | 0.3–0.5 | 94–97 | 3, 20[†] |
| Chlormethiazole | 3.2 | 3.1–5 | 5.4 | 63 | |
| Chlorpheniramine | 9.2 | 12–15 | | 72 | 0.5, 1[†] |
| Chlorpromazine | 9.3 | 16–31 | 40–50 | 91–99 | 0.5, 3[†] |
| Clonazepam | 1.5, 10.5 | 20–60 | 3.1 | 86 | 0.069 |
| Clozapine | | | | | 0.6, 3[†] |
| Codeine | 8.2 | 2–3 | 5–10 | 7 | 0.2, 1.6[†] |
| Dantrolene | 7.5 | 8.7 | | | |
| Dextromethorphan | | | | | 0.1, 3[†] |
| Diazepam | 3.3 | 20–96 | 0.7, 2.6* | 98 | 1.5, 10[†] |
| Diclofenac | | | | | 60 |
| Dihydrocodeine | | | | | 0.3,0.8[†] |
| Diphenhydramine | 8.3 | 5–8 | | 72 | 0.6, 8[†] |
| Diphenoxylate | 7.07 | 2.5 | 4.6 | | |
| Doxylamine | | | | | 0.2, 0.7[†] |
| Droperidol | 7.6 | 2 | | 85–90 | |
| Estazolam | | | | 93 | |
| Ethchlorvynol | | 35 | 5–10 | | 85 |
| Ethosuximide | 9.3 | 60 | 0.7,* 0.9 | 0 | 150 |
| Fentanyl | | | | | 0.003, 0.017[†] |
| Fluphenazine | 3.9, 8.05 | 14 | | | |
| Flurazepam | 1.9 | 47–100? | | 97 | 0.2, 0.5[†] |
| Glutethimide | 9.2 | 10–100 | 10–20 | 54 | 6 |
| Haloperidol | 8.7 | 14–21 | 17–30 | 92 | 42 |
| Hexobarbital | 8.2 | 3–7 | 1.1 | | 8, 50[†] |
| Hydrocodone | | | | | 0.1, 0.2[†] |
| Hydromorphone | | | | | 0.1, 0.1[†] |
| Hydroxyzine | | | | | 0.1, 4[†] |
| Ketamine | 7.5 | 3–4 | | | |
| Levorphanol | | | | | 0.1, 2.7[†] |

*Continued*

*Pharmacokinetics and toxic concentrations (continued)*

| | p$K_a$ | $T_{1/2}$ (h) | $V_d$ (l/kg) | % Bound | Toxic concentration (mg/ml) |
|---|---|---|---|---|---|
| Loperamide | 8.6 | 9–14 | | | |
| Lorazepam | 1.3, 11.5 | 10–24 | 0.9 | 90 | 0.3, 0.5[†] |
| Loxapine | 6.6 | 3–4 | | | |
| Magnesium | | | | | 48.6, 150[†] |
| Meclastine | 8.1 | 35 | 1.14 | 96 | |
| Meperidine | 8.7 | 2.4–4 | 4.3 | 64 | 0.5, 1[†] |
| Meprobamate | | 6–17 | | | 10, 43[†] |
| Methadone | 8.6 | 18–97 | 5–10 | 85 | 1, 0.4[†] |
| Methapyrilene | | | | | 12 |
| Methaqualone | 2.4 | 20–60 | 6 | 80 | 2, 5[†] |
| Methsuximide | | 10 | | | |
| Methyprylon | | | | | 30 |
| Midazolam | | 2-5 | 0.8-6.6 | 95[+] | 1 |
| Morphine | 8.05 | 10–44? | 2.8 | 35 | 0.1, 0.1[†] |
| Naloxone | | 1–2 | | | |
| Nitrazepam | 3.2, 10.8 | 28–30 | 2.1 | 85 | 0.2, 1[†] |
| Normeperidine | | 15–20 | | | |
| Norpropoxyphene | | 30–36 | | | |
| Orphenadrine | 8.4 | 10 | | 20 | |
| Oxazepam | 1.7, 11.6 | 10–14 | 1.6 | 90 | 2, 3[†] |
| Oxycodone | | | | | 0.2, 5[†] |
| Paraldehyde | | 4–10 | | | |
| Pentazocine | 9.0 | 2–3 | 3 | 60–70 | 1, 3[†] |
| Pentobarbital | 7.6 | 23–30 | 0.9–1 | 40–65 | 10, 15[†] |
| Perphenazine | 7.8 | 21 | | | |
| Phenobarbital | 7.4 | 48–144 | 1 | 40–60 | 15, 50[†] |
| Phenytoin | 8.3 | 10–42 | 1 | 89 | 20, 50[†] |
| Pimozide | 8.6 | 29 | | 97 | |
| Prazepam | | 78 | | 85 | |
| Primidone | | 3.3–12.5 | 1 | 0 | 18 |
| Prochlorperazine | 8.1 | 23 | | | |
| Promethazine | 9.1 | | | 7.5 | 1, 2[†] |
| Propoxyphene | 6.3 | 3–12 | 1 | 78 | 0.6, 2[†] |
| Pyrilamine | | | | | 0.12, 11[†] |
| Quazepam | | 25-41 | 5 | 95[+] | |
| Quinalbarbital | 7.9 | 40 | | 65–75 | |
| Secobarbitel | | 29 | | | 30 |
| Temazepam | | 10–15 | 1.4 | 96 | 1, 0.8[†] |
| Thiopental | 7.6 | 3–8 | | 75–90 | 14 |
| Thioridazine | 9.5 | 16–24 | | | 18[†] |
| Triazolam | | 2.3 | 0.8–1.3 | 90 | |
| Tripelennamine | | | | | 10[†] |
| Valproate | | 8–15 | 0.15–0.4 | 90 | 200+ |
| Zolpidem | | | | | 0.5, 1[†] |

[†]Fatal

# 24 Drugs affecting the autonomic nervous system

## ATROPINE, HYOSCYAMINE, BELLADONNA, SCOPOLAMINE, AND SYNTHETIC SUBSTITUTES

Atropine, scopolamine, related alkaloids, and synthetic substitutes are sold both in prescriptions and in a number of proprietary mixtures for the treatment of gastrointestinal diseases, colds, hay fever, Parkinsonism, and asthma. Plants containing atropine and related alkaloids are also occasionally eaten by children. The plants *Atropa belladonna* (deadly nightshade, English nightshade), *Hyoscyamus niger* (henbane), and *Datura stramonium* (jimsonweed) contain 0.25–0.5% atropine or related alkaloids. Tincture of belladonna contains 30 mg of atropine alkaloids per 100 ml. Synthetic atropine substitutes are as follows:

| | |
|---|---|
| Benztropine (Cogentin) | Methantheline (Banthine) |
| Biperiden (Akineton) | Mepenzolate (Cantil) |
| Clidinium (Quarzan) | Methscopolamine (Pamine) |
| Cyclopentolate (Cyclogyl) | Oxybutynin (Ditropan) |
| Dicyclomine (Bentyl) | Procyclidine (Kemadrin) |
| Flavoxate (Urispas) | Propantheline (Pro-Banthine) |
| Glycopyrrolate (Robinul) | Tolterodine (Detrol) |
| Homatropine | Trihexyphenidyl (Artane) |
| Ipratropium (Atrovent) | |

The fatal dose of atropine or scopolamine in children may be as low as 10 mg. Death has occurred from dicyclomine (60 mg/kg) with doxylamine. The fatal dose for other synthetic substitutes would be 10–100 mg/kg. The fatality rate in cases of atropine or scopolamine poisoning is less than 1%.

Atropine and scopolamine paralyze the parasympathetic nervous system by blocking the action on effector cells of the acetylcholine released at nerve endings. Atropine and the various synthetic substitutes also stimulate the central nervous system. Since atropine is almost entirely eliminated by the kidneys, abnormalities of kidney function may lead to toxic reactions in patients receiving atropine. Kidney function must be normal to eliminate the drug.

The pathologic findings are not characteristic. The internal organs may be congested.

## Clinical findings

The principal manifestations of poisoning with these drugs are delirium, fast pulse, and fever.

*Acute poisoning* (from ingestion, injection, or application to mucous membranes)

Therapeutic doses of atropine, scopolamine, or other anticholinergic drugs may cause dilated pupils, blurring of vision, rise in intraocular tension, and increased heart rate. Toxic doses (5–10 mg or higher) may cause hot, dry, red skin; dry mouth; disorientation; hallucinations; aggressive behavior; delirium; rapid pulse and respiration; urinary retention; muscular stiffness; fever; convulsions; and coma. Synthetic substitutes in doses of 0.1–1 g may cause similar symptoms. Some synthetic substitutes are similar to antihistamines and are more likely to cause convulsions. In doses above 10 mg scopolamine also causes respiratory depression and coma.

*Chronic poisoning* (from ingestion, injection, or application to mucous membranes)

The above symptoms may occur after repeated therapeutic doses.

## Prevention

The dosage of atropine or related compounds must be lowered during periods of hot weather for patients who are taking maximum tolerated amounts, since such patients are most susceptible to heat exhaustion. Do not give atropine or related drugs to patients with glaucoma. Reduction of dosage is necessary if urinary retention occurs.

**Treatment**

*Acute poisoning*

(1) Emergency measures – Maintain airway and respiration. Remove poison from mucous membranes by washing. Delay absorption of ingested material by giving activated charcoal and then remove by gastric lavage (see pp. 29–30). Follow with saline catharsis. Efforts to remove these agents are useful for several hours after ingestion, since they depress gastrointestinal motility.

(2) Antidote – To reverse life-threatening central and peripheral effects of atropine and substitutes, give physostigmine salicylate intravenously, 1–5 ml of a solution containing 1 mg in 5 ml of saline. The smaller dose is for children, and injection should take not less than 2 min. Electrocardiographic control is advisable. Dosage can be repeated every 5 min up to a total dose of 2 mg in children and 6 mg in adults every 30 min (see Table 24.2). Physostigmine is contraindicated in hypotensive reactions. Atropine, 1 mg, should be available for immediate injection if physostigmine causes bradycardia, convulsions, or severe bronchoconstriction.

(3) General measures:
   (a) Monitor ECG.
   (b) Reduce rectal body temperature to 38°C by applying wet towels. Dexamethasone, 1 mg/kg slowly intravenously, has been suggested for pyrexia.
   (c) Control convulsions by giving diazepam.
   (d) Give fluids orally or intravenously to maintain urine output.
   (e) If patient does not void catheterization may be necessary to avoid bladder rupture.

*Chronic poisoning*

Discontinue medication and treat as for acute poisoning.

**Prognosis**

A patient who survives for 24 h will probably recover. Whether physostigmine increases the survival rate in patients poisoned with anticholinergic agents has not been determined.

## References

Beaver KM, Gavin TJ. Treatment of acute anticholinergic poisoning with physostigmine. *Am J Emerg Med* 1998;16:505

Burns MJ, *et al*. A comparison of physostigmine and benzodiazepines for the treatment of anticholinergic poisoning. *Ann Emerg Med* 2000;35:374

Martin B, Howell PR. Physostigmine: going…going…gone? Two cases of central anticholinergic syndrome following anaesthesia and its treatment with physostigmine. *Eur J Anaesth* 1997;14:467

Myers JH, *et al*. Anticholinergic poisoning in colicky infants treated with hyoscyamine sulfate. *Am J Emerg Med* 1997;15:532

Perrone J, *et al*. Laboratory confirmation of scopolamine co-intoxication in patients using tainted heroin. *J Toxicol Clin Toxicol* 1999;37:491

Ramirez M, *et al*. Fifteen cases of atropine poisoning after honey ingestion. *Vet Human Toxicol* 1999;41:19

Shannon M. Toxicology reviews: Physostigmine. *Pediatr Emerg Care* 1998;14:224

Thabet H, *et al*. Stramonium poisonings in humans. *Vet Human Toxicol* 1999;41:320

Weiner AL, *et al*. Anticholinergic poisoning with adulterated intranasal cocaine. *Am J Emerg Med* 1998;16:517

Yang C-C, Deng D-F. Clinical experience in acute overdosage of diphenidol. *J Toxicol Clin Toxicol* 1998;36:33

## SYMPATHOMIMETIC AGENTS: EPINEPHRINE, EPHEDRINE, AMPHETAMINE, NAPHAZOLINE, AND RELATED DRUGS

Epinephrine, ephedrine, and related agents are widely sold on prescription and in proprietary mixtures for the treatment of nasal congestion, asthma, and hay fever.

From 1 to 10% of users of epinephrine or related drugs have reactions from overdose. See Table 24.1 for estimated fatal doses. Fatalities are rare.

Epinephrine and related drugs stimulate muscle and gland cells innervated by the sympathetic nervous system. They also produce variable stimulatory effects on the central nervous system.

The pathologic findings are not characteristic.

**Table 24.1** Sympathomimetic agents: epinephrine and related drugs (see treatment on p. 428)

| Drug | MLD* drug (mg) | Method of administration |
|---|---|---|
| Albuterol (salbutamol) | 200 | Oral |
| Amphetamine (Benzedrine) | 10 | Oral |
| Apraclonidine (Iopidine) | 10 | Oral |
| Bitolterol (Tornalate) | 10 | Oral |
| Brimonidine (Alphagan) | 10 | Oral |
| Carbidopa | 1000? | Oral |
| Dextroamphetamine | 20 | Oral |
| Dipivefrin (Propine) | 10 | Topical |
| Dobutamine (Dobutrex) | 200 | IV |
| Dopamine (Intropin) | 200 | IV |
| Ephedrine | 200 | Oral |
| Epinephrine | 10 | IM or subcut |
| Isoetharine (Bronkosol) | 20 | Oral |
| Isometheptene (Midrin) | 200 | Oral |
| Isoproterenol (Isuprel) | 100 | Topical |
| Isoxsuprine (Vasodilan) | 100 | Oral |
| Levodopa (Sinemet) | 1000? | Oral |
| Metaproterenol (Alupent) | 20 | Oral |
| Metaraminol (Aramine) | 60 | Intranasal, IM |
| Methamphetamine | 100 | Oral |
| Methoxamine (Vasoxyl) | 60 | IM, subcut |
| Methylphenidate (Ritalin) | 200 | Oral |
| Midodrine (ProAmatine) | 200 | Oral |
| Naphazoline (Privine) | 10 | Intranasal |
| Norepinephrine (levarterenol, Levophed) | 10 | IM or subcut |
| Pemoline (Cylert) | 200 | Oral |
| Phendimetrazine (Plegine) | 200 | Oral |
| Phenylephrine | 100 | Intranasal |
| Phentermine (Fastine) | 200 | Oral |
| Pirbuterol (Maxair) | 4 | Intranasal, oral |
| Pseudoephedrine (Afrinol) | 200 | Oral |
| Ritodrine (Yutopar) | 200 | Oral |
| Salmeterol (Serevent) | 10 | Oral |
| Terbutaline (Bricanyl) | 50 | Oral |
| Tetrahydrozoline (Tyzine) | 5 | IntranasalTizanidine |
| Tizanidine (Zanaflex) | 10 | Oral |

*Estimated for children up to age 2 years. Adult MLD at least 10 times as high

## Clinical findings

The principal manifestation of poisoning with these drugs is convulsions.

*Acute poisoning* (from injection, ingestion, inhalation, or application to mucous membranes)

Nausea and vomiting, nervousness, irritability, tachycardia, cardiac arrhythmias, dilated pupils, blurred vision, chills, pallor or cyanosis, fever, suicidal behavior, mania, opisthotonos, spasms, convulsions, pulmonary edema, gasping respiration, coma, and respiratory failure. A child died with convulsions, hyperthermia, tachycardia, and cardiac arrest after taking diethylpropion, 30 mg/kg. The blood pressure is markedly raised initially but may be below normal later with persistent anuria. Inhalation or injection of decomposed (pink) epinephrine will cause a psychosis-like state with hallucinations and morbid fears. Perivascular or subcutaneous injection of norepinephrine or other epinephrine substitutes causes cutaneous necrosis or slough. Naphazoline, and tetrahydrozoline can cause hypotension and central nervous system depression. Terbutaline given as a uterine relaxant in threatened abortion has caused maternal pulmonary edema when given with corticosteroids, and death of the fetus when given in 10 times the usual dose. Dopamine (Intropin) can increase cardiac irritability, with paroxysmal supraventricular tachycardia and other arrhythmias, and can cause hypotension. Gangrene of the extremities has occurred after administration of dopamine. Intra-arterial injection of dopamine can cause severe pain, ischemia, and gangrene in the arterial distribution area.

*Chronic poisoning*

Prolonged nasal use of epinephrine or substitutes leads to nasal congestion. Prolonged oral use of amphetamine or ephedrine or similar drugs in large doses by emotionally unstable individuals may lead to personality changes with a psychic craving to continue the use of the drug. Use of these compounds can also cause reactions of tension and anxiety progressing to psychosis. Abuse of methylphenidate has caused fever with eosinophilia. Long-term use of dextroamphetamine or methylphenidate for control of hyperactivity in children has caused growth retardation. Pemoline is suspected of causing liver damage. Isoxsuprine can cause skin rash. Dobutamine has caused anginal pain and dyspnea.

Levodopa can cause anorexia, nausea, tachycardia, ventricular extrasystoles, depression or agitation, hypotension or hypertension, choreiform or dystonic movements, hallucinations, and toxic psychosis. The maximum dose should not exceed 8 g/d. A combination of carbidopa with levodopa (Sinemet) can cause psychosis, depression, convulsions, nausea, cardiac irregularity, hypotension, gastrointestinal ulceration, and hypertension. Continued use of vasopressors such as norepinephrine to maintain blood pressure in the presence of hypovolemia can lead to acidosis.

### Laboratory findings

These are noncontributory.

### Prevention

Parents should be warned of the dangers of incautious administration of potent nose drops to infants. Nasal inhalers and amphetamine preparations should be stored safely. Administration of epinephrine or substitutes during or after surgery may lead to ventricular arrhythmias and cardiac arrest.

### Treatment

### Acute poisoning

(1) Emergency measures:
   (a) If respiration is shallow or if cyanosis is present, give artificial respiration. Maintain adequate arterial $O_2$ concentration. Minute volume of respiration should be 1–1.5 l/10 kg. Vasopressors are contraindicated.
   (b) Remove drug by ipecac emesis followed by activated charcoal. Airway-protected gastric lavage is necessary in hyperactive patients or those with depressed respiration (see pp. 29–32).
   (c) Maintain blood pressure in cardiovascular collapse (see p. 57).
(2) Antidote – For cutaneous or perivascular injection of norepinephrine, infiltrate the area with 5 mg of phentolamine (Regitine). For hypertensive reactions to epinephrine or substitutes, give phentolamine, 5 mg

diluted in saline slowly intravenously, or 100 mg orally. Chlorpromazine is contraindicated except in amphetamine poisoning. In pure amphetamine poisoning, give chlorpromazine, 0.5–1 mg/kg every 30 min as needed. Droperidol, 2.5 mg/min intravenously to a total of 10–15 mg, has been suggested for amphetamine and methamphetamine poisoning.

(3) General measures – Control convulsions (see p. 60). Diazepam is probably safe. Control pyrexia with cooling blanket and dexamethasone, 1 mg/kg slowly intravenously. Acid diuresis may be useful for amphetamine and methamphetamine poisoning.

*Chronic poisoning*

Discontinue use.

**Prognosis**

If the patient survives the first 6 h, recovery is likely. In psychotic reactions resulting from prolonged use, recovery may require weeks or months.

**References**

Guharoy R, *et al*. Methamphetamine overdose: experience with six cases. *Vet Human Toxicol* 1999;41:28.

Harris CR, *et al*. Fatal bupropion overdose. *J Toxicol Clin Toxicol* 1996;35:321

James LP, *et al*. Sympathomimetic drug use in adolescents presenting to a pediatric emergency department with chest pain. *J Toxicol Clin Toxicol* 1998;36:321

LoVecchio F, Curry SC. Dexfenfluramine overdose. *Ann Emerg Med* 1998;32:102

Ooosterbaan R, Burns MJ. Myocardial infarction associated with phenylpropanolamine. *J Emerg Med* 2000;18:55.

Perez JA Jr, *et al*. Methamphetamine-related stroke: four cases. *J Emerg Med* 1999;17:469

Richards JR, *et al*. Methamphetamine abuse and rhabdomyolysis in the ED: a 5-year study. *Am J Emerg Med* 1999;17:681

Sauder KL, *et al*. Visual hallucinations in a toddler: accidental ingestion of a sympathomimetic over-the-counter nasal decongestant. *Am J Emerg Med* 1997;15:521

Stork CM, Cantor R. Pemoline induced acute choreoathetosis: case report and review of the literature. *J Toxicol Clin Toxicol* 1996;35:105

Zaacks SM, *et al*. Hypersensitivity myocarditis associated with ephedra use. *J Toxicol Clin Toxicol* 1999;37:485

Zahn KA, *et al*. Cardiovascular toxicity after ingestion of 'herbal Ecstacy'. *J Emerg Med* 1999;17:289. (Ephedrine)

## PARASYMPATHOMIMETIC AGENTS: PHYSOSTIGMINE, PILOCARPINE, NEOSTIGMINE, AND RELATED DRUGS

Physostigmine, pilocarpine, neostigmine, and methacholine are used for the treatment of myasthenia gravis, for atonic conditions of the gastrointestinal tract and urinary bladder, and for certain cardiac irregularities.

More than 20 fatalities from these compounds have been reported in the literature. Physostigmine, benzpyrinium, and neostigmine inhibit the esterase responsible for hydrolyzing the parasympathetic effector acetylcholine. Pilocarpine, bethanechol, and methacholine act at the same point as does acetylcholine. As a result of these actions these drugs stimulate muscles and glands innervated by the parasympathetic nervous system.

The pathologic findings are congestion of the brain, lungs, and gastrointestinal tract. Pulmonary edema may occur.

### Clinical findings

The principal manifestation of poisoning with these drugs is respiratory difficulty.

*Acute poisoning* (from ingestion, injection, or application to mucous membranes)

Tremor, marked peristalsis with involuntary defecation and urination, pinpoint pupils, vomiting, cold extremities, hypotension, bronchial constriction with difficult breathing and wheezing, twitching of muscles, fainting, slow pulse, convulsions, and death from asphyxia or cardiac slowing. Life-threatening ventricular arrhythmias have occurred after use of physostigmine. Esophageal rupture has occurred from the use of carbachol, a drug similar to bethanechol. Metoclopramide can cause drowsiness, dizziness, and extrapyramidal signs.

**Table 24.2** Parasympathomimetic agents: Physostigmine and related drugs

| Drug | Fatal dose* (mg) | Method of administration |
|---|---|---|
| Acetylcholine | 20 | Injection |
| Bethanechol (Urecholine) | 20 | Injection |
| Carbachol (Miostat) | 10 | Injection or topical |
| Cisapride (Propulside)** | 1000 | Oral |
| Demecarium (Humorsol) | 20 | Topical |
| Donepazil (Aricept) | 100 | Oral |
| Echothiophate (Phospholine) | 10 | Topical |
| Edrophonium (Tensilon) | 100 | Injection |
| Isoflurophate (Floropryl) | 10 | Topical |
| Metoclopramide (Reglan) | 200 | Oral |
| Neostigmine (Prostigmin) | 60 | Oral |
| Neostigmine (Prostigmin) | 10 | Injection |
| Physostigmine (Antilirium) | 6 | Injection or oral |
| Pilocarpine (Salagen) | 60 | Topical |
| Pyridostigmine (Mestinon) | 300 | Oral |
| Tacrine (Cognex) | 1000 | Oral |

*Estimated for adult; **cardiac arrhythmias

### Chronic poisoning

Repeated small doses may reproduce the syndrome described under Acute poisoning.

## Prevention

When physostigmine and related drugs are used atropine should be readily available for immediate use. Do not use physostigmine in the presence of asthma, gangrene, diabetes, cardiac or vascular disease, or mechanical obstruction of the intestines or urogenital tract; in vagotonic states; or in patients receiving choline esters or depolarizing neuromuscular blocking agents such as decamethonium or succinylcholine.

## Treatment of acute or chronic poisoning

### Emergency measures

Maintain artificial respiration until antidote can be given.

*Antidote*

Give atropine, 2 mg slowly intravenously. Repeat this dose intramuscularly every 2–4 h as necessary to relieve respiratory difficulty. For echothiophate only, pralidoxime (see p. 96) is also useful.

**Prognosis**

If atropine can be given, recovery is immediate.

## MISCELLANEOUS BLOCKING AGENTS (Table 24.3)

Sympatholytic agents are used to reduce blood pressure and for other therapeutic purposes. Most of these agents produce postural hypotension, with faintness and tachycardia, dry mouth, cardiac irregularities, and failure of erections. Toxic reactions are controlled by reducing the dosage or discontinuing the drug. Abrupt withdrawal of clonidine may cause hyperexcitability, psychosis, cardiac arrhythmias, and rapid rise of blood pressure. Deaths have occurred.

**Treatment**

In acute toxic reactions to any of the blocking agents discontinue use. Maintain respiration. Remove overdoses with lavage and activated charcoal (see pp. 31–32). Use sympathomimetic agents cautiously, since their effects may be intensified. Mechanical ventilation and cardiac pacing may be necessary. Atropine may also be helpful. For clonidine overdose the administration of atropine, diazoxide for hypertension or dopamine infusion for hypotension, and maximum diuresis with furosemide and mannitol have been successful.

**Table 24.3** Sympathetic, histamine ($H_2$), etc., blocking agents (see p. 435)

| Drug | Safe dose | Toxic effects |
|------|-----------|---------------|
| Acrivastine (Semprex-D) | 50 mg orally | Sedation, headache |
| Bretylium (Bretylol) | 100 mg orally | Nasal congestion, muscular weakness, parotid pain, confusion, ventricular tachycardia and fibrillation |
| Cimetidine (Tagamet), Famotidine (Pepcid), Nizatidine (Axid), Roxatidine (Roxin) | 300 mg orally or IV<br>40 mg orally<br>300 mg orally<br>150 mg orally | Diarrhea, headache, fatigue, dizziness, muscle pain, rash, confusion, phytobezoar, delirium, psychosis, gynecomastia, elevated serum creatinine or liver enzymes, leukopenia, agranulocytosis, thrombocytopenia, erythema annulare centrifugum, ulcer perforation on withdrawal. Hepatitis and interstitial nephritis with renal failure have occurred |
| Clonidine (Catapres) | 0.1 mg orally | Bradycardia, drowsiness, gastrointestinal upset, possible hepatitis, heart failure, rash, coma, arrhythmia, hypotension, depressed respiration, apnea, increased sensitivity to alcohol. Hypertensive crisis on abrupt withdrawal |
| Dapiprazol | 0.5% topical | Irritation, edema, headache, blurring of vision |
| Emadastine, levocabastine | 0.1% topical<br>0.05% topical | Headache, irritation |
| Entacapone, tolcapone | 200 mg orally | Hypotension, diarrhea, depression |
| Guanabenz, Guanadrel, Guanethidine, Guanfacine | 5 mg orally<br>10 mg orally<br>10 mg orally<br>1 mg orally | Diarrhea, mydriasis, constipation, polyarteritis nodosa |
| Methyldopa (Aldomet) | 0.5 g orally | Fluid retention, fever, diarrhea, mental depression, hepatic toxicity, Parkinsonism, arthralgia, leukopenia, hypertension, breast enlargement, amenorrhea, galactorrhea, pancreatitis, myocarditis, hemolytic anemia |
| Metyrosine (Demser) | 500 mg orally | Sedation, extrapyramidal signs, anxiety, psychosis, diarrhea |

*Continued*

*Table 24.3 (continued)*

| Drug | Safe dose | Toxic effects |
|------|-----------|---------------|
| Olopatidine | 0.1% topical | Irritation, headache, local edema |
| Ondansetron (Zofran) | 8 mg orally | Headache, diarrhea, cramps, fever |
| Phenoxybenzamine, Phentolamine | 10 mg orally 100 mg orally | Nasal congestion, miosis, tachycardia, vertigo, indigestion, weakness, vasomotor collapse |
| Pindolol (Visken) | 5 mg orally | Bradycardia, cardiac failure. 5 mg has caused bronchospasm |
| Ranitidine (Zantac) | 100 mg orally | Leukopenia, headache, nausea, possible liver and kidney damage, increased intraocular pressure |
| Sibutramine | 15 mg orally | Insomnia, dry mouth. Rare: interstitial nephritis |
| Tamsulosin | 0.4 mg orally | Hypotension, headache |
| Tolazoline (Priscoline) | 100 mg orally or IV | Pilomotor reactions, formication, tingling, chilliness, nausea, epigastric distress, severe cardiac pain |

## References

Bosek V, *et al*. Acute myocardial ischemia after administration of ondansetron hydrochloride. *Anesthesiology* 2000;92:895

Hirayama K, *et al*. Famotidine-induced acute interstitial nephritis. *Nephrol Dial Transplant* 1998;13:2636

Holm KJ, Spencer CM. Entacapone: A review of it use in Parkinson's disease. *Drugs* 1999;58:159

Lusthof KJ, *et al*. Use of clonidine for chemical submission. *J Toxicol Clin Toxicol* 2000;38:329

Odeh M, Oliven A. Central nervous system reactions associated with famotidine. *J Clin Gastroenterol* 1998;27:253

Schoenwald PK, *et al*. Complete atrioventricular block and cardiac arrest following intravenous famotidine administration. *Anesthesiology* 1999;90:623

Smith GN, Piercy WN. Methyldopa hepatotoxicity in pregnancy: a case report. *Am J Obstet Gynecol* 1995;172:222

Zarifis J, *et al*. Poisoning with anti-hypertensive drugs: methyldopa and clonidine. *J Hum Hypertens* 1995;9:787

# BETA-SYMPATHETIC BLOCKING AGENTS: PROPRANOLOL, ATENOLOL, PINDOLOL, AND OTHERS

Propranolol (Inderal) and other $\beta$-sympathetic blocking agents are used in a wide variety of conditions ranging from migraine to cardiac arrhythmias and narcotic withdrawal.

Initial doses of these drugs (per 70 kg) should not exceed the following (in mg):

Acebutolol (Sectral), 200;
Atenolol (Tenormin), 50
Betaxolol (Kerlone), 10
Bisoprolol (Zebeta), 5
Carteolol (Cartrol), 2.5
Carvedilol (Coreg), 3
Esmolol (Brevibloc), 3.5/min
Labetalol (Trandate, Normodyne), 200

Levobunolol (Betagan ophthalmic)
Metipranolol (Optipranolol ophthalmic)
Metoprolol (Lopressor), 50
Nadolol (Corgard), 40
Penbutolol (Levotol), 20
Pindolol (Visken), 5
Propranolol (Inderal), 10
Sotalol (Betapace), 80
Timolol (Blocadren), 10

Serious symptoms can occur after administration of 1 g of propranolol in adults or 10 mg/kg in children. Several fatalities have occurred.

The effects of propranolol are typical of this group of drugs: propranolol reduces or blocks cardiac and bronchial response to $\beta$-sympathetic stimulation, produces a quinidine-like reduction in myocardial contractility, and has central nervous system effects. A metabolite, 4-hydroxypropranolol, has similar effects.

## Clinical findings

The principal manifestation of poisoning with these agents is hypotension and bradycardia.

### *Acute poisoning* (from ingestion)

Overdoses cause dizziness, slow pulse, arrhythmias, fall in blood pressure, hypoglycemia (in children), respiratory depression, convulsions, bronchospasm, coma, catatonia, and delirium.

*Chronic poisoning* (from ingestion)

Continued administration of therapeutic doses has caused nausea and vomiting, diarrhea, constipation, insomnia, jaundice, fatigue, impotence, alopecia, agranulocytosis, systemic lupus erythematosus (SLE) syndrome, pulmonary edema, pulmonary fibrosis, and thrombocytopenia. Myocardial infarction can occur after abrupt withdrawal.

*Laboratory findings*

Electrocardiographic findings include intraventricular conduction defects including first-degree atrioventricular block, widened QRS complex, and absent P waves.

**Treatment**

*Acute poisoning*

(1) Emergency measures – Maintain respiration, adequate airway, blood pressure, and blood glucose. Monitor ECG. Control convulsions with diazepam. Remove drug by ipecac emesis and gastric lavage with activated charcoal (see pp. 31–32). Efforts to remove the drug are probably useless after 1 hour. Arrhythmias may require pacing.

(2) Antidote – Give isoproterenol, 1–4 µg/min by intravenous infusion, or glucagon, 50 µg/kg immediately followed by 50 µg/kg hourly by infusion. Atropine, 0.01–0.02 mg/kg, is sometimes useful to treat bradycardia. Maintenance of blood pressure may require trial of epinephrine, L-norepinephrine, dopamine, dobutamine, and calcium chloride, 1 g as a bolus and 125 mg/h.

(3) General measures:
    (a) Treat bronchospasm with intravenous aminophylline, 5 mg/kg as a loading dose, then 0.5–1 mg/kg/h to maintain serum aminophylline level just below 20 µg/ml.
    (b) Control convulsions with diazepam, 0.01 mg/kg intravenously over 10 min or magnesium sulfate, 250 mg/h.
    (c) Use sodium bicarbonate, 1 mEq/kg, to control metabolic acidosis and potassium chloride, 10 mEq/h for hypokalemia.

*Chronic poisoning*

Discontinue use of the beta-blocking drug.

**Prognosis**

If blood pressure can be maintained for 24 h, recovery is likely.

**References**

Berthault F, *et al*. A fatal case of betaxolol poisoning. *J Anal Toxicol* 1997;21:228

Love JN, *et al*. Acute beta blocker overdose: factors associated with the development of cardiovascular morbidity. *J Toxicol Clin Toxicol* 2000;38:275

Love JN, *et al*. Characterization of fatal beta blocker ingestion: a review of the American Association of Poison Control Centers data from 1985 to 1995. *J Toxicol Clin Toxicol* 1996;35:353

Love JN. Acebutolol overdose resulting in fatalities. *J Emerg Med* 2000;18:341

Pertoldi F, *et al*. Electromechanical dissociation 48 h after atenolol overdose: usefulness of calcium chloride. *Ann Emerg Med* 1998;31:777

Reith DM, *et al*. Relative toxicity of beta blockers in overdose. *J Toxicol Clin Toxicol* 1996;34:273

Salhanick SD, Wax PM. Treatment of atenolol overdose in a patient with renal failure using serial hemodialysis and hemoperfusion and associated echocardiographic findings. *Vet Human Toxicol* 2000;42:224

# ERGOT, ERGOTAMINE, AND ERGONOVINE

Ergot is a fungus that grows on rye. The derivatives, including ergotamine, methysergide (Sansert), ergoloid (Hydergine), and dihydroergotamine, are used in the treatment of headaches; ergonovine and methylergonovine are used as uterine stimulants, pergolide (Permax) and bromocriptine are used in the treatment of Parkinson's disease. Bromocriptine and cabergoline (Dostinex) are used to suppress prolactin production. Rye flour is sometimes contaminated by the ergot fungus.

The fatal dose of ergot may be as low as 1 g. Fatalities from ergotamine or other purified derivatives have not been reported; presumably the fatal dose is high in relation to the therapeutic dose. However, a dose of 40 mg of ergotamine tartrate over a 5-day period has caused impending gangrene of all 4 extremities.

Ergot and some of its alkaloids stimulate smooth muscles of the arterioles, intestines, and uterus. The pathologic findings include congestion and inflammatory changes in the gastrointestinal tract and kidneys. Gangrene of the fingers and toes may be present.

## Clinical findings

The principal manifestations of poisoning with these drugs are convulsions and gangrene.

*Acute poisoning* (from ingestion, injection, or application to mucous membranes)

Vomiting, diarrhea, dizziness, rise or fall in blood pressure, slow, weak pulse, dyspnea, convulsions, loss of consciousness. The dose necessary to produce abortion may cause fatal poisoning. Bromocriptine causes nausea, headache, dizziness, fatigue, hypertension, pulmonary infiltration, pleural effusion, and thickening of the pleura.

*Chronic poisoning* (from ingestion, injection, or application to mucous membranes)

Ergotism includes two types of manifestations, which may occur together or separately.
(1) Those resulting from contraction of blood vessels and reduced circulation include numbness and coldness of the extremities, tingling, pain in the chest, heart valve lesions, alopecia, oliguria from reduced renal blood flow, and gangrene of the fingers and toes. Hypercoagulability has also been reported.
(2) Those resulting from nervous system disturbances include vomiting, diarrhea, headache, tremors, contractions of the facial muscles, and convulsions.
(3) Methysergide, cabergoline, and pergolide have caused retroperitoneal, pericardial, and pleural fibrosis. Cabergoline has caused interstitial pneumonitis.

## Prevention

Do not give more than 3 mg of purified ergot derivatives (including ergot-amine) daily; higher doses are likely to result in peripheral vascular distur-bances. Ergot preparations are contraindicated in pregnancy, obliterative vascular disease, hypertension, infections, and kidney or liver disease.

## Treatment

### Acute poisoning

(1) Emergency measures – Remove drug by ipecac emesis followed by acti-vated charcoal. Gastric lavage may be necessary (see pp. 29–32).
(2) Antidote – Give a vasodilator such as IV nitroprusside starting at 1–2 mg/kg/min or IV phentolamine starting at 0.5 mg/min; control the rate of administration by monitoring pulse rate and blood pressure.
(3) General measures – Treat convulsions with diazepam (see p. 60). Con-trol hypercoagulability by the administration of heparin; maintain the blood clotting time at approximately twice normal. Do not use vasopressors. If coronary spasm occurs, use sublingual or IV nitroglyc-erin or nefedipine.

### Chronic poisoning

Discontinue the use of ergot preparations. Gangrene will require surgical amputation.

## Prognosis

In acute poisoning from ergot death may occur up to 1 week after poisoning. Complete recovery usually occurs in chronic poisoning if the use of ergot derivatives is discontinued prior to the appearance of gangrene. Hemodialysis is not effective.

## References

Frank W, et al. Low dose cabergoline induced interstitial pneumonitis. *Eur Respir J* 1999;14:968

Liaudet L, et al. Severe ergotism associated with interaction between ritonavir and ergotamine. *BMJ* 1999;318:771

Ling LH, *et al*. Constrictive pericarditis and pleuropulmonary disease linked to ergot dopamine agonist therapy (cabergoline) for Parkinson's disease. *Mayo Clin Proc* 1999;74:371

Nall KS, Feldman B. Postpartum myocardial infarction induced by methergine. *Am J Emerg Med* 1998;16:502

Shaunak S, *et al*. Pericardial, retroperitoneal, and pleural fibrosis induced by pergolide. *J Neurol Neurosurg Psychiatry* 1999;66:79

## INTERACTIONS (see p. 20)

Propranolol and other beta-blocking agents enhance the effects of quinidine, procainamide, antihypertensives, insulin, muscle relaxants, and sulfonylureas and possibly increase the serum level of lidocaine. Levodopa can cause hypertension, especially in the presence of monoamine oxidase inhibitors. Levodopa also augments hypotensive effects of anesthetic agents. The action of levodopa is antagonized by pyridoxine and papaverine. Methyldopa and guanethidine deplete catecholamines and increase the possibility of hypotension during anesthesia. Interaction of methyldopa and phenoxybenzamine can cause urinary incontinence. Propantheline increases absorption of digoxin. Neostigmine potentiates succinylcholine and antagonizes tubocurarine.

Parasympathetic block is enhanced by all of the following: atropine and congeners, antihistamines, tricyclic antidepressants, phenothiazines, and meperidine.

The pressor response from norepinephrine is increased by guanethidine, methyldopa, and tricyclic antidepressants; the pressor response from metaraminol, methoxamine, mephentermine, and phenylephrine is increased by guanethidine, monoamine oxidase inhibitors, and tricyclic antidepressants.

Methyldopa can cause severe hypertension with pargyline.

Atropine-like compounds delay absorption of drugs.

# PHARMACOKINETICS AND TOXIC CONCENTRATIONS (see p. 100)

| | $pK_a$ | $T_{\frac{1}{2}}$ (h) | $V_d$ (l/kg) | % Binding | Toxic concentration (µg/ml) |
|---|---|---|---|---|---|
| Acebutolol | | 3–4 | | | 35[†] |
| Albuterol | 9.3, 10.3 | 2–4 | | | |
| Amphetamine | 9.9 | 10–30 | | | 0.2, 0.5[†] |
| Atenolol | 9.6 | 6–9 | 0.7 | 6–16 | 2, 30[†] |
| Atropine | 9.8 | 13–38 | | 50 | 0.1, 0.2[†] |
| Betaxolol | | 14–22 | | | |
| Bethanidine | | 7–11 | 7 | | |
| Bisoprolol | | 9–12 | | | |
| Bretylium | | 4–17 | | | |
| Bromocriptine | | 48 | 6 | 90–96 | |
| Carteolol | | 6 | | | |
| Carvedilol | | 6–10 | | | |
| Chlorphentermine | 9.6 | 35–40 | | | |
| Ephedrine | | 7 | | | 1,5[†] |
| Esmolol | | 0.15 | | | |
| Fenfluramine | 9.9 | 13–30 | 12–16 | 34 | 0.3, 6[†] |
| Guanethidine | 9, 12 | 216–240 | | | |
| Hyoscine | | 7 | | 10 | |
| Isoxsuprine | 8.0, 9.8 | 1.25 | | | |
| Labetalol | | 5–8 | | | 0.5 |
| Levodopa | 2.3–9.9 | 2.5 | | | |
| Mazindol | 8.5 | 33–55 | | | |
| Metaproterenol | 8.8, 11.8 | 1.5 | | 10 | |
| Methamphetamine | 10.1 | | | | 0.2, 0.23[†] |
| Methyldopa | 2.2–12 | 8 | 0.29 | < 20 | 7, 9[†] |
| Methylphenidate | | | | | 0.5, 2.3[†] |
| Metoclopramide | 7.32 | 2–4 | 1.7–2.9 | | |
| Metoprolol | | 10–12 | | | 1, 10[†] |
| Nadolol | | 9.6–14.2 | 1.4–3.4 | | |
| Penbutolol | | 5 | | | |
| Phentermine | 10.1 | 19–24 | | | 0.2, 1[†] |
| Pindolol | | 3–15 | | | 0.7, 0.01[†] |
| Phenylpropanolamine | | 4 | | | 2, 2[†] |
| Propantheline | | 9 | 1.5 | | |
| Propranolol | 9.45 | 2–16 | 3.6, 4.6 | 90 | 1, 2–4[†] |
| Pseudoephedrine | | 5–16 | | | 1.4, 19[†] |
| Reserpine | 6.1 | 46–168 | | | |
| Salbutamol | | | | | 0.03, 0.16[†] |
| Sotalol | | 12 | | | 5, 40[†] |
| Terbutaline | 10.1 | 3–4 | | 25 | 0.04[†] |
| Timolol | | 4 | | | |

[†]Fatal

# 25  Antiseptics*

## BORIC ACID AND BORON DERIVATIVES

Boric acid ($H_3BO_3$) is a white compound that is soluble to the extent of 5% in water at 20°C. Sodium borate, or borax ($Na_2B_4O_7 \cdot 10H_2O$), is a white compound that is soluble to the extent of 14% in water at 55°C. Sodium perborate ($NaBO_3 \cdot 4H_2O$) is a white compound that is slightly soluble in cold water and decomposes in hot water. Boron oxide is used in industry. Pentaborane, decaborane, and diborane are used as propellants.

Boric acid was formerly used as an antiseptic and to make talcum powder flow freely. Current use is to prevent vaginal yeasts infections (capsules of boric acid are placed intravaginally). Sodium borate (borax) is used as a cleaning agent. Sodium perborate is used as a mouthwash and dentrifice.

The fatal dose of boric acid, sodium borate, or sodium perborate is 0.1–0.5 g/kg. The exposure limits for boron compounds are as follows: boron oxide, 10 mg/m³; anhydrous sodium borate, 1 mg/m³; sodium borate decahydrate, 5 mg/m³; sodium borate pentahydrate, 1 mg/m³; boron tribromide, 1 ppm; decaborane, 0.05 ppm; pentaborane, 0.005 ppm; diborane, 0.1 ppm.

Boric acid and borates are toxic to all cells. The effect on an organ is dependent on the concentration reached in that organ. Because the highest concentrations are reached during excretion, the kidneys are more seriously damaged than other organs. Renal excretion of toxic doses requires one week. The pathologic findings in fatal cases are gastroenteritis, fatty degeneration of the liver and kidneys, cerebral edema, and congestion of all organs.

### Clinical findings

The principal manifestations of poisoning with these compounds are skin excoriations, fever, and anuria.

---

*See also Table 25.2

*Acute poisoning* (from ingestion, skin absorption, or absorption from mucous membranes)

Boron oxide dust is irritating to mucous membranes. Decaborane and penta-borane cause excitability and narcosis, which may be delayed up to 48 hours. Diborane is a pulmonary irritant. After ingestion of boric acid or borates emesis usually occurs immediately, limiting toxicity of these substances. If they are retained progressive development of the following occurs:

(1) Vomiting and diarrhea of mucus and blood.
(2) Erythroderma, followed by desquamation, excoriations, blistering, bullae, and sloughing of epidermis.
(3) Lethargy.
(4) Twitching of facial muscles and extremities, followed by convulsions.
(5) Hyperpyrexia, jaundice, and kidney damage with oliguria or anuria.
(6) Cyanosis, fall in blood pressure, collapse, coma, and death.

*Chronic poisoning* (from ingestion, skin absorption, or absorption from body cavities or mucous membranes)

(1) Prolonged absorption causes anorexia, weight loss, vomiting, mild diar-rhea, skin rash, alopecia, convulsions, and anemia.
(2) Local use of sodium perborate in high concentrations in the mouth may cause chemical burns, low resistance to trauma, and retraction of gums.

*Laboratory findings*

(1) The urine contains protein, epithelial casts, and red blood cells.
(2) One drop of urine acidified with hydrochloric acid and applied to tur-meric paper produces a brownish-red color in the presence of boric acid or borate.
(3) Blood urea nitrogen may be elevated.
(4) Hepatic cell function may be impaired as revealed by appropriate tests (see p. 75).

**Prevention**

Because deaths occur frequently following the improper use of boric acid powder or solution, and because this substance has no therapeutic function that cannot be served equally well by less toxic preparations, it should be removed from home and hospital.

## Treatment

### *Acute poisoning*

(1) Emergency measures:
- (a) Establish airway and maintain respiration.
- (b) Remove boric acid from skin or mucous membranes by washing.
- (c) Remove poison by ipecac emesis followed by activated charcoal. Gastric lavage may be useful (see pp. 29–32).

(2) General measures:
- (a) Maintain urine output by giving liquids orally; if patient is vomiting, give 5% dextrose, 10–40 ml/kg intravenously daily, plus electrolyte replacement as necessary.
- (b) Control convulsions by cautious administration of diazepam, 0.1 mg/kg intravenously (see p. 60).
- (c) Remove boric acid or borates from the circulation by peritoneal dialysis or hemodialysis or by exchange transfusion in infants. Diuresis is hazardous if renal function is impaired.

(3) Special problems – Treat anuria (see p. 66). Treat skin infection with organism-specific chemotherapy.

### *Chronic poisoning*

Discontinue use of boric acid or borate products.

## Prognosis

In the past more than 50% of infants with symptomatic boric acid poisoning died. This type of poisoning is now rare.

## References

Culver, BD, *et al*. Boron and its compounds. *Biol Trace Elem Res* 1997;66:1

Ishii Y, *et al*. A fatal case of acute boric acid poisoning. *J Toxicol Clin Toxicol* 1993;31:345

Restuccio A, *et al*. Fatal ingestion of boric acid in an adult. *Am J Emerg Med* 1992;10:545

Von Burg V. Boron, boric acid, borates, and boron oxide. *J Appl Toxicol* 1992;12:149
Wegman DH, *et al*. Acute and chronic respiratory effects of sodium borate particulate exposures. *Env Health Perspectives* 1994;102:S119

# IODINE, IODOFORM, IODOCHLORHYDROXYQUIN, CHINIOFON, AND IODIDES

Iodine occurs as dark violet plates that are soluble in alcohol but only slightly soluble (0.03%) in water. Tincture of iodine contains 2% iodine and 2.4% sodium iodide in alcohol; strong iodine solution contains 5% iodine and 10% potassium iodide in water.

The fatal dose of iodine and iodoform is estimated to be 2 g. Fatalities have not been reported from iodochlorhydroxyquin or iodide. Organically bound iodine compounds such as iodinated glycerol, povidone-iodine, undecoylium chloride-iodine (Virac), iodoquinol (diiodohydroxyquin, Yodoxin, Diodoquin), clioquinol (Vioform), tetraglycine hydroperiodide (60% iodine), and chiniofon release iodine slowly and have a toxicity equivalent to about one-fifth of their iodine content. The exposure limit for iodine in air is 0.1 ppm; for iodoform, 0.6 ppm.

Iodine acts directly on cells by precipitating proteins. The affected cell may be killed. The effects of iodine are thus similar to those produced by acid corrosives (see p. 242). Iodoform in large doses depresses the central nervous system.

The pathologic findings are excoriation and corrosion of mucous membranes of the mouth, esophagus, and stomach. The kidneys show glomerular and tubular necrosis.

## Clinical findings

The principal manifestations of acute poisoning with these agents are vomiting, collapse, and coma.

### *Acute poisoning*

(1) Ingestion of iodine causes severe vomiting, frequent liquid stools, abdominal pain, thirst, metallic taste, shock, fever, anuria, delirium, stupor, and death in uremia. A patient who recovers from the acute stage

may have esophageal stricture. Iodides may cause temporary enlargement of salivary glands or lymph glands.

(2) Application of iodine to the skin may cause weeping, crusting, blistering, and fever. Individual susceptibility to such reactions is greatly varied; some will react after momentary contact with weak solutions, whereas others will not react after repeated contact with strong solutions.

(3) Application of iodoform to skin or mucous membranes may cause vesiculation and oozing with intense itching, burning pain, tenderness, and irritability.

(4) Injection of iodine compounds may cause sudden fatal collapse (anaphylaxis) as a result of hypersensitivity. Symptoms are dyspnea, cyanosis, fall in blood pressure, unconsciousness, and convulsions.

(5) Ingestion of overdoses of organic iodine compounds causes nausea and vomiting and diarrhea. Respiratory distress, coma, and circulatory collapse have also been reported.

### Chronic poisoning

(1) Prolonged ingestion of iodine or iodine compounds leads to iodism, with erythema, conjunctivitis, stomatitis, acne, rhinorrhea, urticaria, parotitis, anorexia, weight loss, sleeplessness, and nervous symptoms. Myxedema can occur from prolonged administration of iodide.

(2) Iodine and iodine compounds are potent sensitizers. For this reason repeated contact may be followed by sensitivity dermatitis (see p. 80), laryngeal edema, serum sickness with lymph node enlargement, and joint pain and swelling.

(3) Clioquinol, iodoquinol, and other organic iodine compounds can cause nausea, vomiting, diarrhea, neurotoxicity, optic neuritis, peripheral neuropathy, and iodism.

### Laboratory findings

Urine may contain protein, epithelial casts, and red blood cells.

### Prevention

Patients should be tested for sensitivity to iodine or iodine compounds before these substances are used. A suitable test for drugs to be used on the skin is to

place a drop of the solution on the skin and leave the area uncovered for
30 min. Any reaction contraindicates the further use of the drug in question. If
injection of the drug is contemplated, a drop of the solution may be placed in
the conjunctival sac and the presence of irritation noted after 30 min.

## Treatment

### *Acute poisoning*

(1) Emergency measures:
   (a) Establish airway and maintain respiration.
   (b) Give milk; then adsorb remaining iodine with starch solution made
       by adding 15 g of cornstarch or flour to 500 ml of water. Emesis and
       lavage are not indicated in the presence of esophageal injury.
   (c) Give milk orally every 15 min to relieve gastric irritation.
   (d) Treat anaphylaxis (hypotension and bradycardia) by giving
       epinephrine, 0.3–1 ml of 1:1000 solution subcutaneously or intra-
       muscularly, to maintain pulse and blood pressure. Give positive-
       pressure artificial respiration. Give diphenhydramine (Benadryl),
       50 mg slowly intravenously. Give hydrocortisone, 50 mg/h intrave-
       nously until symptoms abate.
   (e) After eye contact wash thoroughly with saline.
(2) Antidote – Sodium thiosulfate will immediately reduce iodine to iodide.
    Give 100 ml of 1% solution orally.
(3) General measures – If urine output is reduced regulate fluid and electro-
    lyte intake (see p. 67). Saline diuresis is useful if renal function is ade-
    quate.
(4) Special problems:
   (a) Treat skin eruptions by applying mild astringent wet dressings (see
       p. 83).
   (b) Treat esophageal stricture (see p. 245).

### *Chronic poisoning*

Discontinue use of iodine or iodides. High sodium chloride intake will speed
recovery. For iodism characterized by skin or mucous membrane reactions,
give cortisone or equivalent corticosteroid, 25–100 mg every 6 h orally until
symptoms abate.

## Prognosis

If the patient survives 48 hours after the ingestion of iodine, recovery is likely, although stricture of the esophagus may be a complication. In sensitivity reactions following the injection of iodine compounds, survival is likely if the patient lives for 1 hour.

## References

Kubota Y, *et al.* Iodine allergy induced by consumption of iodine-containing food. *Contact Dermatitis* 2000;42:286

Kurt TL, *et al.* Fatal iatrogenic iodine toxicity in a nine-week-old infant. *J Toxicol Clin Toxicol* 1996;34:231

Nishioka K, *et al.* The results of ingredient patch testing in contact dermatitis elicited by povidone-iodine preparations. *Contact Dermatitis* 2000;42:90

## PHENOL AND DERIVATIVES

Pure phenol (carbolic acid) is a white solid that liquefies (liquefied phenol) upon the addition of 5% water. Creosotes (wood tar or coal tar) are mixtures of phenolic compounds and other compounds obtained by the destructive distillation of wood or coal.

A large number of phenol derivatives have been used in the past as antiseptics, disinfectants, caustics, germicides, surface anesthetics, antioxidants, and preservatives.

The antioxidants di-tertiary-butyl-*p*-cresol (BHT, DBPD) and 4,4′-thio-bis(6-tertiary-butyl-*m*-cresol) have exposure limits of $10 \, mg/m^3$ and estimated fatal doses of 30 g. The fatal doses of other phenols are listed in Table 25.1. Even a weak phenolic compound such as tannic acid has caused fatalities when given rectally in excessive doses. For this reason 'universal antidote', which contains tannic acid, should never be used. To protect aquatic life, the level of pentachlorophenol in natural water should never exceed $3 \, \mu g/l$.

Phenol denatures and precipitates cellular proteins and thus poisons all cells. In small amounts it has a salicylate-like stimulating effect on the respiratory center. This causes respiratory alkalosis followed by acidosis, which results partly from uncompensated renal loss of base during the stage of alkalosis, partly from the acidic nature of the phenolic radical and partly from

**Table 25.1** Phenol and phenol derivatives

|  | Exposure limit | Fatal dose (g or ml) |
|---|---|---|
| Amyl phenol |  | 5 |
| Benzyl chlorophenol |  | 5 |
| o-sec-Butyl phenol | 5 ppm | 10 |
| Carvacrol |  | 2 |
| Catechol* | 5 ppm |  |
| p-Chloro-m-cresol |  | 5 |
| Chlorophenols |  | 5 |
| Chloroxylenol |  | 5 |
| Creosote (coal tar) |  | 10 |
| Cresol, o-, m-, or p- | 5 ppm | 2 |
| Dichlorophene* |  | 10 |
| Gallic acid |  | 20 |
| Guaiacol |  | 2 |
| Hexachlorophene* |  | 5 |
| Hexylresorcinol[†] |  | 5 |
| Hydroquinone | 2 mg/m$^3$ | 2 |
| Menthol |  | 2 |
| 4-Methoxyphenol | 5 mg/m$^3$ | 10 |
| Monobenzone (Benzylhydroquinone) |  | 5 |
| Naphthol ($\alpha$ or $\beta$) |  | 5 |
| Pentachlorophenol | 0.6 mg/m$^3$ | 1[‡] |
| Phenol | 5 ppm | 2 |
| o-Phenyl phenol |  | 10 |
| Pyrogallol* |  | 2 |
| Resorcinol | 10 mg/m$^3$ | 2 |
| Saponated solution of cresols |  | 10 |
| Tannic acid |  | 20 |
| Tetrachlorophenol |  | 5 |
| Thiocresol |  | 5 |
| Thymol |  | 2 |
| Wood tar |  | 10 |

*May cause sensitivity dermatitis, photosensitivity, or stomatitis; [†]contraindicated in peptic ulcer; [‡]serum 46 µg/ml

derangements in carbohydrate metabolism. Methemoglobinemia may also occur, especially after administration of hydroquinone. The trichlorophenols and 2,4-dimethyl phenol may be carcinogens.

Pathologic findings in deaths from phenol or related compounds are necrosis of mucous membranes, cerebral edema, and degenerative changes in the liver and kidney. Bladder necrosis may also be present.

## Clinical findings

The principal manifestations of poisoning with these agents are vomiting, collapse, and coma.

*Acute poisoning* (from ingestion or application of phenolic compounds to skin or mucous membranes)

Local findings are painless blanching or erythema. Corrosion may occur. General findings are profuse sweating, intense thirst, nausea and vomiting, diarrhea, cyanosis from methemoglobinemia, hyperactivity, stupor, fall in blood pressure, hyperpnea, abdominal pain, hemolysis, convulsions, coma, and pulmonary edema followed by pneumonia. If death from respiratory failure is not immediate, jaundice and oliguria or anuria may occur. Skin absorption of hexachlorophene can cause central nervous system damage, cerebral edema, and muscle contractions.

*Chronic poisoning* (from ingestion or absorption from skin or mucous membranes)

Repeated use may cause symptoms described for acute poisoning. Skin sensitivity reactions occur occasionally. Prolonged skin contact with $\beta$-naphthol may cause bladder tumors, hemolytic anemia, and lens opacities.

*Laboratory findings in acute or chronic poisoning*

(1) Test urine with a few drops of ferric chloride. A violet or blue color indicates the presence of a phenolic compound.
(2) Urine contains red blood cells, protein, and casts.
(3) The blood bicarbonate level may be below 20 mEq/l. The urea nitrogen level is elevated. Methemoglobinemia may be present.
(4) Hepatic cell function may be impaired as revealed by appropriate tests (see p. 75).

## Prevention

Phenol and derivatives must be stored safely. Phenolic ointments or solutions of derivatives such as hexachlorophene should not be used over large areas of the body.

**Treatment**

*Acute poisoning*

(1) Emergency measures:
    (a) Establish airway and maintain respiration.
    (b) Ingestion – In the absence of corrosive injury remove poison by ipecac emesis. Activated charcoal is also useful (see pp. 31–32). Follow with 240 ml of milk. Gastric lavage and emesis are contraindicated in the presence of esophageal injury.
    (c) Surface contamination – Remove poison by washing skin or mucous membranes with large amounts of water for at least 15 min. Follow by repeated application of castor oil.
(2) General measures:
    (a) If blood bicarbonate level is below 20 mEq/l treat as for salicylate poisoning (see p. 371).
    (b) Control convulsions by cautious use of diazepam, 0.1 mg/kg slowly intravenously.
    (c) Treat methemoglobinemia (see p. 78).
(3) Special problems – Treat liver damage (see p. 76). Treat anuria (see p. 66).

*Chronic poisoning*

Discontinue further use of phenol, and treat as for acute poisoning.

**Prognosis**

If the patient survives for 48 hours, recovery is likely.

**References**

Bentur Y, *et al*. Prolonged elimination half-life of phenol after dermal exposure. *J Toxicol Clin Toxicol* 1998;36:707

DeCaprio AP. The toxicology of hydroquinone – relevance to occupational and environmental exposure. *CRC Crit Reviews in Toxicol* 1998;29:283

Durback-Morris LF, Scharman EJ. Accidental intranasal administration of phenol. *Vet Human Toxicol* 1999;41:157

Kamijo Y, *et al*. Rabbit syndrome following phenol ingestion. *J Toxicol Clin Toxicol* 1999;37:509

Wu M-L, *et al*. Concentrated cresol intoxication. *Vet Human Toxicol* 1998;40:341

## CATIONIC DETERGENTS

Cationic detergents are a group of alkyl- or aryl- substituted quaternary N compounds with an ionizable halogen, such as bromide, iodide, or chloride. Cationic detergents are characterized by the fact that the hydrophobic part of the molecule is a cation rather than an anion, as in ordinary soaps.

These compounds – benzethonium chloride (Phemerol), benzalkonium chloride (Zephiran), methylbenzethonium chloride (Diaparene), and cetyl-pyridinium chloride (Ceepryn) – are used to destroy bacteria on skin, surgical instruments, cooking equipment, sickroom supplies, and diapers. Cationic detergents with two long-chain substituents are less toxic than those with short-chain substituents.

The fatal dose by ingestion is estimated to be 1–3 g. At least three fatalities have occurred from accidental ingestion.

Concentrated solutions of cationic detergents are readily absorbed and interfere with many cellular functions. Concentrations down to 1% are injurious to mucous membranes. Cationic detergents are rapidly inactivated by tissues and by ordinary soaps. After prolonged heating (e.g. autoclaving or boiling), cationic detergents can break down to compounds capable of causing methemoglobinemia when they are absorbed by skin or mucous membranes.

The pathologic findings are not characteristic.

### Clinical findings

The principal manifestations of poisoning with these agents are vomiting, collapse, and coma.

The symptoms and signs from ingestion are nausea and vomiting, corrosive damage to the esophagus, collapse, hypotension, convulsions, coma, and death within 1–4 h. Concentrations of 10% are corrosive to the esophagus and mucous membranes. Chronic poisoning has not been reported.

## Prevention

Cationic detergent solutions should be stored in distinctive bottles (never in soft drink bottles) in a safe place.

## Treatment

### *Emergency measures*

(1) Establish airway and maintain respiration.
(2) Give milk or activated charcoal (see pp. 31–32) and remove by catharsis with Fleet's Phospho-Soda, 15–60 ml diluted 1:4 with water. Lavage and emesis are contraindicated in the presence of esophageal injury.

### *Antidote*

Ordinary soap is an effective antidote for unabsorbed cationic detergent. No antidote is known for the systemic effects following absorption.

### *General measures*

Maintain respiration and treat convulsions (see p. 60). Treat hypotension by giving fluids or transfusions (see p. 57). Dialysis and diuresis are not effective. Treat methemoglobinemia (see p. 78).

## Prognosis

If the patient survives for 48 hours recovery is likely.

## CHLORATES

Sodium chlorate ($NaClO_3$) and potassium chlorate ($KClO_3$) are frequent ingredients in mouthwashes and gargles and are also used in matches and weed killers. The heads of 20 large wooden matches contain 300 mg. The chlorates are water-soluble and act as strong oxidizing agents, forming explosive mixtures with organic material.

The fatal dose is about 15 g for adults and 2 g for children, but no fatalities have been reported in recent years. Chlorate ion is irritating to mucous membranes in concentrated solution; after absorption it produces methemoglobinemia by virtue of its oxidizing properties. However the chlorate is not reduced in the process but acts as a catalyst, so that a small amount of chlorate can produce a large amount of methemoglobin.

Pathologic findings in deaths from chlorate are gastrointestinal congestion and corrosion, kidney injury, liver damage, and chocolate color of the blood.

### Clinical findings

The principal manifestations of poisoning with these agents are vomiting and cyanosis.

*Acute poisoning* (from ingestion)

Nausea, vomiting, diarrhea, abdominal pain, hemolysis, cyanosis, anuria, confusion, convulsions.

*Chronic poisoning* (from ingestion)

Continued use in doses less than that necessary to produce the symptoms described for acute poisoning may lead to loss of appetite and weight loss.

*Laboratory findings*

(1) Methemoglobinemia, anemia of the hemolytic type, or elevation of serum potassium level.
(2) Urine contains red blood cells, protein, casts, and hemoglobin products.

### Prevention

Chlorates should never be taken internally. They should be replaced in mouth-washes and gargles by less harmful drugs.

### Treatment

*Acute poisoning*

(1) Emergency measures – Establish airway and maintain respiration. Remove ingested poison by ipecac emesis followed by activated char-coal (see pp. 31–32). Airway-protected gastric lavage is necessary in patients with depressed respiration (see pp. 29–32).

(2) Antidote – Give sodium thiosulfate, 2–5 g in 200 ml of 5% sodium bicarbonate orally, to decompose chlorates. Methylene blue is not useful for reversing chlorate methemoglobinemia and may be hazardous. Ascorbic acid acts slowly (see p. 78).

(3) General measures – Give milk to relieve gastric irritation. Keep patient warm and quiet until cyanosis disappears. If urine output is adequate, force fluids to 2–4 l/d to remove chlorate. Remove chlorate by peritoneal dialysis or hemodialysis.

(4) Special problems – Treat anuria (see p. 66).

*Chronic poisoning*

Discontinue use of drug and treat as for acute poisoning.

**Prognosis**

Death may occur up to 1 week after poisoning, but if symptoms are mild or absent after the first 12 hours recovery is to be expected.

## SILVER AND SILVER SALTS: SILVER NITRATE, SILVER PROTEINATES, AND SILVER PICRATE

Silver nitrate is a water-soluble salt that reacts with chloride to form a precipitate of the insoluble and non-toxic silver chloride. It is used as a local styptic and antiseptic. The colloidal silver proteinates are used as antiseptics on skin and mucous membranes. 'Mild silver protein' contains 19–23% silver; although 'strong silver protein' contains less silver (7.5–8.5%) it is more powerful in its action. Silver picrate (Picragol) is used as 1% powder in kaolin, and in suppositories as an antiseptic on mucous membranes.

The fatal dose of silver nitrate may be as low as 2 g, although recovery has occurred following ingestion of larger doses. No fatalities have been reported in recent years. The silver proteinates and silver picrate have not produced fatal poisoning. The exposure limit for silver and its compounds is 0.01 mg/m$^3$.

Silver nitrate causes a local corrosive effect but is not likely to produce systemic effects because silver ion is precipitated by proteins and chloride. Pathologic findings involve local corrosive damage to the gastrointestinal tract, and there may be degenerative changes in the kidneys and liver.

Repeated use of silver in any form will eventually cause argyria. Excessive use of silver picrate may cause renal damage.

## Clinical findings

The principal manifestations of poisoning with these agents are blackening of mucous membranes, vomiting, and collapse.

*Acute poisoning* (from ingestion of silver nitrate)

Pain and burning in the mouth; blackening of the skin and mucous membranes, throat, and abdomen; salivation; vomiting of black material; diarrhea; anuria; collapse; shock; and death in convulsions or coma. Treatment of burns with silver nitrate has caused methemoglobinemia from absorption of nitrate ion.

*Chronic poisoning* (from application of silver compounds to skin or mucous membranes)

Repeated application or ingestion of silver nitrate or silver proteinates causes argyria, which is a permanent bluish-black discoloration of the skin, conjunctiva, and other mucous membranes. The discoloration first appears in areas most exposed to light, usually the conjunctiva. If silver is not immediately discontinued the discoloration will spread over the entire body.

## Prevention

Silver nitrate sticks should be stored safely. Silver proteinates should not be used repeatedly for the treatment of mucous membrane or skin diseases.

## Treatment

*Acute poisoning*

(1) Emergency measures:
   (a) Dilute ingested silver nitrate by giving water containing sodium chloride, 10 g/l, repeatedly to precipitate silver ion as silver chloride. Follow with catharsis using 30–60 ml of Fleet's Phospho-Soda

diluted 1:4 in water containing 5 g of sodium chloride to precipitate and remove silver from the intestines.
   (b) Treat shock (see p. 56).
   (c) Treat methemoglobinemia (See p. 78).
(2) General measures – Give milk to relieve gastric irritation. Give meperidine (Demerol), 100 mg, or codeine, 60 mg, to relieve pain.

### *Chronic poisoning*

No method is known that will bleach the pigmentation of argyria.

### Prognosis

If treatment with sodium chloride can be started shortly after the ingestion of silver nitrate recovery is likely. The pigmentation of argyria is permanent.

### Reference

Fung MC, Bowen DL. Silver products for medical indications: risk-benefit assessment. *J Toxicol Clin Toxicol* 1996;34:119

**Table 25.2** Miscellaneous antiseptics (for mercurial antiseptics, see p. 294)

| Drug | Findings | Treatment |
|---|---|---|
| Anthralin (Anthra-derm) | Irritation, desquamation | Discontinue |
| Benzoic acid | Ingestion of 50 g causes gastric upset | None |
| Benzyl benzoate | Ingestion of 1 g/kg causes unco-ordination, excitement, convulsions | Remove by gastric lavage |
| Carbamide peroxide (Debrox) | Irritation, pain | Discontinue |
| Chlorhexidine (Peridex, Hibiclens) | Irritation, staining | Discontinue |
| Crotamiton (Eurax) | Burning in mouth. Lethal dose over 0.5 g/kg | Wash skin and give fluids |
| Hydrogen peroxide, up to 90% solutions (exposure limit = 1 ppm) | Concentrated solutions (20–30%) of hydrogen peroxide are strong irritants to the skin or mucous membranes. 6% is a weak irritant; it releases 20 vol% $O_2$ on contact with skin or mucous membranes. When used as colonic lavage, hydrogen peroxide has caused gas embolism and gangrene of the intestine at concentrations down to 0.75%. Treatment for ingestion: give water to dilute; use gastric tube to prevent increased pressure | |
| Oxyquinoline sulfate | Gastrointestinal irritation. Lethal dose is 1 g/kg | Remove by gastric lavage or emesis |
| Parabens (p-hydroxy-benzoic acid, alkyl esters) | Dermatitis | Discontinue |
| Pyridinethione zinc | Gastrointestinal irritation | Remove by gastric lavage or emesis |
| Selenium sulfide (Selsun) | Diffuse hair loss, sensitivity reactions | Discontinue |
| Undecylenic acid and salts | Exudative dermatitis, nausea, fever, headache after ingestion. Lethal dose is 2 g/kg | Discontinue |

## References

Henry MC, *et al*. Hydrogen peroxide 3% exposures. *J Toxicol Clin Toxicol* 1996;34:323

Mullins ME, Beltran JT. Acute cerebral gas embolism from hydrogen peroxide ingestion successfully treated with hyperbaric oxygen. *J Toxicol Clin Toxicol* 1998;36:253

# 26  Cardiovascular drugs

## DIGITALIS AND DIGITALIS PREPARATIONS

Digitalis and cardiac glycosides are used for the treatment of heart failure.

Other digitalis preparations include deslanoside (Cedilanid-D), Digilanid, digoxin, gitalin (Gitaligin), and lanatoside C (Cedilanid). Squill and strophanthus have similar effects.

The fatal dose of digitalis or squill is approximately 2–3 g. All parts of the foxglove (*Digitalis purpurea*, *Digitalis lanata*) have similar toxicity. The dangerous dose of digitoxin is 3–5 mg. For other digitalis-like preparations, the fatal dose is 20–50 times the maintenance dose of the preparation. The fatal amount of the rodenticide scilliroside is 0.7 mg/kg.

Digitalis and the cardiac glycosides increase the force of contraction of the myocardium. In excessive doses they increase the irritability of the ventricular muscle, resulting first in extrasystoles, then in ventricular tachycardia, and eventually in ventricular fibrillation. Digitalis and digitalis-like preparations also stimulate the central nervous system. Potassium loss by vomiting, diarrhea, or diuresis increases the toxicity.

### Clinical findings

The principal manifestations of digitalis poisoning are vomiting and irregular pulse.

*Acute poisoning* (from injection, ingestion, or diuresis in a fully digitalized patient)

Headache, nausea and vomiting, diarrhea, blurred vision, loss of visual acuity, delirium, slow or irregular pulse, fall in blood pressure, aberrant color vision, and death, usually from ventricular fibrillation. In infants cardiac arrhythmias are the most common manifestation of toxicity, and in children severe central nervous system depression sometimes occurs. Elderly patients are likely to have bizarre mental symptoms.

*Chronic poisoning* (from injection or ingestion)

The above symptoms will come on gradually if overdoses are taken. The occurrence of nausea and vomiting tends to limit dosage. Because renal function declines with age, the elderly are more likely to be maintained on too high a dose. Reduce dosage upon the occurrence of anorexia, nausea, and headache to prevent more serious symptoms.

### *Laboratory findings*

(1) The ECG may show heart block, nodal tachycardia, atrial tachycardia, premature ventricular contractions or ventricular extrasystoles, ventricular tachycardia, depressed ST segment, and lengthened PR interval.
(2) Eosinophilia may be present.
(3) Serum potassium is often elevated in acute overdose.
(4) Toxic effects begin to occur at digoxin levels above 1.7 ng/ml and digitoxin levels above 25 ng/ml.

### Prevention

Store digitalis safely. Reduce dosage of digitalis at the first sign of intoxication. Determine digitalis levels before giving large doses. Use extreme care in the administration of digitalis concomitantly with *rauwolfia* alkaloids such as reserpine. *Rauwolfia* apparently sensitizes the heart to the toxic effects of digitalis. The toxicity of digitalis is increased by potassium loss or calcium administration.

Numerous drugs interact to increase digoxin levels (verapamil), diltiazem, bepridil, etc.

### Treatment

### *Acute poisoning*

(1) Emergency measures – Establish airway and maintain respiration. Remove ingested drug by ipecac emesis followed by activated charcoal (see pp. 31–32). Determine serum potassium and magnesium levels hourly. Monitor ECG. Be prepared for transvenous cardiac pacing. Do not give epinephrine or other stimulants – these may induce ventricular fibrillation.

(2) Antidote

    (a) Give digoxin-specific antibodies (Digibind). Follow directions in package insert. Each vial (38 mg) will bind 0.5 mg of digoxin or digitoxin. An estimation of digoxin body burden can be calculated if a steady state serum level can be obtained (drawn 12–16 h after last dosage). In general, 5–10 vials of Digibind are needed to treat chronic and acute poisoning, respectively. Calculations to determine the number of vials needed are based on a volume of distribution ($V_d$) for digoxin of 5–7 l/kg; because $V_d$ is variable, some patients may require more vials than anticipated.

Number of digoxin-Fab vials =

$$\frac{\text{(Steady state serum digoxin ng/ml)} \times \text{(Body weight kg)}}{100}$$

    (b) To reduce a potassium level over 5.5 mEq/l give Kayexalate, 20 g orally or by enema every 4 h. For potassium levels above 6 or 7 mEq/l, administer 50% dextrose, 50 ml plus regular insulin, 0.1 unit/kg IV. In children, give 25% dextrose, 2 ml/kg with 0.1 unit/kg regular insulin. Rapid reduction of serum potassium can be achieved by infusing 1–2 mEq/kg sodium bicarbonate. If necessary hemodialysis can be used to lower potassium levels. Replace low serum potassium or magnesium under laboratory control.

    (c) For atrial and ventricular irregularities give phenytoin, 0.5 mg/kg slowly intravenously at 1- to 2-h intervals. The maximum dose should not exceed 10 mg/kg/24 h. Alternatively, give lidocaine, 1 mg/kg bolus followed by an infusion of 1–4 mg/min to maintain a serum level of 1.5–5 mg/l. If the initial bolus is not effective, a second bolus of 0.5 mg/kg can be given. Maximum bolus dose is 3 mg/kg. Avoid using quinidine, procainamide or bretylium. Propranolol, quinidine, and procainamide are more hazardous.

    (d) Cholestyramine resin given orally reduces the half-life of digitoxin from 6 days to 4.5 days or prevents absorption of digitalis glycosides.

    (e) Atropine, 0.01 mg/kg intravenously, can increase the heart rate in the presence of digitalis heart block.

(3) General measures – If renal function is impaired enforce complete quiet and inactivity until signs of digitalis-induced ventricular abnormalities disappear from the ECG. If renal function is normal give 2–3 liters of fluids orally each 24 h. Do not give diuretic agents or calcium in the presence of digitalis toxicity.

*Chronic poisoning*

Discontinue the drug temporarily and then regulate dosage according to the needs of the patient.

**Prognosis**

Recovery is likely if the patient survives 24 hours.

**References**

Abad-Santos F, *et al*. Digoxin level and clinical manifestations as determinants in the diagnosis of digoxin toxicity. *Therap Drug Mon* 2000;22:163

Gittelman MA, *et al*. Acute pediatric digoxin ingestion. *Pediatr Emerg Care* 1999;15:359

Hauptmann PJ, Kelly RA. Digitalis. *Circulation* 1999;99:1265

Schmitt K, *et al*. Massive digitoxin intoxication treated with digoxin-specific antibodies in a child. *Pediatr Cardiol* 1994;15:48

# QUINIDINE

Quinidine, a white water-soluble alkaloid obtained from cinchona bark, is used for the treatment of cardiac irregularities. The fatal dose of quinidine may be as low as 0.2 g as a result of hypersensitivity. The mortality rate from the use of quinidine in cardiac arrhythmias is 1%.

Quinidine depresses the metabolic activities of all cells, but its effect on the heart is most pronounced. Doses within the therapeutic range may cause slowing of conduction, prolonged refractory period, and even heart block. Larger doses may cause ventricular fibrillation. The pathologic findings in acute fatalities are not characteristic. In some cases petechial hemorrhages may be seen throughout the body as a result of thrombocytopenia.

## Clinical findings

The principal manifestations of quinidine poisoning are fall in blood pressure and nausea.

### *Acute poisoning* (from ingestion)

Overdoses and sometimes doses within the therapeutic range cause tinnitus, headache, nausea, diarrhea, dizziness, severe fall in blood pressure with disappearance of pulse, nystagmus, bradycardia, and respiratory failure.

### *Chronic poisoning* (from ingestion)

Thrombocytopenic purpura may develop after a short course of quinidine. After recovery single doses of 0.05–0.1 g will cause return of the purpuric manifestation. Drug fever, urticaria, exfoliation, and anaphylactoid reactions may also result.

### *Laboratory findings*

(1) In purpura from quinidine the blood thrombocytes are reduced in number.
(2) Electrocardiographic findings may include a notched T wave, T wave inversion, depression of the ST segment, widening of the QRS complex, lengthened QT interval, appearance of premature ventricular beats, lengthened PR interval, ventricular tachycardia, and ventricular fibrillation.
(3) The blood level of quinidine in severe toxicity is 10 µg/ml.

## Prevention

Store quinidine safely. Begin administration of quinidine gradually. Dosage should begin with a test dose of 0.1 g. If no reaction occurs a second dose of 0.1 g can be given after 2 h. Maximum dosage should not exceed single doses of 0.2 g at intervals of not less than 1 hour. In some patients fatal ventricular arrhythmias have occurred as late as 12 h after the last dose of quinidine. Reduce dosage upon the appearance of therapeutic response or signs of toxicity as described above. Discontinue the administration of quinidine if the QRS complex widens by more than 25%. Do not give quinidine in the presence of complete heart block. Patients must be on digoxin before intitiation of quinidine if quinidine is used to treat atrial fibrillation.

## Treatment

### Acute poisoning

(1) Emergency measures – Establish airway and maintain respiration. Discontinue medication at the first sign of toxicity. Remove ingested overdoses of quinidine by ipecac emesis followed by activated charcoal (see inside front cover and pp. 31–32). Raise blood pressure by intravenous saline (see p. 57). Norepinephrine with electrocardiographic control can be used in the absence of arrhythmias. Treat ventricular arrhythmias with phenytoin (see p. 461). Be prepared for transvenous cardiac pacing.

(2) Antidote – Intravenous administration of sodium bicarbonate solution increases serum binding of quinidine, lowers the serum potassium level, and reverses the sodium-channel dependent membrane effects of quinidine.

(3) General measures – Normalize the serum potassium level (see p. 461). As with digitalis overdoses, dialysis is useless.

(4) For torsades des pointes, administer magnesium sulfate 1–2 g, or use overdrive pacing.

### Chronic poisoning

Discontinue quinidine. Treat thrombocytopenic purpura by repeated small transfusions. Do not repeat administration of quinidine in such patients.

## Prognosis

If the patient survives for 24 hours after acute poisoning recovery is probable.

## References

Adornato MC. Toxic epidermal necrolysis associated with quinidine administration. *NY State Dent J* 2000;66(3):38

Grace AA, Camm AJ. Quinidine. *N Engl J Med* 1998;338:35

Kim SY, Benowitz NL. Poisoning due to class IA antiarrhythmic drugs quinidine, procainamide and disopyramide. *Drug Safety* 1990;5:393

## PROCAINAMIDE HYDROCHLORIDE

Procainamide is used for the treatment of cardiac irregularities. As little as 200 mg (2 ml of 10% solution) intravenously has caused death as a result of either hypersensitivity or rapid injection. At least four fatalities have been reported from procainamide poisoning. The rapid administration of procainamide causes irregularities of ventricular contraction, including tachycardia or fibrillation. Agranulocytosis from procainamide is apparently a hypersensitivity reaction.

The pathologic finding in death from agranulocytosis is a lack of myeloid elements in the bone marrow. In sudden deaths following intravenous procainamide administration the pathologic findings are not characteristic.

### Clinical findings

The principal manifestations of procainamide poisoning are irregular pulse and fall in blood pressure.

*Acute poisoning* (from injection)

Rapid intravenous administration of procainamide may cause the pulse to become suddenly irregular or disappear entirely, with collapse and fall in blood pressure and almost immediate onset of convulsions and death.

*Chronic poisoning* (from ingestion)

Continued use of procainamide has led to fever, chills, pruritus, urticaria, malaise, reversible lupus erythematosus-like syndrome including pericarditis but without central nervous system or renal involvement, and agranulocytosis.

*Laboratory findings*

(1) In acute poisoning the ECG shows PR, QRS, QT prolongation, bradycardia, sinus tachycardia, polymorphous ventricular tachycardia (torsades des pointes), asystole.
(2) In chronic poisoning the blood count may reveal diminished or absent granulocytes.

## Prevention

Do not give procainamide at a rate greater than 20 mg/min intravenously and only with ECG control. A complete blood count should be taken repeatedly when a patient develops an infectious illness during the administration of procainamide.

## Treatment

### *Acute poisoning*

(1) Emergency measures – Treat cardiac arrest (see p. 59) following intravenous injection of procainamide.
(2) Special problems – For cardiac arrhythmias, give sodium bicarbonate, 1–2 mEq/kg IV bolus. Repeat to maintain arterial pH at 7.45 to 7.5. Infusion of sodium bicarbonate is not as effective as bolus administration. Give $MgSO_4$, 2 g IV for torsades des pointes. Consider pacemaker in the presence of conduction block. Use normal saline for hypotension before resorting to dopamine or norepinephrine. These may induce ventricular irregularities.

### *Chronic poisoning*

(1) Immediate measures – Discontinue use of the drug at the first sign of symptoms.
(2) General measures – Treat agranulocytosis (see p. 79).

## Prognosis

At least 90% of patients with agranulocytosis from procainamide are likely to recover.

## References

Bizjak ED, *et al.* Procainamide-induced psychosis: case report and review of the literature. *Ann Pharmacother* 1999;33:948

Erdem S, *et al.* Procainamide-induced chronic inflammatory demyelinating polyradiculoneuropathy. *Neurology* 1998;50:824

McLaughlin K, *et al*. Rapid development of drug-induced lupus nephritis in the absence of extrarenal disease in a patient receiving procainamide. *Am J Kidney Dis* 1998;32:698

Murray KD, Vlasnik JJ. Procainamide-induced postoperative pyrexia. *Ann Thorac Surg* 1999;68:1072

## NITRITES AND NITRATES

Nitroglycerin (glyceryl trinitrate), amyl nitrite, sodium nitrite, isosorbide mononitrate, and isosorbide dinitrate are used medically to dilate coronary vessels and to reduce blood pressure. Ethylene glycol nitrite, ethyl nitrite, mannitol hexanitrate, pentaerythritol tetranitrite, trolnitrite phosphate, and nitroglycerin are industrial chemicals. In some instances nitrates such as bismuth subnitrate or nitrate from well water may be converted to nitrite by the action of intestinal bacteria. The nitrites then may cause nitrite poisoning. Nitrites are also used to preserve the color of meat in pickling or salting processes.

Fatal doses have been recorded as follows: ethyl nitrite, 4 g in a 3-year-old child, nitroglycerin, 2 g; sodium nitrite, 2 g. The allowable residue of nitrite in food is 0.01%. More than 10 ppm of nitrogen as nitrate in well water may induce methemoglobinemia in infants. The exposure limit for nitroglycerin, propylene glycol dinitrate, and ethylene glycol dinitrate in air is 0.05 ppm, but concentrations above 0.02 ppm may cause headache.

Nitrates and nitrites can interact with amines either alone or in biological systems to form nitrosamines, which are carcinogenic in animals and are suspected of being carcinogenic in humans (e.g. *N*-nitrosodimethylamine; see p. 167). These nitrosamines occur in surface water as a result of fertilizer contamination, in industrial cutting fluids, in plastics and plasticizers, in toiletries, and in pesticides.

The nitrites dilate blood vessels throughout the body by a direct relaxant effect on smooth muscles. Some nitrites will also cause methemoglobinemia.

The pathologic findings are chocolate-colored blood due to conversion of hemoglobin to methemoglobin and congestion of all organs.

### Clinical findings

The principal manifestations of poisoning with nitrites and nitrates are fall in blood pressure and cyanosis.

*Acute poisoning* (from ingestion, injection, inhalation, or absorption from skin or mucous membranes)

Effects include: headache, flushing of the skin, vomiting, dizziness, collapse, marked fall in blood pressure, cyanosis, convulsions, coma, and respiratory paralysis.

### Chronic poisoning

Repeated administration may lead to the above findings. Nitroglycerin workers show marked tolerance to repeated exposure, but since this tolerance disappears rapidly, a short absence from exposure may lead to severe poisoning from amounts that were previously safe.

### Laboratory findings

Determine blood methemoglobin level in presence of cyanosis. Examination must be made quickly because methemoglobin disappears in standing blood.

### Prevention

Use water free of nitrates for preparing infant formulas. Curing salts containing nitrites must be used in quantities no greater than those allowed by the US Department of Agriculture. Such salts should not be used in other foods or as table salt.

### Treatment

### Acute poisoning

(1) Emergency measures – Establish airway and maintain respiration. Remove ingested overdoses of nitrites by ipecac emesis followed by activated charcoal. Gastric lavage may be useful (see pp. 29–32). Maintain blood pressure by fluid administration (see p. 57). Remove poison from the skin by scrubbing with soap and water.
(2) General measures – Treat methemoglobinemia over 30% with dyspnea by injection of methylene blue (see p. 78).

*Chronic poisoning*

Depending on the severity of the symptoms, treat as for acute poisoning.

**Prognosis**

If the blood pressure is maintained recovery is likely.

**Reference**

Knobeloch L, *et al*. Blue babies and nitrate-contaminated well water. *Environ Health Perspect* 2000;108:675

## ANTICOAGULANTS: HEPARIN, WARFARIN, ETC.

The various anticoagulant drugs are used medically to inhibit the clotting mechanism. Warfarin and a number of chemicals with similar action are also used as rodenticides: dicumarol (bishydroxycoumarin), difenacoum, chloro-phacinone, bromadiolone, brodifacoum (Talon), coumatetryl (Racumin), coumachlor, diphacinone, and pindone.

Single doses of these compounds are not dangerous. Fatalities have been recorded after the following repeated daily doses of anticoagulants: dicumarol, 100 mg; ethyl biscoumacetate, 0.6 g; phenindione, 200 mg. The dangerous dosage of warfarin and diphacinone is 10–100 mg daily. The exposure limit for warfarin and pindone is 0.1 mg/m$^3$. The single-dose LD50 for brodifacoum in rats is 0.67 mg/kg. The single dose of brodifacoum that would be dangerous in humans is unknown.

Lepirudin (Refludan) and heparin and its substitutes – ardeparin (Normiflo), dalteparin (Fragmin), danaparoid (Organan), enoxaparin (Lovenox) – are only effective after injection. Tirofiban inhibits platelet aggregation.

The coumarin and indandione anticoagulants inhibit formation in the liver of a number of clotting factors, the formation of which is dependent on vitamin K. These anticoagulants also increase capillary fragility, an effect which is increased by repeated dosage. Heparin prevents the conversion of prothrombin to thrombin and the action of thrombin on fibrinogen. Numerous gross and microscopic hemorrhages are found at autopsy.

## Clinical findings

The principal manifestation of poisoning with anticoagulants is bleeding.

### Acute poisoning

Hemoptysis, hematuria, bloody stools, hemorrhages in organs, widespread bruising, and bleeding into joint spaces. Heparin or its substitutes can cause pain and bleeding at the injection site or elsewhere.

### Chronic poisoning

Repeated use leads to findings as in acute poisoning. Necrosis of the skin is a rare complication. Heparin or its substitutes cause thrombocytopenia, sensitivity reactions, anaphylaxis, and 'white clot syndrome' with thrombosis and necrosis of skin, myocardial infarction, stroke or pulmonary embolism. Prolonged use of heparin has led to osteoporosis. Phenindione has caused severe renal and liver injuries, of which at least five cases have been fatal.

### Laboratory findings

The prothrombin concentration is lowered after coumarin and indandione anticoagulants. The clotting time is prolonged after heparin. Gross or microscopic hematuria may be present. The white blood count may be decreased after phenindione administration. The red blood count may be reduced. Hemoglobin levels should be determined and the presence of blood in the stools noted.

## Prevention

Anticoagulant drugs are dangerous in blood dyscrasias; kidney, liver, or gastrointestinal diseases; hypertension; subacute infective endocarditis; and pregnancy. Administration of many other drugs enhances the effect of anticoagulants.

The use of coumarin anticoagulants must be controlled by repeated reliable prothrombin determinations. Heparin dosage is controlled by clotting time determinations. These drugs should be used only under daily supervision by a physician.

**Treatment**

*Emergency measures*

(1) Discontinue the drug at the first sign of bleeding or at the appearance of any skin rash.
(2) Give transfusions of fresh blood or plasma if hemorrhage is severe.

*Antidotes*

(1) For heparin overdose give protamine sulfate, 1% slowly intravenously. This drug will antagonize an equal weight of heparin.
(2) For overdose of coumarin anticoagulants give phytonadione (Mephyton), 0.1 mg/kg intramuscularly.

*General measures*

Absolute bed rest must be maintained to prevent further hemorrhage.

**Prognosis**

Death may occur up to 2 weeks after discontinuing the drug. However, adequate therapy with vitamin K will bring the prothombin level back to normal in 24–48 h.

**References**

Shorten GD, Comunale ME. Heparin-induced thrombocytopenia. *J Cardiothor Vasc Anesth* 1996;10:521
Zimbelman J, *et al.* Unusual complications of warfarin therapy: skin necrosis and priapism. *J Pediatr* 2000;137:266

# HYDRALAZINE

Hydralazine (Apresoline) is a synthetic drug used for the treatment of hypertension.

Deaths following hydralazine medication have been rare, but the incidence of serious reactions following continued administration is 10–20%. Pathologic findings in reactions to hydralazine include rheumatic nodules, collagenous necrosis of the skin, and proliferative and necrotizing involvement of the arterioles and arteries of the myocardium, kidney, spleen, jejunum, and ileum.

### Clinical findings

The principal manifestations of hydralazine poisoning are fall in blood pressure and joint swelling.

*Acute poisoning* (from ingestion or injection)

Headache, severe hypotension, coronary insufficiency, and anuria.

*Chronic poisoning* (from ingestion)

Fever, headache, nausea and vomiting, fast pulse, anemia, blood dyscrasias, diffuse erythematous facial dermatitis, lymph gland enlargement, and splenomegaly, progressing to severe arthralgia simulating rheumatoid arthritis or disseminated lupus erythematosus. Joint involvement varies from vague generalized stiffness and aching to severe pain, swelling, and redness of one to several joints. Pericarditis with pleural effusion, polyneuritis, and activation of peptic ulcer have also been reported. Fatal intestinal bleeding has occurred as a result of vascular changes with accompanying ulcerations.

*Laboratory findings*

(1) The urine may show protein or red blood cells.
(2) The complete blood count may show microcytic or normocytic anemia, leukopenia, or lupus erythematosus cells.
(3) Serum proteins may show an increase in the globulin fraction.
(4) The ECG may show arrhythmias.

### Prevention

Patients must be warned to discontinue the use of hydralazine upon the appearance of any reaction.

**Treatment**

*Acute poisoning*

(1) Emergency measures – Establish airway and maintain respiration. Cautious reduction of dosage is indicated in severe hypotensive reactions. Overdoses should be removed by gastric lavage or emesis (see pp. 29–32). Treat hypotension with fluids (see p. 57). Vasopressors are hazardous. Dopamine, 5 µg/kg/min as an infusion to maintain blood pressure at 90 mmHg and adequate renal perfusion, is probably safest.

(2) Special problems – Treat anuria (see p. 66).

*Chronic poisoning*

Discontinue use. Give aspirin, 1–3 g daily, until symptoms regress.

**Prognosis**

If the patient lives for 24 hours after a severe hypotensive reaction survival is likely. Complete recovery from rheumatoid reactions has always occurred.

**References**

Hari CK, *et al*. Hydralazine-induced lupus and vocal fold paralysis. *J Laryng Otology* 1998;112:875

Hofstra AH. Metabolism of hydralazine: relevance to drug-induced lupus. *Drug Metab Rev* 1994;26:485

## CALCIUM CHANNEL BLOCKING AGENTS

**Table 26.1** Calcium channel blocking agents

| | |
|---|---|
| Amlodipine (Norvasc) | Mibefradil (Posicor) |
| Bepridil (Vascor) | Nicardipine (Cardene) |
| Diltiazem (Cardizem) | Nifedipine (Adalat, Oricardua) |
| Felodipine (Plendil) | Nimodipine (Nimotop) |
| Isradipine (DynaCirc) | Nisoldipine (Sular) |
| | Verapamil (Calan, Isoptin, Verelan) |

These drugs block the re-entry of calcium into muscle fibers and are used in the treatment of many conditions in which reduction of muscle contractility would be useful.

Toxicity occurs as a result of the expected actions of these drugs and by interactions with other drugs used at the same time. Verapamil, 1.4 g, has been fatal.

## Clinical findings

The principal manifestations of overdose from these agents are bradycardia and hypotension.

### Acute poisoning (from ingestion)

Bradycardia, hypotension, atrioventricular block, metabolic acidosis, and hyperglycemia.

### Chronic poisoning (from ingestion)

Effects are as for acute poisoning plus gastrointestinal distress with nausea and constipation, skin rash, flushing, dependent edema, weakness, and dizziness. Of these drugs verapamil appears to be most likely to seriously weaken cardiac contractility, especially when used in combination with $\beta$-sympathetic blocking agents. Pre-existing atrioventricular conduction abnormalities are enhanced by verapamil and diltiazem. Nifedipine is most likely to produce hypotension.

### Laboratory findings

(1) Hyperglycemia, hyperkalemia, elevated blood lactate level, reduced blood bicarbonate level, reduced arterial pH.
(2) Verapamil and nifedipine increase digoxin blood levels.
(3) Galactorrhea and prolactinemia with altered liver function have been noted after administration of verapamil.

## Prevention

Combination of these drugs with propranolol or other $\beta$-sympathetic blocking agents should be avoided, since it is more likely to produce serious hypotension. Many drugs increase calcium blocker serum concentration.

## Treatment

### *Emergency measures*

Remove ingested overdose with emesis followed by gastric lavage using activated charcoal (see pp. 31–32).

### *Antidote*

Calcium chloride or calcium gluconate, 10–20 mg/kg as 10% solution diluted in normal saline, should be given intravenously over 30 min and repeated as necessary to control symptoms.

### *General measures*

(1) Atrioventricular block and bradycardia usually respond to atropine or isoproterenol. Intracardiac pacing may be necessary.
(2) Treat hypotension by placing the patient in the supine position and giving intravenous fluids. Pressor agents should be used cautiously; dopamine (3–20 μg/kg/min) is possibly the safest.
(3) Administration of insulin may be necessary. Glucagon, 5–10 mg/h by infusion, has been used.

## Prognosis

Survival for 24 hours has been followed by complete recovery.

## References

Adams BD, Browne WT. Amlodipine overdose causes prolonged calcium channel blocker toxicity. *Am J Emerg Med* 1998;16:527

Brass BJ, *et al*. Massive verapamil overdose complicated by noncardiogenic pulmonary edema. *Am J Emerg Med* 1996;14:459

Evans JSM, Oram MP. Neurological recovery after prolonged verapamil-induced cardiac arrest. *Anaesth Intensive Care* 1999;653:653

Haddad LM. Resuscitation after nifedipine overdose exclusively with intravenous calcium chloride. *Am J Emerg Med* 1996;14:602

Holzer M, *et al*. Successful resuscitation of a verapamil-intoxicated patient with percutaneous cardiopulmonary bypass. *Crit Care Med* 1999;27:2818

Moser LR, *et al*. The use of calcium salts in the prevention and management of verapamil-induced hypotension. *Ann Pharmacotherap* 2000;34:622

Szekely LA, *et al*. Use of partial liquid ventilation to manage pulmonary complications of acute verapamil-sustained release poisoning. *J Toxicol Clin Toxicol* 1999;37:475

Yuan TH, *et al*. Insulin-glucose as adjunctive therapy for severe calcium channel antagonist poisoning. *J Toxicol Clin Toxicol* 1999;37:463

**Table 26.2**  Other cardiovascular drugs*

| Drugs | Clinical findings |
|---|---|
| Abciximab (ReoPro), anagrelide (Agrylin), clopidogrel (Plavix), dipyridamole (Persantine), eptifibatide (Integrilin), ticlopidine (Ticlid), tirofiban (Aggrastat) | Bleeding, headache, dizziness, nausea, flushing, weakness, syncope, gastrointestinal irritation, skin rash, hypersensitivity, exacerbation of chest pain. Ticlopidine: neutropenia, thrombocytopenia, liver damage |
| Alteplase (Activase), anistreplase (Eminase), bivalirudin (Angiomax), cilostazol (Pletal), reteplase (Retavase), streptokinase (Streptase), tenecteplase (TNKase), urokinase (Abbokinase) | Fever, kidney damage, vascular collapse, localized bleeding, sensitivity reactions |
| Amiloride (Midamor) | Hyperkalemia, nausea, vomiting, diarrhea, abdominal pain, constipation, cough, impotence |
| Amiodarone (Cordarone) | Pneumonitis, liver damage, exacerbated arrhythmias |
| Ammonium chloride (Exposure limit, 10 mg/m$^3$) | Nausea, vomiting, profound acidosis. Treat acidosis |
| Amrinone (Inocor) | Thrombocytopenia, arrhythmias, hypotension, nausea and vomiting, diarrhea, hepatotoxicity, pericarditis, pleuritis |
| Angiotensin-converting enzyme inhibitors (ACEI): captopril (Capoten), benazepril (Lotensin), enalapril (Vasotec), fosinopril (Monopril), lisinopril (Prinivil, Zestril), moexipril (Univase), perindopril (Aceon), quinapril (Accupril), ramipril (Altace), trandolapril (Mavik) | Hypotension, edema, lymphadenopathy, proteinuria, renal failure, hemolytic anemia, pancytopenia |

*Continued*

*Table 26.2 (continued)*

| Drugs | Clinical findings |
|---|---|
| Angiotensin II receptor blockers (ARBS): (same effects as ACEI) candesartan, cilexetil (Atacard), eprosartan (Teveten), irbesartan (Avapro), losartan (Cozaar), valsartan (Diovan), telmisartan (Micardis) | Hypotension, edema, lymphadenopathy, proteinuria, renal failure, hemolytic anemia, pancytopenia |
| Atorvastatin (Lipitor), cerivastatin (Baycol), fluvastatin (Lescol), lovastatin (Mevacor), pravastatin (Pravachol), simvastatin (Zocor) | Pain, constipation, nausea, distension, muscle pain, weakness, rash |
| Bumetanide (Bumex) | Muscle cramps, dizziness, hypotension, headache, encephalopathy, ototoxicity |
| Carbonic anhydrase inhibitors: acetazolamide (Diamox), brinzolamide (Azopt), dichlorphenamide (Daranide), dorzolamide (Trusopt), methazolamide (Neptazane) | Papular or erythematous skin eruptions, drowsiness, paresthesias, fatigue, nausea, acidosis, blood dyscrasias similar to those produced by sulfonamides (see p. 485) |
| Clofibrate (Atromid-S), fenofibrate (Tricor), gemfibrozil (Lopid) | Elevation of serum transaminase, nausea, vomiting, diarrhea, abdominal discomfort, headache, dizziness, fatigue, weakness, skin rash, and stomatitis. These drugs increase the risk of gallbladder disease and potentiate coumarin anticoagulant. Leukopenia, agranulocytosis, and Bromsulphalein retention have been reported |
| Dextran, hetastarch (Hextend) | Excessive bleeding, sensitivity reactions, hypertension, pulmonary edema |
| Diazoxide (Hyperstat) | Sodium and water retention, hyperglycemia, myocardial and cerebral ischemia, rash, hyperuricemia, arrhythmias, convulsions, shock, and mental depression; hypertension is rare |
| Disopyramide (Norpace) | Hypotension, cardiac decompensation, heart block, anticholinergic effects |

*Continued*

Table 26.2 (continued)

| Drugs | Clinical findings |
|---|---|
| Diuretics (K depleting): Chlorothiazide (Diuril), chlorthalidone (Hygroton), hydrochlorothiazide, hydroflumethiazide (Saluron), indapamide (Lozol), methyclothiazide (Enduron), metolazone (Zaroxolon), polythiazide (Renese), trichlormethiazide (Naqua, Indapamide) | Chloride loss, potassium loss, lethargy, muscle cramps, acidosis, gastric upset, skin rash, salivary gland obstruction, psychosis, convulsions, hyperuricemia, leukopenia, jaundice, hepatic decompensation in hepatic cirrhosis, photosensitization, precipitation or aggravation of diabetes mellitus, ulceration of small intestine from combined therapy with potassium chloride, hypercalcemia, and, rarely, acute glomerulonephritis, pancreatitis, thrombocytopenic purpura, or agranulocytosis. Acute overdose may cause coma. Infants born of mothers receiving thiazide diuretics may show jaundice or thrombocytopenia. Severe pancreatitis has also occurred during pregnancy. Treatment: give sodium or potassium chloride for measured deficits |
| Diuretics (K sparing): spironolactone (Aldactone), triamterene (Dyrenium), amiloride (Midamor) | Hyperkalemia. Risk increased if used with angiotensin inhibitors. Spironolactone associated with drug fever, gastric ulcers, menstrual irregularity, gynecomastia, rash and confusion |
| Doftilide (Tikosyn) | Prolonged QT interval, contraindicated in long QT syndromes, severe renal impairment, and with cimetidine, verapamil, or ketoconazoles: chest pain, torsades des pointes, dyspnea, flu syndrome, sudden death |
| Epoprostenol (Fiolan) | Flushing, hypotension, headache |
| Ethacrynic acid (Edecrin) | Hyperuricemia, anorexia, abdominal pain, nausea, vomiting, diarrhea, acute pancreatitis, jaundice, agranulocytosis, thrombocytopenia, deafness, ventricular fibrillation resulting from potassium loss. Treatment: give potassium chloride orally for hypokalemia |
| Fenoldopam (Corlorpam) | Reflex tachycardia, increased intraocular pressure |
| Flecainide (Tambocor) | Exacerbated arrhythmias, cardiac arrest, liver damage |
| Furosemide (Lasix), torsemide (Demadex), bumetanide (Bumex) | Skin rash, pruritus, paresthesia, deafness, blurring of vision, hypotension, tetany, dehydration, electrolyte loss, nausea, vomiting, diarrhea. Leukopenia, thrombocytopenia, and acute pancreatitis have occurred. Not in sulfa allergy. Treatment: give potassium chloride orally for hypokalemia |

Continued

*Table 26.2 (continued)*

| Drugs | Clinical findings |
|---|---|
| Ganglionic blocking agents: mecamylamine | Prolonged fall in blood pressure, failure of renal function, myocardial infarction, intestinal obstruction, tremor, psychosis and urine retention. Treatment: maintain blood pressure |
| Ibutilide (Corvert) | Hypotension, exacerbated arrhythmias |
| Mannitol | Headache, nausea, vomiting, chills, dizziness, lethargy, confusion, chest pain, heart failure, pulmonary edema. Fatalities have occurred |
| Metolazone (Zaroxolyn) | Severe electrolyte disturbances (hypokalemia), syncope, hyperglycemia |
| Mexilitene (Mexitil) | Nausea, vomiting, ataxia, tremor, arrhythmias |
| Milrinone (Primacor) | Cardiac arrhythmias, hypotension, headache |
| Minoxidil (Loniten) | Sodium and water retention, hirsutism, pericardial effusion, Stevens–Johnson syndrome |
| Moricizine (Ethmozine) | Arrhythmias, hypotension, ataxia, liver injury, bone marrow effects |
| Nitroprusside, sodium (Nipride) (See p. 312) | Severe hypotension, vomiting, apprehension, hyperventilation, tachycardia, muscular twitching, and reversible hypothyroidism |
| Potassium chloride (coated tablets) | Ulceration, hemorrhage, obstruction, perforation of the small intestine, and cardiac arrest |
| Prazosin (Minipress), doxazosin (Cardura), terazosin (Hytrin) | Dizziness, headache, drowsiness, gastrointestinal disturbances, tachycardia, dyspnea, paresthesias, rash, dysuria, sweating |
| Probenecid (Benemid) | Nausea, skin rash; rarely, liver necrosis, nephrotic syndrome |
| Propafenone (Rythmol) | Liver effects, cardiac conduction defects, agranulocytosis, apnea |
| Quinethazone (Hydromox) | Gastrointestinal upset, skin rash, weakness, dizziness |
| *Rauwolfia* preparations: deserpidine (Enduronyl), rescinnamine (Moderil), reserpine (Serpasil, Diupres) | Diarrhea, nasal stuffiness, anginal pain, extrasystoles, edema, congestive failure, thrombocytopenia, tremors, muscular stiffness, severe hypotension in conjunction with general anesthetic administration, emotional depression |

*Continued*

*Table 26.2 (continued)*

| Drugs | Clinical findings |
|---|---|
| Resins: cholestyramine (Questran, Prevalite), colestipol (Colestid) | Constipation, malabsorption, bleeding due to hypoprothrombinemia (binding of vitamin K), hypersensitivity, headache, vertigo, altered electrolytes, transient elevation of liver enzymes, osteoporosis |
| Sodium morrhuate, sodium psylliate, sodium tetradecylsulfate | Injection causes pain, sensitivity reactions, sloughing, pulmonary embolism, paraplegia. Occlude vein prior to injection |
| Sotalol (Betapace) | Dyspnea, bradycardia, chest pain, asthma, lightheadedness, hypotension, fatigue, caution in congestive heart failure |
| Tocainide (Tonocard) | Blood dyscrasias, pulmonary fibrosis |
| Triamterene (Dyrenium) | Gastrointestinal upset, dry mouth, weakness, tachycardia, hypotension, hyperkalemia, hypokalemia, rise in BUN, leukopenia |

*Treatment: reduce dosage or discontinue drug

## INTERACTIONS (see p. 20)

Coumarin anticoagulants enhance the effects of clofibrate and thyroid hormone. Anabolic steroids, clofibrate, glucagon, phenylbutazone, chloramphenicol, phenyramidol, quinidine, chloral hydrate, tetracyclines, allopurinol, ethacrynic acid, disulfiram, sulfonamides, and thyroid drugs enhance the effects of coumarin anticoagulants by displacing them from protein binding.

Probenecid reduces clearance of penicillins, dapsone, indomethacin, sulfinpyrazone, and *p*-aminosalicylic acid.

In the presence of elevated potassium, digitalized patients given succinylcholine have ventricular arrhythmias.

Antihypertensives enhance the effects of central nervous system depressants, anesthetics, diuretics, monoamine oxidase inhibitors, and tranquilizers.

Quinidine enhances the effects of muscle relaxants.

Antidepressant or antihypertensive drugs (except thiazide diuretics) have enhanced adverse effects when they are combined with pargyline.

Calcium blocker serum concentration is increased by clarithromycin, erythromycin, fluvoxamine, grapefruit juice, itraconazole, ketoconazole, nefazodone. If carbamazepine, phenytoin, primidone, rifampin, or barbiturates are discontinued, monitor for calcium blocker toxicity.

The risk of toxicity from digitalis glycosides is increased by administration of sympathomimetics, reserpine, succinylcholine, or calcium and potassium loss induced by diuretics, carbenoxolone, amphotericin B, corticosteroids, or laxative abuse.

Furosemide can cause tachycardia, hypertension, flush, and sweating in the presence of chloral hydrate.

Salicylates enhance the risk of bleeding when heparin is given.

Thiazide diuretics enhance potassium loss and increase the effect of curare drugs but have no effect on succinylcholine.

Reserpines deplete catecholamines, with resulting hypotension during anesthesia. Patients are then more sensitive to vasopressors.

Hydralazine potentiates anesthetic agents, makes hypotension more likely during anesthesia, and reduces pressor response to drugs.

Quinidine and procainamide increase susceptibility to curare.

Anticoagulants increase susceptibility to bleeding following injection procedures or intratracheal intubation.

Cyclopropane, halothane and other anesthetic agents, neostigmine, atropine, and $d$-tubocurarine trigger arrhythmias in digitalized patients.

## PHARMACOKINETICS AND TOXIC CONCENTRATIONS (see p. 100)

| | $pK_a$ | $T_{1/2}$ (h) | $V_d$ (l/kg) | % Binding | Toxic concentration (µg/ml) |
|---|---|---|---|---|---|
| Acebutolol | | | | | 35[†] |
| Acenocoumarol | | | | | 0.1 |
| Acetazolamide | 7.2 | 2.4–5.8 | | 90–95 | 25 |
| Ajmaline | | | | | 0.15, 5.5[†] |
| Amiodarone | | | | | 2.5 |
| Captopril | | | | | 6, 60[†] |
| Chlorothiazide | 6.7, 9.5 | 0.75–2 | | 20–80 | |
| Clofibrate | 2.95 | 8–54* | 0.09 | 95–98 | |
| Diazoxide | 8.74 | 21–36 | | 90–93 | 50 |
| Dicumarol | 5.7 | 7–100 | | 95 | |
| Digitoxin | | 96–144 | 40.9 | 90–97 | 0.03, 0.1[†] |
| Digoxin | | 3–40 | 5.3, 16* | 20–23 | 0.003, 0.005[†] |

*Continued*

*Pharmacokinetics and toxic concentrations (continued)*

| | p$K_a$ | $T_{1/2}$ (h) | $V_d$ (l/kg) | % Binding | Toxic concentration (µg/ml) |
|---|---|---|---|---|---|
| Diltiazem | | | | | 0.8,1.3[†] |
| Dipyridamole | | | | | 4 |
| Disopyramide | 9.6 | 5 | 0.6–1.3 | 35–95 | 4[†] |
| Ethacrynic acid | 3.5 | 0.5–1 | | | |
| Ethyl biscoumacetate | 3.1 | 3.1 | 2–3.5 | | 90 |
| Felodipine | | | | | 0.01 |
| Flecainide | | | | | 2-3, 10[†] |
| Furosemide | 3.8 | 1–3.5 | 0.1 | 95–97 | 25 |
| Heparin | | 1–2 | 0.06 | 0 | |
| Hydralazine | 7.1 | 2–7.8 | 0.45 | 87 | |
| Hydrochlorothiazide | | 2–15 | | | |
| Isosorbide dinitrate | | 0.3 | | | |
| Isradipine | | | | | 0.01 |
| Lanatoside C | | 33–36 | | 23–25 | |
| Mannitol | | 1.5 | | | |
| Mexiletine | | | | | 2–4, 10[†] |
| Milrinone | | | | | 0.3 |
| Nifedipine | | | | | 0.1, 0.15[†] |
| Nitroglycerin | | 0.3 | | | |
| Nitroprusside | | 150 | | | |
| Phenindione | | 5–10 | | | |
| Prazosin | | | | | 0.9 |
| Probenecid | 3.4 | 4–12 | 0.12–0.18 | 83–94 | |
| Procainamide | 9.2 | 2.2–4 | 1.7–2.2 | 15 | 8-10, 20[†] |
| Propafenone | | | | | 2, 7.7[†] |
| Quinidine | 4.3, 8.4 | 3–16 | 2.1–2.6 | 73–96 | 5-15, 15[†] |
| Reserpine | | 50–100 | | | |
| Spironolactone | | 13–24 | | 98 | |
| Thiocyanate | | | | | 120 |
| Triamterene | 6.2 | 2 | | 67 | |
| Verapamil | | 3–7 | | 6.5 | 1, 2.5[†] |
| Warfarin | 5.05 | 15–70 | 0.1 | 97 | 10, 100[†] |

*For children; [†]fatal

## References

Auzinger GM, Scheinkestel CD. Successful extracorporeal life support in a case of severe flecainide intoxication. *Crit Care Med* 2001;29:887

Chiu T-F, *et al*. Rapid life-threatening hyperkalemia after addition of amiloride HCl/hydrochlorothiazide to angiotensin-converting enzyme inhibitor therapy. *Ann Emerg Med* 1997;30:612

Donovan KD, *et al*. Acebutolol-induced ventricular tachycardia reversed with sodium bicarbonate. *J Toxicol Clin Toxicol* 1999;37:481

Fonck K, *et al*. ECG changes and plasma concentrations of propafenone and its metabolites in a case of severe poisoning. *J Toxicol Clin Toxicol* 1998;36:247

Gershon T, Olshaker JS. Acute pancreatitis following lisinopril rechallenge. *Am J Emerg Med* 1998;16:523

LoVecchio F, *et al*. Hypertonic sodium bicarbonate in an acute flecainide overdose. *Am J Emerg Med* 1998;16:534

Odeh M. Exfoliative dermatitis associated with diltiazem. *J Toxicol Clin Toxicol* 1996;35:101

Rambourg-Schepens M-O, *et al*. Recurrent convulsions and cardiac conduction disturbances after propafenone overdose. *Vet Human Toxicol* 1999;41:153

Silverman AJ, *et al*. Adenosine-induced atrial fibrillation. *Am J Emerg Med* 1996;14:300

Yasui RK, *et al*. Flecainide overdose: is cardiopulmonary support the treatment? *Ann Emerg Med* 1997;29:680

# 27 Anti-infective drugs*

## SULFONAMIDES

Fatalities have occurred following therapeutic doses of almost all sulfonamides.

Sulfonamide compounds or their acetyl derivatives frequently precipitate in the kidney tubules or the ureters, causing renal damage and blocking the secretion of urine. The sulfonamides may affect the function of the bone marrow, liver, or heart by as yet unknown mechanisms. Some reactions are on the basis of hypersensitivity (Stevens–Johnson syndrome). Hemolytic anemia following the administration of sulfonamide apparently occurs, at least in some cases, on the basis of a deficiency of glucose-6-phosphate dehydrogenase (G6PD) activity in erythrocytes.

The pathologic findings are crystalline deposits in the kidney tubules, calices, and ureters. In deaths from sulfonamides necrotic or inflammatory lesions may be found in the liver, heart, kidneys, bone marrow, or other organs. The bone marrow may be lacking in myeloid elements or may be completely aplastic. The liver may show degenerative changes.

**Table 27.1** Sulfonamide and sulfone derivatives

Diaminodiphenylsulfone (DDS, dapsone)*†
Mafenide (Sulfamylon)
Sulfabenzamide (Triple Sulfa)
Sulfacetamide (Sulamyd)
Sulfadiazine (Microsulfon)‡
Sulfadoxine (Fansidar)
Sulfamethoxazole (Gantanol)
Sulfanilamide*
Sulfasalazine (Azulfidine)‡
Sulfinpyrazone (Anturane)
Sulfisoxazole (Gantrisin)

*Causes methemoglobinemia (in addition to clinical findings listed on p. 486); †also causes restlessness and coma; ‡agranulocytosis has been reported in at least seven cases

*See also Table 27.2

## Clinical findings

The principal manifestation of sulfonamide poisoning is hematuria.

*Acute poisoning* (from ingestion or injection)

Gastrointestinal irritation, maculopapular erythematous skin eruptions, fever, mental and visual disturbances, sensitivity reactions, urticaria, hematuria, pain on urination, oliguria or anuria with azotemia, agranulocytosis, hemolytic anemia, thrombocytopenia purpura, conjunctival infection, bullous lesions of the skin, petechiae, jaundice, and increased erythema or injury from sunlight beginning days or weeks after institution of therapy. Such reactions are more frequent after repeated courses of therapy. In addition sulfasalazine has caused irreversible neuromuscular and central nervous system changes and fibrosing alveolitis. Peripheral neuropathy has occurred from long-term dapsone therapy. The combination of trimethoprim and sulfamethoxazole (co-trimoxazole, Bactrim, Septra) has caused anemia, reduction in renal function, thrombocytopenia, nausea and vomiting, diarrhea, mental depression, confusion, facial swelling, headache, bone marrow depression, and liver impairment. Sulfonamides have also caused Stevens–Johnson syndrome: skin eruption, fever, pneumonitis, myocarditis, and renal damage.

*Chronic poisoning*

Findings are the same as those described for acute poisoning.

*Laboratory findings*

(1) The complete blood count may reveal thrombocytopenia and diminution or absence of leukocytes. The red blood cell count may also be diminished.
(2) The urine may contain crystals, red blood cells, and protein.
(3) Blood sulfonamide levels above 10 mg/dl are considered toxic.
(4) In jaundice from sulfonamide administration hepatic cell damage is revealed by appropriate tests (see p. 75).

## Prevention

Do not prescribe sulfonamides unnecessarily. Use the minimum doses necessary to cure the disease. Use of sulfonamides in patients with G6PD deficiency or renal impairment is hazardous. Discontinue long-acting sulfonamides immediately if skin rash occurs.

Renal complications can be minimized if the urine is kept slightly alkaline with sodium bicarbonate, 5–15 g daily, and if the 24-h urine volume is maintained above 1 liter with oral fluids to 2 liters daily. Blood sulfonamide levels should be determined frequently if maximum doses are being given.

## Treatment

### *Acute poisoning*

(1) Emergency measures – Discontinue use at the first sign of skin rash or other untoward reaction. Remove swallowed overdoses by gastric lavage or emesis (see pp. 29–32).
(2) General measures – If renal function is normal force fluids to 4 liters daily to speed excretion of sulfonamides.
(3) Special problems – Hemodialysis is useful if renal function is depressed. Treat agranulocytosis (see p. 79). Treat aplastic anemia by repeated blood transfusions. Methemoglobinemia from sulfonamides does not appear to respond to methylene blue administration. Treat disturbed central nervous system function as for depressant drugs (see p. 394).

### *Chronic poisoning*

Treat as for acute poisoning.

## Prognosis

Renal function may return after 2 weeks of anuria. Agranulocytosis from sulfonamides responds to treatment in 50–75% of cases.

**References**

Dunn RJ. Massive sulfasalazine and paracetamol ingestion causing acidosis, hyperglycemia, coagulopathy, and methemoglobinemia. *J Toxicol Clin Toxicol* 1998;36:239

Northrop CV, *et al*. Sulfonamide-induced iritis. *Am J Emerg Med* 1996;14:577

## ANTIBIOTICS

Most of the deaths that occur as a result of administration of antibiotics are due to hypersensitivity reactions or overgrowth of resistant organisms. It is possible that some fatalities following the injection of insoluble antibiotics have been due to intravenous injection. More than 30 fatalities from aplastic anemia have been reported in patients who had previously taken chloramphenicol.

The pathologic findings in sudden death from hypersensitivity reactions after the injection of antibiotics are constriction of the bronchioles, distension of the lungs, pulmonary edema, congestion of the viscera, and hemorrhages in the lungs. Findings in deaths from overgrowth of resistant organisms are dependent upon the type of organism.

### Clinical findings

*Acute poisoning* (from injection, ingestion, or application to mucous membranes)

The following occur most commonly following parenteral administration of penicillin or streptomycin, less often following administration of other antibiotics: pallor, cyanosis, wheezing, collapse, frothy sputum, pulmonary edema, and death in respiratory failure may occur within seconds to minutes after injection of an antibiotic or its application to mucous membranes. Delayed reactions may consist of fever, skin eruptions, and pharyngeal or laryngeal edema. Oral administration, especially of penicillin, can also cause anaphylactoid reactions characterized by nausea and vomiting, abdominal pain and cramping, localized edema, cyanosis, respiratory distress, convulsions, severe chest pain, and death in respiratory failure.

*Chronic poisoning* (from repeated injection, ingestion, or application to mucous membranes)

The most common untoward reaction to the administration of antibiotics is the overgrowth of organisms not affected by the antibiotic agent, which can occur even after the parenteral injection of antibiotics. In some cases these organisms elaborate toxins that cause severe vomiting, diarrhea, and circulatory collapse. The following antibiotics have additional specific effects:

(1)  Penicillins – Urticaria, fever, rash, peripheral neuritis, wheezing, pruritus, flushing of skin, neutropenia, and fall in blood pressure occur variably after either intermittent or continuous use. Rapid intravenous administration of potassium penicillin can cause cardiac arrhythmia and cardiac arrest. Liver necrosis and hemolytic anemia resulting from anaphylactic reaction have also occurred. Ampicillin has caused reversible impairment of liver function and diarrhea. Methicillin has caused renal damage. Dicloxacillin has caused gastrointestinal upset, skin rash, and possible hepatic dysfunction. Carbenicillin and ampicillin have caused leukopenia. Bacampicillin and amoxicillin are similar to ampicillin. Benzyl penicilloyl polylysine, used as a skin test antigen for penicillin sensitivity, has caused severe sensitivity reactions and does not reveal all penicillin-sensitive individuals. Cloxacillin has caused hepatitis. Mezlocillin has caused thrombocytopenia and cholestatic jaundice. Nafcillin has caused hepatotoxicity. Oxacillin has caused tissue necrosis and liver damage. Piperacillin has caused hypercoagulability and hemolytic anemia. Ticarcillin has caused intrahepatic cholestasis and agranulocytosis.

(2)  Tetracyclines – Chlortetracycline (Aureomycin), oxytetracycline (Terramycin), tetracycline (Tetracyn), doxycycline (Vibramycin), demeclocycline (Declomycin), and minocycline (Minocin) can cause nausea, anorexia, diarrhea, perianal itching, skin eruptions, fever, toxemia, rising levels of blood urea nitrogen, psychotic reactions, anaphylaxis, and collapse from overgrowth of intestinal organisms. Increased intracranial pressure with bulging of fontanels has occurred in infants. A syndrome resembling lupus erythematosus can occur. Chlortetracycline and tetracycline have caused fatal liver damage after large oral or intravenous doses. A similar response is possible with other tetracyclines. It is believed that blood levels for tetracycline that exceed 16 µg/ml of serum

contribute to the development of liver damage. The daily oral dose should not exceed 2 g/d. When left standing, tetracyclines decompose into more toxic products that cause renal damage with polyuria, acidosis, and loss of protein, glucose, amino acids, and potassium. For this reason, a tetracycline should not be used later than the expiration date shown on the package. Tetracycline present during odontogenesis causes hypoplasia and discoloration of teeth; this can occur *in utero* or during childhood. Unless no alternative exists, tetracyclines should not be given for long or indefinite periods to children under 8 years of age. Demeclocycline has caused increased sensitivity to sunlight and reversible diabetes insipidus. Methacycline can cause a parasympathomimetic response.

(3)  Aminoglycosides – Streptomycin, vancomycin (Vancocin), kanamycin (Kantrex), spectinomycin (Trobicin), capreomycin (Capastat), amikacin (Amikin), gentamicin (Garamycin), netilmicin (Netromycin), and tobramycin (Nebcin) can cause paresthesias, lassitude, dizziness, headaches, blurring of vision, fever, and eighth-nerve injury with tinnitus, deafness, loss of sense of balance, renal damage, neuromuscular blockade, and vertigo after parenteral injection. Hearing loss, which may be permanent, occurs most frequently after dihydro-streptomycin, vancomycin, capreomycin, or tobramycin. Infants are especially susceptible. Severe central nervous system and respiratory depression has occurred in infants given streptomycin. Respiratory and cardiac arrest has followed intravenously administered kanamycin. Spectinomycin also causes urticaria, nausea, fever, sleeplessness, and decrease in hemoglobin levels. Skin rash has occurred after topical application of aminoglycosides. Because these drugs are excreted almost entirely by glomerular filtration, periodic evaluation of renal function is essential.

(4)  Chloramphenicol (Chloromycetin) – Nausea and vomiting, diarrhea, mucous membrane lesions, toxemia, hepatitis, and collapse from overgrowth of intestinal organisms; aplastic anemia or agranulocytosis occurs sufficiently often to require blood counts once weekly. Aplastic anemia is believed to result from an idiosyncratic response to excessive blood levels of chloramphenicol. Optic and peripheral neuritis has occurred in conjunction with chloramphenicol therapy. A sudden onset

of vomiting, diarrhea, and irreversible cardiovascular collapse has occurred in premature and newborn infants given more than 25 mg/kg/d. Newborn infants are deficient in the hepatic conjugating enzyme system that ordinarily detoxifies chloramphenicol. Caution should be used in the administration of chloramphenicol to any patient with liver or kidney injury.

(5) Polymyxins – Bacitracin, polymyxin B, and colistin (Coly-Mycin) can cause paresthesias and acute renal damage with proteinuria, nitrogen retention, and oliguria or anuria following injection of these antibiotics. Polymyxin B also causes dizziness, weakness, paresthesias, and severe fall in blood pressure from histamine release. These signs of toxicity from polymyxin B are much more frequent at doses greater than 2.5 mg/kg/d. Colistimethate has also caused leukopenia, neurotoxicity, dizziness, slurred speech, apnea, and fever.

(6) Cycloserine (Seromycin) – Headache, dizziness, lethargy, polyneuritis, psychotic behavior, and convulsions are especially frequent with doses over 0.5 g/d.

(7) Neomycin – Loss of hearing, vestibular damage, skin eruptions, steatorrhea, and kidney damage with proteinuria, edema, and electrolyte disturbances. Large injected doses of neomycin cause respiratory arrest and paralysis of voluntary muscles.

(8) Erythromycin, azithromycin, clarithromycin, dirithromycin – Nausea and vomiting, diarrhea, prostration, skin rash. Jaundice as a result of intrahepatic cholestasis has occurred after administration of erythromycin estolate (Ilosone).

(9) Nystatin (Mycostatin) – Nausea and vomiting, diarrhea, skin rash.

(10) Antifungals – Amphotericin B (Fungizone): therapeutic doses produce fever, anorexia, pain at the injection site, and, if administration is prolonged, gradual reduction of renal function as shown by increased blood urea nitrogen and non-protein nitrogen. Griseofulvin (Fulvicin): urticaria, nausea, diarrhea, headaches, confusion, dizziness, photosensitivity, renal damage, porphyria, and temporary leukopenia have occurred. Griseofulvin markedly potentiates the toxicity of colchicine in experimental animals. Candicidin (Candeptin): rarely, irritation or sensitization of the skin. Terbinafine (Lamisil): hepatic failure, toxic epidermal necrolysis, neutropenia. Azoles – ketoconazole (Nizoral)

fluconazole (Diflucan), itraconazole (Sporanox): hepatic failure, cardiac effects.

(11) Troleandomycin (Cyclamycin) – Skin rash, diarrhea. Liver damage with jaundice has occurred after troleandomycin administration.

(12) Lincomycin (Lincocin) and clindamycin (Cleocin) – Nausea and vomiting, severe inflammation of the colon with diarrhea, skin and mucous membrane reactions, impairment of liver function with jaundice, and reversible leukopenia.

(13) Cephalosporins – Hypersensitivity reactions. Toxic psychosis has occurred when these drugs were used in combination with other drugs. Reduced hemoglobin can occur, especially with cefuroxime. Other reactions:

Cefadroxil (Duricef), cefamandole (Mandole), cefoxitin (Mefoxin), cefotaxime (Claforan), and cefaclor (Ceclor) have caused gastrointestinal disturbances, hypersensitivity reactions, neutropenia, rise in liver enzymes, and a rise in blood urea nitrogen.

Cefdinir: liver and kidney damage, neutropenia.

Cefepime: neurotoxicity, convulsions.

Cefixime: nephrotic syndrome, pseudolymphoma leukemia.

Cefmetazole: asthma, hypoprothrombinemia.

Cefonicid (Monocid), ceftizoxime (Cefizox), cefoperazone (Cefobid), and cefuroxime (Zinacef) have caused pain on injection, skin rash, itching, eosinophilia, diarrhea, vomiting, and possible alterations in liver and kidney function.

Cefotetan: hemolysis.

Cefpodoxime: rash, fever, renal injury.

Cefprozil: rash, leukopenia, cholestasis.

Ceftazidime: encephalopathy.

Ceftibuten: cholestasis.

Ceftriaxone: biliary pseudolithiasis, hemolysis, nephrolithiasis.

Cephalexin: rash, Stevens–Johnson syndrome, toxic epidermal necrolysis, crystalluria after overdose.

Cephalothin (Keflin): skin rash, intense tissue irritation with pain on injection, fever, meningitis, renal failure, thrombocytopenia, and reversible leukopenia.

Cephradine (Anspor), cephapirin (Cefadyl), and cefazolin (Ancef) have caused drug fever, skin rash, elevation of SGOT and other liver enzymes, and eosinophilia.

Loracarbef: liver injury.

(14) Paromomycin (Humatin) – Gastrointestinal disturbances with doses over 3 g daily.

(15) Rifampin (Rimactane) – Gastrointestinal upset, mental effects, exacerbation of previous liver dysfunction, necrologic disturbances, thrombocytopenia and other blood dyscrasias, and renal damage.

(16) Quinolones – ciprofloxacin (Cipro), enoxacin (Penetrex), gatifloxacin (Tequin), levofloxacin (Levoquin), lomefloxacin (Maxaquin), moxifloxacin (Avelox), norfloxacin (Noroxin), ofloxacin (Floxin), sparfloxacin (Zagam), trovafloxacin (Trovan): CNS symptoms, GI disturbances, interstitial nephritis, photosensitivity, liver damage, toxic psychosis.

(17) Imipenem/cilastatin – Convulsions.

(18) Meropenem – Bleeding, liver impairment.

(19) Aztreonam – Convulsions, rash.

(20) Fosfomycin – Rash, gastrointestinal disturbances.

(21) Natamycin – Eye pain, blurred vision.

(22) Rifabutin – Uveitis, polyarthralgia, corneal deposits.

(23) Oxazolidinones – Linezolid (Zyvox): diarrhea, thrombocytopenia, elevated liver enzymes

### *Laboratory findings*

(1) A complete blood count may reveal a decrease in red blood cells, white blood cells, or thrombocytes.

(2) Bacitracin and polymyxin B sulfate may cause proteinuria, hematuria, and increase in blood urea nitrogen.

(3) Administration of amphotericin B, bacitracin, and polymyxin B must be discontinued if blood urea nitrogen rises above 20 mg/dl.

### Prevention

Patients must be carefully questioned concerning previous drug reactions, including rashes, asthma, or local swelling, prior to any injection. Most patients who are susceptible to severe penicillin reactions can be identified beforehand by placing 1 drop of a penicillin preparation (1000 units/ml) on the inner forearm and making a deep scratch in the skin through the drop. If a wheal appears immediately, 1:1000 epinephrine is applied to the scratch and 0.25 ml is given subcutaneously. A tourniquet is applied above the site of the scratch. For patients showing a wheal reaction to the penicillin scratch test, alternative therapy should be used.

## Treatment

### Acute poisoning

(1) Emergency measures for treatment of severe sensitivity reactions (anaphylaxis)
  (a) Give 1 ml of 1:1000 epinephrine intramuscularly. If no response is obtained give 1 ml of 1:10 000 epinephrine slowly intravenously.
  (b) Give positive-pressure artificial respiration.
  (c) Give diphenhydramine (Benadryl), 50 mg slowly intravenously. Give dexamethasone, 1 mg/kg intravenously every 6 h until symptoms abate.
(2) Antidote
  (a) Penicillinase (Neutrapen) will reverse delayed penicillin reactions but is not useful in anaphylaxis. Penicillinase is itself capable of causing serious anaphylactic reactions.
  (b) Respiratory paralysis from neomycin can be antagonized by intravenous administration of 2–10 ml of 10% calcium gluconate.

### Chronic poisoning

(1) Immediate measures – Discontinue drug if there is any untoward change in the patient's condition, and evaluate the possibility of drug reaction.
(2) General measures:
  (a) Treat gastrointestinal distress from oral antibiotics by giving milk every 3 h alternating with bismuth subcarbonate, 5 g every 3 h.
  (b) Treat toxemia from overgrowth of intestinal organisms with an appropriate chemotherapeutic agent after determining the type and sensitivity of the organism. Treat circulatory collapse (see p. 57). Stop antibiotics if possible.

(3) Special problems – Treat aplastic anemia by repeated blood transfusions. Treat anuria (see p. 66).

**Prognosis**

Anaphylactic reactions to antibiotics are frequently fatal. At least 75% of patients with idiosyncratic type aplastic anemia from chloramphenicol have died.

**References**

Czerwenka W, *et al*. Aseptic meningitis after treatment with amoxicillin. *BMJ* 1999;318:1521

Fang C-C, *et al*. Erythromycin-induced acute pancreatitis. *J Toxicol Clin Toxicol* 1996;34:93

Kucukguclu S, *et al*. Multiple-dose activated charcoal in an accidental vancomycin overdose. *J Toxicol Clin Toxicol* 1996;34:83

Norrby SR, Gildon KM. Safety profile of meropenem: a review of nearly 5000 patients treated with meropenem. *Scand J Infect Dis* 1999;31:3

Rolland WA, *et al*. Respiratory distress secondary to both amphotericin B deoxycholate and lipid complex formulation. *Vet Human Toxicol* 2000;42:222

Saryan JA, *et al*. Anaphylaxis to topical bacitracin zinc ointment. *Am J Emerg Med* 1998;16:512

Schatz BS, *et al*. Comparison of cefprozil, cefpodoxime (Proxetil), loracarbef, cefixime, and ceftibuten. *Ann Pharmacotherap* 1996;30:258

Tweddle DA, *et al*. Cyclosporin neurotoxicity after chemotherapy. *BMJ* 1999; 318:1113

# IPECAC AND EMETINE

Ipecac is used as an emetic in the syrup form (see p. 90), never in the fluidextract form; the fluidextract is 14 times as concentrated as the syrup, and 10 ml is hazardous. Emetine, the alkaloid from ipecac (the roots and rhizomes of *Cephaelis ipecacuanha*), is used in the treatment of amebiasis.

The fatal dose of emetine is approximately 1 g. The fatal dose of ipecac cannot be stated, since vomiting prevents estimation of the amount taken.

Emetine weakens cardiac contraction by direct action on the myocardium. The effect is cumulative over a period of 1 month or longer.

The pathologic findings are gastrointestinal congestion and degenerative changes in the kidneys, heart, and liver.

## Clinical findings

The principal manifestations of poisoning with these drugs are fall in blood pressure and vomiting.

*Acute poisoning* (from ingestion or injection of emetine or ingestion of ipecac)

Therapeutic doses of emetine sometimes cause nausea and vomiting, fatigue, dyspnea, tachycardia, low blood pressure, collapse, unconsciousness, and death from heart failure. Ingestion of ipecac fluidextract has caused convulsions and coma as well as esophageal damage with stricture. Doses of emetine above the therapeutic ranges almost always produce toxic effects; syrup of ipecac ordinarily causes only vomiting (see p. 90). If vomiting persists for more than 2–3 h after ipecac administration a search for its cause must be made.

*Chronic poisoning*

The effect of emetine is cumulative over a period of weeks. Cardiomyopathy has occurred from repeated use of syrup of ipecac (see p. 90).

*Laboratory findings*

The ECG reveals depressed T waves and arrhythmias. The urine may contain protein. Leukocytosis is common, and the extent of liver damage should be determined (see p. 75).

## Prevention

Repeated courses of emetine should be avoided. The incidence of myocardial damage is greatly increased when the total dose is over 1 g. Patients should be kept at bed rest during the administration of emetine, and activity should be restricted for several weeks afterward. No more than 30 ml of syrup of ipecac (see p. 90) should be used to induce emesis.

**Treatment**

*Acute poisoning*

(1) Emergency measures – Delay absorption of ingested fluid extract of ipecac by giving activated charcoal, and then remove by gastric lavage (see pp. 31–32).
(2) General measures – The patient should be kept at complete bed rest until recovery is assured. Cautious digitalization may be helpful for myocardial weakness. Replace fluid loss with 5% dextrose in normal saline.

*Chronic poisoning*

Treat as for acute poisoning.

**Prognosis**

Complete recovery after symptomatic myocardial damage from emetine is not likely. Patients with myocardial damage indicated only by electrocardiographic changes may recover completely in 6 months to 1 year.

## QUININE, QUINACRINE, AND CHLOROQUINE

Quinine, quinacrine (mepacrine, Atabrine), chloroquine, and hydroxychloroquine (Plaquenil) are used in the treatment of malaria and for other medical purposes. Quinine is also used (to the extent of 30 mg/500 ml) as the bitter flavoring agent in many tonic drinks. This amount is sufficient to cause severe sensitivity reactions. The fatal dose of any of these drugs can be less than 20 mg/kg in children under 2 years of age. At least three such fatalities have occurred owing to chloroquine, in one instance after 1 or 2 tablets. These drugs depress functions in all cells and especially in the heart. The kidneys, liver, and nervous system may also be affected.

The pathologic findings are degenerative changes in the liver, kidneys, brain, and optic nerve.

**Clinical findings**

The principal manifestations of poisoning with these agents are vomiting and fall in blood pressure.

*Acute poisoning* (from ingestion)

Progressive tinnitus, blurring of vision, weakness, fall in blood pressure, hemoglobinuria, oliguria, and cardiac irregularities. Injection or ingestion of large doses causes sudden onset of cardiac depression. Convulsions and respiratory arrest also occur. Severe sensitivity reactions occur, especially to quinine. These reactions are characterized by edema, erythema, vesiculation, weeping, and bullae and may occur with doses as small as 30 mg. Laryngeal edema and systemic reactions – including headache, fever, dyspnea, nausea, and diarrhea – also occur.

## Chronic poisoning

(1) Repeated ingestion of quinine in large doses causes visual loss associated with bilateral dilated pupils, pallor of optic disks, narrowing of retinal vessels, and papilledema. Late findings include constriction of visual fields.

(2) Quinacrine causes headache, hepatitis, aplastic anemia, psychosis, and jaundice.

(3) Chloroquine causes diarrhea, nausea, headache, deafness, dizziness, porphyria, muscular weakness, blurred vision from corneal lesions, lens opacities, and retinal damage, including macular degeneration. Retinal damage is usually irreversible. Fetal injury has also been reported.

### Laboratory findings

The urine may contain red blood cells, protein, and casts. The pseudo-isochromatic color vision plate (Hardy–Rand–Rittler) can be used as a screening test for the early detection of retinopathy.

## Treatment

### Acute poisoning

(1) Emergency measures – Maintain respiration. Remove swallowed drug by gastric lavage or emesis (see pp. 29–32). Treat fall in blood pressure by injection of norepinephrine. Treat cardiac arrhythmias (see pp. 461–464).

(2) General measures – If urine secretion is adequate give 2–4 liters of fluids daily to promote renal excretion. Acidify urine with 0.5 g of ascorbic acid every 4 h. Exchange transfusion may be useful.
(3) Special problems – Treat anuria (see p. 66).

### *Chronic poisoning*

No treatment appears to be effective for quinine amblyopia.

### Prognosis

If the patient lives for 48 hours recovery is likely. Retinal damage from quinine or chloroquine is likely to be permanent, but other adverse effects are reversible.

### Reference

Jordan P, *et al.* Hydroxychloroquine overdose: toxicokinetics and management. *J Toxicol Clin Toxicol* 1999;37:861

**Table 27.2** Chemotherapy: miscellaneous agents*

| Drug | Clinical findings and contraindications |
| --- | --- |
| Abacavir (Ziagen) | Hypersensitivity, rash, fever, GI symptoms |
| Acyclovir (Zovirax) | Local reactions, transient increase in BUN, encephalopathy, rash, nausea, vomiting, abdominal pain, thrombocytosis, thrombocytopenia, leukopenia |
| Adefovir (Preveon) | Nephrotoxicity, GI symptoms |
| Albendazole (Albenza) | Rash, optic neuritis, liver impariment |
| Amantadine (Symmetrel) | Insomnia, dizziness, ataxia, psychosis, and other CNS signs. Do not use in children. Non-fatal convulsions at 0.5 g/kg |
| 5-Aminosalicylic acid (PAS), mesalamine | Fever, pruritus, erythematous macular or bullous eruptions, acidosis, hypokalemia, crystalluria, nausea, vomiting, anorexia, hepatic necrosis, diarrhea, leukocytosis, laryngeal edema, hemolytic anemia, methemoglobinemia, thrombocytopenia, leukopenia, thyroid suppression |
| Amprenavir (Agenerase) | Increase serum lipids, GI symptoms, paresthesias |
| Atovaquone (Mepron) | Rash, fever, GI effects |
| Bismuth subsalicylate | Exposure 4 weeks to 30 years can cause temporary encephalopathy with mental deterioration and epileptiform convulsions |
| Butenafine (Mentax) | Burning, stinging, rash |
| Ciclopirox (Loprox) | Itching and burning |
| Cinoxacin (Cinobac) | Nausea, vomiting, diarrhea, headache, dizziness, tinnitus, rash, itching |
| Cidofovir (Vistide) | Leukopenia, liver effects, dyspnea |
| Clofazamine (Lamarine) | Renal and GI effects |
| Clotrimazole (Lotrimin) | Irritation to or blistering of skin |
| Crotamiton (Eurax) | Irritant, sensitizer |
| Delavirdine (Rescriptor) | Nausea, cramps, neutropenia, hypotension |
| Didanosine (Zidex) | Pancreatitis, hepatitis, retinal changes |
| Econazole (Spectazole) | Burning, itching, redness |
| Efavirenz (Sustiva) | Photosensitivity, hypersensitivity, rash, mental disturbances |

*Continued*

*Table 27.2 (continued)*

| Drug | Clinical findings and contraindications |
|------|------------------------------------------|
| Ethambutol (Myambutol) | Reversible decrease in visual acuity, anaphylactoid reactions, headache, malaise, anorexia, fever, skin rash, joint pain, numbness and tingling of the extremities, increase in serum uric acid, transient impairment of liver function, toxic epidermal necrolysis |
| Ethionamide (Trecator) | Nausea, diarrhea, skin rash, peripheral neuropathy, toxic psychosis, and liver damage. Injury to the fetus has occurred in experimental animals |
| Famciclovir (Famvir) | CNS effects, GI effects |
| Fluconazole (Difencan) | GI effects, liver damage |
| Flucytosine (Ancobon) | GI effects, blood dyscrasias, elevation of hepatic enzymes and BUN, CNS disturbances |
| Fomivirsen (Vitravene) | Inflammation, abnormal vision |
| Foscarnet (Foscavir) | Renal damage, neurotoxicity |
| Ganciclovir (Citovene) | Leukopenia, thrombocytopenia |
| Indinavir (Crivaxin) | Nephrolithiasis, bilirubinemia |
| Itraconazole (Sporanox) | GI effects, allergic reactions, rash |
| Ketoconazole (Nizoral) | Nausea, vomiting, pruritus, abdominal pain, CNS effects, hepatitis |
| Lamivudine (Epivir) | Pancreatitis, leukopenia, neuropathy |
| Mandelamine | Gastric irritation, nausea, renal irritation, acidosis |
| Mebendazole (Vermox) | Contraindicated in pregnancy. Causes abdominal pain and diarrhea in massive worm infestations |
| Mefloquine (Lariam) | GI and cardiac effects, convulsions |
| Methenamine | Skin rash, kidney and bladder irritation, hematuria, nausea, vomiting |
| Metronidazole (Flagyl) | Nausea, diarrhea, skin rash, dizziness, drowsiness, headache, leukopenia, sensitivity to alcohol. Carcinogenic in rodents. Do not use in early pregnancy |
| Miconazole (Monistat) | Phlebitis, mucous membrane irritation, rash, diarrhea, anorexia, thrombocytopenia |
| Naftifine (Naftin) | Rash |

*Continued*

Table 27.2 (continued)

| Drug | Clinical findings and contraindications |
|------|------------------------------------------|
| Nelfinavir (Viracept) | Leukopenia, joint pain, seizures |
| Nevirapine (Viramune) | Stevens–Johnson syndrome, skin rash, fever, liver effects |
| Nitrofurantoin (Furadantin) | Nausea and vomiting, maculopapular erythematous eruption, anemia, jaundice, bleeding, acute polyneuritis which may be irreversible, leukopenia, cerebellar dysfunction, circulatory collapse, hemolytic anemia of the naphthalene type (see p. 234) |
| Oseltamivir (Tamiflu) | Altered liver function, renal damage, anaphylaxis |
| Penciclovir (Denavir) | Irritation |
| Pentamidine isethionate | Fall in blood pressure, convulsions, neutropenia, bronchospasm, kidney and liver damage. Protect solutions of pentamidine from light |
| Phenazopyridine (Pyridium) | Methemoglobinemia, hemolytic reactions. Unsafe in presence of kidney or liver disease |
| Praziquantel (Biltricide) | Dizziness, drowsiness, headache, malaise, gastrointestinal distress, liver function impairment |
| Pyrazinamide | Hepatic damage, gout, gastric upset, fever |
| Pyrimethamine (Daraprim) | Anemia, leukopenia, thrombocytopenia |
| Ribavirine (Virazole) | Pulmonary effects, cardiac arrest |
| Rifapentine (Priftin) | Hyperuricemia, altered liver enzymes |
| Rimantidine (Flumadine) | GI effects, CNS depression |
| Ritonavir (Norvir), saquinavir (Invirase) | GI and CNS effects |
| Silver sulfadiazine (Silvadene) | Itching, burning, sulfonamide toxicity, leukopenia, possible renal impairment |
| Stavudine (Zerit) | Neuropathy, GI effects, pneumonia |
| Terbinafine (Daskil) | Psoriasis, pustulosis |
| Terconazole (Terazol) | Fever, toxic epidermal necrolysis |
| Thiabendazole (Mintezol) | Vomiting, nausea, dizziness, anorexia, abdominal pain, constipation or diarrhea, headache, skin eruptions, CNS depression and, rarely, crystalluria |
| Trifluridine (Viroptic) | Increased intraocular pressure, corneal damage |

*Continued*

*Table 27.2 (continued)*

| Drug | Clinical findings and contraindications |
|------|------------------------------------------|
| Trimethoprim (Proloprim) | Itching, rash, gastrointestinal distress, anemia, leukopenia, thrombocytopenia, methemoglobinemia, possible renal impairment |
| Trimetrexate (Neutrexin) | GI, hepatic, renal, and bone marrow effects |
| Valacyclovir (Valtrex) | Thrombocytopenia, hemolytic anemia |
| Vidarabine (Vira-A) | Gastrointestinal disturbances, tremor, confusion, psychosis, ataxia, anemia, leukopenia, thrombocytopenia, elevated liver enzymes and bilirubin, corneal changes, sensitivity reactions |
| Zalcitabine (Hivid) | Neuropathy, pancreatitis, hepatic effects |
| Zanamivir (Relenza) | Renal and bone marrow effects, hypoglycemia |
| Zidovudine (Retrovir) | Bone marrow suppression, myopathy, liver effects |

*Treatment: reduce dosage or discontinue

## ISONIAZID

Isoniazid (INH) is used in the treatment of tuberculosis, and patients are often given a supply adequate for several months.

At least some of its toxicity results from relative pyridoxine deficiency induced by isoniazid. Long-term treatment carries a risk of liver damage, especially in patients over 50 years of age.

Pathologic findings in deaths from isoniazid include liver damage with multilobular necrosis.

### Clinical findings

The principal manifestation of acute isoniazid poisoning is convulsions.

### *Acute poisoning* (from ingestion)

Nausea and vomiting, disorientation, lethargy, psychotic behavior, increased reflexes, acidosis, restlessness, muscle twitching, urinary retention, convulsions, coma, cardiorespiratory depression. Hemolysis may occur in patients with glucose phosphate dehydrogenase deficiency.

*Chronic poisoning* (from ingestion)

Peripheral neuropathy and jaundice occur often with long-term administration. The risk of liver damage increases with age.

*Laboratory findings*

(1) Hyperglycemia, reduced blood bicarbonate level, reduced arterial pH.
(2) Abnormal liver function tests.

**Prevention**

Isoniazid should only be dispensed in child-resistant containers. The daily dose should not exceed 10 mg/kg or a total of 300 mg. Each 100 mg of isoniazid should be supplemented with 10 mg of pyridoxine. Patients on long-term therapy should have monthly SGOT determinations and should be warned to see the physician at the first sign of liver toxicity.

**Treatment**

*Acute poisoning*

(1) Emergency measures – Remove ingested isoniazid with emesis or gastric lavage using activated charcoal (see pp. 31–32).
(2) Antidote – Give pyridoxine, 5 g intravenously, to control convulsions; repeat as necessary. The amount of pyridoxine given should at least equal the amount of isoniazid ingested.
(3) General measures:
    (a) Control convulsions with diazepam or phenytoin (see p. 62).
    (b) Dialysis or hemoperfusion is probably not useful.

*Chronic poisoning*

(1) Treat liver damage (see p. 76).
(2) Give pyridoxine, 5 g daily.

**Prognosis**

Patients who survive for 24 hours after acute overdoses will recover completely. In patients who were receiving long-term isoniazid therapy that was discontinued when SGOT levels reached 5 times normal, liver damage was not irreversible.

## INTERACTIONS (see p. 20)

Allopurinol increases the risk of ampicillin rash.

Tetracyclines increase renal toxicity of methoxyflurane.

Furosemide and ethacrynic acid increase nephrotoxicity of cephalosporins and ototoxicity of aminoglycosides. Aminoglycosides enhance nephrotoxicity of cephalosporins.

Sulfisoxazole potentiates thiopental. Sulfonamides potentiate the effects of warfarin, tolbutamide, chlorpropamide, and phenytoin by displacement from protein binding sites. Sulfonamides displace bilirubin from plasma protein binding and drive it into tissues, with increased brain injury in newborn infants (kernicterus).

Quinacrine displaces pamaquine from tissue binding sites and increases pamaquine plasma levels up to 5-fold.

Combination of *p*-aminosalicylate and salicylates gives a mutual increase in toxicity.

Ethanol increases the toxicity of cycloserine.

Aminoglycosides can induce prolonged hypotension during anesthesia.

## PHARMACOKINETICS AND TOXIC CONCENTRATIONS (see p. 100)

| | p$K_a$ | $T_{1/2}$ (h) | $V_d$ (l/kg) | % Binding |
|---|---|---|---|---|
| Amantidine | | 9–15 | | |
| Amikacin | | 2–3 | 0.2–0.3 | 10 |
| Amoxicillin | | 1 | 0.2 | 17 |
| Amphotericin B | | 24 | 4 | 90 |
| Ampicillin | 2.5, 7.2 | 1–1.5, 2* | 0.39 | 23 |
| Benzylpenicillin | 2.8 | 0.5 | 0.3 | 65 |
| Bismuth | | | | 0.05 |
| Carbenicillin | 3.3 | 1–1.5 | 0.17 | 50 |
| Cefalexin | 2.5, 7.3 | 0.5–1 | 0.23 | 15 |
| Cefazolin | | 1.75–2 | 0.14 | 84 |
| Cephaloridine | | 1–1.5 | 0.23 | 20 |
| Cephalothin | 2.5 | 0.5–1 | 0.26 | 50 |
| Cephapirin | | 0.6 | 0.14 | 44–50 |
| Cephradine | 2.6, 7.3 | 0.7 | 0.29 | 10 |
| Chloramphenicol | | 2.1–8.3 | 1.4 | 25–60 |
| Chlorobutanol | | | | 75† |
| Chloroquine | 8.4, 10.8 | 72 | | 55 |
| Clindamycin | 7.45 | 2–4 | 0.5,* 1.14 | 94 |
| Cloxacillin | 2.7 | 0.5 | 0.34 | 95 |
| Colistimethate | | 3–8 | 0.54 | 50 |
| Dapsone | 1.2 | 17–21 | | 72–80 |
| Dicloxacillin | 2.7 | 0.5 | 0.29 | 98 |
| Doxycycline | | 12–20 | | |
| Erythromycin | 8.8 | 1.4 | 0.57 | 12 |
| Ethambutol | | 4–6 | | 6 |
| Floxacillin | 2.7 | 0.8 | | 95 |
| Flucytosine | | 3–8 | | |
| Fusidic acid | 5.35 | 4.8–16.5 | 0.08–0.24 | 97 |
| Gentamicin† | 8.2 | 2.3 | 0.28, 0.56* | 70–80 |
| Griseofulvin | | 22 | | |
| Isoniazid | 3.5 | 0.5–1.5‡ | 0.9 | |
| Kanamycin† | 7.2 | 1.5–3.2 | 0.19, 0.8* | 0–3 |
| Lincomycin | 7.6 | 4.6–5.6 | 0.49 | 72 |
| Methenamine | | 2–6 | | |
| Methicillin | 2.8 | 0.5 | 0.9 | 37 |
| Metronidazole | | 6–14 | | |
| Nafcillin | 2.7 | 0.5 | 0.63 | 90 |
| Nalidixic acid | 6.7 | 1.1–2.5 | 0.26–0.45 | 93–97 |
| Neomycin | | 3 | | |
| Nitrofurantoin | 7.2 | 0.3–0.6 | | 25–60 |
| Oxacillin | 2.9 | 0.5 | 0.41 | 94 |
| Penicillin G | | 0.5 | | |

*Continued*

*Pharmacokinetics and toxic concentrations (continued)*

| | $pK_a$ | $T_{1/2}$ (h) | $V_d$ (l/kg) | % Binding |
|---|---|---|---|---|
| Phenoxymethylpenicillin | 2.7 | 0.5 | 0.73 | 79 |
| Piperazine | | | | 0.5 |
| Polymyxin B | | 4.4 | | |
| Pyrimethamine | 7.2 | 96 | | |
| Quinacrine | 7.7, 10.3 | 120 | | 90 |
| Quinine[†] | 4.3, 8.4 | 8.5 | | 90 |
| Rifampin | | 1.5–5 | | |
| Spectinomycin | | 1.7 | | |
| Streptomycin | | 2–3 | 0.26 | 20–30 |
| Sulfamethoxazole[†] | 5.7 | 8–11 | 0.17 | 62 |
| Sulfasalazine | 0.6–11 | 6–10 | | 99 |
| Sulfisoxazole | | 5–7 | | |
| Tetracycline[†] | 7.7 | 9–11 | 2.5–4 | |
| Tobramycin | | 2–3 | 0.31 | 70–80 |
| Trimethoprim | | 6–17 | | 10 |
| Vancomycin | | 6–8 | | |

*For children. [†]Toxic concentrations (µg/ml): gentamicin 10; kanamycin 25; quinine 10; tetracycline 16; sulfamethoxazole 200; [‡]slow acetylators, 2–4

# References

Adkins JC, Noble S. Efavirenz. *Drugs* 1998;56:1055

Burkhart CN. Ivermectin: an assessment of its pharmacology, microbiology and safety. *Vet Hum Toxicol* 2000;42:30

Foster RH, Faulds D. Abacavir. *Drugs* 1998;55:729

Jarvis B, Lamb HM. Rifapentine. *Drugs* 1998;56:607

McCarty M, *et al*. Hyperkalemic ascending paralysis. *Ann Emerg Med* 1998;32:104 (Trimethoprim)

McNeely W, Spencer CM. Butenafine. *Drugs* 1998;55:405

Noble S, Goa KL. Adefovir dipivoxil. *Drugs* 1999;58:479

Waghorn SL, Goa KL. Zanamavir. *Drugs* 1998;55:721

Watts RG, *et al*. Effect of charcoal hemoperfusion on clearance of pentamidine isethionate after accidental overdose. *J Toxicol Clin Toxicol* 1996;35:89

# 28 Stimulants, antidepressants, antimanics, anticonvulsants, and psychotomimetic agents

## MONOAMINE OXIDASE INHIBITORS: PHENELZINE AND RELATED DRUGS

Tranylcypromine (Parnate) and phenelzine (Nardil) are used in the treatment of depression. Iproniazid, isocarboxazid, pargyline, pheniprazine, and nialamide are no longer marketed in the USA because of hepatitic toxicity. Deaths have occurred with single doses of 25–100 mg/kg, and as little as 50 mg/d has caused fatal liver necrosis. The incidence of symptomatic liver damage from iproniazid has been about 0.1%. Following the ingestion of large doses, the immediate effects result from central nervous system stimulation, whereas the most serious delayed effect of iproniazid and those agents no longer marketed is jaundice from acute liver necrosis.

These compounds are all monoamine oxidase inhibitors (MAOI), and they greatly potentiate the action of compounds such as other sympathomimetic amines. Other agents that interact, sometimes fatally, with the MAOI are barbiturates, dextromethorphan (used in OTC anti-tussives), meperidine, rarely morphine, aminopyrine, isometheptene, metaraminol, phenylpropanolamine, phenylephrine, tricyclic antidepressant; and selective serotonin reuptake inhibitors (SSRIs) such as fluoxetine, nefazodone, tramadol, venlafaxine, and possibly St. John's wort. Symptoms from poisoning due to SSRI drug interactions are likely related to excess serotonin. Serotonin syndrome is characterized by severe hyperthermia, muscular rigidity, disorientation, hypertension, seizures, hypertension followed by hypotension and coma.

### Clinical findings

The principal manifestations of poisoning from the MAOI agents used in medical practice are initial stimulation, hyperthermia, followed by hypotension, coma and death.

*Acute poisoning*

Overdose initially causes symptoms related to catecholamine excess including tremor, ataxia, agitation, flushing, hypertension, diaphoresis, hyperthermia, miosis, increased deep-tendon reflexes, convulsions, tachycardia, and precordial pain. The second phase of toxicity results from catecholamine depletion: profound hypotension, bradycardia, asystole and death from respiratory and circulatory failure.

*Chronic poisoning*

Repeated administration of any of these drugs causes dizziness, weakness, ataxia, hallucinations, mania, agitation, constipation, dry mouth, urine retention, and excessive rise or fall of blood pressure. Iproniazid and pheniprazine may cause liver injury at any time during drug therapy. Symptoms begin with nausea and lethargy; intractable vomiting indicates rapid progression of liver damage. Pheniprazine has caused impaired vision from bilateral optic tract lesions. Combinations of these drugs or these drugs combined with others such as imipramine or opium derivatives have been more likely to cause extreme reactions, including fatal hyperpyrexia. Tranylcypromine, phenelzine, and related drugs have caused severe hypertension following the ingestion of tyramine containing food (cheese, beer, red wine, pickled herring, fermented sausages, fava beans, chocolate, etc.); and drugs such as meperidine, dextromethorphan, phenylpropranolamine, stimulants, other antidepressants (TCA, SSRI, amphetamine.

*Laboratory findings*

Hepatic cell injury is indicated by appropriate tests.

**Prevention**

Drugs with a significant record of hepatic damage should not be used over prolonged periods without close supervision. Avoid administration of these drugs with other stimulant drugs, ephedra, or related alkaloids such as those contained in non-prescription medicines and herbal products advertised as anti-obesity or energy treatments.

*Emergency measures*

(1) Remove ingested drugs by gastric lavage and emesis.
(2) If respiration is depressed, give artificial respiration.
(3) For severe hypertension, avoid any long acting agent as the second phase of toxicity results in profound hypotension. If necessary, use a short-acting beta-blocker (esmolol) or a combination beta/alpha blocker (such as labetalol) or phentolamine (5 mg IV slowly). Methyldopa and guanethidine are contraindicated.
(4) Maintain blood pressure. Place patient in the Trendelenburg position, administer intravenous fluids. Use extreme caution in administering pressor agents. If a pressor must be used, a direct-acting adrenergic agent, such as epinephrine, norepinephrine, or isoproterenol, is preferable because they do not release intracellular amines.
(5) Control convulsions by cautious administration of diazepam slowly intravenously (see p 60).
(6) Treat ventricular arrhythmias with lidocaine or procainamide. Avoid bretylium, as it is associated with increased release of norepinephrine, followed by catecholamine depletion and hypotension.

*General measures*

Discontinue drug at the first appearance of jaundice. Treat liver damage. Dialysis can be effective. Pyridoxine, 200 mg slow IV infusion, has been tried. Control of acidosis may require sodium bicarbonate, up to 3 mEq/kg/h.

**Prognosis**

The fatality rate in acute poisoning has been 1%. About 25% of patients with severe liver damage have died.

# CAFFEINE, THEOPHYLLINE, AND OTHER XANTHINES

Caffeine, aminophylline and are used for the treatment of asthma, chronic obstructive pulmonary disease and apnea. Theophylline has been prescribed as a bronchodilator, diuretic, and respiratory stimulant. Dyphylline is the 7-dihydroxypropyl derivative of theophylline. Theobromine is found in coffee, tea, and chocolate. The derivative pentoxifylline) is used for the treatment of intermittent claudication.

Fatalities have resulted from 0.1 g of aminophylline (theophylline ethylenediamine) intravenously, 25–100 mg/kg by rectal suppository, or as little as 8.4 mg/kg orally in a child. Any oral ingestion exceeding 10 mg/kg requires prompt administration of ipecac. At least four deaths have followed the repeated use of aminophylline rectal suppositories in children. Fatalities from caffeine, 183–250 mg/kg, have been reported. Serum theophylline levels above 20 µg/ml are toxic.

Injection of aminophylline in hypersensitive subjects causes immediate vasomotor collapse and death. Rapid intravenous injection of aminophylline causes cardiac inhibition. In large doses, aminophylline depresses the central nervous system, whereas caffeine stimulates it.

The pathologic findings are not characteristic.

## Clinical findings

The principal manifestations of poisoning with these drugs are intractable seizures, hypotension, and arrhythmias.

### *Acute poisoning*

Intravenous administration of aminophylline is sometimes followed by sudden collapse and death within 1–2 minutes. Oral theophylline can cause vomiting, coma, hyperreflexia, ventricular arrhythmias including fibrillation, hypotension, convulsions, and respiratory arrest. Repeated rectal administration of aminophylline to infants may cause severe vomiting, collapse and death. Doses of caffeine up to 10 g orally have caused gastric irritation, vomiting, and convulsions; complete recovery occurred in 6 h.

### *Chronic poisoning*

Repeated doses of caffeine, theophylline or its salts can cause nausea, vomiting, headache, agitation/anxiety, epigastric pain (gastritis, reflux), fever, tachycardia, arrhythmias, hyperventilation, convulsions, and respiratory failure. Caffeine withdrawal causes severe headaches that may last up to two weeks.

*Laboratory findings*

Urinalysis may show proteinuria.

## Prevention

Test the sensitivity of the patient to intravenous aminophylline by giving 0.1 ml intravenously and waiting 1 min. The rate of injection should not exceed 4 mg/kg every 12 h, especially in infants. The serum concentration of theophylline should not exceed 20 μg/ml. Serum levels must be monitored, as a patient may not exhibit any of the minor toxicity symptoms before onset of seizures. Asymptomatic patients with serum levels greater than 40 should undergo charcoal hemoperfusion before clinical toxicity. Patients who are known to have reduced xanthine clearance are more susceptible to toxicity (neonates, infants less than 6 months, patients with hepatic cirrhosis, pulmonary edema, severe pneumonia, or prolonged fever). Patients started on drugs that inhibit theophylline metabolism are also at increased risk (cimetidine, erythromycin, verapamil, ciprofloxacin, enoxacin, fluvoxamine, tacrine, and troleanomycin).

## Treatment

*Emergency measures*

(1)  Remove ingested drugs by emesis or gastric lavage using activated charcoal (see pp. 31–32) regardless of whether vomiting has occurred.
(2)  Give $O_2$ by non-rebreather mask (bag-valve-mask).
(3)  Maintain blood pressure by administration of fluids. Propranolol antagonizes some of the metabolic and cardiovascular effects of theophylline. Give 0.02 mg/kg by slow IV infusion. Esmolol, which has a half-life of 9 min, is also effective. Give 0.5 mg/kg over 1 min, then 50 μg/kg/min.
(4)  Remove rectally administered aminophylline by enema.

*General measures*

Control convulsions by giving IV diazepam. Treat dehydration with NS or 5% dextrose in water. Charcoal hemoperfusion removes these drugs more effectively than does peritoneal dialysis; the effectiveness of peritoneal dialysis can be increased by adding red blood cells to the dialysate.

**Prognosis**

About 50% of patients with convulsions after theophylline administration have died. Convulsions after caffeine are less likely to be fatal.

**References**

Forman J, *et al*. Myocardial infarction resulting from caffeine overdose in an anorectic woman. *Ann Emerg Med* 1997;29:178

Kamijo Y, *et al*. Severe rhabdomyolysis following massive ingestion of oolong tea: caffeine intoxication with coexisting hyponatremia. *Vet Human Toxicol* 1999; 41:381

Krieger ACC, Takeyasu M. Nonconvulsive status epilepticus in theophylline toxicity. *J Toxicol Clin Toxicol* 1999;37:99

Minton NA, Henry JA. Treatment of theophylline overdose. *Am J Emerg Med* 1996;14:606

Rivenes SM, *et al*. Intentional caffeine poisoning in an infant. *Pediatrics* 1997;99: 736

Shannon M. Life-threatening events after theophylline overdose. *Arch Intern Med* 1999;159:989

# STRYCHNINE

Strychnine is an important component of various tonics and cathartic pills. It is used as a rodenticide. Castrix, another rodenticide, is similar to styrchnine and just as toxic strychnine Derivatives of strychnine and related compounds, such as N-oxystrychnic acid and brucine, have been used as stimulants.

The fatal dose of strychnine is 15–30 mg. The exposure limit for strychnine is 0.15 mg/m$^3$.Strychnine causes markedly increased reflex excitability in the spinal cord; this results in the loss of normal inhibition of motor cell stimulation resulting in simultaneous contraction of all muscles. Rigor mortis occurs immediately after death. Other pathologic findings are not characteristic.

**Clinical findings**

The principal manifestation of acute strychnine poisoning is convulsions. Doses less than necessary to cause acute poisoning are without toxic effect.

*Acute poisoning*

After ingestion, strychnine and related compounds/derivatives cause an increase in deep tendon reflexes. This is followed by stiffening at the knees which is especially noticeable when walking up and down stairs. Next observed are single extensor spasms of the arms and legs. As poisoning progresses, spasms increase in severity and frequency until the patient appears to be in almost continuous opisthotonos. Any sound or movement will elicit a spasm. Death is from respiratory failure.

*Laboratory findings*

Strychnine can be identified in gastric washings or vomitus by appropriate tests. Arterial pH and serum electrolytes will help the physician treat acidosis resulting from hypoxia.

**Prevention**

Strychnine rodent baits are extremely dangerous. Remedies containing strychnine should be discontinued.

**Treatment**

*Emergency measures*

Give artificial respiration with $O_2$ during convulsions. After convulsions and hyperactivity are controlled, remove strychnine by gastric lavage using activated charcoal (see pp. 31–32). No specific antidote is available.

*General measures*

Once symptoms occur, avoid any manipulation such as gastric lavage or emesis. Enforce absolute quiet and absence of stimuli. Control convulsions by inducing paralysis with succinylcholine or a related neuromuscular blocker. Give diazepam, 0.05–0.1 mg/kg IV slowly or midazolam 0.05–0.1 mg/kg IV and repeat as necessary. Control pain with morphine, cautiously monitoring for respiratory depression. Treat acidosis. In severe cases, use a neuromuscular blocker such as succinylcholine, rocuronium, pancuronium, etc.

## Prognosis

If the patient lives for 24 hours, recovery is probable.

## References

Hernandez AF, *et al*. Acute pancreatitis associated with nonfatal strychnine poisoning. *J Toxicol Clin Toxicol* 1998;36:67

Katz J, *et al*. Strychnine poisoning from a Cambodian traditional remedy. *Am J Emerg Med* 1996;14:475

Palatnick W, *et al*. Toxicokinetics of acute strychnine poisoning. *J Toxicol Clin Toxicol* 1996;35:617

# CAMPHOR

Camphor is an ingredient in products that prevent moth-damage and in respiratory/cold remedies (camphorated oil). The fatal dose of camphor is approximately 1 g for a 1-year-old child, the amount contained in 5 ml of camphorated oil or 20 ml of Vicks Vaporub. At least 12 fatal cases of camphor poisoning have occurred. The exposure limit for camphor is 2 ppm. Camphor causes convulsions by stimulating the cells of the cerebral cortex. The pathologic findings include congestion/edema in the gastrointestinal tract, kidneys, and brain.

## Clinical findings

The principal manifestation of acute camphor poisoning is convulsions. Initial symptoms after ingestion include burning in the mouth and throat, epigastric pain, thirst, nausea and vomiting, anxiety, dizziness, irrational behavior, rigidity, rapid pulse, slow respiration, twitching of facial muscles, muscular spasms, and generalized convulsions, and unconsciousness. Poisoning has occurred after intramuscular injection.

## Treatment

### Emergency measures

Establish airway, maintain respiration and control ventilation. After convulsions are controlled, remove swallowed poison by airway-protected gastric lavage followed by 30–60 ml of Fleet's Phospho-Soda diluted 1:4 in water.

*General measures*

Control convulsions with midazolam, diazepam or a neuromuscular blocker such as succinylcholine.

**Prognosis**

If the patient lives for 24 hours recovery will probably occur.

## PICROTOXIN, PENTYLENETETRAZOL, AND NIKETHAMIDE

Picrotoxin is a non-nitrogenous compound of known structure obtained from cocculus indicus (fish berries), the berry of *Anamirta cocculus*, an East Indian plant. The common name is Levant berry. It has been injected as a 'natural remedy' to threat nystagmus and vertigo. The leaves have been inhaled to treat malaria. Picrotoxi, which is present the seeds, has been applied to arrow tips to paralyze fish and animals. Topically, extracts have been applied to treat lice and scabies. Poisoning has occurred from adulteration of beverages with cocculus indicus. Medicinal use has been abandoned in the US. Nikethamide (Coramine) and pentylenetetrazol (Metrazol) are synthetic chemicals no longer available in the USA.

The fatal dose of picrotoxin may be as low as 20 mg or 2–3 cocculus kernals (0.5 g). In the treatment of drug-induced coma in which the convulsive threshold is raised, doses of picrotoxin over 300 mg in 24 h are likely to induce severe toxicity. The fatal dose of pentylenetetrazole may be as low as 1 g. The maximum dose should be limited to 6 g in 24 h. The fatal dose of nikethamide has not been established.

Picrotoxin, pentylenetetrazol, and nikethamide stimulate the spinal cord, medulla, and cerebral cortex. The action persists with picrotoxin for 12–24 h; with pentylenetetrazol, from 5 min to 3 h, and with nikethamide, from 5 to 60 min.

The pathologic findings in fatal cases consist of congestion (edema) of all organs.

## Clinical findings

The principal manifestation of acute poisoning is convulsions. Chronic poisoning has not been reported.

Serious poisoning from therapeutic administration has only occurred after injection. Picrotoxin in fish berries can be absorbed after ingestion. Symptoms and signs include nausea, vomiting, tachypnea, headache, twitching, convulsions, and coma. The stimulant effect of Picrotoxin begins about 20 min after injection, reaches a maximum in about 1 hour, and persists for 6–24 h. Stimulation following injection of pentylenetetrazol or nikethamide begins almost immediately, and the maximum effect is reached in 5–10 min and persists up to 3 h.

When picrotoxin, pentylenetetrazol, or nikethamide were used historically as stimulants for barbituric acid poisoning, the dose necessary to produce stimulation was greatly increased. Smaller dosages were used to treat epilepsy. The large amount given to awaken the patient in a coma caused toxic effects such as hyperthermia, cardiac irregularities, anuria, cerebral injury, pulmonary edema, and liver injury. Convulsions induced by these stimulants in the treatment of drug-induced coma may be followed by severe central nervous system depression.

## Prevention

Sale of cocculus indices (fish berries) should be strictly controlled. Picrotoxin, pentylenetetrazol, and nikethamide are too dangerous to be used therapeutically.

## Treatment

### Emergency measures

(1) Establish airway, maintain respiration and control ventilation.
(2) Delay absorption by giving activated charcoal (see pp. 31–32); then remove by gastric lavage
(3) Slow absorption rate of poison that is injected intramuscularly or subcutaneously by application of ice packs.

### General measures

(1) Treat convulsions. Give diazepam, 2–10 mg intravenously at a rate not greater than 1 mg/min, or use midazolam. If seizures are not controlled, try other anticonvulsants.
(2) Treat hyperthermia by application of wet towels.
(3) Maintain fluid and electrolyte balance. Treat acidosis and hypoxia.
(4) Treat pulmonary edema and cardiac arrhythmias.

### Prognosis

Convulsions which occurring after poisoning with these agents are followed by central nervous system depression, frequently with fatal outcome. Hyperthermia and cardiac arrhythmias induced by picrotoxin, pentylene-tetrazol, or nikethamide are often fatal.

## POLYCYCLIC ANTIDEPRESSANTS: AMITRIPTYLINE, IMIPRAMINE, AND RELATED DRUGS

Amitriptyline (Elavil), clomipramine (Anafranil), imipramine (Tofranil, Janimine), desipramine (Norpramin, Pertofrane), protriptyline (Vivactil), doxepin (Sinequan), maptrotiline (Ludiomil), trimipramine (Surmontil), and nortriptyline (Aventyl) are related drugs used as antidepressants. Cyclo-benzaprine (Flexeril) is chemically related and used as a muscle relaxant. Amoxapine (Asendin) is the demethylated metabolite of the antipsychotic loxapine. Bupropion (Wellbutrin, Zyban) is related to the CNS stimulant diethylproprion. Trazodone is a triazolopyridine antidepressant. Venlafaxine (Effexor), nefazodone (Serzone), and mirtazapine (Remeron) are newer, chemically distinct antidepressants.

This group of drugs has a narrow therapeutic index. Dosages less than ten times a therapeutic dosage can result in death. In general, dosages 10–20 mg/kg cause serious intoxication, and those over 30 mg/kg are life threatening. Plasma levels of these agents and their metabolites can be measured to determine whether a patient's level is in the toxic range. Therapeutic concentrations of parent drug plus metabolite are usually less than 300 ng/ml. Levels that exceed 1000 ng/ml result in serious toxicity. Deaths have occurred following doses as little as 250 mg in a 2-year-old child, and 500–750 mg in a

16-year-old child. One gram of amitriptyline was fatal in a one year old and 1.5 g of desipramine was fatal in a 4-year-old child.

The tertiary or dimethylated TCA's (amitriptyline, imipramine, doxepin and trimipramine) primarily block serotonin reuptake and are more potent anticholinergic and alpha blocking agents than the secondary or mono-methylated amine TCA's (nortriptyline, desipramine and protriptyline). The secondary amines primarily block reuptake of norepinephrine, with less anticholinergic and alpha blocking activity. Thus, the tertiary amines cause more sedation, anticholinergic delirium, orthostatic hypotension, urinary retention, weight gain, blurred vision and antihistaminic activity. Both groups exhibit enhanced toxicity if given with or immediately after stopping monoamine oxidase inhibitors.

## Clinical findings

The principal manifestations of poisoning with these drugs are central nervous system stimulation and cardiac arrhythmias.

### Acute poisoning

Overdoses cause hyperthermia, flushing, mydriasis, dry skin, ataxia, followed by clonic movements or convulsions, hypotension, respiration depression, and delirium, cardiac dysrrhythmias, atrioventricular or intraventricular block, multifocal extrasystoles, and ischemia. Ventricular fibrillation immediately precedes death and may occur after apparent recovery.

### Chronic poisoning

Dryness of the mouth, constipation, excessive sweating, orthostatic hypotension, drowsiness, blurred vision, and tremor, are common expected side effects. Hypersensitive reactions, such as cutaneous vasculitis, photo-toxicity and urticaria are indications to stop therapy. Excessive dosage or serum concentration is associated with agitation, urinary retention, severe orthostatic hypotension, tachycardia, increased intraocular pressure, jaundice with acute liver necrosis, cardiac arrhythmias, paresthesias, confusion, agitation, abdominal pain, and ataxia. Lethargy, convulsions, anticholinergic psychosis, and leukopenia have occurred rarely. Renal damage has been reported after overdose of imipramine, amoxapine, and maprotiline. Amoxapine, maprotiline and bupropion are more likely to cause seizures which can result in rhabdomyolysis, acute tubular necrosis, and renal failure. Pulmonary edema has been reported after amitriptyline. Abrupt withdrawal results in nausea, headache, vertigo, nightmares, and malaise. A slow taper off medication can prevent this withdrawal syndrome. In rare circumstances, acute psychosis has been observed following abrupt cessation of therapy.

### Laboratory findings

The ECG may reveal atrioventricular or intraventricular block, prolonged PR and QT intervals, widened QRS complex, flat or inverted T waves, supraventricular or ventricular tachycardia, ventricular fibrillation or asystole.

## Prevention

These drugs should not be used in conjunction with monoamine oxidase inhibitors. When changing therapy from a polycyclic antidepressant to a MAOI (or vice versa) at least 2 weeks must elapse after discontinuation of the initial drug before starting the new agent in order to avoid toxicity. Levels of the tricyclic agents increase when enzyme inhibitors are ingested (cimetidine, fluconazole, fluoxetine, fluvoxamine, paroxetine, phenothiazines, propoxyphene and quinidine). Nefazodone should not be administered with terfenadine (off US market) or astemizole.

## Treatment

### Emergency measures

(1) Observe all patients with a history of ingestion for 6 h regardless if symptoms are present.
(2) Establish airway and maintain respiration and ventilation. Monitor ECG for 24 hours *after* any cardiac rhythm has resolved.
(3) Remove ingested drug by gastric lavage after giving activated charcoal.
(4) Maintain blood pressure by giving IV fluids. Avoid vasoconstrictor agents.
(5) Patients with hypotension, QRS widening or metabolic acidosis may quickly deteriorate into an abnormal cardiac rhythm. Treat acidosis with

sodium bicarbonate because hyperventilation results in a *temporary* respiratory alkalosis.

(6) Control convulsions by giving diazepam, 0.05–1.0 mg/kg IV slowly. Diazepam is currently preferred for initial management of convulsions. Once the patient is intubated and on a ventilator, succinylcholine administration may be used.

(7) Control arrhythmias by giving phenytoin, 0.5 mg/kg/min intravenously. Give a loading dosage of 15–20 mg/kg IV at a rate not to exceed 50 mg/min (1 mg/kg/min in children). The total dosage should not exceed of 5 mg/kg. In children, phenytoin can be administered by intraosseous injection. Never administer by intramuscularly. Maintaining serum pH above 7.40–7.45 by infusing sodium bicarbonate, 2–3 mEq/kg may help prevent arrhythmias. Do NOT give physostigmine, quinidine, procainamide, disopyramide, corticosteroids, propranolol, or atropine. In the past, physostigmine was used to treat TCA poisoning; however, it may induce arrhythmias, exacerbate hypotension or cause seizures.

### General measures

Osmotic diuresis and dialysis are *not* effective. Treat cardiac arrest.

### Prognosis

Patients have died as late as 72 hours after ingestion of an overdose.

### Drug interactions increasing antidepressant toxicity

Paralytic ileus and central nervous system depression from tricyclic antidepressants is increased by ethanol.

Blood levels of and possible toxicity from tricyclic antidepressants are increased by aspirin, chloramphenicol, haloperidol, chlorpromazine, perphenazine, and diazepam.

The risk of cardiac arrhythmias from tricyclic antidepressants is increased by the presence of levodopa, guanethidine, bethanidine, and debrisoquine and by prior administration of thyroid hormone. The effect of nortriptyline is enhanced by hydrocortisone and perphenazine. Amitriptyline increases absorption of coumarin anticoagulants.

Tricyclic antidepressants are atropine-like and quinidine-like, therefore they potentiate the anticholinergic hypotensive effects of agents with similar pharmacologic effects. Tricyclics alter catecholamine levels in the brain and interact dangerously with monoamine oxidase inhibitors.

If given meperidine, furazolidone, or a monoamine oxidase inhibitor is administered in combination with an antidepressant, increased risk occurs to develop agitation, tremor, pyrexia, and coma.

Monoamine oxidase inhibitors can potentiate anesthetic and pressor agents.

In the presence of monoamine oxidase inhibitors or isoniazid, the amino acid tyramine present in beer, wine, aged cheese, and other fermented foods can cause hypertension. Monoamine oxidase inhibitors enhance the effects of hypoglycemic drugs.

## References

Ayers S, Tobias JD. Bupropion overdose in an adolescent. *Peditr Emerg Care* 2001;17:104

Bennett JA, *et al*. A risk-benefit assessment of pharmacological treatments for panic disorder. *Drug Safety* 1998;18:419

Burda A, *et al*. Nefazadone-induced acute dystonic reactions. *Vet Human Toxicol* 1999;41:321

Girault C, *et al*. Syndrome of inappropriate secretion of antidiuretic hormone in two elderly women with elevated serum fluoxetine. *J Toxicol Clin Toxicol* 1996;35:93

Graudins A, *et al*. Fluoxetine-induced cardiotoxicity with response to bicarbonate therapy. *Am J Emerg Med* 1997;15:501

Harrigan RA, Brady WJ. ECG abnormalities in tricyclic antidepressant ingestion. *Am J Emerg Med* 1999;17:387

Henry JA. Epidemiology and relative toxicity of antidepressant drugs in overdose. *Drug Safety* 1997;16:374

Iwersen S, Schmoldt A. Three suicide attempts with meclobemide. *J Toxicol Clin Toxicol* 1996;34:223. (MAO-A)

Klein-Schwartz W, Anderson B. Analysis of sertraline-only overdoses. *Am J Emerg Med* 1996;14:456

McFee RB, *et al*. A nationwide survey of the management of unintentional – lowdose tricyclic antidepressant ingestions involving asymptomatic children. *J Toxicol Clin Toxicol* 2000;38:15

Paris PA, Saucier JR. ECG conduction delays associated with massive bupropion overdose. *J Toxicol Clin Toxicol* 1998;36:595.

Partridge SJ, *et al*. A depressed myocardium. *J Toxicol Clin Toxicol* 2000;38:453. (venlafaxine, paroxetine)

Personne M, *et al*. Citalopram overdose – review of cases treated in Swedish hospitals. *J Toxicol Clin Toxicol* 1996;35:237

Spigset O. Adverse reactions of selective serotonin reuptake inhibitors. *Drug Safety* 1999;20:277

Taboulet P, *et al*. Cardiovascular repercussions of seizures during cyclic antidepressant poisoning. *J Toxicol Clin Toxicol* 1995;33:205

## SELECTIVE SEROTONIN REUPTAKE INHIBITORS (SSRIs)

Citalopram (Celexa), fluoxetine (Prozac), fluvoxamine (Luvox), paroxetine (Paxil), and sertraline (Zoloft) are used in the treatment of depression, senile dementia, obsessive–compulsive disorders, and in nicotine and alcohol addiction.

In one series, SSRIs were at least partially implicated as follows: fluoxetine, 60 deaths; fluvoxamine, 5 deaths; sertraline, 75 deaths; paroxetine, 28 deaths. In this series the lowest blood concentrations of drug resulting in death were as follows: fluoxetine, 0.63 mg/l; paroxetine, 0.4 mg/l; sertraline, 1.5 mg/l. Patients have survived overdoses as follows: citalopram, 5200 mg; fluoxetine, 300 mg; fluvoxamine, 9000 mg; paroxetine, 850 mg; sertraline, 8400 mg.

These drugs inhibit the reuptake of serotonin (5-hydroxytryptamine) and toxicity is the result of excessive stimulation of serotonin receptors. They increase the risk of arrhythmias and convulsions when used with other drugs.

### Clinical findings

The principal manifestations of poisoning with these drugs are cognitive changes (agitation, confusion, coma, delirium, hallucinations, headache, insomnia), autonomic dysfunction (arrhythmias, diaphoresis, diarrhea, hypertension, hyperthermia, mydriasis, nausea and vomiting, shivering) and neuromuscular abnormalities (ataxia, convulsions, hyperreflexia and clonus, nystagmus, tremor, rhabdomyolysis).

*Acute poisoning*

Serotonin syndrome is characterized by the symptoms listed above. Rhabdomyolysis and kidney failure can follow hypoxia and seizures.

*Chronic poisoning*

Memory loss, dyspnea, insomnia, ECG changes, rash, water retention with hyponatremia, impotence. Altered liver function has been associated with fluvoxamine. Possible increased risk of falling, especially in elderly patients.

*Laboratory findings*

The ECG may reveal widened QRS and prolonged QT interval. Serum creatine kinase and liver enzymes may be elevated.

**Prevention**

These drugs should not be used in conjunction with monoamine oxidase inhibitors. Use cautiously with other agents having a stimulant or MAOI effects (St. John's wort). If a change from one type of drug to another is contemplated at least 4 weeks must elapse between the administration of the two drugs.

**Treatment**

(1) Observe all patients with a history of ingestion for 6 h.
(2) Establish airway, maintain respiration and ventilation. Monitor ECG until the patient is free of arrhythmias for 24 h.
(3) Remove ingested drug by gastric lavage after giving activated charcoal (see pp. 31–32).
(4) Avoid vasoconstrictor agents.
(5) Control convulsions by giving diazepam, 0.05–1.0 mg/kg slowly intravenously.
(6) If serotonin syndrome is suspected, give cyproheptadine, 0.1 mg/kg, maximum dose, 0.25 mg/kg/day.

**Prognosis**

Fatalities are rare.

## References

Barbey JT, Roose SP. SSRI safety in overdose. *J Clin Psychiatry* 1998;59(Suppl 15):42

Brendel DH, *et al*. Massive sertraline overdose. *Ann Emerg Med* 2000;36:524

Edwards JG, Anderson I. Systematic review and guide to selection of selective serotonin reuptake inhibitors. *Drugs* 1999;57:507

Girault C, *et al*. Syndrome of inappropriate secretion of antidiuretic hormone in two elderly women with elevated serum fluoxetine. *J Toxicol Clin Toxicol* 1996;35:93

Goeringer KE, *et al*. Postmortem forensic toxicology of selective serotonin reuptake inhibitors: review of pharmacology and report of 168 cases. *J Foren Sci* 2000;45:633

Graudins A, *et al*. Fluoxetine-induced cardiotoxicity with response to bicarbonate therapy. *Am J Emerg Med* 1997;15:501

Graudins A, *et al*. Treatment of the serotonin syndrome with cyproheptadine. *J Emerg Med* 1998;16:615

Horowitz BZ, Mullins ME. Cyproheptadine for serotonin syndrome in an accidental pediatric sertraline ingestion. *Pediatr Emerg Care* 1999;15:325

Klein-Schwartz W, Anderson B. Analysis of sertraline-only overdoses. *Am J Emerg Med* 1996;14:456

Partridge SJ, *et al*. A depressed myocardium. *J Toxicol Clin Toxicol* 2000;38:453 (venlafaxine, paroxetine)

Personne M, *et al*. Citalopram overdose – review of cases treated in Swedish hospitals. *J Toxicol Clin Toxicol* 1996;35:237

Rothenhaeusler HB, *et al*. Suicide attempt by pure citalopram overdose causing long-lasting severe sinus bradycardia, hypotension and syncopes: successful therapy with a temporary pacemaker. *Pharmacopsychiatry* 2000;33:150

Sleeper R, *et al*. Psychotropic drugs and falls: new evidence pertaining to serotonin reuptake inhibitors. *Pharmacotherapy* 2000;20:308

Spigset O. Adverse reactions of selective serotonin reuptake inhibitors. *Drug Safety* 1999;20:277

## ANTIMANIC AGENTS – LITHIUM

Lithium carbonate is used to treat acute mania and depression as well as for prophylaxic treatment for patients with recurrent affective disorders. Non-psychiatric uses include cluster headaches. Other drugs used as mood stabilizers include carbamazepine, valproate (see anticonvulsants, and verapamil. Lithium is excreted by the kidney. It is teratogenic.

## Clinical findings

### Acute poisoning

Symptoms of toxicity occur at serum levels over 2 mEq/l. Acute toxicity can occur from (1) overdose, (2) too large of dose given to someone with renal dysfunction, or (3) giving the drug to someone who is sodium depleted (fever, low-salt diet, diuretic use). Mild symptoms include lethargy, fine tremors, anorexia, sedation, nausea, vomiting and diarrhea. Severe intoxication causes impaired consciousness, hyperreflexia, fasciculations, myoclonic and choreoathetoid movements, ataxia, seizures, and coma. ECG abnormalities are rarely seen.

### Chronic poisoning

Symptoms and signs include: diarrhea, bloating and abdominal pain, nausea, weight gain, acne, hypothyroidism, muscle weakness, tremor, cognitive complaints, renal tubular dysfunction, polyuria, polydipsia, (diabetes insipidus), nephrotic syndrome, thrombocytosis, leukocytosis without left shift. Serum levels greater than 1.5 mEq/l are associated with neurotoxicity.

### Laboratory findings

Large urine volumes are observed. To avoid acute toxicity, serum lithium levels can be measured. Because chronic ingestion can cause hypothyroidism, thyroid stimulating hormone (THS) is measured to detect any change in thyroid function. Lithium can raise serum calcium and parathyroid hormone levels and decrease serum phosphorous, yet most changes in serum calcium are without clinical significance. Platelet and white blood counts are often increased.

## Treatment

### Emergency measures

Begin treatment with respiratory support if indicated and intravenous access. Clinical data indicates activated charcoal is of value in treating lithium toxicity. However, in the case of intentional overdose other drugs are often ingested, therefore activated charcoal is given under these circumstances.

Sodium polystyrene given by repeated oral route may useful in lowering lithium serum levels. Saline diuresis (150–300 cc/h IV of 0.9% sodium chloride) may enhance lithium excretion if total body sodium load is low. Osmotic diuresis with mannitol increases lithium clearance by 30–60%, but because it may cause dehydration, it is not recommended. In severe cases, such as when the level is >4 mEq/l, the patient is comatose or is exhibiting significant neurologic findings, hemodialysis is indicated.

## References

Favin FD, *et al.* In vitro study of lithium carbonate adsorption by activated charcoal. *J Toxicol Clin Toxicol* 1988;256:443–50

Roberge RJ, *et al.* Use of sodium polystyrene in a lithium overdose. *Ann Emerg Med* 1993;22:1911–15

Vestergaard P, *et al.* Clinically significant side effects of lithium treatment: a survey of 237 patients in long-term treatment. *Acta Psychiatr Scand* 1980;62: 193–200

## PHENCYCLIDINE

Phencyclidine (PCP) is one of the most common 'recreational' drugs (angel dust, peace pill, hog, goon, krystal, animal tranquilizer). It is available under a variety of 'street names'. It can be smoked, snorted, ingested, or injected. The fatal dose is about 1 mg/kg in adults. Children are more susceptible. Several deaths have occurred. Phencyclidine is related to the dissociative anesthetic ketamine. It has both excitatory and depressant effects. Symptoms may persist for several days, with a cyclic course that is a result of excretion and reabsorption from the intestine. Pathologic findings are non-specific.

### Clinical findings

The principal manifestations of phencyclidine poisoning are sympathomimetic excess manifested by psychosis, convulsions, and respiratory depression.

### *Acute poisoning*

Doses <5 mg in adults cause hyperactivity, euphoria, rigidity, peripheral anesthesia, nystagmus, incoordination, and wild movements. Doses of 5–10 mg cause hallucinations, stupor or coma, fever, muscle rigidity, and salivation. Doses over 10 mg cause hypertension, convulsions, decreased or absent reflexes, laryngeal stridor, respiratory depression, hyperthermia, and sweating. Death occurs from hyperthermia, acute rhabdomyolysis, or from dangerous behavior while intoxicated.

### Laboratory findings

Urinalysis dipstick reveals myoglobinuria. Qualitative urine screen detects PCP. Serum CPK may be increased. At dosages above 10 mg, the EEG reveals a slowed delta rhythm and rhythmic to dysrrhythmic theta activity. Fatalities have occurred at drug blood levels above 2 µg/ml. Increased BUN/serum creatinine indicate renal failure.

## Treatment

### Emergency measures

In the presence of respiratory difficulty, intubate and ventilate with oxygen. Remove drug by gastric lavage. Activated charcoal is useful (see pp. 31–32), and, if indicated, saline cathartic (30 ml of Fleet's Phospho-Soda diluted to 200 ml) is used after charcoal.

### General measures

(1) Monitor vital signs including temperature, prevent injuries, and restrict sensory input. Resume gastric suction one hour after the administration of any oral drug.

(2) Intubate and give oxygen to patients with coma, convulsions, or respiratory depression. Control convulsions by giving diazepam, 2–5 mg slowly intravenously (or lorazepam/ midazolam). Repeat every 30 min as necessary.

(3) In the presence of myoglobinuria, maintain urine volume with intravenous fluids and mannitol. Alkalinization of the urine with sodium bicarbonate will minimize deposition of myoglobin in the kidney. Although urinary acidification increases the urinary concentration of PCP, there is no evidence that this enhances systemic elimination and acidification aggravates myoglobinuric renal failure.

**Prognosis**

Patients ordinarily recover consciousness in 24–48 h, but a week may be necessary for complete recovery.

**References**

Deutsch SI, *et al.* Neurodevelopmental consequences of early exposure to phencyclidine andrelated drugs. *Clin Neuropharm* 1998;21:320

Mvula MM, *et al.* Relationship of phencyclidine and pregnancy outcome. *J Reprod Med* 1999;44:1021

Rumack BH. Phencyclidine overdose: an overview. *Ann Emerg Med* 9:595, 1980

## PSYCHOTOMIMETIC AGENTS

Psychotomimetic agents can be classified as follows:

(1)   LSD (lysergic acid diethylamide): semi-synthetic, from ergot.

(2)   DMT (dimethyltryptamine): Synthetic and from a South American plant (*Piptadenia peregrina*).

(3)   DET (diethyltryptamine): synthetic.

(4)   'STP,' DOM (2,5-dimethoxy-4-methylamphetamine): synthetic.

(5)   MDA (methylene dioxyamphetamine): synthetic.

(6)   MDMA, Ecstasy (3,4-methylene dioxymethamphetamine): synthetic.

(7)   GHB, GBL, 1,4-BD (gamma hydroxybutyrate, gamma butyrolactone, 1,4-butanediol): synthetic.

(8)   Psilocybin and psilocin: derivatives of 4-hydroxytryptamin: synthetic; also from a mushroom (*Psilocybe mexicana*).

(9)   Bufotenine (dimethyl serotonin): synthetic; also from *Piptadenia peregrine*, *Amanita muscaria*, and the skin of a toad (*Bufo marinus*).

(10)  Ibogaine: from the plant *Tabernanthe iboga*.

(11)  Harmine and harmaline: from plants (*Peganum harmala* and *Banisteria caapi*).

(12)  Ditran: synthetic.

(13)  Marihuana: From the plant C*annabis sativa*.

(14)  Mescal (peyote): from the plant *Lophophora williamsii*. Contains mescaline; also available in synthetic form.

(See also Amphetamine, p. 415)

## Clinical findings

Manifestations requiring medical intervention are hyperexcitability, agitation, ataxia, hypertension or hypotension, convulsions, coma, and prolonged psychotic states. In addition, LSD causes mydriasis, tremor, exaggerated reflexes, fever, psychopathic behavior, increased homicidal or suicidal risk, and prolonged mental dissociation.

## Treatment

Give diazepam, 0.1 mg/kg orally, to control agitation and/or convulsions. In the presence of coma or respiratory difficulty intubate and maintain ventilation. Prevent extubation and aspiration. Administer naloxone, 0.4 mg and repeat up to a total dose of 2 mg to counteract effects of opioids. Give thiamine 100 mg IV. Treat arrhythmias, hypotension, and prevent patient from self-injury.

## PHARMACOKINETICS AND TOXIC CONCENTRATIONS (see p. 100)

| | $pK_a$ | $T_{1/2}$ (h) | $V_d$ (l/kg) | Percentage binding | Toxic concentration ($\mu$g/ml) |
|---|---|---|---|---|---|
| Amitriptyline | 9.4 | 32–40 | | 83–96 | 1 |
| Caffeine | | 3 | | | 15, 80[†] |
| Desipramine | 9.5 | 12–54 | 22–59 | 73–92 | 1 |
| Fluoxetine | | | | | 2[†] |
| Imipramine | 9.5 | 8–16 | 20–40 | 75–96 | 1 |
| LSD | | | | | 0.002, 0.005[†] |
| Maprotiline | | | | | 0.3, 1[†] |
| MDA | | | | | 1.5 , 6[†] |
| MDMA (Ecstasy) | | | | | 0.5, 0.42[†] |
| Nortriptyline | 9.7 | 15–90 | 20–57 | 90–94 | 1 |
| Phencyclidine | 8.6–9.4 | 48–168 | 6 | | 0.02, 0.3[†] |
| THC | | | | | 0.002[†] |
| Theophylline | 8.75 | 3–7 | 0.33, 0.74* | 15 | 15, 45[†] |

*For children; [†]fatal

# References

Brust JCM. Other agents: phencyclidine, marijuana, hallucinogens, inhalants, and anticholinergics. *Neurol Clin* 1993;11:555

Chin RL, *et al*. Clinical course of gamma-hydroxybutyrate overdose. *Ann Emerg Med* 1998;31:716

Craig K, *et al*. Severe gamma-hydroxybutyrate withdrawal: a case report and literature review. *J Emerg Med* 2000;18:65

Garbino J, *et al*. Ecstasy ingestion and fulminant hepatic failure: liver transplantation to be considered as a last therapeutic option. *Vet Human Toxicol* 2001;43: 99

Li J, *et al*. A tale of novel intoxication: a review of the effects of gamma-hydroxybutyric acid with recommendations for management. *Ann Emerg Med* 1998;31:729

Li J, *et al*. A tale of novel intoxication: seven cases of gamma-hydroxybutyric acid overdose. *Ann Emerg Med* 1998;31:723

Louagie HK, *et al*. A sudden awakening from a near coma after combined intake of gamma-hydroxybutyric acid (GHB) and ethanol. *J Toxicol Clin Toxicol* 1996;35:591

Malav M. Unintentional methamphetamine intoxication. *J Emerg Nursing* 2001;27:13

Mueller PD, Korey WS. Death by "Ecstasy": the serotonin syndrome? *Ann Emerg Med* 1998;32:377

Okun MS, *et al*. GHB toxicity: what you need to know. *Emerg Med* 2000(Dec); 32(12):10

Over JE, *et al*. Gamma-hydroxybutyrate withdrawal syndrome. *Ann Emerg Med* 2001;37:147

Ramcharan S, *et al*. Survival after massive ecstasy overdose. *J Toxicol Clin Toxicol* 1998;36:727. (3,4-methylenedioxymethamphetamine)

Sanchez-Ramos JR. Psychostimulants. *Neurol Clin* 1993;11:535

Solowij N. *Cannabis and Cognitive Functioning*. CRC Press, 1998

Tunnicliff G. Sites of action of gamma-hydroxybutyrate (GHB) – a neuroactive drug with abuse potential. *Clin Toxicol* 1997;35:581

Walter FG, *et al*. Marijuana and hyperthermia. *J Toxicol Clin Toxicol* 1996;34:217

# 29  Irritants and rubefacients*

## CANTHARIDIN

Cantharidin, the most important active principle of *Cantharis vesicatoria* (Spanish fly), is used as a skin irritant or vesicant and has an undeserved reputation as an aphrodisiac. The fatal dose may be as small as 10 mg. Cantharidin is an extremely potent irritant to all cells and tissues. The pathologic findings are necrosis of the esophageal and gastric mucosa and intense congestion of the genitourinary tract, with free blood in the renal pelves, ureters, and bladder. The cells of the renal tubules are damaged. Hemorrhagic changes are also found in the ovaries.

### Clinical findings

The principal manifestations of cantharidin poisoning are vomiting and collapse.

*Acute poisoning* (from ingestion or application to skin or mucous membranes)

Severe irritation of skin or mucous membranes with formation of bullae, abdominal pain, nausea, diarrhea, vomiting of blood, severe fall in blood pressure, hematuria, uremia, coma, and death in respiratory failure.

*Chronic poisoning*

Repeated small amounts may cause the findings described for acute poisoning.

*Laboratory findings*

Microscopic or gross hematuria, erythrocytosis, leukocytosis, and hemoglobinemia.

---

*See also Table 29.1

**Prevention**

As cantharidin has no use that cannot be achieved by less dangerous substances, it should not be prescribed or sold for any purpose.

**Treatment**

Remove swallowed poison by gastric lavage or emesis with activated charcoal (see pp. 31–32). Treat cardiovascular collapse and shock by blood transfusions and intravenous administration of saline (see p. 57). Prevent renal damage by maintaining maximal diuresis with intravenous fluids, mannitol, and diuretics.

**Prognosis**

If the patient is asymptomatic at the end of 72 hours recovery is likely. Death may occur, however, up to 1 week after poisoning.

## METAL SALTS: ALUMINUM, COPPER, TIN, NICKEL, AND ZINC SALTS

Salts of metals are used as astringents, deodorants, and antiseptics. The most used salts are copper sulfate ($CuSO_4$), zinc sulfate ($ZnSO_4$), aluminum acetate ($[CH_3COO]_3Al$), aluminum subacetate ($[CH_3COO]_2AlOH$), stannous chloride ($SnCl_2$), nickel ammonium sulfate ($NiSO_4[NH_4]_2SO_4$), potassium alum ($KAl[SO_4]_2$), aluminum chloride ($AlCl_3$), and ammonium alum ($NH_4Al[SO_4]_2$). Soluble salts with similar toxicities are formed by the action of acids on galvanized or copper-lined utensils. These salts are all water-soluble. Their precipitating effect on proteins forms the basis of their astringent and antiseptic effects. Zinc oxide, which is insoluble, has no acute toxicity. The exposure limit for these salts is $2\,mg/m^3$. Zinc acetate (Galzin) is used to reduce the absorption of copper in the treatment of Wilson's disease.

Fatalities have been reported following the ingestion of 10 g of zinc or copper sulfate. Copper sulfate poisoning is a leading cause of death in some parts of the third world. It is used orally as an emetic and as 'cleansing agent' in religious ceremonies. It has been found in children's 'toy chemistry sets' to grow crystals. Acidic water can leach copper from pipes and one outbreak of poisoning has been reported due to this mechanism of exposure. Copper sulfate is contained in herbicides: the fumes cause 'vineyard sprayer's lung'. No fatalities from aluminum salts have been reported in recent years, but excessive aluminum loading can occur as a result of dialysis, intravenous therapy, or administration of aluminum hydroxide in the presence of renal impairment. The pathologic findings in deaths from astringent salts include hemorrhagic gastroenteritis and kidney and liver damage.

**Clinical findings**

The principal manifestations of poisoning with metal salts are vomiting and collapse. The vomitus is often green or blue, however other body secretions (urine) are not colored as they would be if methylene blue had been ingested. This finding can help differentiate between ingestion of these two chemicals.

*Acute poisoning* (from ingestion)

Burning pain in the mouth and throat, vomiting, water or bloody diarrhea, tenesmus, retching, hemolysis, hematuria, anuria, liver damage with jaundice, hypotension, collapse, and convulsions. Hyperglycemia – from which the patient subsequently died – has been reported after a dose of zinc sulfate.

*Chronic poisoning*

Repeated application of solutions to the skin may cause erythematous, papular, and granulomatous reactions in susceptible individuals. Lotions containing zirconium are especially likely to produce granulomatous reactions; the amount that must enter the skin to produce such a reaction is extremely small. Copper poisoning has occurred from the application of copper sulfate to extensive areas of burned skin. Inhalation of copper-containing sprays is reported to be associated with an increased incidence of lung cancer and – possibly – hepatic injury. Symptoms of aluminum poisoning include encephalopathy, weakness, osteomalacia, and elevated serum calcium level. Excessive intake of zinc is reported to affect immune responses. Excessive zinc absorption from toys is reported to cause refractory anemia.

## *Laboratory findings*

(1) Urinalysis may reveal hematuria and proteinuria. Urine volume may be reduced.
(2) Blood urea nitrogen and creatinine levels are elevated in the presence of renal damage.

## Prevention

Solutions of astringent salts should be stored safely. Chemistry sets for children should be checked for copper sulfate and adults must supervise the experiments.

## Treatment

### *Emergency measures*

Dilute the poison immediately with water or milk and remove by gastric lavage unless the patient is already vomiting.

### *Antidote*

For copper and zinc poisoning, give calcium disodium edetate orally and intravenously (see p. 88). Penicillamine has been used in copper poisoning, however results of efficacy are conflicting (see p. 94).

### *General measures*

(1) Treat hypotension (see p. 57).
(2) To relieve irritation give milk or starch drinks made by dissolving 10 g of cornstarch or flour in 1 liter of water.
(3) Replace fluids lost by vomiting or diarrhea with 5% dextrose in saline.
(4) Keep the patient warm and quiet.
(5) If vomiting is protracted (after poison has been expelled), then treat with anti-emetic (metoclopramide, ondansetron, etc.).

### *Special problems*

Treat anuria (see p. 66) and liver damage (see p. 76).

**Prognosis**

The patient is likely to recover if symptoms are mild after the first 6 h. In severe poisoning death may occur up to 1 week after ingestion.

## VOLATILE OILS

Volatile or essential oils are colorless liquids consisting of mixtures of saturated or unsaturated cyclic hydrocarbons, ethers, alcohols, esters, and ketones. Natural oil of bitter almonds contains 4% hydrogen cyanide, and artificial oil of bitter almonds contains mandelonitrile (see p. 312). These liquids all evaporate readily at room temperature. Volatile oils or the plants containing them – turpentine, citronella, sassafras, anise, cinnamon, apiol, pepper, clove, pine, absinthe, pennyroyal, savin, rue, tansy, and eucalyptus – are used as skin irritants. Some volatile oils or the plants from which they are derived have undeserved reputations as abortifacients. The plants contain 1–5% of volatile oil.

Ingestion of 15 g of a volatile oil such as turpentine has caused death, although many patients have survived ingestion of much larger doses with minimal symptoms. The exposure limit for turpentine is 100 ppm.

The poisonous effect of volatile oils is to some extent related to volatility, since the less volatile substances are more slowly absorbed. For example pine oil, the less volatile residue after the removal of turpentine, is about one-fifth as poisonous as turpentine. The effects of the less volatile and poorly absorbed volatile oils resemble those of kerosene, and systemic effects are far less pronounced than the local effects resulting from aspiration. Volatile oils irritate all tissues intensely.

The pathologic findings in fatalities from ingestion of volatile oils include renal degenerative changes and intense congestion and edema in the lungs, brain, and gastric mucosa.

### Clinical findings

The principal manifestations of acute poisoning with the volatile oils are vomiting and circulatory collapse. Aspiration causes a pneumonitis like that due to kerosene.

## Symptoms and signs

Symptoms from ingestion are abdominal burning, nausea and vomiting, diarrhea, dysuria, hematuria, unconsciousness, shallow respiration, and convulsions. Inhalation causes dizziness, rapid, shallow breathing, tachycardia, bronchial irritation, and unconsciousness or convulsions. Anuria, pulmonary edema, and bronchial pneumonia may complicate recovery after either type of exposure. An amount of volatile oil capable of inducing abortion is likely also to produce irreversible renal damage.

## Chronic poisoning

No cumulative effects have been reported.

## Laboratory findings

The urine may contain hemoglobin, red blood cells, protein, casts, and reduced sugar. Anemia may be present.

## Prevention

Medications containing turpentine or other volatile oils must be labeled *for external use only*; after use, any remaining medication should be discarded.

A mask capable of absorbing organic vapors may be used for short periods if atmospheres containing high concentrations of volatile oils must be entered.

## Treatment

### Emergency measures

(1) Give 120–240 ml of milk; then remove by gastric lavage or emesis, taking care to prevent aspiration (see pp. 29–32). Follow these procedures by administering 30–60 ml of Fleet's Phospho-Soda diluted 1:4 in water.
(2) Give artificial respiration if necessary.

### General measures

(1) Give milk, 250 ml, as necessary to allay gastric irritation.
(2) Give atropine, 1 mg, to decrease bronchial secretions.

(3) If kidney function is normal give fluids to 3–4 liters daily to maintain maximum urinary output after the danger from pulmonary edema has passed (after the first 24 hours).

(4) Keep the patient warm and quiet.

### Special problems

Treat pulmonary edema (see p. 55) and anuria (see p. 66). Control convulsions (see p. 60).

### Prognosis

If the patient lives for 48 hours complete recovery is likely; laboratory evidence of renal damage may persist for several months.

## ACONITE

Aconite consists of the dried tuberous root of *Aconitum napellus* (monkshood). The most active principle, aconitine, is an alkaloid which stimulates and then depresses myocardium, smooth muscles, skeletal muscles, central nervous system, and peripheral nerves.

Tincture of aconite is used in liniments as a skin irritant. Monkshood or aconite (*Aconitum columbianum* or *A. napellus*) has caused poisoning when eaten in a salad or when mistaken for radishes. Larkspur (*Delphinium* species) has similar toxicity and contains a number of alkaloids, including delphinine and aconitine. All parts of the plants are poisonous. The fatal dose of aconite may be as small as 1 g of the plant, 5 ml of the tincture, or 2 mg of aconitine. Fatalities have been rare in recent years.

### Clinical findings

The principal manifestations of aconite poisoning are low blood pressure and slow respiration.

*Acute poisoning* (from ingestion or absorption through the skin)

Nausea and vomiting; burning followed by numbness and tingling of the mouth, throat, and hands; blurred vision; slow, weak pulse; fall in blood pressure; chest pain; shallow respiration; convulsions; and death due to respira-

**Table 29.1** Miscellaneous irritants*

| Irritant | Clinical findings |
| --- | --- |
| Anthralin (Anthra-derm) | Irritation, desquamation. Avoid in renal disease |
| Arnica | Irritating to skin and mucous membranes |
| Capsicum | Ingestion of more than 30 mg causes vomiting, diarrhea, and pain on urination. Drowsiness and coma can occur |
| Cashew nut oil | Blisters skin, causes vomiting and diarrhea |
| Cocillana | Vomiting, diarrhea, collapse, headache and rhinorrhea |
| Oil of mustard | Blistering and corrosion of skin or gastrointestinal tract. A single drop in the eye has caused blindness |

*Treatment: for ingestion, gastric lavage: for skin contamination, wash in running water for at least 15 min, then apply wet dressings (see p. 83)

tory failure or ventricular fibrillation. In one case cardiac infarction was apparently related to excessive application of aconite liniment over 2 weeks.

### Chronic poisoning

Repeated application or ingestion causes the symptoms described for acute poisoning.

### Laboratory findings

The ECG may reveal changes associated with myocardial infarction.

## Prevention

Any use of tincture of aconite as a liniment should be avoided. Children should be warned against eating wild plants that may be aconite.

## Treatment

### Emergency measures

Delay absorption of ingested aconite by giving activated charcoal, then remove by gastric lavage (see pp. 31–32). Give artificial respiration or $O_2$ as necessary.

### General measures

Keep the patient warm and quiet. Digitalization may counteract cardiac depression. Treat convulsions (see p. 60). Manage cardiac arrhythmias (see pp. 461–464).

### Prognosis

Survival for 24 hours is usually followed by recovery.

### References

Brown L, *et al*. Corneal abrasions associated with pepper spray exposure. *Am J Emerg Med* 2000;18:271

Gulbransen G, Esernio-Jenssen D. Aspiration of black mustard. *J Toxicol Clin Toxicol* 1998;36:591

Karras DJ, *et al*. Poisoning from "Spanish Fly" (cantharidin). *Am J Emerg Med* 1996;14:478

Lewis MR, Kokan L. Zinc gluconate: acute ingestion. *J Toxicol Clin Toxicol* 1998;36:99

Sontz E, Schwieger J. The 'green water' syndrome: copper-induced hemolysis and subsequent acute renal failure as consequence of a religious ritual. *Am J Med* 1995;9:311

Witherell LE, *et al*. Outbreak of acute copper poisoning due to soft drink dispenser (letter). *Am J Pub Health* 1980;70:1115

# 30  Cathartics*

## MAGNESIUM SULFATE AND OTHER MAGNESIUM SALTS

Magnesium sulfate ($MgSO_4$) is a water-soluble salt that is used orally as a cathartic and intravenously as an anticonvulsant and antihypertensive agent in managing toxemia.

The fatal dose of absorbed magnesium ion is approximately 30 mg/kg, an amount that would raise the serum magnesium to the lethal level of 13–15 mEq/l. The fatal dose by oral or rectal administration has been as low as 30 g in the presence of inadequate renal function. Fatalities are rare.

Elevated serum levels of magnesium depress or paralyze nerves and muscles, an action which is antagonized by calcium. Systemic effects are ordinarily absent after ingestion of magnesium sulfate, since the normal kidney is able to remove magnesium ion more rapidly than it can be absorbed from the gastrointestinal tract. However, if renal function is impaired, dangerous serum magnesium levels may be reached.

Pathologic findings in poisoning with magnesium salts are hemorrhagic gastroenteritis and congestion of the lungs.

### Clinical findings

The principal manifestations of acute poisoning with magnesium salts are watery diarrhea and respiratory failure.

#### Acute poisoning

Ingestion of a large quantity of a concentrated solution of magnesium sulfate will cause gastrointestinal irritation, vomiting, abdominal pain, watery or bloody diarrhea, tenesmus, and collapse.

Rectal administration of magnesium sulfate has caused flushing, thirst, coma, respiratory depression, flaccid paralysis, fall in blood pressure, and death. Intravenous administration causes these same symptoms depending on

---

*See also Table 30.1

the rapidity of the injection. Symptoms of restlessness, flushing, and slight fall in blood pressure begin at serum magnesium levels of 4 mEq/l and progress to coma, flaccid paralysis, and failure of respiration at serum magnesium levels of 13–15 mEq/l.

### Chronic poisoning

Long-term use of magnesium-containing antacid (Gelusil) has caused renal failure from precipitation of magnesium ammonium phosphate in the kidney.

### Laboratory findings

Serum magnesium levels should be determined if magnesium poisoning is suspected. Levels above 4 mEq/l indicate dangerous retention of magnesium.

## Prevention

Do not give concentrated magnesium sulfate solutions orally or by enema. Intravenous magnesium sulfate must be given cautiously and with continuous supervision, since the therapeutic margin is small and respiratory paralysis may occur suddenly.

## Treatment

### Emergency measures

Establish airway and maintain respiration. Dilute orally or rectally administered magnesium sulfate by giving tap water. Give artificial respiration if necessary.

### Antidote

Give calcium gluconate, 1 ml of 10% solution per kilogram, slowly intravenously up to a total of 10 ml.

### General measures

Keep the patient warm. If renal function is normal give adequate fluids to allow the removal of magnesium ion. If renal function is impaired, dialysis may be necessary to reduce serum magnesium level.

**Prognosis**

The patient will recover if the initial effect is survived.

**Reference**

Nordt SP, *et al*. Hypermagnesemia following an acute ingestion of Epsom salt in a patient with normal renal function. *J Toxicol Clin Toxicol* 1996;34:735

## CROTON OIL, COLOCYNTH, PODOPHYLLUM, ELATERIN, BRYONIA, AND GAMBOGE

Croton oil is a non-volatile oil obtained from the seeds of *Croton tiglium*. The oil contains about 10% of a resin that is responsible for the effects of the oil. The active principles of colocynth (from *Citrullus colocynthis*), bryonia (from *Bryonia alba*), and elaterin (from the fruit of *Ecballium elaterium*) are mixtures of alkaloids, resins, and glycosides. Podophyllum resin (from *Podophyllum peltatum*, mayapple) and gamboge (from *Garcinia hanburyi*) are gum resins. Podophyllum resin (podofilox, Condilox) is used as a keratolytic.

These drugs are all extremely potent irritants and cathartics. The fatal dose of any may be as low as 1 ml or 1 g, but fatalities have not been reported in recent years. The resinous principles are irritating to all cells and tissues and can be dangerous even when applied to the intact skin. The pathologic findings in fatalities from these drugs include congestion and degenerative changes in the gastrointestinal tract, liver, kidneys, and brain.

**Clinical findings**

The principal manifestations of acute poisoning are vomiting, diarrhea, and collapse. Chronic poisoning does not occur.

*Symptoms and signs* (from ingestion or application to the skin)

Burning pain in the mouth and stomach, tenesmus, vomiting, watery or bloody diarrhea, pallor, collapse, fall in blood pressure, tachycardia, coma, and death.

*Laboratory findings*

Gross or occult blood in the stools; proteinuria and gross or microscopic hematuria.

**Prevention**

All these irritant resinous cathartics are too dangerous for medicinal use and should be abandoned.

**Treatment of acute poisoning**

*Emergency measures*

(1) Delay absorption and reduce gastrointestinal irritation by giving tap water, milk, or liquid petrolatum. Remove by gastric lavage or emesis (see pp. 29–32). These measures are of little use after symptoms occur.
(2) Treat shock (see p. 56).

*General measures*

(1) Give milk, 250 ml, every hour to relieve gastrointestinal irritation.
(2) Maintain hydration by giving fluids orally or intravenously.
(3) Relieve pain with morphine 1–2 mg IV as necessary.
(4) Give atropine, 1 mg every 4 h, to reduce gastrointestinal secretions.

**Prognosis**

Recovery is likely if the patient lives for 48 h.

**Table 30.1** Miscellaneous cathartics*

| Drug | Clinical findings or effects |
|------|------------------------------|
| Mineral oil, liquid petrolatum | Dissolves and prevents the absorption of vitamin A from the intestinal contents; deposition of mineral oil can be found in the lymph glands of chronic users, but a deleterious effect from this deposition has not been noted. Aspiration, with subsequent pulmonary infiltration, has also occurred. Use of mineral oil nose drops has led to pulmonary deposition of mineral oil |
| Aloe, aloin | Purging, gastrointestinal distress, collapse, blood in the stools |
| Senna (ExLax), cascara sagrada | Purging, collapse, blood in the stools |
| Phenolphthalein | Two types of reactions have been reported rarely, characterized by (1) purging, collapse, and fall in blood pressure, or (2) an erythematous, itching skin rash that may progress to persistent ulceration |
| Castor oil (ricinoleic ester) | Self-limited irritation of small intestine |
| Bisacodyl (Dulcolax), Casanthranol | Abdominal cramps, skin rash, prolonged diarrhea |
| Etulos, karaya, methylcellulose, psyllium hydrophilic mucilloid (Metamucil), *Sterculia* gum | If insufficient water is taken these drugs could cause intestinal obstruction |
| Sodium sulfate | Purging, fluid loss, blood in stools, fall in blood pressure, hypernatremia |
| Sodium phosphate | See p. 257 |

*Treatment: reduce dosage or discontinue use

# 31 Endocrine drugs*

## ANTITHYROID DRUGS (see also Iodides, p. 445)

Methimazole (Tapezole) and propylthiouracil are used in the treatment of hyperthyroidism. They act by interfering with the formation of thyroxine by the thyroid gland.

An accurate estimate of the number of fatalities from antithyroid drugs is not possible, but several deaths have been reported from their side-effects. The incidence of leukopenia or agranulocytosis from these drugs may be 0.5–1% of users, but over 90% of these recover.

The antithyroid drugs may depress formation of granulocytes in the bone marrow, apparently as a hypersensitivity reaction. Pathologic findings in deaths from antithyroid drugs include ulcerations in the pharynx and gastro-intestinal tract, bronchial pneumonia, and aplasia of the bone marrow.

### Clinical findings

The principal manifestations of antithyroid drug poisoning are skin rash and leukopenia. Acute poisoning has not been reported.

### *Symptoms and signs* (from ingestion)

Adverse reactions usually appear in the first few weeks of therapy and may consist of skin rash, urticaria, joint pains, fever, sore throat, anorexia, malaise, and agranulocytosis. Toxic neuropathy has been reported in one case after methimazole therapy had been continued for 40 days. The patient suddenly developed difficulty in walking, which progressed rapidly to left foot drop, absent knee and ankle reflexes, and inability to stand. Hypoprothrombinemia with purpura has been reported during propylthiouracil therapy, and hepatic injury has been reported during methimazole and propylthiouracil therapy.

---

*See also Table 31.1

*Laboratory findings*

A complete blood count (cbc) reveals decrease in or absence of granulocytes.

**Prevention**

Patients being started on antithyroid drug therapy should receive a weekly complete blood count for the first month, since the incidence of agranulocytosis or leukopenia appears to be highest in the first few weeks. After this period patients should be warned to discontinue antithyroid drugs and report for examination upon the appearance of fever, sore throat, purpura, malaise, loss of appetite, or other illness.

**Treatment**

*General measures*

(1) Give organism-specific chemotherapy to control concomitant infections during agranulocytosis.
(2) Good oral hygiene should be maintained.
(3) Exposure to infectious diseases should be avoided during the period of leukopenia or agranulocytosis.

*Special problems*

Treat toxic neuropathy by physiotherapy.

**Prognosis**

Only about 1–5% of patients developing leukopenia or agranulocytosis from antithyroid drugs have died; in one patient having a toxic neuropathy during methimazole therapy, leg weakness persisted for over a year.

# CORTICOSTEROIDS: ADRENAL CORTEX HORMONES AND SUBSTITUTES

Cortisone, hydrocortisone, desoxycorticosterone acetate, fludrocortisone, prednisolone, prednisone, triamcinolone, methylprednisolone, other synthetic substitutes, and corticotropin (the adrenal-stimulating hormone of the pituitary) are used in replacement therapy for adrenal insufficiency and in the treatment of many other diseases. Glycyrrhizin, the active principle of licorice, in large doses acts in a manner similar to cortisone.

Fatalities following administration of the adrenal hormones or corticotropin are rare and have occurred as complications of existing disease. Anaphylaxis has followed injection of corticotropin. These hormones cause salt and water retention, electrolyte imbalance, increase in blood volume, negative nitrogen balance, and decrease in resistance to micro-organisms. Pathologic findings in deaths following cortisone, hydrocortisone, or corticotropin administration have not indicated specific organ damage.

**Clinical findings**

The principal manifestations of poisoning with these drugs are hypertension and edema.

*Acute poisoning* (from injection of corticotropin)

Anaphylaxis with prostration, rigor, weak pulse, loss of consciousness, and death. Other acute reactions have not developed, although aggravation of peptic ulcer, edema, hypokalemia, or infection may occur.

*Chronic poisoning*

Hypertension; edema; nervousness; sleeplessness; skin eruptions; depression; cataracts; amenorrhea; alkalosis; euphoria; decrease in pain sensation; psychosis; weakness; deafness; convulsions; hirsutism in women; intestinal perforation in ulcerative colitis; activation of peptic ulcer with bleeding or perforation; modification of immune responses with activation of a tuberculous, fungal, or other infection; increase in severity of diabetes; thrombotic episodes; hypokalemia with muscular weakness progressing to muscle degeneration; acute pancreatitis; rupture of the Achilles tendon; osteoporosis; aseptic bone necrosis; pseudotumor cerebri; and cardiac conduction defect. Repeated intra-articular injection has caused destruction of the joint. Abrupt withdrawal of adrenal cortex hormones may cause symptoms of adrenal cortex deficiency: hypotension, coma, weakness, and tremors. Death from steroid therapy ordinarily results from either acute adrenal insufficiency or gastric ulcer with hemorrhage or perforation. Application of corticosteroids to the eye causes an increase in intraocular pressure. Application of corticosteroids to the skin can cause atrophic changes in the skin, secondary infections, burning, itching, irritation, dryness, folliculitis, hypertrichosis, acne, and pigmentation. Absorption can cause pituitary suppression and potassium depletion.

### *Laboratory findings*

Serum electrolyte studies may indicate hypernatremic, hypokalemic alkalosis.

### Prevention

Use minimal effective doses of corticosteroids or corticotropin. Decrease dosage or discontinue the drug at the first sign of toxicity. If prolonged therapy is needed, serum sodium and potassium levels should be monitored to prevent severe electrolyte imbalance. Restriction of sodium intake and administration of supplementary potassium may be necessary. When treating children increase the dosage gradually.

### Treatment

### *Acute poisoning* (anaphylaxis due to corticotropin)

Emergency measures – Give epinephrine, 1 mg of 1:1000 solution subcutaneously.

### *Chronic poisoning*

(1)  Immediate measures – Reduce dosage of cortisone or related compounds to minimal maintenance dose at the first sign of toxicity.
(2)  General measures – Intestinal perforation will require surgical closure. Treat convulsions (see p. 60).
    Observe caution in the systemic administration of steroids during bacterial or viral infections. Do not use steroids on the eye in such cases.

### Prognosis

Recovery is likely if the patient survives for 24 hours.

## ANTIDIABETES DRUGS

Insulin and a number of synthetic drugs are used to treat diabetes:

(1) *Sulfonylureas*: acetohexamide (Dymelor), chlorpropamide (Diabinese), glimepiride (Amaryl), glipizide (Glucotrol), glyburide (Diabeta, Glynase, Micronase), tolazamide (Tolinase), tolbutamide (Orinase).

(2) *Biguanides*: metformin (Glucophage).

(3) *Alpha-glucosidase inhibitors*: acarbose (Precose), miglitol (Glyset).

(4) *Thiazolidinediones*: pioglitazone (Actos), rosiglitazone (Avandia).

(5) *Meglitinide analog*: repaglinide (Prandin).

Troglitazone has been removed from the USA market due to hepatotoxicity.

### Clinical findings

The principal manifestation of antidiabetes drug poisoning is hypoglycemia.

*Acute poisoning*

Insulin and the sulfonylureas cause hypoglycemia. The other synthetic agents are unlikely to cause hypoglycemia but they may cause nausea, vomiting, and dizziness.

*Chronic poisoning*

Sulfonylureas can cause the following: hypoglycemia, nausea and vomiting, weakness, intolerance to alcohol, skin eruptions, and, rarely, leukopenia, thrombocytopenia, thyroid suppression, hyperlipemia, increased BUN, or gastrointestinal bleeding from ulceration.

Acarbose and miglitol can cause diarrhea and abdominal discomfort. Hepatitis and erythema multiforme have occurred with acarbose. Do not combine acetaminophen with acarbose.

Pioglitazone and rosiglitazone can cause edema with weight gain. Troglitazone and rosiglitazone have caused liver damage.

Metformin causes lactic acidosis and hemolytic anemia. A possible increased risk of cardiovascular disease has been suggested. Gastrointestinal disturbance may occur early during therapy and diarrhea may occur late.

## *Laboratory findings*

Elevated liver transaminases and possibly BUN with acarbose and miglitol. Check liver enzymes frequently during administration of thiazolidinediones.

## Prevention

Avoid sulfonylureas and metformin in alcoholic patients. Do not use any of the synthetic antidiabetes agents in the presence of liver disease, kidney disease, pregnancy, or lactation. Metformin should not be used in the presence of heart disease, vascular disease, or inflammatory diseases.

## Treatment

### *General measures*

Give dextrose; in sulfonylurea hypoglycemia that is refractory to the administration of dextrose, give octreotide, 1 μg/kg SC. Repeat 0.5 μg/kg every 12 h as necessary.

## Prognosis

Hypoglycemia from these agents responds readily to dextrose and octreotide therapy and other symptoms disappear promptly on discontinuing medication.

## References

Ciechanowski K, *et al*. Chlorpropamide toxicity with survival despite 27-day hypoglycemia. *J Toxicol Clin Toxicol* 1999;37:869

Lalau J-D, Race J-M. Lactic acidosis in metformin-treated patients. *Drug Safety* 1999;20:377

McLaughlin SA, *et al*. Octreotide: an antidote for sulfonylurea-induced hypoglycemia. *Ann Emerg Med* 2000;36:133

Quadrani DA, *et al*. Five year retrospective evaluation of sulfonylurea ingestion in children. *J Toxicol Clin Toxicol* 1996;34:267

Spiller HA, *et al*. Multicenter case series of pediatric metformin ingestion. *Ann Pharmacother* 2000;34:1385

Szlatenyi CS, *et al*. Delayed hypoglycemia in a child after ingestion of a single glipizide tablet. *Ann Emerg Med* 1998;31:773

Turner RC, Holman RR. Metformin and risk of cardiovascular disease. *Cardiology* 1999;91:203

## INTERACTIONS (see p. 20)

The hypoglycemic effect of the sulfonylureas (tolbutamide, chlorpropamide) may be increased by ethanol, dicumarol, sulfafenazole, oxyphenbutazone, aspirin, phenylbutazone, and chloramphenicol.

The following drugs reduce the effectiveness of hypoglycemic agents: thiazide diuretics, diazoxide, corticosteroids, oral contraceptives, furosemide, and ethacrynic acid.

Anabolic steroids potentiate vitamin K.

The effect of insulin may be increased by ethanol, propranolol, levodopa, and monoamine oxidase inhibitors.

Phenytoin increases the effects of thyroid drugs.

Methandrostenolone enhances plasma levels of oxyphenbutazone.

One week of adrenal steroid administration can impair pituitary adrenal control for 9–10 months, resulting in marked hypotension during anesthesia or other procedures.

## PHARMACOKINETICS (see p. 100)

| | $pK_a$ | $T_{1/2}$ (h) | $V_d$ (l/kg) | % Binding |
|---|---|---|---|---|
| Acetohexamide | | 3.5–11 | | |
| Chlorpropamide | 4.8 | 24–42 | 0.09–0.27 | 88–96 |
| Cortisone | | 0.5–2 | | |
| Dexamethasone | | 3–4.5 | | 77 |
| Fludrocortisone | | 0.5 | 70–79 | |
| Glibenclamide | 5.3 | 10–16 | 0.3 | 99 |
| Glibornuride | | 5–12 | 0.25 | 97 |
| Glipizide | | 3–7 | 0.16 | 92–99 |
| Hydrocortisone | | 1.5–2 | | >90 |
| Insulin | | 2 | 0.66 | |
| Levothyroxine | | 150 | | |
| Liothyronine | | 35–60 | | >99 |
| Methimazole | | 6–7 | | |
| Methylprednisolone | | 3.5 | 1.5 | |
| Phenformin | | 11 | | 19 |
| Prednisolone | | 2.5–3 | | 90 |
| Propylthiouracil | 7.8 | 2–4 | | |
| Thyroxine | | 80–180 | | >99 |
| Tolazamide | 3.1, 5.7 | 7 | | |
| Tolbutamide | 5.3 | 4–10 | 0.14 | 95–97 |
| Triamcinolone | | >5 | | |

**Table 31.1** Miscellaneous drugs used for endocrine effects*

| Drug | Clinical findings |
| --- | --- |
| Alprostadil (Prostin VR) | Apnea, bradycardia, fever, convulsions, hypothermia, diarrhea |
| Aminoglutethimide (Cytandren) | Skin rash, nausea, anemia, pancytopenia |
| Androgens and anabolic steroids: Danazol, dehydroepi-androsterone (DHEA), fluoxymesterone, nandrolone, oxandrolone, oxymetholone, stanozolol, testosterone | Abnormal liver function tests, salt and water retention, and masculinization, particularly of the female fetus |
| Methyltestosterone (Metandren) | Jaundice from bile stasis, enlarged liver, fatal biliary cirrhosis |
| Becaplermin (Regranex) | Redness, ulceration, infection |
| Calcitonin (Calcimar) | Nausea, vomiting, sensitivity reactions, local inflammation, and facial flushing |
| Carboprost (Hemabate), dinoprostone (Cervidil), latanoprost (Xalatan) | Vomiting, bronchospasm, hypotension, chest pain, abdominal cramps, visual disturbances from local application |
| Clomiphene (Clomid) | Hot flashes, abdominal discomfort, nausea, vomiting, nervous tension and insomnia, headache, and dizziness; contraindicated in liver disease |
| Contraceptives, oral: Desogestrel-ethinyl estradiol, ethynodiol-ethinyl estradiol, levonorgestrel-ethinyl estradiol, norethindrone-ethinyl estradiol, norethindrone-mestranol, norethynodrel-mestranol, norgestrel-ethinyl estradiol, norgestimate-ethinyl estradiol | Nausea, vomiting, fluid retention, jaundice, menstrual irregularities. Thrombophlebitis with episodes of thromboembolic disease, as well as fatal embolism and eye changes (including papilledema, paralysis of eye muscles, and temporary diminution of vision), have occurred in rare cases |
| Cosyntropin (Cortrosyn) | Hypersensitivity |
| Epoetin alfa (Epogen, Procrit) | Hypertension, weakness, local reactions, joint pain |
| Epoprostenol, prostacyclin, Flolan | Flushing, headache, vomiting, fever, slow pulse, muscle pain |

*Continued*

*Table 31.1 (continued)*

| Drug | Clinical findings |
|---|---|
| Estrogens: chlorotrianisene, dienestrol, diethylstilbestrol, estradiol, conjugated estrogens, estropipate, ethinyl estradiol | Headache, nausea and vomiting, and excessive vaginal bleeding; breasts enlarged from inhalation during manufacture or application to skin as hormone cream. Genital abnormalities in male offspring and genital cancer in female offspring of mothers exposed to diethylstilbestrol during pregnancy. Chlorotrianisene has caused alteration in corneal curvature |
| Finasteride (Propecia, Proscar) | Impotence, gynecomastia, anemia, possible liver function abnormalities |
| Follitropins (Gonal-F, Fertinex) | Rash, injection site reactions, GI disturbance, hot flash, calcium loss, menopause symptoms |
| Glucagon | Nausea, vomiting, hypotensive reaction or other sensitivity reaction |
| Gonadorelin (Factrel, Lutrepulse), human chorionic gonadotropin, menotropins | Headache, nausea, abdominal discomfort, flushing, local swelling and pain, possible hypersensitivity reactions |
| Histrelin (Supprelin) | Hypotension, rash, pain, bleeding |
| Human growth hormone (somatropin) | Pain and swelling at injection site, lipodystrophy, muscle pain, headache, hypercalcuria |
| Hydroxyprogesterone | Edema, exacerbation of epilepsy, migraine, asthma |
| Insulin | Hypoglycemia, anaphylaxis |
| Nafarelin (Synarel) | Bone density loss, paresthesias, memory loss, chest pain, rash, muscle pain, headache |
| Norethindrone (Norlutate) | Jaundice and death from liver damage have occurred. Masculinization can be irreversible in the female fetus |
| Oxytocin | Uterine rupture, fetal damage |
| Progestins: progesterone, medroxyprogesterone, hydroxy-progesterone, levonorgestrel, norgestrel | Porphyria, masculinization of the female fetus, embolism, thrombosis |
| Raloxifene (Evista) | Chest pain, fever, muscle pain, cramps |
| Repaglinide (Prandin) | Hypoglycemia, gastrointestinal effects |
| Sermorelin (Geref) | Flushing |

*Continued*

*Table 31.1 (continued)*

| Drug | Clinical findings |
| --- | --- |
| Somatropin | Pain and swelling at injection site, lipodystrophy, muscle pain, headache, hypercalcuria |
| Tamoxifen (Nolvadex) | Menopausal induction, hypercalcemia, edema; teratogenic |
| Thyroid preparations: dextrothyroxine (Choloxin), levothyroxine, liothyronine, liotrix | Increased metabolism, cardiac arrhythmia, myocardial infarction, tachycardia. Potentiates the effect of the coumarin anticoagulants |
| Thyroid | Ingestion of desiccated thyroid, 0.3 g/kg, has caused fever, tachycardia, hypertension, hyperactivity, and cardiovascular collapse; recovery followed |
| Yohimbine (Yocon) | Edema, elevated blood pressure, irritability, tremors, sweating, nausea and vomiting, dizziness |

*Treatment: reduce dosage or discontinue. [†]give glucose and octreotide for hypoglycemia

## References

Cather JC, *et al*. Finasteride – an update and review. *Cutis* 1999;64:167

Cumming RG, Mitchell P. Inhaled corticosteroids and cataract: prevalence, prevention and management. *Drug Safety* 1999;20:77

Hack JB, *et al*. Severe symptoms following a massive intentional L-thyroxine ingestion. *Vet Human Toxicol* 1999;41:323

Kachhi PN, Henderson SO. Priapism after androstenedione intake for athletic performance enhancement. *Ann Emerg Med* 2000;35:391

Kruse JA. Metformin-associated lactic acidosis. *J Emerg Med* 2001;20:267

Lowe CE, *et al*. Upper gastrointestinal toxicity of alendronate. *Am J Gastroenterol* 2000;95:634

Meinhardt W, *et al*. Comparative tolerability and efficacy of treatments for impotence. *Drug Safety* 1999;20:133

Mrvos R, *et al*. Carboprost exposure in a newborn with recovery. *J Toxicol Clin Toxicol* 1999;37:865

Seifert SA, *et al*. Accidental, intravenous infusion of a peanut oil-based medication. *J Toxicol Clin Toxicol* 1998;36:733 (Progesterone)

Sullivan ML, *et al*. Atrial fibrillation and anabolic steroids. *J Emerg Med* 1999;17:851

Zeitoun K, Carr BR. Is there an increased risk of stroke associated with oral contraceptives? *Drug Safety* 1999;20:467

# 32 Miscellaneous therapeutic and diagnostic agents

## DISULFIRAM AND THIOCARBAMATES

Disulfiram (Antabuse) is used in the treatment of alcoholism. It is thought that this drug interferes with the enzymatic breakdown of ethanol at the acetaldehyde level and allows acetaldehyde to accumulate. Another possible explanation is that the toxicity of disulfiram is much greater in the presence of ethanol because ethanol alters the body's ability to detoxify disulfiram. Severe toxic reactions occur at blood acetaldehyde levels greater than 0.5 mg/dl. Fatalities may occur at blood ethanol levels of 1 mg/ml (0.1%) after the ingestion of as little as 0.5–1 g of disulfiram. At least 6 such fatalities have been reported. No fatalities have been reported from the ingestion of disulfiram without the ingestion of ethanol. Disulfiram is not known to increase the toxicity of isopropyl alcohol. Animal experiments indicate that ingestion by an adult of 30 g of disulfiram as a single dose would produce serious toxic effects.

A large number of thiocarbamates and dithiocarbamates (Table 32.1) are used in agriculture and veterinary medicine. These agents probably have toxic effects similar to those of disulfiram, although poisoning has not been reported. The exposure limit for ferbam is 10 mg/m$^3$; for disulfiram, 2 mg/m$^3$; and for thiram, 5 mg/m$^3$.

Disulfiram is absorbed slowly, reaching a peak level 24 h after a single dose. Excretion is slow, only about 50% of the drug in the body being excreted in 1 week. Thus a severe reaction to ethanol may occur several weeks after discontinuation of disulfiram.

The effects of disulfiram on the body have not been studied extensively. Slight effects on the central nervous system have been noted after ordinary doses, but the mechanism of their production is unknown.

The pathologic findings in deaths from disulfiram–ethanol reactions are not characteristic.

---

*See also Tables 32.2, 32.3, 32.4

**Table 32.1** Thiocarbamates and dithiocarbamates

| | Exposure limit (mg/m$^3$) | LD50 (mg/kg) |
|---|---|---|
| Avadex BW, triallate, Far-Go | | 1675 |
| Benthiocarb, Saturn, Bolero | | 560 |
| Butylate, Sutan | | 4650 |
| Cycloate, Ro-Neet, hexylthiocarbam | | 3160 |
| Dimepiperate, yukamate | | 946 |
| Drepamon | | 10 000+ |
| Eptam, EPTC | | 1650 |
| Esprocarb | | 3700 |
| Ferbam | 10 | 17 000 |
| Maneb | | 6750 |
| Metam, Vapam, Sistan, carbam | | 820 |
| Metiram, Polyram | | 10 000+ |
| Nabam | | 400 |
| Pebulate, Tillam | | 1120 |
| Propineb, Antracol | | 8000 |
| Prosulfocarb | | 1820 |
| Pyributicarb | | 5000+ |
| Thiobencarb | | 560 |
| Thiram | 5 | 780 |
| Urbacid | | 100 |
| Vernolate | | 1625 |
| Zineb | | 5200 |
| Ziram | | 1400 |

## Clinical findings

The principal manifestations of ethanol ingestion while under treatment with disulfiram are hypotension and hyperventilation.

### Acute poisoning

(1) From ingestion of ethanol in any form or inhalation of ethanol while under treatment with disulfiram – as little as 10 ml of ethanol can be dangerous.
  (a) Mild symptoms – flushing, sweating, tachycardia, breathlessness, hyperventilation, fall in blood pressure, nausea and vomiting, and drowsiness.
  (b) Severe symptoms – severe fall in blood pressure, cardiac arrhythmias, air hunger, and chest pain or cardiac infarction.

(2) From ingestion of disulfiram, carbamate, or thiocarbamates without ethanol – central nervous system depression, headache, rash, optic or peripheral neuropathy, psychotic behavior. Corrosive injury to mucous membranes is possible. Skin exposure to Vegadex (2-chloroallyl diethyl dithiocarbamate) has caused pain on washing hands in hot or cold water for up to 48 hours. Some of these agents cause convulsions in animals.

*Chronic poisoning* (from ingestion of disulfiram or thiocarbamates)

Fatigue, weakness, impotence, and headache may occur, but these symptoms disappear with continued use. Toxic psychosis, hepatitis, and central nervous system depression have been reported.

### *Laboratory findings*

Blood ethanol levels above 50 mg/dl (0.05%) are extremely dangerous during the administration of disulfiram. Determine AST/ALT levels before and during use of disulfiram to monitor liver function.

### Prevention

The dose of disulfiram should not exceed 0.5 g daily.

Disulfiram–ethanol reactions are extremely dangerous in the presence of heart disease, diabetes mellitus, pregnancy, arteriosclerosis, or hyperthyroidism. Disulfiram should not be given to patients with cirrhosis of the liver or nephritis or to patients taking paraldehyde. Test drinks of ethanol for a patient under disulfiram therapy should not exceed 10 ml.

Do not begin disulfiram therapy until the patient has abstained from drinking ethanol for at least 24 hours.

### Treatment

### *Acute poisoning*

Give artificial respiration and $O_2$, and maintain blood pressure (see p. 57). Administration of ascorbic acid has been reported to ameliorate disulfiram–ethanol reactions; the suggested dose is 0.1–1 g.

*Chronic poisoning*

Mild symptoms tend to disappear on continued use. Neuropsychologic symptoms may require discontinuance of disulfiram therapy.

**Prognosis**

In a patient receiving disulfiram therapy, sudden death may occur up to 24 hours after ingesting ethanol.

## IRON SALTS

Iron for the treatment of anemia is in either the ferrous ($Fe^{2+}$) or the ferric ($Fe^{3+}$) form. Ferric iron is not absorbed as such but must be converted to ferrous iron for absorption.

The dangerous dose of iron can be as small as 30 mg/kg. Ferrous sulfate (hydrous) is 20% iron and ferrous fumarate is 33% iron. At least 30 children have died from ingestion of iron compounds. No significant toxic reactions have occurred after overdoses of any children's-size multiple vitamins containing iron. The toxic effect of iron is due to unbound iron in the serum. Soluble ferric or ferrous iron salts also cause corrosive damage to the stomach and small intestine.

The pathologic findings in fatal cases include pulmonary edema and hemorrhages, dilatation of the heart, and hemorrhagic and necrotic gastroenteritis. Iron pigment may be found in the stomach, liver, lungs, and kidneys. Degenerative changes may be found in the lymph nodes, liver, and kidneys. Venous thromboses are found in the mucosa of the small intestine.

**Clinical findings**

The principal manifestations of poisoning with iron compounds are vomiting, diarrhea, and circulatory collapse.

*Acute poisoning* (from ingestion)

Lethargy, nausea and vomiting, upper abdominal pain, tarry stools, diarrhea, fast and weak pulse, hypotension, dehydration, acidosis, and coma occur within one-half to one hour following ingestion of iron salts. All symptoms may clear in a few hours and the patient may be asymptomatic for 24 hours, after which symptoms return, with cyanosis, pulmonary edema, shock, convulsions, acidosis, anuria, hyperthermia, and death in coma within 24–48 h. Liver necrosis may occur 2 days after ingestion.

Injection of iron–dextran has caused fever, tachycardia, enlargement of lymph nodes, skin rash, back pain, and, in some cases, anaphylactoid reactions.

### Chronic poisoning

Administration of parenteral iron preparations in excess dosage causes exogenous hemosiderosis with damage to the liver and pancreas. Injection of large amounts of iron–dextran complex (Imferon) intramuscularly in experimental animals has caused sarcoma. However, injection of 953 ml of iron–dextran in one patient did not result in sarcoma.

### Laboratory findings

(1) Increased red blood cell count and hemoglobin indicate hemoconcentration.
(2) Stools may contain gross or occult blood.
(3) Serum iron levels above 400–500 μg/dl are a cause for concern; iron levels over 500 μg/dl in a symptomatic patient are an indication for chelation therapy with deferoxamine (see below).
(4) Measurements of iron-binding capacity are not usually helpful.
(5) Iron medications are opaque in X-rays of the abdomen, but an absence of opaque material on X-ray does not exclude the possibility of iron ingestion.

### Prevention

Iron medications must be stored safely. Parenteral iron preparations are contraindicated in hemochromatosis and in the presence of renal or hepatic damage. Slow-release iron tablets are especially hazardous.

### Treatment

### Emergency measures

(1) Establish airway and maintain respiration.

(2) If the serum iron determination will be delayed and the patient has a history of excessive iron ingestion and symptoms more serious than nausea and vomiting, consider giving deferoxamine, 40 mg/kg intravenously (see below).

(3) Draw blood for determination of hemoglobin level, white blood cell count, serum iron level, electrolyte concentrations, and blood typing.

(4) In patients not in shock or coma, induce emesis with syrup of ipecac (see p. 90) if the patient has not vomited. If gastric lavage is performed as well, add sodium bicarbonate, 20 g/l, and leave sodium bicarbonate solution in the stomach.

(5) Start an infusion of isotonic saline or dextrose solution to correct electrolyte disturbances and dehydration.

(6) Order an abdominal X-ray only if large numbers of ferrous sulfate tablets were ingested.

### Antidote

If there are iron tablets visible on X-ray, symptoms or signs of iron poisoning, or pink ('vin rosé') urine with good urine output, give chelation therapy with deferoxamine, 15 mg/kg/h by continuous intravenous infusion to a maximum of 80 mg/kg in each 12-h period. Monitor blood pressure during administration of deferoxamine, and reduce the rate of administration if the blood pressure falls. Single doses should not exceed 1 g and the maximum in 24 h should not exceed 6 g. Deferoxamine is hazardous in patients with severe renal disease or anuria, and dialysis is necessary in such cases. Injected deferoxamine is associated with a high risk and should be reserved for serious poisoning. Continue deferoxamine therapy until the patient is free from symptoms and signs for 24 h.

### General measures

Treat shock (see p. 56) and acidosis (see p. 71). Maintain adequate intravascular volume and tissue perfusion by intravenous therapy. Exchange transfusion has also been used in small infants. Maintain urine output at 1 ml/kg/h. Gastrotomy may be necessary to remove a bolus of iron tablets.

**Prognosis**

If the patient is asymptomatic at the end of 48 hours recovery is likely.

# LITHIUM

Lithium salts (Eskalith, Lithane, Lithobid, Lithonate) are used in the treatment of bipolar affective disorders, depression, alcoholism, schizoaffective disorders, and headaches. Lithium has a narrow therapeutic index and useful plasma levels range between 0.6 and 1.2 mEq/l with toxicity beginning at 1.5 mEq/l. Toxicity includes central and peripheral neurologic effects, cardiac effects, and renal effects. Pathologic findings are cerebellar, olivary, and red nucleus degeneration and interstitial nephritis.

One 300 mg tablet of lithium carbonate supplies 8 mEq of lithium. A single 1800 mg dose (6 tablets) of lithium carbonate will produce a plasma lithium level of 1.4 mEq/l in a 60 kg patient but in acute ingestion clinical signs do not correlate with plasma level.

## Clinical findings

The principal manifestations of poisoning are tremor, ataxia, and convulsions.

### Acute poisoning

Overdose causes nausea, vomiting, tremor, diarrhea, drowsiness, muscular weakness, lack of co-ordination, slurred speech, confusion, hyperthermia, athetotic movements, convulsions, coma, and fall in blood pressure.

### Chronic poisoning

Memory deficits, myocarditis, psychosis, skin eruptions, thyroid enlargement and hypothyroidism, interstitial nephritis, diabetes insipidus, renal failure, and bone marrow depression.

### Laboratory findings

Plasma level should not exceed 1.6 mEq/l. Plasma concentrations and chronic toxicity: 2 mEq/l, hyperreflexia, dysarthria; 2.5 mEq/l, ataxia, confusion, involuntary movements; 3 mEq/l, delirium, coma, seizures.

## Prevention

Lithium is dangerous in the presence of anorexia, diabetes, cirrhosis, congestive heart failure, renal insufficiency, other medications, and restricted sodium intake.

## Treatment

### *Emergency measures*

(1) Remove ingested lithium overdose by ipecac emesis and gastric lavage. Charcoal is useless.
(2) If respiration is depressed or in the presence of convulsions, establish airway and give artificial respiration.
(3) Do bowel irrigation with polyethylene glycol–electrolyte solution especially in presence of sustained-release lithium. Give 25 ml/kg/h orally or by nasogastric tube.
(4) Replace fluid deficit with normal saline or 5% dextrose to maintain normal serum sodium.

### *General measures*

Consider hemodialysis if serum lithium is above 4 mEq/l after chronic administration, above 6 mEq/l after acute overdose, or above 2.5 mEq/l in the presence of renal impairment or serious neurologic symptoms. Hemodialysis can reduce plasma lithium by 1 mEq/l in 4 h.

## Prognosis

In acute poisoning complete recovery is likely. Overdoses during chronic administration are more hazardous.

## References

Dawson AH, Whyte IM. Therapeutic drug monitoring in drug overdose. *Br J Clin Pharmacol* 1999;48:278 (Lithium.)
Gitlin M. Lithium and the kidney. *Drug Safety* 1999;20:231
Kores B, Lader MH. Irreversible lithium neurotoxicity: an overview. *Clin Neuropharmacol* 1997;20:283

Lee DC, Klachko MN. Falsely elevated lithium levels in plasma samples obtained in lithium containing tubes. *J Toxicol Clin Toxicol* 1996;34:467

Mangano WE, *et al.* Pathologic assessment of cerebellar atrophy following acute lithium intoxication. *Clin Neuropathol* 1997;16:30 (level 3.2 mEq/l)

Oakley PW, *et al.* Lithium: thyroid effects and altered renal handling. *J Toxicol Clin Toxicol* 2000;38:333

Sadosty AT, *et al.* The use of lithium levels in the emergency department. *J Emerg Med* 1999;17:887

Scharman EJ. Methods used to decrease lithium absorption or enhance elimination. *J Toxicol Clin Toxicol* 1996;35:601

Timmer RT, Sands JM. Lithium intoxication. *J Am Soc Nephrol* 1999;10:666

**Table 32.2** Miscellaneous drugs and chemicals*

| Agent | Clinical findings |
|-------|-------------------|
| Acetohydroxamic acid (Lithostat) | Headache, depression, nausea and vomiting, diarrhea, hemolytic anemia, alopecia, rash, phlebitis, palpitation |
| Acitretin (Soriatane), adapalene (Differin), alitretinoin (Panretin), etritinate (Tegison), isotretinoin (Accutane) | Birth defects, cheilitis, desquamation, hair loss, fatigue, hypertriglyceridemia, joint and muscle pain, possible depression leading to suicide |
| Adenosine phosphate | Local erythema, rash, flushing, palpitation, anaphylaxis |
| Alendronate (Fosamax), pamidronate (Aredia), risedronate (Actonel), tiludronate (Skelid) | Hypocalcemia, pain, GI ulceration, rash, ECG changes, liver damage, esophageal injury |
| Allopurinol (Zyloprim) | Rash, fever, nausea, vomiting, diarrhea, leukopenia, eosinophilia, reversible liver impairment. The possibility of cataract formation has been suggested |
| Aluminum hydroxide | Delays absorption of drugs |
| p-Aminobenzoic acid (10 g or more daily), octyl dimethyl p-aminobenzoic acid | Nausea, vomiting, acidosis, methemoglobinemia, and sensitivity reactions, including fever and rash, to any quantity |
| Aminocaproic acid (Amicar) | Rash, hypotension, nausea, diarrhea, delirium, thrombotic episodes or cardiac and hepatic necrosis |
| Aminolevulinic acid (Levulan) | Photosensitivity: itching, burning, desquamation |
| Amlexanox (Aphthasol) | Irritation, dermatitis |
| Aprotinin (Trasylol) | Fibrillation, infarction, tachycardia, renal or liver damage |
| Arginine (R-Gen) | Flushing, nausea and vomiting, headache, abdominal pain, decreased platelet count, thrombocytopenia, acrocyanosis, elevated BUN, sensitization |
| Basiliximab (Simulect) | GI upset, neuropathy, hematuria, rash, hypotension |
| Beractant (Survanta), calfactant (Infasurf), poractant (Curosurf) | Bradycardia, apnea, decreased oxygen saturation, pulmonary effects |
| Betaine (Cystadane) | Nausea, vomiting, diarrhea |
| Calcium carbonate | Increased gastric acid secretion |

*Continued*

*Table 32.2 (continued)*

| Agent | Clinical findings |
|-------|-------------------|
| β-Carotene (Solatene) | Diarrhea |
| Cellulose sodium phosphate (Calcibind) | Diarrhea, hyperoxaluria, hypomagnesemia |
| Chenodiol (Chenix) | Elevated serum liver enzyme levels, hepatitis, diarrhea, leukopenia, increased serum cholesterol |
| Cholestyramine (Questran) | Constipation, vitamin K deficiency, rash, mucous membrane irritation, osteoporosis, eosinophilia |
| Chymopapain (Chymodiactin, Diskase) | Hypersensitivity, anaphylaxis, transverse myelitis, rash, back pain |
| Chymotrypsin (Chymar, Cytolav, Enzeon) | Anaphylactic reactions; ulceration, pain, and swelling at injection site |
| Colfosceril (Exosurf) | Apnea, bleeding, bronchial plugging |
| Collagenase (Biozyme-C) | Burning, pain, erythema, hypersensitivity |
| Cromolyn (Intal) | Bronchospasm, laryngeal edema, irritation, rash, dysuria |
| Cyclamate | Diarrhea. A breakdown product found in human urine, cyclohexylamine, has caused chromosome breaks in experimental animals |
| Cyclosporin A | Hypertension, kidney and liver damage |
| Cysteamine (Cystagon) | Hypotension, fever, weakness, rash, encephalopathy |
| Daclizumab (Zenapax) | Hyperglycemia, raised or lowered blood pressure, depression, rash, pain, possible sensitivity reactions |
| Deoxyribonuclease (dornase, Pulmozyme) | Sensitivity reactions |
| Dexpanthenol (Ilopan) | Hypersensitivity reactions, potentiation of parasympathomimetic agents |
| Dexrazoxane (Zinecard) | Myelosuppression, rash, extravasation |
| Digalloyl trioleate | Sensitivity reactions |
| Dimethyl sulfoxide | Irritant, narcotic, convulsant. Visual disturbances. Large IV doses cause kidney and liver damage and hemolysis |

*Continued*

*Table 32.2 (continued)*

| Agent | Clinical findings |
|-------|-------------------|
| Etanercept (Enbrel) | Injection reaction, sensitivity, GI upset, infection |
| Etidronate (Didronel) | Nausea, vomiting, diarrhea, hypocalcemia |
| Fibrinolysin-desoxyribonuclease (Elase) | Skin irritation |
| Folic acid | Sensitivity reactions, rash, bronchospasm, anaphylaxis after injection |
| Fructose | Metabolic acidosis after injection |
| Glatiramer (Copaxone) | Pain, tachycardia, possible sensitivity, rash |
| γ-Globulin | Cardiac arrhythmias, hypotension, fever, renal impairment, sensitivity reactions, including anaphylaxis |
| Guaifenesin | Emesis |
| Hyaluronate (Hyalgan, Synvisc) | Pain, rash, itching, cramps |
| Hyaluronidase (Wydase) | Sensitivity reactions |
| Imiglucerase (Cerezyme), alglucerase (Ceredase) | Hypotension, sensitivity reactions, rash, local reactions |
| Imiquimod (Aldara) | Ulceration, pain |
| Infliximab (Remicade) | Infections, pain, injection reactions, headache |
| Lactulose | Potassium depletion |
| Leflunomide (Arava) | Diarrhea, hypertension, infections, fetal, liver, and kidney damage |
| Levocarnitine (Carnitor) | Hypertension, edema, pain, hypercalcemia |
| Magnesium trisilicate | Silicate urinary stones |
| Masoprocol (Actinex) | Redness, burning, rash, paresthesias, sensitizer |
| Methylene blue | Quadriplegia after intrathecal injection |
| MSG (monosodium glutamate) | Feeling of pressure in head, tightness of face; seizures |
| Montelukast (Singulair), zafirlukast (Accolate) | Fever, rash, GI symptoms, pain, eosinophilia, polyneuropathy |
| Muromonab-CD3 (Orthoclone OKT3) | Fever, dyspnea, pain, tachycardia, pulmonary edema, kidney damage, encephalopathy |

*Continued*

*Table 32.2 (continued)*

| Agent | Clinical findings |
|---|---|
| Mycophenolate (CellCept) | Pain, fever, thrombosis, hypertension, anemia |
| Octreotide (Sandostatin) | Hepatitis, edema, GI disturbances, pain |
| Oprelvelkin (Neumega) | Fever, rash, edema, CNS effects |
| Orlistat (Xenical) | Diarrhea, rash, pain, hypertension, depression |
| Palivizumab (Synagis) | Altered liver function, infections |
| Pancrelipase (Pancrease) | Gastrointestinal distress, hyperuricemia |
| Pegademase (Adagen) | Possible sensitivity |
| Pemirolast (Alamast) | Fever, upper respiratory symptoms, burning |
| Pentosan polysulfate (Emiron) | Rash, diarrhea, altered liver tests, possible bleeding, thrombocytopenia |
| Poison ivy extract, alum-precipitated | Gastrointestinal upset, joint swelling, purpura |
| Protamine sulfate | Hypertension, sensitivity |
| Protein hydrolysates | Brain damage in animals. Sudden death has occurred in those on restricted protein hydrolysate diets, possibly from potassium or magnesium deficiency |
| Renacidin | Injurious to kidney and other organs. Not to be used above the ureterovesical junction |
| Saccharin | 5 g has caused nausea, vomiting, diarrhea |
| Sacrosidase (Sucraid) | Diarrhea, pain |
| Sevelamer (Renagel) | GI effects, changed blood pressure |
| Sildenafil (Viagra) | Flushing, headache, fall in blood pressure |
| Sirolimus (Rapamune) | Rash, hyperlipidemia, raised blood pressure |
| Sodium chloride | In infants excessive amounts cause coma and convulsions that may be persistent owing to vascular injury. Dialysis is lifesaving |
| Sodium polystyrene sulfonate (Kayexalate) | Gastrointestinal upset, fecal impaction, hypokalemia |
| Sucralfate (Carafate) | Gastrointestinal distress, rash, itching |

*Continued*

*Table 32.2 (continued)*

| Agent | Clinical findings |
| --- | --- |
| Tacrolimus (Prograf) | Hypertension, edema, hyperglycemia, kidney injury, paresthesias, hemolysis, angiopathy |
| Tartrazine (FD and C yellow No. 5) | Life-threatening allergic reactions, cross reaction to aspirin |
| Tazarotene (Tazorac) | Irritation |
| Terpin hydrate | Liver injury from excessive use |
| Tazarotene (Tazorac), mequinol (Solage), tretinoin (Retin-A) | Topical: skin or mucous membrane irritation |
| Trientine (Cuprid) | Anemia, pain, lupus erythematosus |
| Trioxsalen (Trisoralen), Methoxsalen | Nausea and epigastric discomfort; possible increased sensitivity to sun or ultraviolet light after overdose |
| Thalidomide | Neuropathy, edema. Not for fertile females |
| Trastuzumab (Herceptin) | Fever, pain, CNS symptoms, upper respiratory symptoms |
| Tromethamine (THAM) | Sloughs from perivascular injection. May depress respiration |
| Ursodiol (Actigall) | Pain, diarrhea, rash |
| Zileuton (Zyflo) | Pain, altered liver enzymes, GI effects |

*Treatment: withdraw drug

**Table 32.3** Natural medicines and dietary additives*

| Agent | Clinical findings |
| --- | --- |
| Black cohosh (*Cimicifuga, Actaea*) | GI effects, bradycardia, convulsions, visual effects |
| Bladderwrack (*Fucus*) | High in Na, I |
| Burdock (*Arctium*) | Sensitizer |
| Chromium picolinate | Trivalent form if ingested in excess causes thrombocytopenia, renal failure and hepatitis |
| Comfrey (*Symphytum*) | Possible liver damage |
| Damiana (*Turnera diffusa*) | Convulsions in excess |
| Dong quai (*Angelica sinensis*) | Photodermatitis, possible carcinogen, mutagen |
| Echinacea | Fever, dizziness, pain, rash, sensitivity, weakness |
| Ephedra (Ma Huang and other diet aids) | Hypertension, palpitations, tachycardia |
| Feverfew (*Tanacetum*) | GI effects, irritation, ulceration, contact dermatitis |
| Gingko | Nausea, vomiting, diarrhea, seizures, rash, bleeding |
| GMB, GLB (gamma hydroxy-butyric acid, gamma butyro-lactone) see Table 23.7 | Coma |
| Golden seal (*Hydrastis*) | GI and cardiac effects, convulsions, local irritation |
| Gotu kola (*Centella asiatica*) | Itching, photosensitivity, raised blood pressure |
| Guarana (*Paullinia cupana*) | GI spasms, vomiting, arrhythmias, caffeine-like effect |
| Hawthorn leaves (*Crataegus*) | GI and cardiac effects, rash, agitation |
| Kava kava (*Piper methysticum*) | GI disturbances, headache, psychomotor difficulties, drowsiness, skin changes |
| Nicotinic acid, nicotinamide | Depressed liver function, activation of peptic ulcer. After IV administration, fall in blood pressure may be severe, and anaphylactic reactions occur rarely |
| St John's wort (*Hypericum*) | Insomnia, mania, neuropathy, sedation, possible serotonin syndrome and photosensitivity |
| Saw palmetto (*Serenoa repens*) | Dizziness, GI effects, possible hepatitis and male sexual dysfunction |
| Uva ursi (*Arctostaphylos*) | GI effects, cyanosis, convulsions, kidney and liver damage |
| Valerian (*Valeriana*) | Headache, tremor, cramps, possible liver damage |

*Continued*

*Table 32.3 (continued)*

| Agent | Clinical findings |
| --- | --- |
| Vitamin A (20–100 times daily requirement) | Painful nodular periosteal swelling, osteoporosis, itching, skin eruptions and ulcerations, anorexia, increased intracranial pressure, irritability, drowsiness, alopecia, liver enlargement (occasionally); and diplopia, papilledema, and other symptoms suggesting brain tumor |
| Vitamin B$_1$ (thiamine) | Drug fever and anaphylaxis after IV administration |
| Vitamin B$_{12}$ (cyanocobalamin) | Sensitivity reactions, gastrointestinal distress, thrombosis, itching, rash |
| Vitamin C | Amounts up to 10 g or more daily may cause diarrhea |
| Vitamin D, calcitriol, calciferol, calcifidiol, calcipotriene (Dovonex), doxercalciferol (Hectorol), ergocalciferol, paricalcitol (Zemplar) (150 000 units or more daily) | Weakness, nausea, vomiting, diarrhea, anemia, and decrease in renal function with polyuria, increase in potassium loss, acidosis, proteinuria, and moderate elevation of blood pressure. Serum calcium and BUN (blood urea nitrogen) are raised. Calcium deposits are seen in the cornea and conjunctiva; less commonly, strabismus, epicanthal folds, papilledema, slow pupillary reaction to light, iritis, and cataract occur. X-rays show metastatic calcification in the kidney, heart, aorta, blood vessels, and skin. Excessive doses during pregnancy are suspected of causing retardation and congenital heart defects in children. Skin application: irritation, peeling. Give disodium edetate orally to increase fecal loss of calcium |
| Vitamin E (α-tocopherol) | Gastrointestinal distress, fatigue, rash, increased serum cholesterol. IV injection in premature infants can cause pulmonary deterioration, thrombocytopenia, liver failure, ascites, kidney damage, sepsis, and necrotizing enterocolitis: these effects may be due to the polysorbate contained in the preparation |
| Vitamin K | Hemolytic anemia, hyperbilirubinemia, icterus, impairment of function and enlargement of liver; deaths in newborn infants from excessive doses. Total dose should not exceed 3 mg of menadiol or 1 mg of menadione. Excessive doses have caused decreased liver function and hypoprothrombinemia in adults |
| Vitamin K$_1$ (phytonadione) | IV administration is hazardous. Deaths have occurred at injection rates greater than 1 mg/min |
| Wild yam (*Dioscorea*) | Emesis in excess |
| Wormwood (*Artemesia absinthum*) | GI disturbances, convulsions, renal damage |

# OXYGEN

$O_2$ therapy is used in the treatment of many medical conditions in which inadequate circulation, $O_2$ transport, or respiration is present or suspected.

$O_2$ concentrations above 40% in the newborn increase the incidence of retrolental fibroplasia. A suggested mechanism is the induction of retinal vasoconstriction. Oxygen therapy is also believed to play a role in infant respiratory distress syndrome.

In adult humans, concentrations over 21% cause damage related to the duration of exposure; 100% $O_2$ causes pulmonary irritation and reduced vital capacity in about 50% of those exposed for 8–24 h. Pure $O_2$ at pressures of 2–3 atmospheres causes almost immediate adverse effects by means of direct central nervous system injury.

## Pathologic findings

### Retrolental fibroplasia

The earliest change is the appearance of new blood vessels in the nerve fiber layer of the retina. Later changes include the spreading of these vessels through the retina into the vitreous humor. Evidence of hemorrhage from these new blood vessels is present, and this is later organized by fibrosis. As this fibrosed tissue contracts, it becomes detached and folded and forms the membrane behind the lens that is called 'retrolental fibroplasia'.

### Pulmonary damage in adults

Administration of $O_2$ in concentrations above 20% at or above atmospheric pressure causes pulmonary damage characterized by capillary congestion, alveolar proteinaceous exudate, intra-alveolar hemorrhage, hyaline membrane, edema, fibroblastic proliferation, and hyperplasia of alveolar cells. Damage is proportionate to the concentration and duration of exposure.

## Clinical findings

The principal manifestations of exposure to elevated $O_2$ concentrations are blindness and pulmonary changes.

### Retrolental fibroplasia

Concentrations of $O_2$ over 40% may cause visible vasoconstriction and even obliteration of retinal vessels in premature infants. Two to 6 weeks after birth, dilatation and tortuosity of the retinal vessels begin to appear. The lesions may progress rapidly to hemorrhages and edema followed by membrane formation through retinal detachment, or they may regress without impairment of vision.

### Pulmonary irritation

$O_2$ concentrations above 60% cause irritation of the respiratory tract, cough, decrease in vital capacity, and substernal distress in a high percentage of subjects when exposure is continued for 24 hours. As the concentration of $O_2$ is increased above 60%, the incidence of symptoms increases rapidly. One patient developed irreversible pulmonary damage after about 16 h of exposure to hyperbaric $O_2$.

### Oxygen poisoning

Inhalation of pure $O_2$ at elevated pressures, such as those that occur during marine diving, causes the rapid development of nervousness, hilarity, impaired judgment, paresthesias, muscular twitching or spasms, unconsciousness, and even convulsions. The latent period prior to the onset of symptoms depends on the pressure: at 3 atmospheres (20 m or 66 feet of sea water), the latent period is about 2 h; at 4 atmospheres (30 m or 100 feet of sea water), it is 30 min. The interval is shortened by exercise.

## Prevention

### Retrolental fibroplasia

Prolonged $O_2$ therapy at concentrations above 40% should be avoided by the use of equipment that allows adequate dilution of $O_2$ with air. Reliable methods include the use of tanks containing 60% nitrogen and 40% oxygen and the use of devices that mix $O_2$ from a high-pressure tank with sufficient air so that the final concentration of $O_2$ is 40%. $O_2$ should be given to premature infants only when it is definitely indicated by cyanosis and respiratory distress. Irregular respiration is not an indication for $O_2$ therapy. When $O_2$ therapy is necessary, use should be based on frequent arterial $O_2$ measurements. The $O_2$ concentration under operating conditions should be tested at least every 30 min by a reliable $O_2$ analyzer.

If proper control of $O_2$ therapy cannot be maintained, the use of $O_2$ for premature infants must be discontinued until reliable control can be instituted.

### Oxygen poisoning

Pure $O_2$ should not be breathed at pressures higher than atmospheric pressure. $O_2$ should not be used for diving equipment or submarine escape equipment unless the partial pressure of $O_2$ can be kept below 200 mmHg.

## Treatment

### Retrolental fibroplasia

No specific treatment is effective.

### Pulmonary irritation

Reduce the concentration of $O_2$ to 60% or less. Interrupt $O_2$ therapy frequently.

### Oxygen poisoning

Reduce the $O_2$ concentration below a partial pressure of 200 mmHg.

## Prognosis

Complete blindness may result in as many as 10% of premature infants who show evidence of retrolental fibroplasia.

## References

Leach RM, *et al*. Hyperbaric oxygen therapy. *BMJ* 1998;317:1140

Phelps DL, *et al*. Supplemental therapeutic oxygen for prethreshold retinopathy of prematurity (STOP-ROP), a randomized, controlled trial. *Pediatrics* 2000; 105:295

Sheridan RL, Shank ES. Hyperbaric oxygen treatment: a brief overview of a controversial topic. *J Trauma* 1999;47:426

**Table 32.4** Diagnostic agents

| Agent | Clinical findings |
|---|---|
| Diatrizoate (Hypaque)*, iocetamic acid (Cholebrine), iodamide (Renovue), iodipamide* (Cholografin), iopanoic acid*, iothalamate (Conray)*, metrizamide (Amipaque), tyropanoate | Reactions include a feeling of generalized warmth, nausea, and vomiting. Other side-effects include flushing of the face and neck, urticaria, fall in blood pressure, hyperpnea, generalized itching and weakness, lacrimation, salivation, edema of the glottis, bouts of coughing, choking sensations, and cyanosis. Although these symptoms usually disappear in 15–30 min, they may progress rapidly and result in death from bronchial constriction or cardiovascular collapse. Prior to injection of a water soluble organic iodine compound, epinephrine, 1:1000, should be prepared in a syringe for injection in case of a reaction. After injecting the first 1 ml of iodine compound, wait 30–60 s to observe any immediate reactions. The rest of the injection should then be given slowly. Doses of contrast media exceeding 3 ml/kg have sometimes caused renal medullary necrosis |
| *p*-Aminohippurate | Nausea, vomiting, sudden warmth |
| Ethiodized oil* | Irritation or sensitivity reactions of skin or mucous membranes |
| Ipodate* | Nausea, vomiting, diarrhea, dysuria, urticaria, headache, increase in serum bilirubin, and, rarely, hypotension |
| Sodium tyropanoate (Bilopaque) | Gastrointestinal upset, allergic skin reactions, laryngotracheal edema |

*For treatment, see p. 447.

# ANTICANCER AGENTS

Overdose with many of the agents listed in Table 32.5 causes leukopenia, granulocytopenia, thrombocytopenia, hypoplasia of all elements of bone marrow, nausea and vomiting, and anorexia.

Treatment of poisoning with these agents consists of discontinuing the drug, giving blood transfusions, and treating bone marrow depression. Treat overdoses of methotrexate by giving leucovorin calcium (folinic acid), 3–6 mg intramuscularly daily. Sodium thiosulfate can be used to antagonize immediately the effects of mechlorethamine.

**Table 32.5** Anticancer agents

| Name | Clinical findings (In addition to those on p. 575) |
| --- | --- |
| Aldesleukin (Proleukin) | Hypotension, infarction, anuria, capillary leakage |
| Altretamine (Hexalen) | Neuropathy |
| Amifostine (Ethyol) | Hypotension, hypocalcemia |
| Anastrozole (Arimidex) | Hypertension, CNS effects |
| Asparaginase (Elspar) | Sensitization, depressed liver function, reductions in clotting factors, elevated BUN, pancreatitis, depression, fever |
| Azathioprine (Imuran) | Mouth lesions, skin rash, fever, alopecia, arthralgia, steatorrhea, jaundice, shock, plasmacytosis, anemia |
| BCG vaccine | Bladder irritation |
| Bexarotene (Targretin) | Altered liver function, rash, CNS effects |
| Bicalutamide (Casodex) | CNS effects, anemia |
| Bleomycin (Blenoxane) | Pulmonary fibrosis with 1% mortality. Fever, chills, vesiculation, hyperpigmentation |
| Busulfan (Myleran) | Depression of erythropoiesis leading to aplastic anemia, diffuse pulmonary fibrosis, precipitation of uric acid in kidney tubules, hemorrhages |
| Capecitabine (Xeloda) | Skin effects, fever |
| Carboplatin (Paraplatin) | Neuropathy |
| Carmustine, lomustine (CeeNu). | Liver function alteration, ataxia, dysarthria, CNS depression, renal damage, pulmonary damage |
| Chlorambucil (Leukeran) | Interstitial pneumonia. Convulsions and coma after administration of 5 mg/kg orally, followed by recovery |
| Cisplatin (Platinol) | Renal damage, hemolysis, tetany |
| Cladribin (Leustatin) | Renal damage, neuropathy |
| Cyclophosphamide (Cytoxan) | Alopecia, myocardial damage, interstitial pneumonitis |
| Cytarabine (Cytosar) | Nausea, vomiting, megaloblastosis |
| Dacarbazine (DTIC-Dome) | Diarrhea |
| Dactinomycin (Cosmegen) | Cheilosis, glossitis, oral ulceration |

*Continued*

*Table 32.5 (continued)*

| Name | Clinical findings (In addition to those on p. 575) |
|------|-----------------------------------------------------|
| Daunorubicin (DaunoXome) | Stomatitis, myocardial damage |
| Denileukin (Ontak) | Respiratory symptoms, edema, hypotension, rash, pain |
| Docetaxel (Taxotere) | Hypersensitivity, hypertension, uremia, neuropathy |
| Doxorubicin (Doxil), epirubicin (Ellence) | Irreversible myocardial toxicity |
| Estramustine (Emcyt) | Edema, embolism, infarction |
| Etoposide (VePesid) | Diarrhea, hypotension, sensitivity reactions, alopecia, fever |
| Exemestane (Aromasin) | CNS effects, pain, fever |
| Fludarabine (Fludara) | Neuropathy, hemolysis |
| Floxuridine, 5-Fluorouracil | Diarrhea, alopecia, dermatitis, hyperpigmentation |
| Fluorescein | Sensitivity reactions |
| Flutamide (Eulexin) | Liver effects |
| Gemcitabine (Gemzar) | Liver and kidney damage, neuropathy |
| Goserelin (Zoladex) | Cardiac and renal effects |
| Hydroxyurea | Maculopapular rash, facial erythema, dysuria, alopecia, fever, drowsiness, disorientation, hallucinations, convulsions, impairment of renal tubular function |
| Idarubicin (Idamycin) | Cardiac effects |
| Ifosfamide (Ifex) | Renal effects |
| Infliximab (Remicade) | CNS effects, infections, pain |
| Interferons | Bleeding, suicidal ideas, respiratory symptoms, psychosis, necrosis of femoral head |
| Irinotecan (Camptosar) | Diarrhea |
| Letrozol (Femara) | Hypercalcemia, fetal damage |
| Leucovorin | Hypersensitivity |
| Leuprolide (Lupron) | Cardiac effects |
| Levamisole (Ergamisol) | Fever, gastrointestinal upset. Fatal at 15 mg/kg |

*Continued*

*Table 32.5 (continued)*

| Name | Clinical findings (In addition to those on p. 575) |
|---|---|
| Megestrol (Megace) | Neuropathy |
| Mechlorethamine (nitrogen mustard, Mustargen) | Thrombosis at site of injection, necrosis following extravascular injections, precipitation of uric acid in kidney tubules |
| Melphalan (Alkeran) | Hypocalcemia, reversible lung damage |
| 6-Mercaptopurine (Purinethiol) | Hepatic necrosis |
| Methotrexate | Anemia, diarrhea, ulcerative stomatitis, melena, dermatitis, alopecia, liver injury. Neurotoxocity after intrathecal injection |
| Mitomycin (Mutamycin) | Alopecia, pulmonary damage |
| Mitoxantrone (Novantrone) | Cardiac effects |
| Nilutamide (Nilandrone) | CNS effects |
| Paclitaxel (Taxol) | Hypersensitivity, hypertension, neuropathy |
| Pegaspargase (Oncaspar) | Hypersensitivity, neuropathy |
| Pentostatin (Nipent) | Renal damage |
| Plicamycin (Mithracin) | Bleeding, fever, abnormal liver function |
| Porfimer (Photofrin) | Pulmonary and cardiac effects, photosensitivity |
| Procarbazine (Matulane) | Myalgia, arthralgia, fever, weakness, dermatitis, alopecia, paresthesias, hallucinations, tremors, convulsions, coma |
| Rituximab (Maxalt) | Pain, fever, CNS effects, neutropenia |
| Sargramostim (Filgrastim) | Fever, hypotension, rash |
| Streptozocin (Zanosar) | Possible liver and kidney damage |
| Temozolomide (Temodar) | Edema, CNS effects |
| Teniposide (Vumon) | Hypersensitivity, hypertension |
| Testolactone (Teslac) | Paresthesias |
| Thioguanine | Jaundice |
| Thiotepa (triethylenethiophosphoramide) | Precipitation of uric acid in kidney tubules |

*Continued*

Table 32.5 (continued)

| Name | Clinical findings (In addition to those on p. 575) |
| --- | --- |
| Topotecan (Hycamtin) | Dyspnea |
| Toremifene (Fareston) | Induced menopause |
| Tretinoin (Vesanoid) | Fever, pulmonary effects, leucocytosis, arrhythmias, edema, cardiac failure |
| Uracil mustard | Rash, alopecia |
| Valrubicin (Valstar) | Local effects |
| Vinblastine (Velban) | Ileus, mental depression, paresthesias, loss of deep reflexes, and even permanent CNS damage |
| Vincristine (Oncovin) | Alopecia, paresthesias, neuritic pain, motor difficulties, loss of tendon reflexes |
| Vinorelbine (Navelbine) | Neuropathy |

## COLCHICINE AND COLCHICUM

Colchicine and colchicum are used in the treatment of gout. The alkaloid colchicine is present in all parts of the meadow saffron (*Colchicum autumnale*). Another alkaloid, demecolcine, has also been isolated from the plant. Tincture of colchicum is made from the seeds.

The fatal dose of colchicine for adults is 20 mg. The fatal dose of tincture of colchicum may be as small as 15 ml. Fatalities occur in about 50% of those seriously poisoned. Colchicine has also caused thrombocytopenia with hemorrhages, leukopenia, or liver damage.

Colchicine is apparently converted in the body to oxydicolchicine, which, in excessive doses, is extremely irritating to all cells. The pathologic findings in fatal cases are congestion and degenerative changes in the gastrointestinal tract and kidneys.

### Clinical findings

The principal manifestations of poisoning with these compounds are vomiting, diarrhea, and collapse.

## Acute poisoning

After 3–6 h, overdose causes burning in the throat, vomiting, watery to bloody diarrhea, abdominal pain, oliguria, fall in blood pressure, anuria, cardiovascular collapse, delirium, convulsions, and muscular weakness with respiratory failure. Sudden death may occur after rapid intravenous administration of 2 mg of colchicine.

## Chronic poisoning

Repeated administration of demecolcine and colchicine sometimes causes pancytopenia, thrombocytopenia with hemorrhages, leukopenia, malabsorption, oliguria, and hepatitis.

## Laboratory findings

Urinalysis may show hematuria, proteinuria, or hemoglobin casts. In demecolcine poisoning all formed elements of the blood are decreased.

## Prevention

Begin gout therapy with doses of colchicine no larger than 0.5 mg, and do not repeat doses oftener than every hour. Discontinue at onset of diarrhea or other toxic manifestations. Keep colchicine away from children. Since effective doses are approximately 80% of toxic doses, cautious use is imperative.

## Treatment

### Emergency measures

(1) Discontinue medication if any symptoms of poisoning occur.
(2) Delay absorption of ingested poison by giving tap water, milk, or activated charcoal and then remove by gastric lavage or emesis (see pp. 31–32).
(3) Treat shock by intravenous administration of saline, and glucose (see p. 56).
(4) Give artificial respiration if muscular weakness is present. Give $O_2$ for cyanosis.

(5) An experimental colchicine antibody has been used in Europe, but it is not available in the USA.

## *General measures*

Admit any patient with suspected colchicine toxicity to an intensive care unit for fluid volume volume replacement and cardiac monitoring.

## Prognosis

If the administration of fractional doses of colchicine is discontinued at the onset of nausea and vomiting, recovery ordinarily occurs. Single doses of 4–8 mg orally or 2 mg intravenously may lead to fatalities in spite of therapy.

## References

Milne ST, Meek PD. Fatal colchicine overdose: report of a case and review of the literature. *Am J Emerg Med* 1998;16:603

Mullins ME, *et al*. Fatal cardiovascular collapse following colchicine ingestion. *J Toxicol Clin Toxicol* 2000;38:51

## INTERACTIONS (see p. 20)

Vitamin K displaces bilirubin from plasma protein binding and drives bilirubin into tissues, with increased brain injury in newborn infants (kernicterus).

Lithium increases the toxicity of haloperidol.

Combination of vinblastine and bleomycin causes Raynaud's disease.

Allopurinol enhances the effects of azathioprine and 6-mercaptopurine.

Sodium restriction and diuretics that induce sodium loss increase the toxicity of lithium.

## PHARMACOKINETICS AND TOXIC CONCENTRATIONS (see p. 100)

| | $pK_a$ | $T_{1/2}$ (h) | $V_d$ (l/kg) | % Binding |
|---|---|---|---|---|
| Allopurinol | 9.4 | 2–30 | | 0–4.5 |
| Azathioprine | | 3 | | 30 |
| Colchicine | 1.7, 12.4 | 0.32 | 2.19 | |
| Cyclophosphamide | | 3–11 | | 0–10 |
| Cytarabine | 4.3 | 1.9–2.6 | | |
| Daunorubicin | | 6–63 | | |
| 5-Fluorouracil | 8.1 | 0.17–0.33 | | |
| Lithium[†] | | 7–35 | 0.4–1.4 | 14 |
| 6-Mercaptopurine | 7.6 | 1.5 | | |
| Methotrexate | 4.3, 5.5 | 3.5, 27 | | 50 |
| Vinblastine | 5.4, 7.4 | 3 | 1.4–1.7 | |
| Vincristine | 5.0, 7.4 | 1.5 | | |

[†]Toxic concentrations lithium; 1 mmol/l

## References

### Disulfiram and thiocarbamates

Chick J. Safety issues concerning the use of disulfiram in treating alcohol dependence. *Drug Safety* 1999;20:427

Saxon AJ, *et al.* Disulfiram use in patients with abnormal liver function test results. *J Clin Psychiatry* 1998;59:313

### Iron salts

Fine JS. Iron poisoning. *Curr Probl Pediatr* 2000;30:71

Howland MA. Risks of parenteral deferoxamine for acute iron poisoning. *J Toxicol Clin Toxicol* 1996;34:491

Palatnick W, Tenenbein M. Leukocytosis, hyperglycemia, vomiting, and positive X-rays are not indicators of severity of iron overdose in adults. *Am J Emerg Med* 1996;14:454

Tenenbein M. Benefits of parenteral deferoxamine for acute iron poisoning. *J Toxicol Clin Toxicol* 1996;34:485

Tran T, *et al.* Intentional iron overdose in pregnancy – management and outcome. *J Emerg Med* 2000;18:225

Wu M-L, *et al.* A fatal case of acute ferric chloride poisoning. *Vet Human Toxicol* 1998;40:31

## Anticancer agents

Gibbon BN, Manthey DE. Pediatric case of accidental oral overdose of methotrexate. *Ann Emerg Med* 1999;34:98

Jaskiewicz K, *et al.* Increased matrix proteins, collagen and transforming growth factor are early markers of hepatotoxicity in patients on long-term methotrexate therapy. *J Toxicol Clin Toxicol* 1996;34:301

Larouche G, *et al.* Corticosteroids and serious cytarabine-induced pulmonary edema. *Pharmacotherapy* 2000;20:1396

Meggs WJ, Hoffman RS. Fatality resulting from intraventricular vincristine administration. *J Toxicol Clin Toxicol* 1998;36:243

## Diagnostic agents

Guharoy R, *et al.* Fatal adverse event secondary to high osmolality agent. *Vet Human Toxicol* 1998;40:285 (Iothalamate)

Mikkonen R, *et al.* Seasonal variation in the occurrence of late adverse skin reactions to iodine-based contrast media. *Acta Radiol* 2000;41:390

Srinivasan R, Dean HA. Thorotrast and the liver – revisited. *J Toxicol Clin Toxicol* 1996;35:199

## Dietary additives, vitamins, natural medicines

Barrett B, *et al.* Assessing the risks and benefits of herbal medicine: an overview of scientific evidence. *Altern Therap* 1999;5(4):40

Boullata JI, Nace AM. Safety issues with herbal medicine. *Pharmacotherapy* 2000;20:257

Cerulli J, *et al.* Chromium picolinate toxicity. *Ann Pharmacother* 1998;32:428

Ernst E, *et al.* Adverse effects profile of the herbal antidepressant St. John's wort (*Hypericum perforatum*). *Eur J Clin Pharmacol* 1998;54:589

Gaster B, Holroyd J. St. John's wort for depression. *Arch Intern Med* 2000;160: 152

Lee DC, Lee GY. the use of pamidronate for hypercalcemia secondary to acute vitamin D intoxication. *J Toxicol Clin Toxicol* 1998;36:719

Sunner S, *et al.* Pediatric gamma hydroxybutyrate intoxication. *Acad Emerg Med* 1997;4:1041

Viera AJ, Yates SW. Toxic ingestion of gamma hydroxybutyric acid. *South Med J* 1999;92:404

## Miscellaneous

Burgess JL, *et al.* Sulfhemoglobinemia after dermal application of DMSO. *Vet Human Toxicol* 1998;40:87

Collins MD, Mao GE. Teratology of retinoids. *Annu Rev Pharm Toxicol* 1999;39: 399

Farrell SE, Epstein SK. Overdose of *Rogaine Extra Strength for Men* topical minoxidil preparation. *J Toxicol Clin Toxicol* 1999;37:781

Gerard JM, Luisiri A. A fatal overdose of arginine hydrochloride. *J Toxicol Clin Toxicol* 1996;35:621

Kloner RA. Cardiovascular risk and sildenafil. *Am J Cardiol* 2000;86(suppl):57F

Mrvos R, *et al.* Tacrolimus (FK 506) overdose: a report of five cases. *J Toxicol Clin Toxicol* 1996;35:395

Pham P-TT, *et al.* Cyclosporine and tacrolimus-associated thrombotic micro-angiopathy. *Am J Kidney Dis* 2000;36:844

Taler SJ, *et al.* Cyclosporin-induced hypertension: incidence, pathogenesis and management. *Drug Safety* 1999;20:437

Valvano MN, Martin TP. Periorbital urticaria and topical fluorescein. *Am J Emerg Med* 1998;16:525

Wechsler ME, *et al.* Churg–Strauss syndrome in patients receiving montelukast as treatment for asthma. *Chest* 2000;117:708

# VI.  Animal and plant hazards

# 33 Reptiles

## SNAKES (Tables 33.1, 33.2, 33.3, and 33.4)

Poisonous snakes occur throughout most parts of the tropical and temperate zones of the world, though they are more numerous in tropical or semitropical areas.

The degree of toxicity resulting from snakebite depends on the potency of the venom, the amount of venom injected, and the size of the person bitten. Table 33.1 shows the smallest dose by intraperitoneal or intravenous injection that kills 50% of a group of experimental mice (LD50) and the amount of dried venom in the venom glands of an adult specimen. The amount of venom injected by the snake may vary from 0 to 75% of the total stored in the gland.

In 1991 there were five deaths from venomous reptile bites in the USA; each year several thousand patients receive antiserum. Worldwide, deaths have been estimated at 30 000–40 000.

### Pathologic physiology

Poisoning may occur from injection or absorption of venom through cuts or scratches.

Snake venoms are complex and include proteins, some of which have enzymatic activity. The effects produced by venoms include neurotoxic effects with sensory, motor, cardiac, and respiratory difficulties; cytotoxic effects on red blood cells, blood vessels, heart muscle, kidneys, and lungs; defects in coagulation; and effects from local release of substances by enzymatic action.

### Pathology

The pathologic findings in nervous tissue include changes in Nissl granules, fragmentation of the reticulum of the nerve cells, opacity of the nuclei, and fragmentation and swelling of the nucleoli. Acute granular degeneration may be seen in the cells of the anterior medulla. Loss of staining characteristics is also present. Other findings are widespread gross and petechial hemorrhages, necrosis and desquamation of the renal tubules, cloudy swelling and granular changes in the cells of other organs, and extensive local hemorrhages at the site of the wound.

**Table 33.1** Venoms of important poisonous snakes

| Snake | Average length of adult (inches) | Approximate yield, dry venom (mg) | LD50 (mg/kg) |
|---|---|---|---|
| **North America:** | | | |
| Rattlesnakes (*Crotalus*) | | | |
|   Eastern diamondback (*Crotalus adamanteus*) | 33–65 | 370–720 | 1.68 |
|   Western diamondback (*Crotalus atrox*) | 30–65 | 175–325 | 3.71 |
|   Timber (*Crotalus horridus horridus*) | 32–54 | 95–150 | 2.63 |
|   Prairie (*Crotalus viridis viridis*) | 32–46 | 25–100 | 1.61 |
|   Great Basin (*Crotalus viridis lutosus*) | 32–46 | 75–150 | 2.20 |
|   Southern Pacific (*Crotalus viridis helleri*) | 30–48 | 75–160 | 1.29 |
|   Red diamond (*Crotalus ruber ruber*) | 30–52 | 125–400 | 3.70 |
|   Mojave (*Crotalus scutulatus*) | 22–40 | 50–90 | 0.21 |
|   Sidewinder (*Crotalus cerastes*) | 18–30 | 18–40 | 4.00 |
| Moccasins (*Agkistrodon*) | | | |
|   Cottonmouth (*Agkistrodon piscivorus*) | 30–50 | 90–148 | 4.00 |
|   Copperhead (*Agkistrodon contortrix*) | 24–36 | 40–72 | 10.50 |
|   Cantil (*Agkistrodon bilineatus*) | 30–42 | 50–95 | 2.40 |
| Coral snakes (*Micrurus*) | | | |
|   Eastern coral snake (*Micrurus fulvius*) | 16–28 | 2–6 | 0.97 |
| **Central and South America:** | | | |
| Rattlesnakes (*Crotalus*) | | | |
|   Cascabel (*Crotalus durissus terrificus*) | 20–48 | 20–40 | 0.30 |
| American lance-headed vipers (*Bothrops*) | | | |
|   Barba amarilla (*Bothrops atrox*) | 46–80 | 70–160 | 3.80 |
| Bushmaster (*Lachesis mutus*) | 70–110 | 280–450 | 5.93 |
| **Asia:** | | | |
| Cobras (*Naja*) | | | |
|   Asian cobra (*Naja naja*) | 45–65 | 170–325 | 0.40 |
| Kraits (*Bungarus*) | | | |
|   Indian krait (*Bungarus caeruleus*) | 36–48 | 8–20 | 0.09 |
| Vipers (*Vipera*) | | | |
|   Russell's viper (*Vipera russellii*) | 40–50 | 130–250 | 0.08 |
| Pit vipers (*Agkistrodon*) | | | |
|   Malayan pit viper (*Agkistrodon rhodostoma*) | 25–35 | 40–60 | 6.20 |

*Continued*

*Table 33.1 (continued)*

| Snake | Average length of adult (inches) | Approximate yield, dry venom (mg) | LD50 (mg/kg) |
|---|---|---|---|
| **Africa**: | | | |
| Vipers | | | |
| Puff Adder (*Bitis arietans*) | 30–48 | 130–200 | 3.68 |
| Saw-scaled viper (*Echis carinatus*) | 16–22 | 20–35 | 2.30 |
| Mambas (*Dendroaspis*) | | | |
| Eastern green mamba (*Dendroaspis augusticeps*) | 50–72 | 60–95 | 0.45 |
| **Australia**: | | | |
| Tiger snake (*Notechis scutatus*) | 30–56 | 30–70 | 0.04 |
| **Europe**: | | | |
| European viper (*Vipera berus*) | 18–24 | 6–18 | 0.55 |
| **Indo Pacific**: | | | |
| Beaked sea snake (*Enhydrina schistosa*) | 30–48 | 7–20 | 0.01 |

*All tables in this chapter are modified from *Poisonous Snakes of the World*. Navmed P-5099. US Department of the Navy, Bureau of Medicine and Surgery, 1968. US Government Printing Office, Washington, DC 20402

**Table 33.2** Symptoms and signs of crotalid bites

| Symptoms and signs | North American rattlesnakes (Crotalus) | Central and South American rattlesnakes (Crotalus) | North American moccasins (Agkistrodon) | American lance-headed vipers (Bothrops) | Asian lance-headed vipers (Trimeresurus) | Malayan pit viper (Agkistrodon) |
|---|---|---|---|---|---|---|
| Swelling and edema | +++ | + | ++ | +++ | +++ | +++ |
| Pain at site of bite | ++ | ++ | + | +++ | ++ | ++ |
| Discoloration of skin | +++ | + | + | +++ | +++ | ++ |
| Vesicles | +++ | | + | +++ | ++ | ++ |
| Ecchymosis | +++ | + | ++ | +++ | +++ | +++ |
| Superficial thrombosis | ++ | | | ++ | | |
| Necrosis | ++ | | + | +++ | + | + |
| Sloughing of tissue | ++ | | | +++ | + | + |
| Lassitude | ++ | +++ | + | ++ | ++ | ++ |
| Thirst | ++ | ++ | + | +++ | + | ++ |
| Nausea or vomiting (or both) | ++ | ++ | + | ++ | | |
| Weak pulse and changes in rate | +++ | +++ | + | +++ | ++ | ++ |
| Hypotension or shock | +++ | + | + | +++ | ++ | ++ |
| Sphering or destruction of red cells | +++ | | | +++ | | |
| Increased bleeding time | ++ | + | | ++ | + | + |
| Increased clotting time | +++ | + | | +++ | ++ | +++ |
| Hemorrhage | +++ | | + | +++ | ++ | ++ |

*Continued*

Table 33.2 (continued)

| Symptoms and signs | North American rattlesnakes (Crotalus) | Central and South American rattlesnakes (Crotalus) | North American moccasins (Agkistrodon) | American lance-headed vipers (Bothrops) | Asian lance-headed vipers (Trimeresurus) | Malayan pit viper (Agkistrodon) |
|---|---|---|---|---|---|---|
| Anemia | ++ | | | ++ | + | + |
| Glycosuria | ++ | | + | ++ | | |
| Proteinuria | ++ | + | + | ++ | + | + |
| Tingling or numbness | ++ | +++ | + | ++ | + | |
| Fasciculations | + | ++ | | + | | |
| Muscular weakness or paralysis | + | +++ | | + | | |
| Ptosis of lids | + | ++ | | + | | |
| Blurring of vision | + | +++ | | + | | |
| Respiratory distress | ++ | +++ | + | ++ | | |
| Swelling of regional lymph nodes | ++ | + | + | ++ | + | |

**Table 33.3** Symptoms and signs of elapid bites

| Symptoms and signs | Cobras (Naja) | Kraits (Bungarus) | Mambas (Dendroaspis) | Taipan (Oxyuranus) | Coral snakes (Micurus) |
|---|---|---|---|---|---|
| Pain at site of bite | ++ | + | + | + | ++ |
| Localized edema | + | | | | + |
| Drowsiness, lassitude | +++ | +++ | ++ | +++ | +++ |
| Feeling of thickened tongue and throat, slurring of speech, difficulty in swallowing | +++ | +++ | +++ | +++ | ++ |
| Ptosis | +++ | +++ | ++ | +++ | ++ |
| Changes in respiration | ++ | +++ | ++ | +++ | ++ |
| Headache | ++ | ++ | ++ | +++ | ++ |
| Blurring of vision | ++ | ++ | +++ | +++ | ++ |
| Weak pulse and changes in rate | ++ | ++ | ++ | + | ++ |
| Hypotension or shock | ++ | +++ | ++ | + | + |
| Excessive salivation | +++ | +++ | +++ | + | +++ |
| Nausea and vomiting | + | ++ | +++ | +++ | + |
| Abdominal pain | + | +++ | +++ | +++ | + |
| Pain in regional lymph nodes | + | ++ | +++ | +++ | + |
| Localized discoloration of skin | ++ | | | | + |
| Localized vesicles | + | | | | |
| Localized necrosis | + | | | | |
| Muscle weakness, paresis, or paralysis | ++ | +++ | ++ | +++ | + |
| Muscle fasciculations | + | + | + | + | + |
| Numbness of affected area | ++ | +++ | + | + | +++ |
| Convulsions | + | + | | | |

**Table 33.4** Symptoms and signs of viperid bites

| Symptoms and signs | Russell's viper (Vipera russellii) | Saw-scaled viper (Echis carinatus) | Levantine viper (Vipera labetina) and related species | European viper (Vipera berus) | Puff adder (Bitis arientans) |
|---|---|---|---|---|---|
| Swelling and edema | +++ | +++ | ++ | ++ | + |
| Pain at site of bite | +++ | +++ | ++ | ++ | +++ |
| Discoloration of skin | +++ | ++ | ++ | ++ | +++ |
| Weakness | ++ | ++ | + | ++ | ++ |
| Nausea or vomiting (or both) | ++ | + | +++ | ++ | ++ |
| Abdominal pain | ++ | + | +++ | + | ++ |
| Diarrhea | ++ | + | +++ | + | ++ |
| Thirst | ++ | +++ | + | ++ | + |
| Chills or fever | ++ | ++ | ++ | | + |
| Swelling of regional lymph nodes | + | + | ++ | ++ | ++ |
| Facial edema | + | | ++ | + | + |
| Dilation of pupils | ++ | + | + | + | + |
| Weak pulse and changes in rate | ++ | + | ++ | + | + |
| Proteinuria | ++ | ++ | ++ | | |
| Hypotension | ++ | ++ | ++ | + | ++ |
| Shock | ++ | ++ | ++ | + | ++ |
| Hemorrhage* | ++ | +++ | ++ | + | ++ |
| Anemia | ++ | ++ | + | | |
| Vesicles | ++ | ++ | ++ | + | ++ |
| Ecchymosis | ++ | ++ | ++ | + | ++ |
| Necrosis | ++ | + | + | | ++ |
| Decreased platelets | + | + | + | | + |
| Prolonged clotting time | +++ | +++ | ++ | | + |

*Usually limited to area of wound in puff adder and European viper bites. However, bleeding from the gums, intestine, and urinary tract may occur, particularly in saw-scaled viper and Russell's viper envenomizations

## Clinical findings

The diagnosis of a poisonous snakebite depends on finding one or more puncture wounds or tooth marks and any one of the following signs of envenomization: local swelling, local pain, ecchymosis, blurring of vision, any evidence of muscular weakness, drowsiness, nausea, vomiting, salivation, or sweating. (See Tables 33.1, 33.2, 33.3, and 33.4.)

### Crotalid envenomization

Swelling, edema, and local pain beginning within 10 min. Discoloration of skin and ecchymosis develop over several hours and progress to petechiae and hemorrhagic vesiculations. Weakness, sweating, faintness, nausea, tender lymph nodes, and tingling or numbness of tongue, mouth, or scalp are common. Hemoglobin, blood volume, and platelets decrease. Cranial nerve paralysis, respiratory difficulty, and sensitivity reactions occur.

### Viperid envenomization

Local pain, swelling, edema, skin discoloration, and ecchymosis occur. Bleeding from the wound and from the gums is common in severe Russell's and saw-scaled viper bites. The blood may fail to clot. Severe poisoning is indicated by swelling extending above the elbows or knees within 2 h or by hemorrhages.

### Elapid envenomization

Cobra bites are characterized by pain within 10 min, but onset of swelling is slow. General symptoms include drowsiness, weakness, excessive salivation, and paralysis of the facial muscles, lips, tongue, and larynx. Blood pressure falls and respiration becomes difficult. Ptosis, blurring of vision, convulsions and headache also occur. The kraits, mambas, and taipan and coral snakes cause less local reaction, but abdominal pain is more intense. Severe poisoning is indicated by neurotoxic signs occurring within 1 h.

### Envenomization by sea snakes

Bites cause little local pain, but there is pain in skeletal muscles, especially during motion. Paresthesias of the tongue and mouth, difficulty with swallowing, trismus, weakness of extraocular muscles, papillary dilation, and ptosis also occur. Myoglobinuria is diagnostic.

## Laboratory findings

The levels of prothrombin, fibrinogen, fibrin products, hematocrit, hemoglobin, and platelets should be determined.

## Prevention

People in snake-infested areas should wear shoes and heavy canvas leggings because more than half of all bites are on the lower parts of the legs.

Snake venom antiserum for snakes of the region should be readily available in areas where snakebites are frequent.

Avoid walking at night or in grass and underbrush. Do not climb rocky ledges without visual inspection. Do not kill snakes unnecessarily; many people are bitten in such attempts.

## Treatment

Treatment of snakebite requires immediate identification, and administration of appropriate antiserum. Bring the dead snake in with the patient, if possible.

### *Emergency measures*

(1) Immobilize the patient and the bitten part in a horizontal position. Wash the bitten area with water to remove surface venom. Avoid any manipulation of the bitten area. Do not allow the patient to walk, run, or take alcoholic beverages or stimulants. Transport the patient without delay to a medical facility for definitive treatment.

(2) If symptoms develop rapidly and antiserum cannot be given, apply constricting bands just proximal and distal to the bite. A $\frac{1}{2} \times 24$ inch thin rubber band or $\frac{1}{8}$-inch-diameter thin-walled gum rubber tubing is satisfactory. (Bands are not helpful if they are applied more than 30 min after the bite or after giving antiserum.) The bands should occlude lymph drainage but not veins or arteries. Move the bands as swelling progresses. The bands should be left in place until antiserum can be given. Be prepared to cope with severe fall in blood pressure when the bands are

released. Remove constricting bands completely 4–8 h after antiserum is given.

(3) Incision through the fang marks by untrained persons as an emergency measure is not advisable; it is too hazardous to underlying structures and at best removes only 20% of the venom.

*Antidote* (check antiserum availability at local poison center)

(1) Give specific antiserum intravenously after testing for serum sensitivity (see below). Since antiserum can be dangerous to life, wait for clear evidence of systemic venom toxicity beyond nausea and vomiting before beginning administration. In coral snake bite, 1–5 vials of antivenom should be given as soon as possible, since the venom is fixed in neural tissues before symptoms occur. If there are any signs of envenomization, give 3–5 vials. The size of the initial dose of *Micrurus fulvius* antiserum depends on the extent of initial pain and the certainty that the bite actually injected venom. Overtreatment is common but preferable. In crotalid envenomization with minimal systemic symptoms and signs, give 3–5 vials of antivenom. If there is progressive swelling, paresthesia around the mouth, or any other systemic symptoms, an initial dose of up to 10 vials may be needed depending on the severity of symptoms. Dilute the initial dose of antiserum with 500 ml of 5% dextrose in saline and start a slow intravenous drip if the patient is not sensitive or has been desensitized. Cardiorespiratory resuscitation measures, including epinephrine, must be available. If no sensitivity reaction occurs in the first 5 min, increase the flow rate in order to inject the total dose in 1 h. If swelling does not progress and paresthesias disappear, give a second 500 ml of saline with 3–5 vials of antiserum over the next 4 h. If swelling progresses and systemic symptoms increase, a total dose of antiserum up to 300 ml in the first 4 h may be necessary. Antiserum is less useful after a delay of 4 h and probably useless after 24 h. A dose of 30 ml or more will ordinarily produce serum reactions.

Serum sensitivity is determined by injecting into the skin (intradermally) 0.02 ml of antiserum diluted 1:100 in 0.9% saline solution with control injection of 0.9% saline for comparison. Examine in 10 min. A positive reaction is indicated by a wheal or swelling surrounded by redness. The test can also be done by placing a drop of diluted antiserum in the conjunctival sac. Congestion, lacrimation, and itching indicate a positive reaction. Apply 1:1000 epinephrine locally to limit the reaction.

If the sensitivity test is positive, desensitize the patient by injecting 0.05 ml of 1:100 dilution subcutaneously. Double the amount injected every 5 min until 1 ml of 1:10 dilution is given; then, if no reaction occurs, begin a slow intravenous drip of 1:50 dilution as above. Reactions are controlled by the repeated injection of epinephrine, 1:1000 solution, and administration of diphenhydramine, 50 mg intravenously, as necessary.

(2) Even in the absence of a skin sensitivity reaction to a test injection, serum sickness occurs in about 30% of patients given 3 vials of antiserum and in more than 90% of those given 6 vials or more.

## *General measures*

(1) Monitor blood pressure, pulse, respiration, central venous pressure, hematocrit, hemoglobin products in urine, and catheterized urine output. Repeat the blood coagulation profile every 4 h as necessary. Measure the circumference of the affected extremity at several places every 15 min to monitor progression of swelling and to determine the need for additional antivenom.

(2) In antiserum reactions, give prednisone, 45–60 mg daily in divided doses, but avoid giving corticosteroids for 24 h after antivenom administration, if possible.

(3) Maintain blood pressure (see p. 57). Central venous pressure should exceed 5 cm of water. Intravenous fluid needs may reach 1 liter/h. If the hemoglobin level falls below 10 g/dl, give packed red blood cells or whole blood to raise the hemoglobin level to 12 g/dl.

(4) If the fibrinogen level is low, give human fibrinogen intravenously. Platelet transfusion may be necessary. Other coagulopathies require replacement with specific factors, fresh whole blood, or plasma. Exchange transfusion should be considered.

(5) For convulsions or respiratory paralysis, give artificial respiration. Respiratory paralysis for up to 10 days is compatible with recovery after elapid envenomization.

(6) Treat renal failure by fluid and electrolyte restriction or hemodialysis.

(7) Give tetanus antitoxin or, if the patient has already been immunized, tetanus toxoid.

(8) For infection in the bitten area, give organism-specific chemotherapy.

(9) Control pain by the use of aspirin or codeine. Avoid depressant narcotics.

## Prognosis

Adequate, early, specific antiserum treatment will reduce the mortality rate from all snakebites below 10%.

## GILA MONSTER

The Gila monster (*Heloderma* species), the only poisonous lizard, lives in desert areas of the south-western USA and northern Mexico. This lizard does not have fangs like many poisonous snakes. Instead, grooves in the front teeth carry the poison. The fatal dose of the venom is not known, but toxicity is presumably comparable to some snake venoms, since severe injury may follow a scratch from the teeth of the Gila monster. The venom causes enzymatic tissue destruction. The pathologic findings are similar to those from rattlesnake bite.

Fatal poisoning is rare, since the lizard is uncommon and is not likely to bite unless handled.

### Clinical findings

Symptoms and signs (from a bite or tooth-scratch from a Gila monster) include nausea and vomiting, local swelling and pain that spreads rapidly, cyanosis, respiratory depression, and weakness. The laboratory findings are not characteristic.

### Treatment

*Emergency measures*

If, in biting, the lizard is tenacious, cut the muscles at the angle of the lizard's jaw to loosen it. Enforce complete inactivity of the victim, as for snakebite (see p. 595).

*Antidote*

No specific antiserum is available.

*General measures*

See p. 597 for the general measures used in the treatment of snakebite.

## Prognosis

The mortality rate is about 1% in adults and about 5% in children.

## References

Bentur Y, *et al*. Delayed administration of *Vipera xanthina palaestinae* antivenin. *J Toxicol Clin Toxicol* 1996;35:257

Bond GR, Burkhart KK. Thrombocytopenia following timber rattlesnake envenomation. *Ann Emerg Med* 1997;30:40

Boyer DM. *Antivenom Index*. American Zoo and Aquarium Association and American Association of Poison Control Centers, 1994 (available through local poison center)

Boyer LV, *et al*. Recurrent and persistent coagulopathy following pit viper envenomation. *Arch Intern Med* 1999;159:706

Britt A, Burkhart K. *Naja naja* bite. *Am J Emerg Med* 1997;15:529

Carroll RR, *et al*. Canebrake rattlesnake envenomation. *Ann Emerg Med* 1997;30:45

Caywood MJ. Near-fatal rattlesnake envenomation. *J Emerg Nursing* 2001;27: 113

Chen J-C, *et al*. Risk of immediate effects from F(ab)$_2$ bivalent antivenin in Taiwan. *Wilderness Env Med* 2000;11:163

Clark RF, *et al*. Successful treatment of crotalid-induced neurotoxicity with a new polyspecific crotalid fab antivenom. *Ann Emerg Med* 1997;30:54

Dart RC, *et al*. Affinity-purified, mixed monospecific crotalid antivenom ovine fab for the treatment of crotalid venom poisoning. *Ann Emerg Med* 1997;30:33

Gibley RL, *et al*. Intravascular hemolysis associated with North American crotalid envenomation. *J Toxicol Clin Toxicol* 1998;36:337

Hawgood BJ. Hugh Alistair Reid OBE MD: Investigation and treatment of snake bite. *Toxicon* 1998;36:431

Jasper EH, *et al*. Venomous snakebites in an urban area: what are the possibilities? *Wilderness Envir Med* 2000;11:168

Keyler DE, Vandevoort JT. Copperhead envenomations: clinical profiles of three different subspecies. *Vet Human Toxicol* 1999;41:149

Kurnik D, *et al.* A snake bite by the burrowing asp, *Atractaspos engaddensis.* *Toxicon* 1999;37:223

Lifshitz M, *et al.* Disseminated intravascular coagulation after *Cerastes vipera* envenomation in a 3-year-old child: a case report. *Toxicon* 2000;38:1593

Moon MD, Galvan TJ. Management of a 36-year-old man with pit viper envenomation. *J Emerg Nursing* 2001;27:108

Moss ST, *et al.* An examination of serial urinalyses in patients with North American crotalid envenomation. *J Toxicol Clin Toxicol* 1998;36:329

Moss ST, *et al.* Association of rattlesnake bite location with severity of clinical manifestations. *Ann Emerg Med* 1997;30:58

Nordt SP. Anaphylactoid reaction to rattlesnake envenomation. *Vet Human Toxicol* 2000;42:12

Rosen PB, *et al.* Delayed antivenom treatment for a patient after envenomation by *Crotalus atrox. Ann Emerg Med* 2000;35:86

Russell FE. When a snake strikes. *Emerg Med* 1990 (Jun 30);22:21

Seifert SA, *et al.* Relationship of venom effects to venom antigen and antivenom serum concentrations in a patient with *Crotalus atrox* envenomation treated with a fab antivenom. *Ann Emerg Med* 1997;30:49

Stipetic ME, *et al.* A retrospective analysis of 96 "asp" (*Megalopyge opercularis*) envenomations in central Texas during 1996. *J Toxicol Clin Toxicol* 1999;37:457

Theakston RDG. An objective approach to antivenom therapy and assessment of first-aid measures in snake bite. *Ann Trop Med Par* 1997;91:857

# 34  Arachnids and insects*

## BLACK WIDOW SPIDER

The black widow spider (*Latrodectus mactans*), also called 'hourglass' spider, may be found throughout the USA and even in Canada but is most numerous in the warmer areas. Other members of the *Latrodectus* genus are common throughout the temperate and tropical zones. These spiders inhabit woodpiles, outhouses, brush piles, and dark corners of barns, garages, and houses. Only the female is dangerous. It is jet black with a globular abdomen that is ordinarily marked with orange or red spots in the shape of an hourglass.

The toxicity of the venom is probably greater than that of the snake venoms, but the spider injects only a minute amount of poison. The bite is ordinarily only dangerous to life in children weighing less than 15 kg. The venom of the black widow spider causes various neurologic effects that have not been completely elucidated. The pathologic findings are not characteristic.

The number of bites is about 500 per year, but the fatality rate is below 1% of those bitten.

### Clinical findings

The principal manifestation of black widow spider bite is immediate muscle spasm. Symptoms and signs consist of slight pain, blanching, and swelling at the site of the bite, progressing rapidly to pain in the chest, abdomen, and joints and to nausea, salivation, and sweating. Breathing later becomes labored, and muscular pain, tightness, and cramping extend throughout the body. The abdominal, chest, or back muscles are rigid, and the patient, in contrast to patients with acute abdominal emergencies, is extremely restless. Recovery begins after 12–24 h and is complete within a week.

---

*See also Tables 34.1 and 34.2

## Prevention

Prevention depends on the destruction of black widow spiders wherever found. The bottoms of outdoor privy seats should be sprayed with creosote every 3 months to repel the spiders. Rubbish and woodpiles should not be moved without the wearing of gloves and a heavy shirt buttoned at the wrists. Shoes, clothing and sleeping accommodation should be inspected for black widow spiders prior to use.

## Treatment

### Emergency measures

(1) Enforce complete rest. Establish airway and maintain respiration.
(2) Apply cold packs to the bite for several hours.
(3) For funnel-web spider bite, apply an arterial tourniquet until a medical facility can be reached.

### Antidote

Give antiserum, 1–2.5 ml diluted in 50 ml of 5% dextrose in saline intravenously over 15 min after testing for sensitivity. To test for sensitivity, inject 0.1 ml of 1:10 dilution in saline intradermally. A positive reaction consists of an urticarial wheal surrounded by a zone of erythema.

### General measures

Avoid overtreatment.
(1) Give aspirin or codeine to control pain. In children, give codeine phosphate, 1 mg/kg subcutaneously.
(2) Give calcium gluconate, 10 ml of 10% solution slowly intravenously to relieve muscular cramping.
(3) Cortisone relieves symptoms but apparently has no effect on the overall mortality rate.
(4) Administration of methocarbamol (Robaxin), 10 ml intravenously over a 5-minute period followed by 10 ml in 250 ml of 5% glucose over 2 h, is reported to relieve muscle spasms.
(5) For funnel-web spider bite, antivenom is effective.

## Prognosis

Death from spider bite in previously well individuals is unlikely. Recovery is usually complete within a week.

## References

Bush SP, *et al.* Green lynx spider (*Peucetia viridans*) envenomation. *Am J Emerg Med* 2000;18:64

Harrington AP, *et al.* Funnel-web spider (*Hadronyche infensa*) envenomations in coastal south-east Queensland. *Med J Austral* 1999;171:651

Pincus SJ, *et al.* Acute and recurrent skin ulceration after spider bite. *Med J Austral* 1999;171:99

Reeves JA, *et al.* Black widow spider bite in a child. *Am J Emerg Med* 1996;14:469

Vetter RS. Envenomation by a spider *Agelenopsis aperta* (Family: *Agelenidae*) previously considered harmless. *Ann Emerg Med* 1998;32:739

Watson J. Spider bites: assessment and management. *J Am Acad Nurse Pract* 1999;11:215

## BROWN RECLUSE SPIDER (Violin Spider)

The brown recluse spider (*Loxosceles recluse*), found in 25 states ranging from Hawaii to New Jersey and Texas to Illinois, has caused more than 10 deaths. It is light yellow to medium dark brown with a darker brown violin-shaped patch on the back. The body is $\frac{3}{8} - \frac{1}{2}$ inch long, $\frac{1}{4}$ inch wide, and $\frac{3}{4} - 1$ inch toe-to-toe. It is found in dark, undisturbed places. The female is more dangerous than the male.

The venom causes necrosis by activating the clotting mechanism to form microthrombotic aggregates that plug arterioles and venules.

## Clinical findings

The principal manifestation of recluse spider bite is cutaneous necrosis. The bite is initially painless, with pain developing in 2–8 h, followed by blisters, redness, swelling, bleeding, or ulceration. The untreated lesion increases in size for up to a week. Systemic symptoms and signs include cyanosis, hemoglobinuria, fever, chills, malaise, weakness, nausea and vomiting, joint pain, skin rash, and delirium. The onset of intravascular hemolysis can be

**Table 34.1** Diagnosis and treatment of poisoning from other spiders

| Scientific and common name | Range | Clinical findings | Treatment |
|---|---|---|---|
| Loxosceles laeta (brown spider) | South America | Cutaneous necrosis, jaundice, hemoglobinuria | Specific antiserum |
| Atrax robustus, Hadronyche sp. (funnel-web spider) | Australia | Erythema, chills, paresthesia, collapse, coma, cholinergic crisis | See p. 602 |
| Phoneutria fera (tarantula spider) | Brazil | See L. mactans, p. 601 | Give antiserum |
| Lycosa erythrognata (tarantula spider), Lycosa raptoria | Brazil | See L. mactans, p. 601 | Give antiserum |
| Ctenus nigriventer | Brazil | Necrosis, muscular cramps, respiratory failure | Give antiserum |

detected early by determining hemoglobin and hematocrit every 6 h for the first 48 h.

## Prevention

Wear gloves when investigating secluded areas, and carefully examine clothing that has been stored before use.

## Treatment

The treatment is controversial. The use of maximum doses of systemic or local adrenocortical steroids, local phentolamine, excision, and exchange transfusion have all been recommended. Most bites resolve without treatment. Skin grafts are rarely necessary. Treat hemolytic reaction (see p. 80).

## Prognosis

Healing of necrotic areas may require 6–8 weeks. Death ordinarily occurs in the first 48 h.

## References

Cacy J, Mold JW. The clinical characteristics of brown recluse spider bites treated by family physicians. *J Fam Pract* 1999;48:536

Jarvis RM, *et al*. Brown recluse spider bite to the eyelid. *Ophthalmology* 2000;107:1492

Wright SW, *et al*. Clinical presentation and outcome of brown recluse-spider bite. *Ann Emerg Med* 1997;30:28

## SCORPIONS

Poisonous scorpions of the USA (*Centruroides gertschii* and *Centruroides sculpturatus*) live mainly in the arid Southwest. In Brazil the poisonous species are *Tityus bahiensis* and *Tityus serrulatus*. In North Africa the poisonous scorpions are *Androctonus australis* and related species, *Buthus occitonus*, and *Buthacus arenicola*.

In areas inhabited by both poisonous scorpions and poisonous snakes, the mortality rate from scorpions may be higher because they live around homes and bites are more common. Scorpion venoms cause local, central nervous system, and cardiac effects.

Approximately 1000 stings in adults and children occur yearly in the south-western USA, with about one fatality per year. Most of the deaths occur in children under 6 years of age. Reliable data on the incidence of stings are not available for other areas.

### Clinical findings

Local evidence of a sting is sometimes minimal or absent. The usual symptoms are a mild tingling or burning at the site of the sting, which may progress up the extremity. In severe cases spasm in the throat, a feeling of thick tongue, restlessness, muscular fibrillation, abdominal cramps, convulsions, incontinence, hypertension, hypotension, oliguria, tachycardia, cardiac arrhythmias, pulmonary edema, and respiratory failure occur. Although the duration of symptoms is ordinarily 24–48 h, neurologic manifestations may persist for up to 1 week. Laboratory tests are noncontributory.

### Prevention

Spaces under houses and boardwalks should be tightly enclosed and sprayed regularly with creosote or other insecticides. Rubbish should not be left scattered where children play. Area treatment with insecticides is apparently ineffective in reducing the number of scorpions for more than a short time.

## Treatment

### *Emergency measures*

(1) Immobilize the patient and the bitten part immediately.
(2) Give artificial respiration with $O_2$ if respiration is depressed.
(3) Apply cold packs (10–15°C) for the first few hours to help slow absorption.

### *Antidote*

(1) The use of specific scorpion antiserum is controversial.
(2) Prazosin, dobutamine, and midazolam have been suggested as antidotes.

### *General measures*

(1) Control convulsions (see p. 60). Diazepam may be useful.
(2) Inject calcium gluconate, 10 ml of 10% solution slowly intravenously, to help relieve muscular cramps.
(3) Treat pulmonary edema with sodium nitroprusside infusion.
(4) Opiate analgesics may cause respiratory depression or potentiate post-ictal depression.

## Prognosis

Fatalities are rare except in children under 6 years of age. Rapid progression of symptoms in the first 2–4 h after a sting indicates a poor outcome. Survival for 48 h is ordinarily followed by recovery, although deaths have occurred 4 days after stinging.

## References

Abroug F, *et al*. High-dose hydrocortisone hemisuccinate in scorpion envenomation. *Ann Emerg Med* 1997;30:23

Bawaskar HS, Bawaskar PH. Management of scorpion sting. *Heart* 1999;82:253 (Prazosin)

Belghith M, *et al*. Efficacy of serotherapy in scorpion sting: a matched pair study. *J Toxicol Clin Toxicol* 1999;37:51

Bush SP. Envenomation by the scorpion (*Centruroides limbatus*) outside its natural range and recognition of medically important species. *Wilderness Envir Med* 1999;10:161

Elatrous S, *et al*. Dobutamine in severe scorpion envenomation. *Chest* 1999;116: 748

Fernandez-Bouzas A, *et al*. Brain infarcts due to scorpion stings in children: MRI. *Paediatr Neurol* 2000;42:118

Ghalim N, *et al*. Scorpion envenomation and serotherapy in Morocco. *Am J Trop Med Hyg* 2000;62:277

Gibley R, *et al*. Continuous intravenous midazolam infusion for *Centruoides exilicauda* scorpion envenomation. *Ann Emerg Med* 1999;34:620

Karnad DR. Haemodynamic patterns in patients with scorpion envenomation. *Heart* 1998;79:485

LoVecchio F, *et al*. Incidence of immediate and delayed hypersensitivity to *Centruroides* antivenom. *Ann Emerg Med* 1999;34:615

**Table 34.2** Diagnosis and treatment of poisoning due to other insects and arachnids

| Name | Clinical findings | Treatment |
|------|-------------------|-----------|
| Ticks: *Amblyomma americanum, Dermacentor* species, *Ixodidae* species | Ataxia, weakness, paralysis coming on 12–24 h after attachment of the tick. Respiratory failure may occur | Remove the tick by applying kerosene or ether, by gentle traction with forceps, or by surgical excision. Apply moist heat |
| Ticks: *Ornithodoros* species | Severe pain and swelling, persisting for 1–2 weeks | |
| Bee, wasp, yellow jacket | Single or multiple stings may cause severe fall in blood pressure, difficult breathing, collapse, optic and peripheral neuropathy, nephritic syndrome, and hemoglobinuria. A sensitivity reaction may cause severe collapse, bronchial constriction, edema of the face and lips, and itching. Death may occur within 1 h | Epinephrine, 0.2–0.5 ml of 1:1000 subcut. or IV. Give diphenhydramine, 50 mg subcut. or IV, cautiously. Give hydrocortisone IV for severe collapse. Sensitive persons should carry treatment kits. Venom desensitization is possible |
| *Epyris californicus* (wasp) | Numbness, itching, diarrhea, wheezing, prostration, sweating, drowsiness, with recovery in 30 min. See above under bee, wasp, and yellow jacket | |
| Caterpillars | Redness, swelling, intense local pain, vomiting, shock, and sometimes convulsions from skin contact | Give meperidine or diphenhydramine IM or calcium gluconate IV. Hydrocortisone may be useful |
| Millipedes | Vesicular dermatitis with intense itching and burning lasting for 1–24 h from skin contact | Relieve itching by cold applications |
| *Scolopendra subspinipes* (centipede) | Pain, redness, swelling | Cold applications |
| *Solenopsis saevissima* (fire-ant) | Pain, swelling, edema, bullae | Steroids may be useful |

## References

deShazo RD, *et al*. Fire ant attacks on residents in health care facilities: a report of two cases. *Ann Intern Med* 1999;131:424

Kolecki P. Delayed toxic reaction following massive bee envenomation. *Ann Emerg Med* 1999;33:114

Maltzman JS, *et al*. Optic neuropathy occurring after bee and wasp sting. *Ophthalmology* 2000;107:193

Revai T, Harmos G. Simvastatin treatment in nephrotic syndrome associated with a bee sting. *J R Soc Med* 1999;92:23

# 35 Marine animals*

## SHELLFISH

Mussels, clams, oysters, and other shellfish growing in many marine locations become poisonous during the warm months (May to October in the northern hemisphere) from feeding on certain dinoflagellates, including *Gonyaulax catenella*. One mussel, clam, or oyster may contain a fatal dose of poison. More than ten deaths have been reported in the literature in the USA from this type of poisoning.

The poisonous principle contained in shellfish is a nitrogenous compound that produces a curare-like muscular paralysis. The pathologic findings in deaths from shellfish poisoning are not characteristic.

### Clinical findings

The principal manifestation of shellfish poisoning is respiratory paralysis.

After ingestion of poisonous shellfish numbness and tingling of lips, tongue, face, and extremities occur and nausea and vomiting follow, progressing to respiratory paralysis. Convulsions may or may not occur.

### Prevention

Do not eat fresh shellfish during the summer months. Check with local health department.

### Treatment

Remove ingested shellfish by gastric lavage or emesis (see pp. 29–32). Tracheal intubation and assisted ventilation with $O_2$ may be necessary if respiration is impaired.

---

*See also Table 35.1

## Prognosis

The fatality rate is 1–10%. If the patient survives for 12 h recovery is likely.

## References

Poli MA, *et al*. Neurotoxic shellfish poisoning and brevetoxin metabolites: a case study from Florida. *Toxicon* 2000;38:981

Todd ECD. Emerging diseases associated with seafood toxins and other water-borne agents. *Ann NY Acad Sci* 1994;740:77

Van Dolah FM. Marine algal toxins: origins, health effects, and their increased occurrence. *Environ Health Perspect* 2000;108(Suppl):133

Whittle K, Gallacher S. Marine toxins. *Br Med Bull* 2000;56:236

## FISH

The flesh of a number of fish found in tropical waters may be poisonous at certain times of the year. They apparently become poisonous by feeding on certain marine organisms. Some fish, such as puffers (family *Tetraodontidae*), triggerfish, and parrot fish, are poisonous during most of the year. Others, such as the moray eel, surgeon fish, moon fish, porcupine fish, filefish, and goatfish, are poisonous for only a part of the year in some localities. The most common type of fish poisoning, known as ciguatera, occurs with fish that are ordinarily considered edible (grouper, surgeon fish, barracuda, pompano, mackerel, butterfly fish, snapper, sea bass, perch, wrasse, etc.) but become sporadically poisonous in certain localities. Scombroid fish poisoning occurs after consumption of improperly prepared tuna and other scombroidei; it is due to the growth of surface organisms in fish stored at ambient temperatures. Some of the toxic effects from scombroid fish poisoning may be the result of liberation of histamine-like amines during bacterial decomposition.

More than 300 species have been reported to cause outbreaks of fish poisoning. The puffer family seems to have the most potent toxin; the mortality rate may be as high as 50%. In other types of fish poisoning the mortality rate ranges from less than 1% to as high as 10%, depending on the physical condition of the individual, the amount of fish eaten, and the potency of the toxin. The incidence of poisoning may be as high as 5–50% of the population in tropical countries where fish forms a large part of the diet. In Hawaii 50–100 cases are reported yearly, with a mortality rate of less than 1%.

The poison present in the flesh or viscera of the fish apparently exerts its primary effect on the peripheral nervous system, but the physiologic mechanism is as yet unknown. The pathologic findings are not characteristic.

**Clinical findings**

The principal manifestations of ciguatera are vomiting and muscular paralysis. Scombroid poisoning causes vomiting.

*Ciguatera*

Symptoms of acute poisoning begin 30 min to 4 h after ingestion and include numbness and tingling of the face and lips that spreads to fingers and toes. This is followed by nausea and vomiting, diarrhea, malaise, dizziness, abdominal pain, and muscular weakness. In severe poisoning, these symptoms progress to foaming at the mouth, muscular paralysis, dyspnea, or convulsions. Death may occur from convulsions or respiratory arrest within 1–24 h. If the patient recovers from the immediate symptoms, muscular weakness and paresthesias of the face, lips, and mouth may persist for weeks. These paresthesias characteristically consist of reversed temperature sensations; thus, cold food or other cold objects cause a searing pain or an 'electric shock' sensation, and hot things feel cold. Laboratory findings are not contributory.

*Scombroid poisoning*

Symptoms include nausea and vomiting, cramps, diarrhea, facial flushing, headache, and burning in the mouth.

**Prevention**

Adequate prophylactic measures have not been developed, since some tropical fish that are considered edible may sometimes be poisonous. The following fish found in tropical waters should never be eaten: puffers, trunk or box fish, triggerfish, thorn fish, filefish, parrot fish, and porcupine fish. Scombroid fish should be refrigerated immediately after being caught.

## Treatment

### Emergency measures

Remove the ingested fish by gastric lavage or emesis (see pp. 29–32). Maintain adequate airway. Treat respiratory failure (see p. 53).

### General measures

Treat convulsions (see p. 60). Treat shock (see p. 56). In scombroid poisoning, give antihistamines, cimetidine, and corticosteroids. In ciguatera, mannitol infusion (1 g/kg in 30 min) is reported to be helpful.

## Prognosis

Mortality rates may vary from less than 1% to more than 50%. The lower rate may be expected when the fish is known to be a common type of edible fish.

## References

Asaeda G. The transport of ciguatoxin: a case report. *J Emerg Med* 2001;20:263

Blomkalns AL, Otten EJ. Catfish spine envenomation: a case report and literature review. *Wilderness Envir Med* 1999;242:242

Eckstein M, *et al*. Out-of-hospital and emergency department management of epidemic scombroid poisoning. *Acad Emerg Med* 1999;6:916

Karalis T, *et al*. Three clusters of ciguatera poisoning: clinical manifestations and public health implications. *Med J Austral* 2000;172:160

Landau M. *Poisonous, Venomous and Electric Marine Organisms of the Atlantic Coast, Gulf of Mexico and the Caribbean*. Plexus Publishing, 1997

Lehane L. Ciguatera update. *Med J Austral* 2000;172:176

**Table 35.1** Venomous fish

| Name | Clinical findings | Treatment |
|------|-------------------|-----------|
| Sting-ray (*Urobatis halleri* and others) | Penetration of the skin by the barb in the tail of the sting-ray causes intense local pain, swelling, nausea and vomiting, abdominal pain, dizziness, weakness, generalized cramps, sweating, fall in blood pressure. Recovery occurs in 24–48 h. Fatalities have occurred when the barb has penetrated the chest or abdomen | 1. Cleanse wound by irrigation and remove foreign material<br>2. Soak wound in hot water (45–60°C) for 30–60 min<br>3. Surgically debride and close wound |
| Scorpion fish (*Scorpaena guttata*) | Spines of the gill covers may penetrate skin and cause severe local pain and swelling, with extension of pain and swelling to involve the entire extremity | 1. Treat as for sting-ray<br>2. For pain, give meperidine, 50–100 mg subcutaneously |
| Jellyfish or Portuguese Man-of-war (*Physalia* species) | Contact with these jellyfish causes urticarial wheals, numbness and pain of the extremities, severe chest and abdominal pain, abdominal rigidity, and dysphagia. Deaths are rare | Inject 10 ml of 10% calcium gluconate IV to relieve muscular cramps. Apply aromatic spirits of ammonia in compress to remove the venom |
| Jellyfish or sea wasp (*Chironex fleckeri, Chiropsalmus quadrigatus*) | Wheals, extreme pain, skin necrosis, respiratory and cardiac depression. Death occurs in minutes | Apply occlusive tourniquet immediately. Give antiserum |
| Stonefish (*Synanceja trachynis, Synanceja horrida*) | Intense radiating pain with blanching, then cyanosis of the affected part, nausea and vomiting, fever, delirium, respiratory distress, and convulsions | Treat as above for sting-ray and scorpion fish. Give specific antiserum |

# 36 Plants*

## AKEE

The unopened unripe fruit and the cotyledons of the tropical akee (*Blighia sapida*) are poisonous. In Cuba and Jamaica, up to 50 cases of poisoning (with some deaths) occur yearly. Approximately 85% of these cases of poisoning are in children. Poisoning has not been reported from Florida, where the akee is also grown. One unripe fruit contains a lethal dose of the poison, which is soluble in boiling water.

The toxic effects produced by akee are as yet poorly understood. The pathologic findings in the brain are congestion and hemorrhages in the subarachnoid space and parenchyma. The lungs show congestion and serous exudate. The liver and kidneys reveal marked fatty degeneration; less marked degenerative changes are seen in the heart and brain.

### Clinical findings

The principal manifestations of akee poisoning are vomiting, circulatory collapse, and hypoglycemia.

### *Symptoms and signs* (from ingestion)

Nausea, vomiting, and abdominal discomfort usually begin within 2 h after ingestion. The patient recovers from this attack and is free of symptoms for 2–6 h. Vomiting or retching may then return, followed shortly by convulsions, coma, hypothermia, hypoglycemia, and fall in blood pressure. In fatal cases death occurs within 24 h after ingestion of the fruit.

### *Laboratory findings*

(1) The blood chloride level is increased and the blood glucose is low.
(2) The red and white blood cell counts are decreased.

---

*See also Tables 36.1 and 36.2

(3) Hepatic cell function may be impaired as revealed by appropriate tests (see p. 75).

## Prevention

Only fully opened fruit should be picked. Fallen, unripe fruit should be burned to prevent children from eating it. The fruit capsule and seeds are both toxic. If fruit is cooked, the water should be discarded and not used for further cooking.

## Treatment

### *Emergency measures*

Remove the poison by gastric lavage or emesis (see pp. 29–32).

### *Antidote*

None is known. Alcohol was at one time thought to be a useful antidote, but experiments indicate that it is not effective.

### *General measures*

Control convulsions (see p. 60). Give carbohydrates as 5% glucose intravenously or as sugar dissolved in fruit juice orally to protect the liver and maintain blood sugar. Treat uremia (see p. 66).

## Prognosis

Recovery is rare after the onset of convulsions or coma. Patients having only the primary attack of vomiting recover completely in a few days.

## CASTOR BEAN AND JEQUIRITY BEAN

The castor bean plant (*Ricinus communis*) is grown for commercial and ornamental purposes. The residue or pomace after castor oil extraction of castor beans gives rise to dust that may cause sensitivity reactions or poisoning.

Jequirity (rosary bean, love beads, *Abrus precatorius*) is grown as an ornamental vine in tropical climates. The beans are 6 mm long and are bright orange with one black end. They are used as rosary beads and as decorations for costumes.

Ingestion of only one castor bean or jequirity bean has apparently caused fatal poisoning when the bean was thoroughly chewed. If the beans are swallowed whole, poisoning is unlikely because the hard seed coat prevents rapid absorption. In a recent report no toxicity was found in three cases of castor bean ingestion.

Ricin, a toxic albumin found in castor beans, and abrin, a similar albumin found in jequirity beans, cause agglutination and hemolysis of red blood cells at extreme dilutions (1:1 000 000). They are also injurious to all other cells and are heat-labile.

The pathologic findings in fatal cases of castor bean or jequirity bean poisoning include hemorrhage and edema of the gastrointestinal tract, hemolysis, and degenerative changes in the kidneys.

## Clinical findings

The principal manifestations of poisoning with these beans are vomiting, diarrhea, and circulatory collapse.

### *Acute poisoning* (from ingestion)

After 2 h to several days, burning of the mouth, nausea and vomiting, diarrhea, abdominal pain, drowsiness, disorientation, cyanosis, stupor, circulatory collapse, retinal hemorrhage, hematuria, convulsions, and oliguria may begin and progress to death in uremia up to 12 days after poisoning. The vomitus and stools may contain blood.

### *Chronic poisoning* (from inhalation of dust from castor bean pomace)

Dermatitis and inflammation of the nose, throat, and eyes. Instances of asthmatic attack have also been reported from exposure to the dust.

### *Laboratory findings*

The urine may contain protein, casts, red blood cells, and hemoglobin. The blood may show an increase in blood urea nitrogen and non-protein nitrogen.

## Prevention

Children should not be allowed access to castor beans or jequirity beans. Dust from handling castor bean pomace should be controlled by proper air exhaust.

## Treatment

### Acute poisoning

(1) Emergency measures – Remove ingested beans by gastric lavage or emesis (see pp. 29–32). Catharsis is also useful. Maintain circulation by blood transfusions (see p. 57).

(2) General measures – Alkalinize the urine by giving 5–15 g of sodium bicarbonate daily to prevent precipitation of hemoglobin or hemoglobin products in the kidneys. Control convulsions with diazepam (see p. 62).

(3) Special problems – Treat anuria (see p. 66). For dehydration, maintain central venous pressure by giving fluids.

### Chronic poisoning

Remove from exposure.

## Prognosis

The fatality rate is approximately 5%. Death may occur up to 14 days after poisoning.

## References

Garcia-Gonzalez JJ, *et al*. Pollinosis to *Ricinus communis* (castor bean): an aerobiological, clinical and immunochemical study. *Clin Exp Allergy* 1999;29: 1265

le Coz C-J, Ball C. Recurrent allergic contact dermatitis and cheilitis due to castor oil. *Contact Derm* 2000;42:114

Palatnich W, Tenenbein M. Hepatotoxicity from castor bean ingestion in a child. *J Toxicol Clin Toxicol* 2000;38:67

## FAVA BEANS

Fava beans (*Vicia faba*), or horse beans, are grown commercially for use as a food.

Severe reactions occur occasionally following ingestion of fava beans or inhalation of the pollen of growing plants.

At least 8 cases of favism have been reported in the USA. Deaths have not been reported in the USA but have occurred in Italy.

Fava beans induce agglutination and hemolysis in individuals who have a deficiency of the enzyme glucose-6-phosphate dehydrogenase. The pathologic findings are hemolysis and hemoglobin precipitation in the kidneys. The beans contain dopamine.

### Clinical findings

The principal manifestations of acute favism are jaundice and oliguria.

*Symptoms and signs* (from ingestion of beans or inhalation of pollen)

Fever, malaise, jaundice, dark urine, oliguria, pallor, enlargement of the spleen and liver beginning 1–2 days after ingesting the beans or 1–8 h after inhaling the pollen from the plant.

*Laboratory findings*

Anemia and increased serum bilirubin (see p. 75). Non-protein nitrogen may be increased if oliguria occurs. Hemoglobinuria may occur.

### Prevention

In order to prevent development of sensitivity, fava beans should not be served as food to children under the age of 1 year.

### Treatment

*General measures*

(1) Alkalinize the urine with sodium bicarbonate, 2 g every 4 h.
(2) In the presence of normal renal function maintain urine output by giving 2–4 liters of fluid daily orally or intravenously.
(3) Hydrocortisone, 4–10 mg/h intravenously, may be used.

**Prognosis**

Recovery is likely with adequate treatment.

**Reference**

Hampl JS, *et al.* Acute hemolysis related to consumption of fava beans: a case study and medical nutrition therapy approach. *J Am Diet Assoc* 1997;97:182

**Table 36.1** Plants commonly involved in poisoning*

| Name | Poisonous part of plant, and active principle if known | Clinical findings | Treatment |
|---|---|---|---|
| Arum family: Calla lily, elephant ear, jack-in-the-pulpit (*Dieffenbachia, Caladium, Alocasia, Colocasia, Philodendron, Arisaema triphyllum*) | All parts (oxalates and other toxins) | Severe irritation of mucous membranes, nausea and vomiting, diarrhea, salivation. Rare systemic effects | Give demulcents: milk, vegetable oil, cooling drinks |
| Oleander (*Nerium oleander*) | All parts (oleandrin) | Same as for digitalis, p. 459 | As for digitalis (See p. 460) |
| Pokeweed (*Phytolacca americana*) | All parts but especially root (saponins), glycoproteins | Burning in the mouth and stomach, persistent vomiting and diarrhea, slowed respiration and weakness | Remove ingested poison as outlined on pp. 29–32 |
| Rhubarb (*Rheum* species) | Leafy part (oxalic acid) | Nausea, vomiting, diarrhea, abdominal pain, reduced urine formation, hemorrhages. See oxalic acid p. 240 | Treat as for oxalic acid, p. 241 |
| Solanaceae: | | | |
| Blue nightshade (*Solanum dulcamara*) | Leaves and fruit (solanine) | Abdominal pain, vomiting, diarrhea, mental and respiratory depression, hypothermia or fever, delirium, slow or fast pulse, shock | Maintain respiration and circulation. Remove ingested poison as outlined on pp. 29–32 |
| Black nightshade (*Solanum nigrum*) | Leaves and unripe berries (solanine) | | |

*Continued*

Table 36.1 (continued)

| Name | Poisonous part of plant, and active principle if known | Clinical findings | Treatment |
|------|-----|------|------|
| Jerusalem cherry (*Solanum pseudocapsicum*) | Leaves and unripe berries (solanine) | | |
| Potato (*Solanum tuberosum*) | Green tubers, new sprouts (solanine) | | |
| Yew (*Taxus*) | Wood, bark, leaves, seeds (taxine) | Nausea, vomiting, diarrhea, abdominal pain, dyspnea, dilated pupils, weakness, convulsions, shock, coma | Remove ingested poison as outlined on pp. 29–32 |

*See also croton oil (*Croton tiglium*, p. 543), deadly nightshade (*Atropa belladonna*, p. 422), foxglove (*Digitalis purpurea, Digitalis lanata*, p. 459). henbane (*Hyoscyamus niger*, p. 422), jimsonweed (*Datura stramonium*, p. 422), larkspur (*Delphinium* species, p. 538), meadow saffron (*Colchicum autumnale*, p. 579), monkshood (*Aconitum napellus, Aconitum columbianum*, p. 538)

## HEMLOCK

The poisonous plants of the parsley family include poison hemlock (*Conium maculatum*), water hemlock (*Cicuta maculata* and other *Cicuta* species), and dog parsley (*Aethusa cynapium*).

Fatalities are reported at intervals of several years. A piece of *Cicuta maculata* 1 cm in diameter may produce fatal poisoning.

*Cicuta* species contain cicutoxin, a central nervous system stimulant like picrotoxin.

*Conium maculatum* and *Aethusa cynapium* contain a number of piperidine derivatives, including coniine, which cause peripheral muscular paralysis similar to that from curare. Nicotine-like ganglionic blockade also occurs.

The pathologic findings in *Cicuta* poisoning are similar to those from picrotoxin (see p. 516). The pathologic findings in *Conium* poisoning are inflammation of the gastrointestinal tract with congestion of the abdominal organs.

## Clinical findings

The principal manifestations of hemlock poisoning are convulsions and respiratory failure.

### Symptoms and signs (from ingestion)

(1) *Cicuta* species (e.g. water hemlock) cause abdominal pain, nausea and vomiting, sweating, hematemesis, diarrhea, convulsions, cyanosis, and respiratory failure or cardiac arrest.
(2) *Conium maculatum* (poison hemlock) and *Aethusa* (dog parsley) cause nausea and vomiting, salivation, fever, and gradually increasing muscular weakness followed by paralysis with respiratory failure.

### Laboratory findings

The urine may reveal temporary proteinuria.

## Prevention

Children and adults should never eat unidentified wild plants.

## Treatment

### Emergency measures

Remove poison by gastric lavage or emesis with activated charcoal (see pp. 31–32). Treat respiratory failure by artificial respiration with $O_2$. Prepare to treat cardiac arrest.

### General measures

Control convulsions (see p. 60). Diazepam may be useful.

## Prognosis

With early and adequate therapy, the death rate should be less than 10%.

**References**

Drummer OH, *et al*. Three deaths from hemlock poisoning. *Med J Austral* 1995;162:592

Frank BS, *et al*. Ingestion of poison hemlock (*Conium maculatum*). *West J Med* 1995;163:573

## MUSHROOMS

Poisonous mushrooms may grow wherever non-poisonous mushrooms grow. The most dangerous species are *Amanita phalloides*, *Amanita verna*, *Amanita virosa*, *Gyromitra esculenta*, and the *Galerina* species.

Ingestion of part of one mushroom of a dangerous species may be sufficient to cause death. Over 100 fatalities occur each year from eating poisonous mushrooms.

*Amanita muscaria* contains, in variable amounts, an atropine-like alkaloid and a substance that causes narcosis, convulsions, and hallucinations. Some mushrooms contain the alkaloid muscarine, which produces the same effect as parasympathetic stimulation on smooth muscles and glands. Chronic poisoning does not occur.

*Amanita phalloides* contains the heat-stable polypeptides amanitin and phalloidin, which damage cells throughout the body. Liver, kidneys, brain, and heart are especially affected. Other mushrooms of the *Amanita* genus as well as of the genus *Galerina* may cause similar poisoning. The toxic principle is rapidly bound to tissues.

The pathologic finding in fatalities from mushroom poisoning is fatty degeneration in the liver, kidneys, heart, and skeletal muscles.

### Clinical findings

The principal manifestations of acute mushroom poisoning are vomiting, respiratory difficulty, and jaundice.

*Symptoms and signs* (from ingestion)

(1) *Amanitin* (amatoxin) type cyclopeptides (*Amanita phalloides*, *Amanita verna*, *Amanita virosa*; *Galerina autumnalis*, *Galerina marginata*, *Galerina venenata*) – After a latent interval of 6–24 h severe nausea and vomiting begin and progress variably to diarrhea, bloody vomitus and

stools, painful tenderness and enlargement of the liver, oliguria or anuria, jaundice, pulmonary edema, headache, mental confusion and depression, hypoglycemia, and signs of cerebral injury with coma or convulsions. The fatality rate is about 50%.

(2) Gyromitrin type (monomethylhydrazine) (*Gyromitra* and *Helvella* species) – Vomiting, diarrhea, convulsions, coma, hemolysis. The fatality rate is 15–40%.

(3) Muscarine type (*Inocybe* and *Clitocybe* species) – Vomiting, diarrhea, bradycardia, hypotension, salivation, miosis, bronchospasm, lacrimation. Cardiac arrhythmias may occur. The fatality rate is 5%.

(4) Anticholinergic type (*Amanita muscaria, Amanita pantherina, Amanita cokeri, Amanita crenulata, Amanita solitaria*) – This type causes a variety of symptoms that may be atropine-like, including excitement, delirium, salivation, wheezing, vomiting, diarrhea, slow pulse, dilated or constricted pupils, and muscular tremors, beginning 1–2 h after ingestion. Fatalities are rare.

(5) Gastrointestinal irritant type (*Boletus, Cantharellus, Clitocybe, Clorophyllum, Hebeloma, Lactarius, Lepiota, Naematoloma, Rhodophyllus, Russula,* and *Tricholoma* species) – Nausea, vomiting, diarrhea, cardiac arrhythmias, and malaise, which may last up to 1 week. Fatalities are rare.

(6) Disulfiram type (*Coprinus* species) – Vomiting, diarrhea, cardiac arrhythmias, and disulfiram-like sensitivity to alcohol that may persist for several days. Fatalities are rare.

(7) Hallucinogenic type (*Psilocybe* and *Panaeolus* species) – Mydriasis, ataxia, weakness, disorientation, abdominal pain, fever, and convulsions. Fatalities are rare.

(8) Renal damage type (*Cortinarius* spp., *Amanita smithiana,* others) – Nausea, vomiting, diarrhea, renal failure.

### *Laboratory findings*

Increase in creatinine and blood urea nitrogen. Effects on the liver are revealed by SGOT, SGPT, lactate dehydrogenase (LDH), and bilirubin levels. The blood sugar level should be monitored daily or oftener. After gyromitrin, the methemoglobin level may be increased.

## Prevention

The frequent occurrence of mushroom poisoning indicates that any ingestion of wild mushrooms is hazardous and not worth the risk.

## Treatment

### Emergency measures

Remove ingested mushrooms by ipecac emesis unless the patient has already vomited. After emesis give activated charcoal (see pp. 31–32) in 70% sorbitol to aid in the removal of any unabsorbed poison.

### Antidote

(1) In amanitin type poisoning, the use of *N*-acetylcysteine has been suggested. Give 200 mg/kg IV then 10 mg/kg/h. Penicillin G in high doses has also been suggested as a receptor site competitor.
(2) For mushrooms producing predominantly muscarinic-cholinergic symptoms, give atropine, 1 mg orally or subcutaneously.
(3) For gyromitrin poisoning, give pyridoxine, 25 mg/kg intravenously.
(4) For cardiac arrhythmias resulting from *Coprinus* or *Clitocybe* ingestion, propranolol may be useful. Avoid alcoholic beverages.

### General measures

(1) Careful control of fluid and electrolyte balance, with avoidance of hypoglycemia, must be continued for 5–10 days. In severely poisoned patients liver function has been known to begin to return 6–8 days after exposure, followed by eventual complete recovery.
(2) The use of hemodialysis or charcoal hemoperfusion for the removal of mushroom toxins is controversial. Hemodialysis is life-saving in renal failure after mushroom ingestion.
(3) Large quantities of carbohydrate appear to help protect the liver from further damage. Give 5–10% dextrose, 4–5 liters intravenously every 24 h, if the urine output is adequate. Give vitamin K for bleeding.
(4) As soon as fluids can be given by mouth give fruit juices fortified by glucose, 120 g/l, up to 4–5 orally daily.

## Special problems

(1) Treat anuria (see p. 66).
(2) Control convulsions (see p. 60).
(3) Reduce fever by active cooling. Dialysis can be used as a rapid means of reducing body temperature.
(4) Maintain respiration but avoid intubation unless necessary.
(5) Forced diuresis to 3–6 ml/kg/h with furosemide, 0.25–1 mg/kg/h, is useful.

## Prognosis

Approximately 50% of individuals poisoned by *Amanita phalloides* or other mushrooms that damage the liver and other internal organs will die. However, in the absence of injury to internal organs and with adequate atropinization, mushroom poisoning is not likely to be fatal.

## References

Borowiak KS, *et al.* Psilocybin mushroom (*Psilocybe semilanceata*) intoxication with myocardial infarction. *J Toxicol Clin Toxicol* 1998;36:47

Leathem AM, *et al.* Renal failure caused by mushroom poisoning. *J Toxicol Clin Toxicol* 1996;35:67 (*Amanita*)

Montanini S, *et al.* Use of acetylcysteine as the life-saving antidote in *Amanita phalloides* (Death cap) poisoning. Case report on 11 patients. *Arzneim Forsch* 1999;49:1044

Mullins ME, Horowitz BZ. The futility of hemoperfusion and hemodialysis in *Amanita phalloides* poisoning. *Vet Hum Toxicol* 2000;42:90

Rohrmoser M, *et al.* Orellanine poisoning: rapid detection of the fungal toxin in renal biopsy material. *J Toxicol Clin Toxicol* 1996;35:63 (*Cortinarius* sp.)

Splendiani G, *et al.* Continuous renal replacement therapy and charcoal plasma perfusion in treatment of amanita mushroom poisoning. *Artif Organs* 2000;24:305

Warden CR, Benjamin DR. Acute renal failure associated with suspected *Amanita smithiana* mushroom ingestions: a case series. *Acad Emerg Med* 1998;5:808

## POISON IVY (POISON OAK) AND POISON SUMAC

Poison ivy (*Rhus radicans*), poison oak (*Rhus toxicodendron*, *Rhus diversiloba*), and poison sumac (*Rhus vernix*) are all related plants that grow widely in the USA.

Fatalities are rare, but at least 50% of those who handle *Rhus* species will have a severe dermatitis, and up to 10% will have temporarily disabling generalized effects.

*Rhus toxicodendron* and related species contain urushiol, which is a mixture of catechols that may be potent sensitizers, since repeated contact appears to increase the severity of the reaction. Renal irritation occurs after severe exposure. In deaths from poison ivy and related plants the pathologic findings include renal and myocardial damage.

### Clinical findings

The principal manifestations of poisoning with these plants are vesiculation and generalized edema.

*Acute poisoning* (from contact, ingestion, or inhalation of smoke of burning plants)

(1) Local effects – These begin 12 h to 7 days after contact and include itching, swelling, papulation, vesiculation, oozing, and crusting.
(2) General effects – These include generalized edema, pharyngeal or laryngeal edema, oliguria, weakness, malaise, and fever.

### Chronic poisoning

Repeated exposure increases the severity of symptoms. Attempts to produce immunity by repeated exposure may lead to severe poisoning.

### Laboratory findings

The urine may contain protein, red blood cells, and casts. Examination of the blood may reveal a high non-protein nitrogen level.

## Prevention

Teach children to recognize and avoid the plants.

Wear heavy clothing and leather gloves if contact with *Rhus* species is unavoidable. The use of silicone base cream appears to give some protection. Avoid touching animals that have been in contact with *Rhus* species. Clean the skin thoroughly with strong soap and water immediately after contact.

Desensitization of hypersensitive individuals may be attempted with commercially available antigens. The use of alum-precipitated antigen is apparently completely ineffective. Do not ingest the plant in an attempt to achieve immunity.

## Treatment

*Emergency measures* (must be done within minutes to be effective)

Remove skin contamination by thorough washing with strong laundry soap and water. Remove ingested poison by gastric lavage or emesis followed by saline catharsis (see pp. 29–32).

*General measures*

(1) Treat the exudative stage by exposure to air or, if the irritation is severe, with mild wet dressings such as aluminum acetate, 1%, or potassium permanganate, 1:10 000.
(2) In severe generalized reactions to poison ivy, systemic administration of cortisone or related steroids will relieve symptoms but will not shorten the course of the disease. The dosage of cortisone is 25–100 mg orally every 6 h.
(3) Give starch or oatmeal baths to allay itching.
(4) Give 2–4 liters of fluids daily if urinary output is normal.
(5) Launder or expose clothing to air and sunlight for 48 h.

*Special problems*

Treat anuria (see p. 66).

## Prognosis

Recovery is usually complete in 2–3 weeks.

## References

Cohen LM, Cohen JL. Erythema multiforme associated with contact dermatitis to poison ivy: three cases and a review of the literature. *Cutis* 1998;62:139

Fisher AA. Poison ivy/oak dermatitis. Part 1: Prevention – soap and water, topical barriers, hyposensitization. *Cutis* 1996;57:384

Lee NP, Arriola ER. Poison ivy, oak, and sumac dermatitis. *West J Med* 1999;171: 354

Stibish AS, *et al*. Cost-effective post-exposure prevention of poison ivy dermatitis. *Int J Dermatol* 2000;39:515

## VERATRUM AND ZYGADENUS

False hellebore (*Veratrum alba*, *Veratrum viride*, or *Veratrum californicum*) is widely distributed in the northern temperate zone; the death camas (*Zygadenus venenosus*) grows in the north-west USA. Both are members of the lily family. A number of cases of poisoning have been reported recently, but fatalities are rare. The fatal dose of the fresh plant may be as small as 1 g.

*Veratrum* and *Zygadenus* species contain nitrogenous compounds which slow the heart rate and lower blood pressure by a vagus reflex that originates in receptors in the heart and lungs. Larger doses raise the blood pressure by a direct effect on the vasomotor center in the brain.

## Clinical findings

The principal manifestations of poisoning with these plants are vomiting and fall in blood pressure.

### *Acute poisoning* (from ingestion)

Nausea, severe vomiting, diarrhea, muscular weakness, visual disturbances, slow pulse (down to 30 or below), and low blood pressure (50 mmHg systolic or less). With excessive amounts the blood pressure may rise to 200 mmHg or higher accompanied by a rapid, thready pulse. Use of *Veratrum* alkaloids in high doses medicinally has caused myotonia, muscular spasms, and neuropathy.

*Chronic poisoning*

Repeated ingestion of small doses may produce tolerance to the blood pressure lowering effect but apparently not to the blood pressure raising effect.

**Prevention**

Children should be warned to avoid eating strange plants.

**Treatment**

*Acute poisoning*

(1) Emergency measures – Remove ingested poison by gastric lavage or emesis (see pp. 29–32).
(2) General measures – Atropine will block the reflex fall in blood pressure and the bradycardia. Give 0.5–2 mg intravenously; repeat every hour until symptoms are controlled. If hypertension is present give sympathetic blocking agents, e.g. phentolamine hydrochloride (Regitine), 5–10 mg intravenously, or hydralazine, 10–20 mg intramuscularly.

*Chronic poisoning*

Discontinue the use of *Veratrum* drugs.

**Prognosis**

If atropine can be given, recovery is likely.

**Table 36.2** Additional poisonous plants

| Name | Poisonous part of plant, and active principle if known | Clinical findings | Treatment |
|---|---|---|---|
| Baneberry (*Actaea* species) | All parts | Nausea, vomiting, diarrhea, shock | * |
| Betelnut (*Areca catechu*) | Seed (arecoline) | Vomiting, diarrhea, difficult breathing, impaired vision, convulsions | *Give atropine, 2 mg subcut.; repeat as necessary |
| Bird of paradise (*Caesalpinia gilliesii*, *Poinciana* species) | Seed pod | Nausea, vomiting, diarrhea | *Give milk, beaten eggs, liquid petrolatum; replace fluids |
| Bleeding heart (*Dicentra* species) | All parts (alkaloids) | Ataxia, respiratory depression, convulsions | * |
| Bloodroot (*Sanguinaria* species) | All parts (sanguinarine) | Vomiting, diarrhea, shock, coma | * |
| Boxwood (*Buxus sempervirens*) | Leaves and twigs | Nausea, vomiting, convulsions | * |
| Buckeye, horse chestnut (*Aesculus* species) | Seed (a glycoside) | Nausea, vomiting, weakness, paralysis | * |
| Burning bush (*Euonymus atropurpureus*), spindle tree (*Euonymus europaea*) | Fruit and leaves | Nausea, vomiting, diarrhea, weakness, chills, coma, or convulsions | * |
| Calabar bean (*Physostigma venenosum*) | Bean (physostigmine; see p. 430) | Dizziness, faintness, vomiting, diarrhea, pinpoint pupils | See p. 431 |
| Celandine (*Chelidonium majus*) | All parts (chelidonine) | Nausea, vomiting, coma | * |

*Continued*

*Table 36.2 (continued)*

| Name | Poisonous part of plant, and active principle if known | Clinical findings | Treatment |
|------|------|------|------|
| Cherry (*Prunus* species) | Seed, leaves (amygdalin) | Stupor, vocal cord paralysis, twitching, convulsions, and coma from chewing seeds. See cyanide poisoning (p. 314) | *Treat cyanide poisoning (see p. 315) |
| Chinaberry (*Melia azedarach*) | Fruit and leaves | Nausea, vomiting, diarrhea, paralysis | * |
| Chrysanthemum | All parts (a resin) | Exudative dermatitis from sensitivity | Wash skin |
| Corn cockle (*Agrostemma githago*) | Seeds (githagin) | Nausea, vomiting, respiratory depression | * |
| Crowfoot family: Christmas rose (*Helleborus niger*) | All parts (helleborin and related alkaloids) | Severe gastrointestinal irritation with vomiting and diarrhea | * |
| Crowfoot or buttercup (*Ranunculaceae*) | All parts | | |
| Marsh marigold (*Caltha palustris*) | All parts | | |
| Daffodil (*Narcissus pseudonarcissus*) | Bulb | Nausea, vomiting, diarrhea | * |
| Daphne | All parts | Stomatitis, abdominal pain, vomiting, bloody diarrhea, weakness, convulsions, kidney damage | |

*Continued*

*Table 36.2 (continued)*

| Name | Poisonous part of plant, and active principle if known | Clinical findings | Treatment |
|------|------|------|------|
| Elderberry (*Sambucus* species) | Leaves, shoots, bark, and roots (cyanogenic glycoside) | Dizziness, headache, nausea, vomiting, respiratory stimulation, tachycardia, convulsions | *Treat cyanide poisoning (see p. 315) |
| Finger cherry (*Rhodomyrtus macrocarpa*) | Fruit | Complete and permanent blindness within 24 h | * |
| Glory lily (*Gloriosa superba*) | All parts (gloriosine, colchicine) | Vomiting, diarrhea, fall in blood pressure, alopecia | *Maintain blood pressure, treat as for colchicine (see p. 580) |
| Holly (*Ilex* species) | Berries | Vomiting, diarrhea, narcosis | * |
| Hyacinth | Bulb | Nausea, vomiting | * |
| Hydrangea | All parts (possibly cyanogenic) | Gastroenteritis. Observe for cyanide symptoms | *Treat cyanide poisoning (see p. 315) |
| Indian tobacco (*Lobelia inflata*) | All parts ($\alpha$-lobeline) | Progressive vomiting, weakness, stupor, tremors, pinpoint pupils, unconsciousness (see Nicotine, p. 138) | *Give artificial respiration. Give atropine, 2 mg subcut |
| Iris (*Iridaceae*) | Root | Nausea, violent diarrhea, abdominal burning | * |
| Jessamine (*Gelsemium sempivirens*) | All parts (gelsemine and related alkaloids) | Muscular weakness, convulsions, sweating, respiratory failure | *Give atropine, 2 mg subcut. every 4 h; artificial respiration |
| Jetberry (*Rhodotypos scandens*) | Berries (cyanogenic glycoside) | Like cherry. See Cyanide, p. 314 | See p. 315 |

*Continued*

*Table 36.2 (continued)*

| Name | Poisonous part of plant, and active principle if known | Clinical findings | Treatment |
|------|------|------|------|
| Jute (*Corchorus olitorius, Corchorus capsularis*) | Fibrous stem | Asthmatic attacks, rhinitis from sensitivity | Avoid further exposure |
| Laburnum, golden chain (*Laburnum anagyroides*), Kentucky coffee berry (*Gymnocladus dioica*) | Leaves, pod, and seeds (cytisine) | Burning in the mouth and abdomen, nausea, severe vomiting, diarrhea, prostration, irregular pulse and respiration, delirium, twitching, unconsciousness. Renal damage may occur | * |
| Lantana (*Lantana camara*) | All parts (lantanin) | Photosensitization with great increase in injury from sunlight | Avoid sunlight |
| | Green fruit | Vomiting, lethargy, cyanosis, coma, dilated pupils, slowed respiration | *Administer $O_2$ |
| Laurel (*Kalmia* species) | All parts (andromedotoxin) | Salivation, increased tear formation, nasal discharge, vomiting, convulsions, slow pulse, low blood pressure, paralysis | Treat as for veratrum (see p. 631) |
| Lily-of-the-valley (*Convallaria* species) | All parts (digitalis-like) | See Digitalis, p. 459 | See p. 460 |
| Locust (*Robinia pseudoacacia*) | Seed (robin) | Same as for castor bean, p. 617 | Same as for castor bean, see p. 618 |
| Lupin, lupine (*Lupinus* species) | All parts but especially in berries (lupinine and related alkaloids) | Paralysis, weak pulse, depressed breathing, convulsions | *Give artificial respiration, treat convulsions (see p. 60) |

*Continued*

*Table 36.2 (continued)*

| Name | Poisonous part of plant, and active principle if known | Clinical findings | Treatment |
|---|---|---|---|
| Manchineel (*Hippomane mancinella*) | Sap | Severe irritation, blistering, peeling of skin from contact with the sap | Wash with soap and water or alcohol |
| Mango (*Mangifera indica*) | Skin of fruit and sap of tree | Dermatitis, nausea, vomiting, diarrhea | Do not eat the peel, and avoid contact with the sap |
| Mexican poppy (*Argemone mexicana*) | Leaves and seeds (alkaloids) | Vomiting, diarrhea, cardiac and visual effects | * |
| Mistletoe (*Phoradendron flavescens*) | All parts but especially in berries | Vomiting, diarrhea, and slowed pulse similar to digitalis (see p. 459) | Treat as for digitalis (see p. 460) |
| Moonseed (*Menispermum canadense*) | Fruit (alkaloid) | Nausea, vomiting, mechanical injury | * |
| Nutmeg (*Myristica fragrans*) | Seeds (myristicin) | Hallucinations, delirium, convulsions | * |
| Physic nut (*Jatropha* species) | Seed | Nausea, vomiting, bloody diarrhea, unconsciousness | * |
| Poinsettia (*Euphorbia pulcherrima*) | Leaves, stems, sap | Irritation, vesication, gastroenteritis | *Wash sap from skin with soap and water |
| Primrose (*Primula* species) | Stems and leaves (primin) | Skin reddening and irritation, itching, swelling, and blistering on contact with the plant | Wash skin with rubbing alcohol after handling the plant |
| Privet (*Ligustrum vulgare*) | Berries and leaves | Gastrointestinal irritation and renal damage, fall in blood pressure | *Treat as for veratrum (see p. 631) |

*Continued*

*Table 36.2 (continued)*

| Name | Poisonous part of plant, and active principle if known | Clinical findings | Treatment |
|------|------|------|------|
| Rayless goldenrod (*Aplopappus heterophyllus*), snakeroot (*Eupatorium rugosum*) | All parts (tremetol) | Drinking milk from animals that have been fed on white snakeroot or rayless goldenrod causes nausea, loss of appetite, weakness, severe vomiting, jaundice from liver damage, constipation, and convulsions. There may be oliguria or anuria from kidney damage | Treat liver damage (see p. 76): treat anuria (see p. 66) |
| Rhododendron | All parts (andromedotoxin) | Salivation, increased tear formation, nasal discharge, vomiting, convulsions, slowing of the pulse, lowering of blood pressure, paralysis | *Treat as for veratrum (see p. 631) |
| Sweet pea (*Lathyrus* species) | All parts but especially seeds | Paralysis, weak pulse, depressed breathing, convulsions | *Give artificial respiration; treat convulsions (see p. 60) |
| Tung nut (*Aleurites fordii*) | Seed (a sapotoxin) | Nausea, vomiting, abdominal pain, weakness, fall in blood pressure, shallow respiration | * |
| Wisteria | All parts. | Gastric upset, vomiting | * |
| Yellow oleander (*Thevetia* species) | All parts (digitalis-like) | See Digitalis, p. 459 | See p. 460 |

*Remove ingested poison by activated charcoal, gastric lavage, or emesis, and treat symptoms

## References

Chang S-S, *et al*. Poisoning by *Datura* leaves used as edible wild vegetables. *Vet Human Toxicol* 1999;41:242

Eray O, *et al*. Severe uvular angioedema caused by intranasal administration of *Ecbalium elaterium*. *Vet Human Toxicol* 1999;41:376

Heath KB. A fatal case of apparent water hemlock poisoning. *Vet Human Toxicol* 2001;43:35

Hung D-Z, Deng J-F. Acute myocardial infarction temporally related to betel nut chewing. *Vet Human Toxicol* 1998;40:25

Ko RJ. Causes, epidemiology, and clinical evaluation of suspected herbal poisoning. *J Toxicol Clin Toxicol* 1999;37:697

Krenzelok EP, *et al*. American mistletoe exposures. *Am J Emerg Med* 1997;15: 516

Krenzelok EP, *et al*. Is the yew really poisonous to you? *J Toxicol Clin Toxicol* 1998;36:219

Lin T-J, *et al*. Calcium oxalate is the main toxic component in clinical presentations of *Alocasis Macrorrhiza* (l) Schott and Endl poisonings. *Vet Human Toxicol* 1998;40:93

Lin T-J, *et al*. Two outbreaks of acute tung nut (*Aleurites fordii*) poisoning. *J Toxicol Clin Toxicol* 1996;34:87

McGrath-Hill CA, Vicas IM. Case series of *Thermopsis* exposures. *J Toxicol Clin Toxicol* 1996;35:659

Mellick LB, *et al*. Neuromuscular blockade after ingestion of tree tobacco (*Nicotiana glauca*). *Ann Emerg Med* 1999;34:101

Pedaci L, *et al*. *Dieffenbachia* species exposures: an evidence-based assessment of symptom presentation. *Vet Human Toxicol* 1999;41:335

Raikhlin-Eisenkraft B, Bentur Y. *Ecbalium elaterium* (squirting cucumber) – remedy or poison. *J Toxicol Clin Toxicol* 2000;38:305

Schneider F, *et al*. Plasma and urine concentrations of atropine after the ingestion of cooked deadly nightshade berries. *J Toxicol Clin Toxicol* 1996;34:113

Tanner TL. *Rhus* (*Toxicodendron*) dermatitis. *Primary Care* 2000;27:493

Wu C-L, *et al*. Lung injury related to consuming *Sauropus androgynus* vegetable. *J Toxicol Clin Toxicol* 1996;35:241

Wu K-D, *et al*. The milk-alkali syndrome caused by betel nuts in oyster shell paste. *J Toxicol Clin Toxicol* 1996;34:741

# Index*

*Cross-references in the index are sometimes to synonymous or chemically similar substances that cause the same toxic manifestations. Treat poisoning as for poisoning due to the substance referred to. For mixtures, the approximate concentration of active ingredient is given in square brackets.

First-aid measures in poisoning. See inside front cover.

10-80 *see* Fluoroacetate 137
A-Rest 160
Aagrano *see* Mercury 294
Aaron's Grease Cleaner *see* Potassium
   hydroxide [9%] 211
Aatrex 152
Abacavir 500
Abamectin 147
Abate 124
Abbokinase 477
Abciximab 477
Abdominal distension 69
Abrasives 328
Abrin 617
*Abrus precatorius*, jequirity bean 616
Absinthe 536
Acacia dust *see* Wood dust 340
Acarbose, interactions 550
Acarol 110
Accolate 567
Accupril *see* Quinapril 477
Accutane 565
ACE inhibitors, congestive heart failure
   59
Acebutolol 435, 441, 482
ACEI 477
Acenaphthalene *see* Naphthalene 234
Acenaphthylene *see* Polycyclic aromatic
   hydrocarbons 236
Acenocoumarol 482
Aceon *see* perindopril 477
Acephate 124
Acetal 224
Acetaldehyde 219
Acetamide 164

Acetaminophen 373
   interactions 378, 550
Acetarsone 271
Acetazolamide 478, 482
Acetic acid 243
Acetic anhydride 243
Acetoarsenite *see* Arsenic 270
Acetohexamide 550, 552
Acetohydroxamic acid 565
Acetomeroctol 295
Acetone 224
Acetone cyanohydrin 312
Acetonitrile 312
Acetophenetidin 373
Acetophenetidin *see* Phenacetin
Acetophenone 224
Acetyl chloride 243
*N*-Acetyl-*p*-aminophenol *see* Phenacetin 373
2-Acetylaminofluorene 164
Acetylarsan *see* Arsenic 270
Acetylcholine 430, 431
Acetylcysteine 375
Acetyldigitoxin *see* Digitalis 459
Acetylene 238
Acetylene dichloride *see* 1,2-
   Dichloroethane 185
Acetylene tetrabromide *see* Tetrabromoethane
   198
Acetylenetetrachloride *see*
   Tetrachloroethane 178
Acetylsalicylic acid 367
Acidosis 71
Acid(s)
   corrosive 240, 242, 243
   *see also specific types*

639

Acifluorfen 110
Acitretin 565
Acme Kwik Slik No.420 *see* Toluene 231
Acne medication *see* Ethanol [40%] 202
Aconite 538
Aconitine 538
*Aconitum* 538
Acrex 135
Acridine 164
Acrivastine 433
Acrolein 224, 236
Acrylamide 164
Acrylic acid 243
Acrylonitrile 311, 312
*Actaea* sp 570, 632
ACTH *see* Corticotropin 547
Actidil 402
Actidione 153
Actigall 569
Actinex 567
Activase 477
Actonel 565
Actos 550
Actril 110
*N*-Actylcysteine, as antidote 626
Acyclovir 500
Adagen 568
Adanon 398
Adapalene 565
Adder, bites 593
Addiction 49
    ethanol 204
    narcotic 399
Adefovir 500
Adenosine phosphate 565
Adhesive, instant *see* Methyl-two-
    cyanoacrylate 312
*Adkistrodon*, moccasin snake 588
Adrenal cortex hormones 547
Adrenal steroids, interactions 552
Adrenalin *see* Epinephrine 425
Advantage 126
Aerocase *see* Cyanide 311
Aerosol propellant 191
*Aesculus* sp 632
*Aethusa cynapium*, dog parsley 622, 623
Afcophene *see* Toxaphene 115
Aflix 124
Afrinol 426
After-shave lotion *see*
    Ethanol [50%] 202
    Isopropyl alcohol 214
Afugan 125
AGE *see* Allyl glycidyl ether 225

Agenerase 500
Aggrastat 477
*Agkistrodon* sp 588
    bites 590, 591
Agoral *see* Phenolphthalein 545
Agranulocytosis 79
Agricultural poisoning, prevention 6
Agricultural poisons **107–160**
Agrosan *see* Phenyl mercury 295
*Agrostemma githago*, corn cockle 633
Agrothion 124
Agrox *see* Organic mercury [2%] 294
Agrylin 477
Air pollution 16, 236, 247, 252, 255, 320, 327
Airway management 52
    equipment 54
Ajmaline 482
Akee 615
Akineton 422
Alachlor 155
Alamast 568
Alanap 151
Alanycarb 126
Alar 160
Albendazole 500
Albenza 500
Albuterol 426, 441
Alclometasone *see* Corticosteroids 547
Alcoholic beverages 202
Alcohol(s) **199–215**
Aldactone 479
Aldara 567
Aldehydes 224, 236
Aldesleukin 576
Aldicarb 126
Aldol *see* Paraldehyde 219
Aldomet 433
Aldoxycarb 126
Aldrin 119
Alendronate 565
*Aleurites fordii*, tung nut 637
Alfenta 398
Alfentanil 398, 420
Algin 347
Alglucerase 567
Aliene 124
Aliphatic hydrocarbons 228
Alitretinoin 565
Alival *see* Iodine 445
Alkalis 257
Alkavervir *see* Veratrum 630
Alkeran 578
Alkron *see* Parathion 123
Alkyl sodium sulfate 358

Alkylquaternary ammonium salts *see* Cationic
   detergents 452
Allantoin 347
Allegra 402
Allethrin 158
Allopurinol 565, 582
   interactions 481, 505, 581
Alloxydim 151
Alltox *see* Toxaphene 115
Allyl alcohol 213
Allyl barbiturates, interactions 415
Allyl bromide 196
Allyl chloride 196
Allyl glycidyl ether 225
Allyl-isothiocyanate *see* Oil of mustard 539
Allylpropyl disulfide 317
Allyxycarb 126
Almond(s), bitter, oil of 311, 536
*Alocasia* 621
Aloe 545
Aloin 545
Alphagan 426
Alprazolam 411, 420
Alprostadil 553
Alsystin 110
Altace *see* Ramipril 477
Alteplase 477
Altretamine 576
Alum *see* Potassium alum 533
Alumi-Glo *see* Fluoride [4%] 263
Aluminum acetate 533
Aluminum alkyls 338
Aluminum ammonium sulfate *see* Aluminum
   salts 533
Aluminum Brite *see* Fluoride [2%] 263
Aluminum chloride 533
Aluminum cleaner *see* Hydrofluoric acid
   [6%] 263
Aluminum hydroxide 347, 534, 565
Aluminum oxide 338
Aluminum powder 338
Aluminum pyro powder 338
Aluminum salts 533
Aluminum sodium sulfate *see* Aluminum
   salts 533
Aluminum subacetate 533
Aluminum sulfide *see* Hydrogen sulfide 316
Aluminum welding fumes 338
Alupent 426
*Amanita* sp 624, 625
   *A. muscaria* 529, 624, 625
Amanitin 624
Amantadine 500, 506
Amaryl 550

Amaryllis *see* Colchicine 579
Amatoxin 624
Amaze 124
Ambien 412
*Amblyomma americanum* 608
Ambush 159
Amcinonide *see* Corticosteroids 547
American lance-headed vipers 588
Ametryn 151
Amex 135, 160
Amiben 110
Amicar 565
Amidate 411
Amidosulfonic acid *see* Sulfamic acid 243
Amifostine 576
Amikacin 490, 506
Amikin 490
Amiloride 477, 479
1-Amino-2-propanol 164
3-Amino-9-ethylcarbazole 164
2-Aminoanthraquinone 164
*p*-Aminobenzoic acid 565
2-Aminobutane 258
Aminocaproic acid 565
4-Aminodiphenyl 164
Aminoglutethimide 553
Aminoglycosides 490
   interactions 415, 505
*p*-Aminohippurate 575
Aminolevulinic acid 565
*p*-Aminophenol 164
Aminophylline 510, 511
2-Aminopropane 258
2-Aminopyridine 164
4-Aminopyridine 164
Aminopyridines 164
Aminopyrine 377
   interactions 378, 508
5-Aminosalicylic acid 500
*p*-Aminosalicylic acid, interactions 481, 505
2-Aminothiazole 164
3-Amino1,2,4-triazol 151
Amiodarone 477, 482
Amipaque 575
Amitraz 158
Amitriptyline 518, 519, 530
   interactions 521
Amitrole 151
Amlexanox 565
Amlodipine 473
Ammate 157
Ammonia 261
Ammonia water *see* Ammonium
   hydroxide 261

Ammoniated mercury 295
Ammonium alum 533
Ammonium bromide 408
Ammonium chloride 477
Ammonium hydroxide 261
Ammonium persulfate 256
Ammonium sulfamate *see* Sulfamate 157
Ammonium sulfhydrate *see* Hydrogen
   sulfide 316
Ammonium tetrachlorozincate *see* Zinc
   salts 533
Ammonium thioglycolate *see*
   Thioglycolates 345
Amobarbital 392, 420
Amodrine *see* Aminophylline [100 mg] 510
Amosite 331
Amoxapine 518, 519
Amoxicillin 489, 506
Amphetamine 425, 426, 441
Amphotericin B 491, 506
   interactions 416, 482
Ampicillin 489, 506
Amprenavir 500
Amrinone 477
Amygdalin 311
Amyl acetate 226
Amyl alcohol 213
Amyl nitrite 467
Amyl phenol 449
Amylene hydrate *see* Amyl alcohol 213
Amytal 392
Anabasine 138
Anabolic steroids 533
   interactions 481, 552
Anacin *see* Aspirin [400 mg] 367
Anafranil 518
Anagrelide 477
Analgemul *see* Methyl salicylate [10%] 367
Analgesic tablets, compound *see* Aspirin 367
Analgesic(s) and antipyretics **367–378**
*Anamirta cocculus* 516
Anastrozole 576
Ancef 493
Ancobon 501
Ancymidol 160
*Androctonus australis* 605
Androgens 553
Anectine 414
Anesthetics **379–389**
   interactions 388
      anti-infective drugs 505
      antidepressants 522
      autonomic nervous system drugs 440
      cardiovascular drugs 481-482

depressants 415
      endocrine drugs 552
Anethole *see* Volatile oils [10%] 536
Angel dust *see* Phencyclidine 527
*Angelica sinesis* 570
Angiomax 477
Angiotensin II receptor blockers 478
Angiotensin-converting enzyme inhibitors 477
Angostura *see* Quinine [1%] 497
Anilazine 154
Aniline 163, 164
Anilofos 124
Animal and plant hazards **585–638**
Animal tranquilizer *see* Phencyclidine 527
Anise 536
Anisic acid *see* Benzoic acid 458
Anisidine, *o-* or *p-* 164
Anistreplase 477
Annmonium sulfide 316
Anoxia *see* Hypoxia 52
Ansaid 377
Anspor 493
Ant control *see*
      Boric acid [2%] 442
      Chlorpyrifos [1%] 124
Ant-Not *see* Thallium [2%] 140
Ant-Stop *see* Thallium [2%] 140
Antabuse 556
Anthio 124
Anthiomaline *see* Antimony 269
Anthophyllite 331
Anthra-derm 458, 539
Anthralin 458, 539
9,10-Anthraquinone 151
Anti-inflammatory agents, non steroidal **367–378**
Anti-rust
      auto radiator *see* Sodium nitrite [10%] 467
      liquid *see* Kerosene [10%] 228
      *see also* Oxalic acid [30%] 240
Antibiotics 488
Anticancer agents 575
Anticoagulants 469
      interactions 482
         coumarin 521
Anticonvulsants 62, 390, **508–531**
Antidepressants **508–532**
      interactions 203, 415, 481
      polycyclic 518
      toxicity, drug interactions 521
      triazolopyridine 518
      tricyclic, interactions 440
Antidiabetic drugs 550
Antiepileptic agents 390, 393

Antifreeze *see* Ethylene glycol 209
Antifungals 491
Antihistamines 402
    interactions 203, 415, 440, 508
Antihypertensives, interactions 440, 481
Antilirium 95
    *see also* Physostigmine 431
Antimanics **508–531**
Antimony 269
Antimony pentasulfide *see* Sulfides 316
Antimony potassium tartrate 269
Antineoplastic agents 575
Antioxidants **366**
Antipyrine 377
Antiseptics 217, **442–458**
    Mercury 295
    *see also* Formaldehyde 217
Antithyroid drugs 547
Antivenoms *see* Antisera 596
Antracol 557
Antrol Ant Killer *see* Boric acid [2%] 442
ANTU 151
Anturane 485
Anzemet 411
Apamide *see* Acetaminophen 373
APC *see* Aspirin [200 mg] 367
Aphthasol 565
Apinol *see* Volatile oils 536
Apiol 536
Aplastic anemia 79
*Aplopappus heterophyllus*, rayless
    goldenrod 637
Apocodeine *see* Apomorphine 398
Apomorphine 398
Appetite suppressant *see* Methamphetamine
    [15 mg] 426
Applaud 158
Apple extract, ferreted *see* Ironsalts 559
Apraclonidine 426
Apresoline 471
Aprocarb *see* Baygon 126
Aprotinin 565
Aquari-Sol *see* Silver salts [0.5%] 455
Aquarium products 359
Aquathol *see* Endothall [20%] 154
Arachnids and insects **601–609**
Aralen phosphate *see* Chloroquine 497
Aramine 426
Arava 567
ARBS 478
*Arctium* 570
*Arctostaphylos* 570
Ardeparin 469
Arduan 414

*Areca catechu*, betelnut 632
Aredia 565
Aresin 155
Aretit *see* Dinoseb 135
*Argemone mexicana*, Mexican poppy 636
Argentic fluoride *see* Fluoride 263
Arginine 565
Argyrol *see* Silver proteinate 455
Aricept 431
Arimidex 576
*Arisaema triphyllum* 621
Arnica 539
Arochlor 189
Aromasin 577
Aromatic compounds 39
Aromatic hydrocarbon(s) 231
Aromatic naptha *see* Benzene 231
Aromatic solvent *see* Benzene 231
Arrestin Cough Medicine *see*
    Dextromethorphan [0.2%] 398
Arsacetin *see* Arsenic 270
Arsan *see* Arsenic 270
Arsanilic acid *see* Arsenic 270
Arsenal 151
Arsenamide *see* Arsenic 270
Arsenate 271
Arsenic 38, 270
Arsenic acid 271
Arsenic trioxide 271
Arsenite 271
Arsine 270
Arsinic-arsonic acid *see* Arsenic 270
Arsphenamine 271
Arsthinol *see* Arsenic 270
Artane 422
*Artemesia absinthum* 571
Artificial respiration 7
    methods 53
Artificial Smoke *see* Volatile oils [50%] 536
Arum family 621
Arylam *see* Carbaryl 126
ASA *see* Aspirin 367
ASA Compound *see* Phenacetin 373
Asafetida *see* Volatile oils 536
Asarum *see* Volatile oils 536
Asbestos 39, 331
Asbestosis 332
Asendin 518
Asian cobra 588
Asparaginase 576
Aspergum *see* Aspirin 367
Asphalt fumes 338
Aspirin 367
    interactions 378, 521, 552

Aspirjen Jr *see* Aspirin [100 mg] 367
Astelin 402
Asthma remedies *see* Aminophylline 510
Astimizole 402
Astringent *see* Aluminum salts 533
Astringent lotion *see* Ethanol [50%] 202
Asulam 151
Asulox 151
Atabrine 497
Atacard 478
Atarax 402
Atenolol 435, 441
Ativan 412
Atlas A *see* Arsenic [25%] 270
Atmospheric particulates **327–340**
Atorvastatin 478
Atovaquone 500
Atracurium 414
*Atrax robustus*, funnel-web spider 604
Atrazine 152
Atridazole 154
Atrinol 160
Atromid-S 478
*Atropa belladonna* 422
Atropine 422, 441, 461
    as antidote 84, 130, 626
    interactions 440, 482
Atropine-like compounds, interactions 440
Atrovent 422
Aureomycin 489
Aurothioglucose 377
Auto corrosion inhibitor *see* Bichromate
    [1%] 280
Auto polish *see* Kerosene [50%] 228
Avadex BW 557
Avandia 550
Avapro 478
Avelox 493
Avenge 145
Aventyl 518
Avermectins 147
Avitrol *see* 4-Aminopyridine 164
Axid 433
Azacyclotin 158
Azathioprine 576, 582
    interactions 581
Azelastine 402
Azide
    sodium 152
        *see also* Hydrazoic acid 166, 243
Azinphos 124
Azinphos-ethyl 124
Azinphos-methyl 124
Azithromycin 491

Azobenzene 164
Azodrin 124
Azoles 491
Azopt 478
Aztreonam 493
Azulfidine 485

Baam 158
Baby oil *see* Mineral oil 545
Baby powder *see*
    Boric acid [5%] 442
    Silica 328
Bacampicillin 489
Bachmann Styrene Solvent *see* 1,1,1-
    Trichloroethane 181
*Bacillis cereus*, food poisoning 350, 351
*Bacillis subtilis*, enzymes 307
Bacitracin 491
Baclofen 411, 420
Bacterial food poisoning 350
Bactine *see* Ethanol [17%] 202
Bactrim 486
Bagasse *see* Sugar cane dust 339
Bagassosis *see* Sugar cane dust 339
Baking powder 359
Baking soda 359
BAL (dimercaprol) 87
Balan 152
Balarsen *see* Arsenic 270
Balata *see* Sugar cane dust 339
Banana oil *see* Amyl acetate 226
Bancol 158
Baneberry 632
*Banisteria caapi* 529
Banthine 422
Bantrol 110
Bantron *see* Lobeline [0.2 mg] 138
Banvel 110
Bap 160
Barba amarilla snake 588
Barbital 392, 420
Barbiturates 392
    interactions 482, 508
Barekil *see* Nicotine [40%] 138
Barium 133
Barium sulfate 133, 338
Barnon 110
Barracuda 611
Barytes 338
Basagran 152
Basalin 154
Basiliximab 565
Basitac 155
Bath salts *see* Borax [10%] 442

Batteries, button *see* Alkalis 257
Battery boxes *see* Lead 282
Battery electrolyte *see* Sulfuric acid [33%] 255
Bauxite 338
Baycol 478
Baycor 152
Baygon 126
Bayleton 157
Bayluscid 160
Bayrusil 125
Baytan 158
Baytex 124
Baythion 125, 126
Baythroid 158
BBC 193
BCG vaccine 576
1,4-BD 529
Beacon All-Brands Wax Remover *see* Ethanolamine [12%] 258
Beaked sea snake 589
Becaplermin 553
Beclomethasone *see* Corticosteroids 441
Bee sting 608
Belladonna 422
Ben-Gay Lotion *see* Methyl salicylate [30%] 367
Benadryl 87, 402, 494
Benalaxyl 152
Benazepryl 477
Benazolin 152
Bendiocarb 126
Benefin 152
Benemid 480
Benfuracarb 126
Benlate 126
Benodanil 152
Benomyl 126
Benoxinate 382
Bensulide 124
Bensultap 158
Bentazone 152
Benthiocarb 557
Bentyl 422
Benzabor *see* Borate 442
Benzalchloride 243
Benzaldehyde 224
Benzalkonium chloride 452
2-Benzanilide 152
Benzedrine 426
Benzene 39, 228, 231
Benzene hexachloride 113
Benzethonium chloride 452
Benzidine 164

Benzine 228
Benzo(α)pyrene 238
Benzocaine 382
Benzoic acid 458
Benzol *see* Benzene 231
Benzomate 158
Benzonatate 411
Benzonitrile 312
Benzoquinone 224
Benzoxinate 158
Benzoyl chloride 196, 243
Benzoyl peroxide 225, 243
Benzpyrinium 430
Benztropine 422
Benztropine mesylate 84
Benzyl acetate *see* Benzyl alcohol 382
Benzyl alcohol 382
Benzyl benzoate 458
Benzyl bromide *see* Benzyl chloride 196
Benzyl chloride 196, 243
Benzyl chlorophenol 449
Benzyl penicilloyl polylysine 489
Benzylamine *see* Diethylamine 258
6-Benzylaminopurine 160
Benzylcyanide 312
Benzylhydroquinone 449
Benzylmorphine hydrochloride *see* Morphine 398
Benzylpenicillin 506
Benzyltrichloride 243
Bepridil 473
Beractant 565
Berylliosis 275
Beryllium 275
Best's Roach Killer *see* Boric acid 442
Beta-blocking agents 435
    congestive heart failure 59
    interactions 378, 440
Betagan 435
Betaine hydrochloride 565
Betamethasone *see* Corticosteroids 441
Betanal 156
Betanex 126
Betapace 435, 481
Betasan 124
Betaxolol 435, 441
Betelnut 632
Bethanechol 430, 431
Bethanidine 441
    interactions 521
Bexarotene 576
Bexton 156
BGE *see* Butyl glycidyl ether 225
BHC *see* Benzene hexachloride 113

BHT 448
Bi-Cal *see* Mercury salts 294
Bicalutamide 576
Bichloride *see* Mercury 294
Bichromate 280
Bidrin 124
Bifenox 117
Bifluoride *see* Fluoride 263
Biguanides 550
Bilirubin, and vitamin K 581
Bilopaque 575
Biltricide 502
Bim 158
Bin Fume *see*
    Carbon tetrachloride [65%] 172
    Ethylene dichloride [30%] 185
Binapacryl 135
Biozyme-C 566
Biperiden 422
Biphenyl 238
    polychlorinated and polybrominated 188
4-Biphenylamine *see* 4-Aminodiphenyl 164
Birch oil *see* Volatile oils 536
Bird of paradise 632
Birlane 124
Bisacodyl 545
Bis(2-chlorethoxy)methane 196
Bis(2-chlorethyl)sulfide 196
Bis(2-chloroisopropyl)ether 196
Bis(chloromethyl)ether 196
Bis(diethoxyphosphinothioylthio) methane 124
Bis(diethylthiocarbamoyl)disulfide *see* Disulfiram 556
Bishydroxycoumarin 469
Bismuth 506
Bismuth subnitrate 467
Bismuth subsalicylate 500
Bismuth telluride 307
Bisoprolol 435, 441
Bitertanol 152
*Bitis arietans*
    bites 593
    puff adder 589
Bitolterol 426
Bitter almonds, oil of 311, 536
Bivalirudin 477
Black cohosh 570
Black nightshade 621
Black widow spider 601
Bladafume 125
Bladderwrack 570
Bladex 152
Blasticidin-S 152

Blazer 110
Bleach(es)
    powdered 359
    *see also*
        Oxalates 240
        Sodium hypochlorite 356
Bleaching solutions 356
Bleeding heart 632
Blenoxane 576
Bleomycin 576
    interactions 581
*Blighia sapida*, akee 615
Blocadren 435
Blocking agents
    histamine 433
    miscellaneous 432
    sympathetic 433
Blood dyscrasias 79
Bloodroot 632
Blue Blazes *see* Copper sulfate 533
Blue nightshade 621
Blue Nitro 411
Blue Ribbon Hand Cleaner *see* Kerosene [50%] 228
Blue Streak Roach Killer *see* Fluoride [63%] 264
Blue vitriol *see* Copper sulfate 533
Body freshener *see* Ethanol [65%] 202
Bol-Maid *see* Hydrochloric acid [8%] 243
Bol-Shine *see* Hydrochloric acid [23%] 243
Bolero 557
*Boletus* sp 625
Bolstar 125
Bonamine *see* Meclizine 402
Bone oil 164
Bonide Ant Killer *see* Diazinon, [1%] 124
Bonine 402
Borascu *see* Borate 442
Borate 442
Borateem *see* Borax 442
Borax 442
Boraxo *see* Borax 442
Bordeaux mixture *see* Copper salts 533
Boric acid 442
Borneol *see* Camphor 515
Bornyl compounds *see* Volatile oils 536
Borocil *see* Borate 442
Boroglycerine *see* Boric acid [25%] 442
Borolin *see* Borate [95%] 442
Boron derivatives 442
Boron oxide 442
Boron tribromide 442
Boron trifluoride 264
Boron trioxide *see* Boric acid 442

*Bothrops* sp 588
  bites 590, 591
Botulin antitoxin 85
Botulinus toxin 348
Botulism 348
Bowes Seal Fast Tube Repair *see* Benzene [95%] 231
Bowl cleaners *see* Hydrochloric acid 243
Boxwood 632
Boxwood dust *see* Wood dust 340
Boyer Brass and Copper Polish *see* Mineral spirits 228
Boyer Drain Opener *see* Sodium hydroxide 257
BPMC 126
Brake fluid *see* Ethylene glycol 209
Brass *see* Lead 282
Bravo 110
Brawn *see* Phosphoric acid [20%] 243
Bretylium 433, 441
Bretylol 433
Brevibloc 435
Brevital 392
Bric-Nu *see* Hydrochloric acid [6%] 243
Bricanyl 426
Brimonidine 426
Brinzolamide 478
Brodifacoum 469
Bromacil 152
Bromadiolone 469
Bromate 343
Bromazil 110
Bromic acid *see* Hydrochloric acid 243
Bromide 408, 420
Brominal 152
Bromine 243
Bromine pentafluoride 264
Bromisovalum 408
Bromo-Seltzer 408
  *see also* Acetaminophen [325 mg] 373
Bromoacetone 196
*p*-Bromoaniline *see* Aniline 163
Bromobenzene *see* Chlorobenzene 196
Bromobenzyl cyanide 193, 312
Bromocriptine 437, 441
Bromodichloromethane 196
Bromofenoxim 152
Bromoform 196
Bromofume *see* Ethylene dichloride 185
Bromopropylate 110
Bromoxynil 152
Brompheniramine 402, 420
Bromural 408
Bronkaid tablets *see* Ephedrine [24 mg] 426

Bronkosol 426
Bronopol 152
Bronze-Powder *see* Copper powder [25%] 307
Broot 126
Brown Patch Control *see* Chloronitrobenzenes [24%] 165
Brown recluse spider 603
Brown spider 604
Brucine 513
Brush cleaner, liquid *see* Xylene [60%] 231
Brush Top Spot Remover *see*
  Naphtha [40%] 228
  Trichloroethane [60%] 181
Bryonia 543
*Bryonia alba* 543
Buchu *see* Camphor 515
Buckeye 632
Budesonide *see* Corticosteroids 547
*Bufo marinus* 529
Bufotenine 529
Bumetanide 478, 479
Bumex 478, 479
Bumintest *see*
  Boric acid [56 mg] 442
  Sulfosalicylic acid [400 mg] 243
*Bungarus* sp 588
  bites 592
Bupirimate 152
Bupivacaine 382, 389
Buprenex 398
Buprenorphine 398, 420
Buprofezin 158
Bupropion 518, 520
Burdock 570
Burning bush 632
Burnley Soldering Paste *see* Zinc salts [28%] 533
Burow's solution *see* Aluminum acetate 533
Bushmaster snake 588
BuSpar 411
Buspirone 411
Busulfan 576
Butabarbital 392, 420
Butacarb 126
Butachlor 152
1,3-Butadiene 238
Butalbital 420
Butamiphos 124
Butane 238
1,4-Butanediol 529
Butanone-2 224
Butenafine 500
Butene *see* Butane 238
*Buthacus arenicola* 605

*Buthus occitonus* 605
Butisan-S 155
Butocarboxim 126
Butorphanol 398
Butoxone 117
2-Butoxy ethanol 213
β-Butoxy-β′-thiocyano-diethyl ether *see*
    Lethane 142
Butoxycarboxim 126
Butoxypolypropylene glycol *see*
    Polypropylene glycol 213
Butralin 160
Buttercup 633
Butterfly fish 611
Butyl acetate 226
Butyl acrylate 226
Butyl alcohol 213
Butyl aminobenzoate 382
Butyl carbitol 213
Butyl cellosolve *see* 2-Butoxy ethanol 213
Butyl chloride 196
n-Butyl glycidyl ether 225
Butyl lactate 226
*n*-Butyl nitrite *see* Amyl nitrite 467
*o*-sec-Butyl phenol 449
*p*-tert-Butyl toluene 238
Butylamine 258
Butylate 126, 557
Butylene *see* Ethylene 385
Butylmercaptan 317
Butyrac 117
n-Butyraldehyde *see* Acetaldehyde 219
γ Butyrolactone 529
γ-Butyrolactone 411, 529, 570
n-Butyronitrile 312
*Buxus sempervirens*, boxwood 632

Cabergoline 437
Cacodylic acid 271
Cadminate *see* Cadmium 278
Cadmium 278
Cadusafos 124
*Caesalpinia gilliesii*, bird of paradise 632
Caffeine 510, 511, 530
Calabar bean 632
Calci-Solve *see* Hydrochloric acid [35%] 243
Calcibind 566
Calciferol 571
Calcifidiol 571
Calcimar 553
Calcipotriene 571
Calcitonin 553
Calcitriol 571
Calcium arsenate *see* Arsenic 270

Calcium blockers 473
Calcium carbimide *see* Cyanamide 311
Calcium carbonate 347, 565
Calcium chloride 85, 243
Calcium cyanamide *see* Cyanamide 311
Calcium disodium edetate 88
Calcium gluconate 85
    as antidote 542
Calcium hydroxide 258
Calcium hypochlorite 359
Calcium oxide 258
Calcium phosphate 347
Calcium polysulfide 316
Calendula *see* Volatile oils [1%] 536
Calfactant 565
Calirus 152
Calixin 158
Calla lily 621
Calo-Chlor *see* Mercuric chloride [30%] 294
Calogran *see* Mercury salts 294
Calomel 294
*Caltha palustris*, marsh marigold 633
Cam Kleen *see* Phosphoric acid [22%] 243
Cambogia *see* Gamboge 543
Camphene, chlorinated 115
Campho-Phenique *see*
    Camphor [10%] 515
    Phenol [5%] 448
Camphor 515
Camphorated oil 515
Camphorated tincture of opium 398
Camptosar 577
Cancer, anticancer agents 575
Cancer prevention 13
Candeptin 491
Candesartan 478
Candicidin 491
*Cannabis sativa* 529
*Cantharellus* sp 625
Cantharides *see* Cantharidin 532
Cantharidin 532
*Cantharis vesicatoria* 532
Cantil 422
Cantil snake 588
Caparol 156
Capastat 490
Capecitabine 576
Capoten 477
Capreomycin 490
Caprolactam 165
Caprylates 347
Caprylic alcohol *see* Amyl alcohol 213
Caps (fireworks) *see* Chlorates 453
Capsebon *see* Cadmium [1%] 278

Capsicum 539
Captafol 152
Captan 156
Captopril 477, 482
Carafate 568
Caragard 157
Carbachol 431
Carbam 557
Carbamate pesticides 126
Carbamazepine 393, 420, 525
  interactions 482
Carbamide peroxide 458
Carbaryl 123, 126
Carbendazim 152
Carbendazime 126
Carbenicillin 489, 506
Carbenoxolone, interactions 416, 482
Carbetamide 126, 152
Carbidopa 426
Carbitol 213
Carbocaine 311
Carbofuran 126
Carbolic acid 448
Carbon black 338
Carbon dioxide 307
Carbon disulfide 317
Carbon monoxide 39, 320
Carbon tetrabromide 196
Carbon tetrachloride 39, 172
Carbona Cleaner see Trichloroethylene 179
Carbonic anhydrase inhibitors 478
Carbonyl fluoride 264
Carboplatin 576
Carboprost 553
Carbosulfan 126
Carbowax 347
Carboxin 152
Carbromal 408
Carburetor cleaner see Xylene [45%] 231
Carcinogens 13
Cardiac arrest 59
Cardiazol see Metrazol 516
Cardiorespiratory system, poison diagnosis 45
Cardiovascular drugs **459–484**
Cardizem 473
Cardura 480
Carisoprodol 391
Carmustine 576
Carnitor 567
β-Carotene 566
Carpet backing 359
Cartap 158
Carteolol 435, 441
Carter's Little Pills see Bisacodyl [5 mg] 545

Cartrol 435
Carvacrol 449
Carvedilol 435, 441
Carzol 126
Casanthranol 545
Cascabel, rattlesnake 588
Cascara sagrada 545
Case hardening see Cyanide 311
Cashew nut oil 539
Casodex 576
Casoron 153
Cassava 311
Cassia see Aloe 545
Castor bean 616
Castor oil 545
Castrix 151, 513
Catapres 433
Catechol 449
Catecholamines, interactions 388, 416, 440, 482
Caterpillars 608
Cathartics 30, **541–545**
Caulking compound see Lead 282
Caustic potash see Potassium hydroxide 257
Caustic soda see Sodium hydroxide 257
Ceclor 492
Cedar dust see Wood dust 340
Cedilanid 459
CeeNu 576
Ceepryn 452
Cefaclor 492
Cefadroxil 492
Cefadyl 493
Cefalexin 506
Cefamandole 492
Cefazolin 506
Cefdinir 492
Cefepime 492
Cefixime 492
Cefizox 492
Cefmetazole 492
Cefobid 492
Cefonicid 492
Cefoperazone 492
Cefotaxime 492
Cefotetan 492
Cefoxitin 492
Cefpodoxime 492
Cefprozil 492
Ceftazidime 492
Ceftibuten 492
Ceftizoxime 492
Ceftriaxone 492
Cefuroxime 492

Celandine 632
Celebrex 377
Celecoxib 377
Celexa 523
CellCept 568
Cellosolve acetate *see* 2-Ethoxy ethanol 213
Cellulose sodium phosphate 566
Celontin 393
Celphos *see* Phosphine 301
Cement
    plastic *see* Ethylene dichloride 185
    polystyrene *see* Toluene [20%] 231
    Portland 258
    rubber *see* Benzene [95%] 231
Cenol Roost Paint *see* Nicotine 138
*Centella asiatica* 570
Centipede 608
Central nervous system, poison diagnosis 43
*Centruroides* sp 605
Cephaeline *see* Emetine 495
*Cephaelis ipecacuanha* 495
Cephalexin 492
    *see also* Cefalexin 506
Cephaloridine 506
Cephalosporins 492
    interactions 505
Cephalothin 492, 506
Cephapirin 493, 506
Cephradine 493, 506
Ceramics glaze *see* Lead [20%] 282
Cercobin 157
Cerebyx 393
Ceredase 567
Ceresan 295
Cerezyme 567
Cerium 307
Cerivastatin 478
Cervidil 553
Cesium hydroxide 258
Cetacaine 382
Cetirazine 402
Cetylpyridinium chloride 452
Charcoal
    activated 31
    use 85
Charcoal starter *see* Kerosene [90%] 228
*Chelidonium majus*, celandine 632
Chem-sen *see* Arsenic 270
Chemical food poisoning 355
Chenix 566
Chenodiol 566
Cherry 633
    finger 634
    Jerusalem 622

Child abuse, poisoning in 104
Chinaberry 633
Chiniofon 445
Chinosol 153
*Chironex fleckeri* 614
*Chiropsalmus quadrigatus* 614
Chlomethoxyfen 110
Chlomethoxynil 117
Chlor-Trimeton 402
Chloral hydrate 390, 391, 420
    interactions 481, 482
Chloramben *see* Amiben 110
Chlorambucil 576
Chloramphenicol 490, 506
    interactions 203, 481, 521, 552
Chlorates 453
Chlorax *see* Sodium chlorate 453
Chlorazepate 420
Chlorbufam 126
Chlordane 119
Chlordecone 119
Chlordiazepoxide 411, 420
Chlorethoxyfos 124
Chlorex *see* 2,2′-Dichloroethyl ether 197
Chlorfenvinphos 124
Chlorflurenol 110
Chlorhexidine 458
Chloric acid *see* Hydrochloric acid 243
Chloridazone 153
Chlorinated camphene 115
Chlorinated diphenyl *see* Polychlorinated
    biphenyls 188
Chlorinated diphenyl oxide 189
Chlorinated insecticides
    polycyclic 119
    *see also* Halogenated insecticides 109
Chlorinated lime 359
Chlorinated terpenes 115
Chlorine 243
Chlorine dioxide 243
Chlorine trifluoride 243, 264
Chlormephos 124
Chlormequat 145
Chlormerodrin 295
Chlormethiazole 420
Chlornaphthalene *see* Polychlorinated
    naphthalene 188
1-Chloro-1-nitropropane 165
2-Chloro-1,3-butadiene 196
*p*-Chloro-*m*-cresol 449
3-Chloro-1,2-propanediol 196
3-Chloro-1,3-propanediol 196
β-Chloro-propionitrile *see* Acrylonitrile 312
Chloroacetaldehyde 196

Chloroacetic acid 196
Chloroacetone *see* Acetyl chloride 243
2-Chloroacetophenone 193
Chloroacetylchloride 243
*p*-Chloroaniline 165
Chlorobenzene 196
    derivatives 110
Chlorobenzene derivatives 109
Chlorobenzilate 110
*o*-Chlorobenzylidene malononitrile 193
Chlorobromomethane 196
Chlorobutane 196
Chlorobutanol 506
Chlorocide *see* Chlordane 119
Chlorodibromomethane 196
Chlorodifluoromethane 192
Chlorodinitrobenzene *see*
    Chloronitrobenzenes 165
Chlorodiphenyl 189
2-Chloroethanol *see* Ethylene chlorohydrin 187
Chloroethylene *see* Vinyl chloride 198
2-Chloroethylvinyl ether 196
Chloroform 385
Chlorohydroxymercuriphenol *see* Mercury 294
ChloroIPC 110
Chloromethylmethyl ether 196
Chloromycetin 490
Chloronaphthalenes 188
Chloroneb 110
Chloronitrobenzenes 165
Chloronitropropane 165
Chloropentafluoroethane 192
Chlorophacinone 469
Chlorophenols 449
Chlorophenyl mercaptan 316
Chlorophyll 347
Chloropicrin 165, 193
Chloroprene *see* 2-Chloro-1,3-butadiene 196
Chloroprocaine 382
3-Chloropropene *see* Allyl chloride 196
Chloroquine 497, 506
*o*-Chlorostyrene 196
*N*-Chlorosuccinamide 359
Chlorothalonil 110
Chlorothene *see* 1,1,1-Trichloroethane 181
Chlorothiazide 479, 482
*o*-Chlorotoluene 196
Chlorotoluidine 165
Chlorotoluron 110
Chlorotrianisene 554
Chlorotrifluoromethane 192
Chloroxine *see* Chinosol 153
Chloroxylenol 449
Chlorpheniramine 402, 420

Chlorphentermine 441
Chlorpromazine 404, 420
    interactions 521
Chlorpropamide 550, 552
    interactions 377, 505, 552
Chlorpropham 110, 126
Chlorpyrifos 124
Chlorpyrifos-methyl 124
Chlorsulfuron 110
Chlortetracycline 489
Chlorthal 110
Chlorthalidone 479
Chlorthiamid 153
Chlorzoxazone 411
Cholebrine 575
Cholestyramine 481, 566
Cholestyramine resin 461
Cholinesterase inhibitor pesticides **123–132**
Cholografin 575
Choloxin 555
Choride 39
Chorionic gonadotrophin 554
Christmas rose 633
Chromate 280
Chrome pigments *see*
    Chromate 280
    Lead 282
Chromic acid 280
Chromite 280
Chromium 39, 280
Chromium picolinate 570
Chromyl chloride 280
Chrysanthemum 633
Chrysene 238
Chrysoidin 360
Chryson 159
Chrysotile 331
Churchill's caustic *see* Iodine 445
Chymar 566
Chymodiactin 566
Chymopapain 566
Chymotrypsin 566
Ciclopirox 500
*Cicuta maculata*, water hemlock 622, 623
Cicutoxin 622
Cidex *see* Glutaraldehyde [2%] 224
Cidial 125
Cidofovir 500
Cidol-roach poison *see* Fluoride [10%] 264
Ciguatera 352
    fish poisoning 611, 612
Cilastatin 493
Cilexetil 478
Cilostazol 477

Cimetidine 433
*Cimicifuga* 570
Cinchona *see* Quinine 497
Cinchonidine *see* Quinine 497
Cinchonine *see* Quinine 497
Cincophen 377
Cineol *see* Volatile oils 536
Cinerin *see* Allethrin 158
Cinnabar *see* Mercury 294
Cinnamon oil 536
Cinnamoyl chloride *see* Benzoyl chloride 196
Cinobac 500
Cinoxacin 500
Cipro 493
Ciprofloxacin 493
Circulatory failure 56
Cisapride 431
Cisatracurium 414
Cisplatin 576
Citalopram 523
Citanest 382
Citovene 501
Citral *see* Volatile oils 536
Citronella 536
*Citrullus colocynthis* 543
Cladribin 576
Claforan 492
Clams 610
Clarithromycin 491
    interactions 481
Claritin 402
Cleaners 360
    chrome *see* Oxalic acid [10%] 240
    coin *see* Phosphoric acid [35%] 243
    electric train *see* Kerosene [90%] 228
    household, powder *see* Sodium carbonate
        [25%] 257
    metal *see* Acids 242
    motor *see* Kerosene 228
    pipe and drain *see* Lye 257
    radiator *see* Sodium phosphates 257
    shoe *see* Trichloroethylene [75%] 179
    solvent type *see* naphtha 228
    typewriter *see* Ethylene dichloride 185
    wall *see* Sodium tripolyphosphate 257
    *see also* Cyanide 311
    *see also* Oxalic acid 240
    *see also* Phosphoric acid 243
Cleaning solutions *see*
    Acids 242, 243
    Alkalis 257
    Ammonium hydroxide (ammonia
        water) 261
    Benzene [50%] 231

Cyanides 311
    Methanol 199
    Oxalic acid (10 240
    Silver nitrate 455
Cleaning solvents 360
Cleansing cream 347
Clemastine 402
Clenzoil *see* Turpentine [20%] 536
Cleocin 492
Clidinium 422
Climbing lily *see* Colchicine 579
Clindamycin 492, 506
    interactions 416
Clinitest *see*
    Copper sulfate 533
    Sodium hydroxide [250 mg] 257
Clinoril 377
Clinquinol 445
*Clitocybe* sp 625
Clobetasol *see* Corticosteroids 547
Clocortolone *see* Corticosteroids 547
Cloethocarb 126
Clofazamine 500
Clofentezine 110
Clofibrate 478, 482
    interactions 481
Clomid 553
Clomiphene 553
Clomipramine 518
Clonazepam 411, 420
Clonidine 433
Clopidogrel 477
Clopidol 165
Clopyralid 110
Clorazepate 411
*Clorophyllum* sp 625
Clorox 356
*Clostridium botulinum* 348
*Clostridium perfringens* 350, 351
Cloth dyes 360
Cloth marking ink 360
Clotrimazole 500
Clout 151
Clove oil 536
Cloxacillin 489, 506
Clozapine 411, 420
Clozaril 411
CN 193
Co-Deltra *see* Prednisone 546
Co-Ral 124
Co-trimoxazole 486
Coal dust 338
Coal oil *see* Kerosene 228
Coal tar 338, 448, 449

Coal tar naphtha 231
Cobalt 307
Cobex 135
Cobra (pesticide) 110
Cobras 588
 bites 592
Coca leaves *see* Cocaine 379
Cocaine 379, 389
 related compounds 379
Cocculus indicus 516
Cocillana 539
Codeine 397, 398, 420
Cogentin 422
Cognex 431
Coke oven emissions 338
Colchicine 579, 582
Colchicum 579
*Colchicum autumnale* 579
Cold remedies *see*
 Antihistamines 401
 Phenacetin [70%] 373
 Salicylates 367
Cold tablets *see* Antihistamines 401
Cold wave lotions 345
Cold wave neutralizer *see* Potassium
 bromate 343
Cold wave permanents *see* Potassium
 bromate 343
CoLena *see* Sulfuric acid [100%] 255
Colestid 481
Colestipol 481
Colfosceril 566
Colistimethate 491, 506
Colistin 491
Collagenase 566
Collodion *see* Ether [50%] 385
Collyrium Lotion *see* Boric acid [3%] 442
*Colocasia* 621
Colocynth 543
Cologne *see* Ethanol, denatured [75%] 202
Coly-Mycin 491
Coma 63
Comet Clear Dope *see* Toluene [40%] 231
Comet Hobby Cement *see* Toluene [62%]
 231
Comfrey 570
Comite 159
Compazine 404
Compound 10-80 *see* Sodium
 fluoroacetate 137
Comtan, see Entacapone 433
Concentration, lethal, defined 35
Condilox 543
Condurangin *see* Strychnine 513

Congestive heart failure 58
Coniine 622
*Conium maculatum*, poison hemlock 622, 623
Conolite Contact Bond *see* Toluene
 [100%] 231
Conray 575
Contac *see* Chlorpheniramine [4 mg] 402
Contraceptives
 oral 553
  interactions 552
*Convallaria* sp 635
Convulsions 60
 anticonvulsants 62
Cooking pots, galvanized *see* Chemical food
 poisoning 355
Cooling system cleanser *see*
 Oxalic acid [50%] 240
 Sodium carbonate 257
Cooling tower treatment *see* Sulfuric acid
 [40%] 255
Copaxone 567
Copon Thinners *see* Toluene [70%] 231
Copper Brite *see* Phosphoric acid [30%] 199
Copper carbonate *see* Copper salts 533
Copper cleaner *see* Sulfamic acid [10%] 199
Copper fumes or powder 307
Copper naphthenate *see* Copper salts 533
Copper oxide *see* Copper salts 533
Copper salts 533
Copper sulfate 533
Copper-lined utensils 533
Copperhead snake 588
*Coprinus* sp 625
Coral snakes 588
 bites 592
Coramine 516
Corbel 154
Corbit 151
*Corchorus* sp 635
Cordarone 477
Coreg 355
Corgard 435
Corlorpam 479
Corn cockle 633
Corn cures *see* Salicylic acid [20%] 367
Correction fluid *see*
 1,1,1-Trichloroethane 181
 Trichloroethylene 179
Correctol *see* Bisacodyl [5 mg] 545
Corrosive sublimate of mercury 294
Corrosives **240–268**
 acid-like 242
Corticaine 382
Corticorelin *see* Corticotropin 547

Corticosteroids 547
    interactions 377, 416, 482, 552
Corticotropin 547
*Cortinarius* sp 625
Cortisone 547, 552
    interactions 378
Cortrosyn 553
Corundum *see* Aluminum oxide 338
Corvert 490
Cosban 126
Cosmegen 576
Cosmetics **343–347**
Cosyntropin 553
Cotoran 154
Cotton dust 338
Cottonmouth snake 588
Cough remedies *see*
    Antibiotics 488
    Antihistamines 402
Coumachlor 469
Coumaphos 124
Coumarin anticoagulants 469
    interactions 203, 378, 415, 481, 521
Coumatetryl 469
Counter 125
Coyden *see* Clopidol 165
Cozaar 478
CPMC 126
*Crataegus* 570
Crayons
    children's *see* Paraffin 347
    industrial 360
    tailor's *see* Lead [5%] 282
Creosote 448, 449
Cresol(s) 449
Crest Toothpaste *see* Fluoride 264
Crimidine *see* Castrix 151, 513
Cristobalite 329
Crivaxin 501
Crocidolite 331
Cromolyn 566
Croneton 126
Crotalid bites 590, 594
*Crotalus* spp 588
    bites 590, 591
Crotamiton 458, 500
Croton oil 543
*Croton tiglium* 543
Crotonaldehyde 224
Crowfoot family 633
Cryolite 263
Crystal Clear Household Cement *see* Toluene
    [26%] 231
CS 193

*Ctenus nigriventer* 604
Cumene 238
Cupric compounds *see* Copper salts 533
Cuprid 569
Cuprimine *see* Penicillamine 94
Cuprous compounds *see* Copper salts 533
Curacron 125
Curare derivatives 413
    interactions 482
Curosurf 565
Curzate 153
Cuticle remover 345
Cyamelide *see* Cyanide 311
Cyanamide 311, 312
Cyanazine 152
Cyanic acid *see* Hydrogen cyanide 311
Cyanide(s) 39, 86, **311–326**
Cyano-methyl-mercuri-guanidine 295
Cyanoacetic acid 312
Cyanocobalamin 86, 571
Cyanogas *see* Cyanide 311
Cyanogen 311, 312
Cyanogen bromide *see* Cyanogen chloride 311
Cyanogen chloride 311, 312
Cyanogenetic glycosides 311
Cyanophos 124
Cyclamate 566
Cyclamycin 492
Cyclizine 402
Cycloate 557
Cyclobenzaprme 518
Cyclogyl 422
Cycloheptanone *see* Cyclohexanone 224
Cyclohexane 238
Cyclohexanesulfamic acid *see* Cyclamate 566
Cyclohexanol 213
Cyclohexanone 224
Cyclohexene 238
Cycloheximide 153
Cyclohexylamine 165, 258
2-Cyclohexyl-4,6-dinitrophenol *see*
    Dinitrophenol 135
Cyclopentadiene 238
Cyclopentane 238
Cyclopentolate 422
Cyclophosphamide 576, 582
Cyclopropane 385
    interactions 482
Cyclorite *see* Tetryl 168
Cycloserine 491
    interactions 505
Cyclosporin A 566
Cycocel 145
Cyflee 124

Cyfluthrin 158
Cyhexatin 158
Cylert 426
Cymag *see* Cyanide 311
Cymarin *see* Digitalis 459
Cymoxanil 153
Cypermethrin 158
Cyprazine 153
Cyprex 153
Cyprofuram 153
Cyproheptadine 402
Cyromazine 158
Cystadane 565
Cystagon 566
Cysteamine 566
Cytandren 553
Cytarabine 576, 582
Cythioate 124
Cytolav 566
Cytosar 576
Cytoxan 576
Cytrolane 125

2,4-D 117
Dacamox 126
Dacarbazine 576
Daclizumab 566
Daconil 110
Dacthal 110
Dactinomycin 576
Daffodil 633
Dalapon 159
Dalgan 398
Dalmane 411
Dalteparin 469
Damiana 570
Daminozide 160
Danaparoid 469
Danazol 553
Dantrium 411
Dantrolene 86, 411, 420
Daphne 633
Dapiprazol 433
Dapsone 485, 486, 506
    interactions 481
Daranide 478
Daraprim 502
Darvin 126
Darvon 398
Daskil 502
*Datura stramonium* 422
Daubentonia *see* Abrin 617
Daunorubicin 577, 582
DaunoXome 577

Daxolin 412
Daycon *see* Phosphoric acid [27%] 243
Daypro 377
Dazomet 153
2,4-DB 117
DBCP *see* Dibromochloropropane 197
DBPD 448
DCNA 110
DDD 109
DDS 485
DDT 109, 110
DDVP 124
Deadly nightshade 422
Death camas 630
Debarking compound *see* Arsenic 270
Debrisoquine, interactions 521
Debrox 458
Decaborane 442
Decahydronaphthalene 238
Decalin *see* Decahydronaphthalene 238
Decanol 213
Decis 159
Declomycin 489
Deet 151
DEF 124
Deferoxamine 86, 561
Dehorning paste *see* Sodium hydroxide
    [40%] 257
Dehydrocorticosterone *see* Corticosteroids 547
Dehydroepiandrosterone 553
Delan 154
Delavirdine 500
Delirium, management of 64
Delphene *see* Deet 151
Delphinine 538
Delphinium 538
Deltamethrin 159
Demadex 479
Demecarium 431
Demeclocycline 490
Demecolcine 579
Demerol 398
Demeton 125
Demosan 110
Demser 433
Demulcents 347
Denatured ethanol 202
Denavir 502
*Dendroaspis* sp 589
    bites 592
Denileukin 577
Deobase *see* Kerosene 228
Deodorants *see*
    Aluminum salts [25%] 533

Ethanol [50%] 202
Formaldehyde 217
Deoxyribonuclease 566
Depakene 393
Depakote 393
Depilatories 345
    see also Sodium hydroxide [5%] 257
    see also Sulfides 316
    see also Thioglycolates [10%] 345
Depos-off see Hydrochloric acid [7.5%] 243
Depressants **390–421**
    interactions 415
    nonbarbiturate 391
    selective 409
*Dermacentor* sp, ticks 608
Dermatitis 81
Derosal 152
Derris see Rotenone 159
Deserpidine 480
Desferal see Deferoxamine 86, 561
Desflurane 385
Desipramine 419, 518, 530
Deslanoside 459
Desmedipham 126
Desmetryn 153
Desogestrel-ethinyl estradiol 553
Desomorphine see Morphine 398
Desoximetasone see Corticosteroids 547
Desoxycorticosterone acetate 547
Destun 156
DET 529
Detergents 357
    anionic 358
    cationic 452
    dishwashing, hand 358
    laundry see Sodium tripolyphosphate
        [30%] 257
Detrol 422
Developer, photographic 362
Devrinol 153
Dexall Wood Bleach see Potassium hydroxide
    [8%] 257
Dexamethasone 494, 552
    see also Corticosteroids 547
Dexedrine see Dextroamphetamine 426
Dexol see Borate [40%] 442
Dexpanthenol 566
Dexrazoxane 566
Dextran 478
Dextroamphetamine 426
Dextromethorphan 398, 420
    interactions 508
Dextrotest P see Sulfosalicylic acid 243
Dextrotest S see Sodium hydroxide 257

Dextrothyroxine 555
Dezocin 398
DGE see Diglycidyl ether 225
DHEA 553
Di-Chlor-Mulsion see Ethylene dichloride
    [90%] 185
Di-Syston 124
Di-tertiary-butyl-*p*-cresol 448
Diabeta 550
Diabetes, antidiabetic drugs 550
Diabinese 550
Diacetone alcohol 213
Diacetylmorphine see Heroin 398
Diagnosis of poisoning **35–51**
    central nervous system 43
    differential 38
    eyes 44
    history 40
    laboratory examination 47
    principles 35
    skin 42
    systems review 41
Diallylamine 165
Dialysis 68, 98
Diaminodiphenylmethane 165
Diaminodiphenylsulfone 485
Diamox 478
Diaparene 452
Diaper Sweet see Sodium perborate [10%] 257
Diarrhea 69
Diatomaceous earth 328, 329
Diatrizoate 575
Diazepam 411, 420
    for convulsions 62
    interactions 415, 521
Diazinon 124
Diazomethane 165
Diazoxide 478, 482
    interactions 415, 552
Dibenzyline see Phenoxybenzamine 433
Diborane 442
Dibrom 124
Dibromochloropropane 197
Dibromoethane 197
Dibucaine 382
Dibutyl phthalate 151
Dibutyl succinate 151
2-*N*-Dibutylaminoethanol 258
Dibutylphosphate 226, 243
Dicamba 110
Dicatrete see Sulfuric acid [40%] 255
*Dicentra* sp 632
Dichlobenil 153
Dichlofluanid 153

Dichlone *see* Dichloronaphthoquinone 197
1,1-Dichloro-1-nitroethane 165
1,3-Dichloro-5,5-dimethylhydantoin 359
1,1-Dichloro-1,2,2,2-tetrafluoroethane 192
Dichloroacetic acid 197
Dichloroacetylene 197
Dichlorobenzene 197
3,3′-Dichlorobenzidine 165
3-amino-2,5-Dichlorobenzoic acid 110
Dichlorodifluoromethane 192
Dichlorodinitrobenzene *see*
    Chloronitrobenzenes 165
Dichlorodiphenyltrichloroethane 110
1,2-Dichloroethane 185
Dichloroethene 197
1,1-Dichloroethane 197
2,2′-Dichloroethyl ether 197
1,1-Dichloroethylene 197
1,2-Dichloroethylene 197
Dichlorofluoromethane 192
Dichloroisocyanurate 359
Dichloromethane 183
Dichloromethyl ether *see* 2,2′-Dichloroethyl
    ether 197
Dichloronaphthalenes 188
2,3-Dichloro1,4-naphthoquinone 197
Dichloronitrobenzene 165
Dichloropbenoxyacetic acid 117
Dichlorophenarsine hydrochloride *see*
    Arsenic 270
Dichlorophene 449
Dichlorophenol *see* Chorophenols 449
2,4-Dichlorophenoxyacetic acid 117
2,4-Dichlorophenoxyethyl sulfate 117
Dichloropropane 197
Dichloropropanol 197
Dichloropropene 197
2,2-Dichloropropionic acid 243
Dichlorotetrafluoroethane 192
Dichlorphenamide 478
Dichlorprop 117
Dichlorvos 124
Diclofenac 377, 420
Diclofop methyl 117
Dicloran 110
Dicloxacillin 489, 506
Dicodid 398
Dicofol 110
Dicrotophos 124
Dicumarol 469, 482
    interactions 552
Dicuran 110
Dicyclomine 422
Dicyclopentadiene 238

Didanosine 500
Didronel 567
*Dieffenbachia* 621
Dieldrin 119
Dienestrol 554
Dienochlor 110, 159
Diesel oil 228
Diet aids 570
Diethanolamine 258
Diethofencarb 126
Diethyl ether 385
    interactions 388
Diethyl ketone 224
Diethyl mercury 294
Diethyl sulfate 250
*N,N*-Diethyl-*m*-toluamide 151
Diethylamine 258
Diethylaminoethanol 258
*N,N*-Diethylbenzamide *see* Deet 151
Diethylene glycol 209
Diethylene triamine 258
Di(2-ethylhexyl) phthallate *see*
    Dioctylphthallate 226
Diethylphthallate 226
Diethylstilbestrol 554
Diethyltryptamine 529
Difenacoum 469
Difencan 501
Difenzoquat 145
Differin 565
Diflorasone *see* Corticosteroids 547
Diflubenzuron 110
Diflucan 492
Diflunisal 377
Difluorodibromomethane 192
1,1-Difluoroethylene 192, 197
Difolatan 152
Digalen *see* Digitalis 459
Digalloyl trioleate 566
Digibind 461
    *see also* Digoxin Immune Fab 86
Digifolin *see* Digitalis 459
Digilanid 459
Digitalis 58, 459
    glycosides, interactions 482
    interactions 481
Digitoxin 459, 482
Diglycidyl ether 225
Digoxin 459, 482
    interactions 440
Digoxin Immune Fab 86
Dihydrazine *see* Hydralazine 471
Dihydrocodeine 398, 420
Dihydroergotamine 437

Dihydroisocodeine *see* Codeine 398
Dihydrostreptomycin 490
Dihydrotachysterol *see* Vitamin D 571
Dihydroxyacetone 346
Diiodohydroxyquin 445
Diisobutyl ketone 224
Diisopropylether *see* Isopropyl ether 225
Dikegulac 160
Dilantin 393
    for convulsions 62
Dilaudid 398
Dilsocarb 126
Diltiazem 473, 483
Dimazine *see* Dimethylhydrazine 165
Dimecron 125
Dimefuron 153
Dimelone 151
Dimenhydrinate 402
Dimepiperate 557
Dimercaprol 87
Dimercaptopropanol *see* Dimercaprol 87
Dimetane 402
Dimethachlor 153
Dimethametryn 153
Dimethenamid 153
Dimethepin 160
Dimethipin 153
Dimethirimol 153
Dimethoate 124
Dimethomorph 153
2,5-Dimethoxy-4-methylamphetamine 529
Dimethoxymethane *see* Methylal 225
*N,N*-Dimethyl aniline 165
Dimethyl carbate 151
Dimethyl mercury 294
Dimethyl serotonin 529
Dimethyl sulfate 250
Dimethyl sulfoxide 566
1,1′-Dimethyl-4,4′-dipyridylium dichloride 145
Dimethyl-*p*-phenylenediamine *see* *p*-
    Phenylenediamine 167
Dimethylacetamide 165
Dimethylamine 258
Dimethylaminoazobenzene 165
Dimethylaniline 163, 165
Dimethylarsinic acid 271
3,3′-Dimethylbenzidine 165
Dimethylcarbamoyl chloride 165
Dimethyl-2,2-dichlorovinyl phosphate 124
Dimethylformamide 165
Dimethylhydrazine 165
Dimethylnitrosamine 165
Dimethylphthalate 151
Dimethyltryptamine 529

Dimethylvinphos 124
Dimethylvinyl chloride *see* Vinyl chloride 198
Dimilin 110
Dimorphone *see* Hydromorphone 398
Dinitramine 135
Dinitro-6-sec-butylphenol 135
Dinitro-*o*-amyl phenol *see* Dinitrophenol 135
Dinitro-*o*-butyl phenol *see* Dinitrophenol 135
Dinitro-*o*-cresol 135
Dinitroaniline *see* Aniline 163
Dinitroanisole *see* Dinitrophenol 135
Dinitrobenzenes 165
Dinitrocyclohexylphenol 135
Dinitronaphthol *see* Dinitrophenol 135
Dinitrophenol 135
Dinitrotoluamide 166
Dinitrotoluene 166
Dinobuton 135
Dinocap 135
Dinoprop 135
Dinoprostone 553
Dinoseb 135
Dinoterb 135
Dioctyl sodium sulfosuccinate 358
Dioctylphthallate 226
Diodoquin 445
Dionin 398
*Dioscorea* 571
Diovan 478
Dioxabenzofos 124
Dioxane 225
Dioxin 109, 117
Diphacinone 469
Diphenamid 153
Diphenex 117
Diphenhydramine 87, 402, 420, 494
Diphenoxylate 398, 420
Diphenyl
    chlorinated *see* Polychlorinated
        biphenyl 188
    *see also* Biphenyl 238
Diphenyl oxide *see* Phenyl ether 225
*N,N*-Diphenylamine 166
Diphenylhydantoin 393
1,2-Diphenylhydrazine 166
Diphenylnitrosamine 166
Dipivefrin 426
Diprivan 412
Dipropyl ketone 224
Dipropylene glycol 213
Dipropylene glycol methyl ether 213
Dipterex 125
Dipyridamole 477, 483
Dipyrone 377

Diquat 145
Dirithromycin 491
Disalcid 367
Disappearance half-life, defined 100
Dishwashing compounds 360
Dishwashing detergent, machine *see* Sodium
    carbonate [50%] 257
Disinfectant, pine oil 536
Disipal 402
Diskase 566
Disopyramide 478, 483
Distension, abdominal 69
Distillates, petroleum 228
Disulfiram 556
    interactions 415, 481
Disulfoton 124
Dithianon 154
2,4-Dithiobiuret 166
Dithiocarbamate 556
Ditran 529
Ditropan 422
Diupres 480
Diuresis, osmotic 98
Diuretics 479
    congestive heart failure 59
    interactions 416, 481, 482, 552, 581
    mercurial 295
    osmotic 98
Diuril 479
Diuron 154
Divalproex 393
Divinyl benzene 238
Divinyl ether 385
Diweevil fumigant *see* Ethylene dichloride
    [70%] 185
Dixon red tailor crayon *see* Lead [1%] 282
DMSA 97
DMT 529
DNOC 135
Dobutamine 426
Dobutrex 426
Docetaxel 577
Docusate 358
Dodemorph 154
Dodine 153
Doftilide 479
Dog parsley 622, 623
Dog repellent *see*
    Naphthalene 234
    Nicotine [6%] 138
Dog-Buttons *see* Strychnine 513
Dolasetron 411
Dolobid 377
Dolophine 398

DOM 529
Domeboro tablets *see* Aluminum acetate 533
Donepazil 431
Dong quai 570
Donnagesic Extentabs *see* Codeine
    [97 mg] 398
Dononex 571
Doodle Oil *see*
    Ethanol [90%] 202
    Volatile oils [10%] 536
Dopamine 426
Doral 412
Doriden 391
Dormethan 398
Dornase 566
Doryl *see* Bethanechol 431
Dorzolamide 478
Dosanex 155
Dose, lethal, defined 35
Dostinex 437
Douche, liquid *see* Ethanol [15%] 202
Dow Oven Cleaner *see* Sodium hydroxide
    [4%] 257
Dowfume *see*
    Carbon tetrachloride [83%] 172
    Dibromoethane [70%] 197
    Methyl bromide 176
Dowgard *see* Ethylene glycol 209
Down the Drain *see* Potassium hydroxide
    [36%] 257
Dowpon 159
Dowtherm A *see* Biphenyl 238
Doxacurium 414
Doxazosin 480
Doxepin 518, 519
Doxercalciferol 571
Doxil 577
Doxorubicin 577
Doxycycline 489, 506
Doxylamine 420
Dr Miles' Nervine 408
Drain cleaners 360
Dramamine 402
Drano 360
    Industrial *see* Sodium hydroxide [10%] 257
    Liquid *see* 1,1,1-Trichloroethane [99%]
        181
Drepamon 557
Dri-Worm *see* Fluoride [10%] 263
Drier, chemical *see* Calcium chloride 243
Dristan *see* Aspirin [324 mg] 367
Dromoran *see* Morphine 398
Droperidol 411, 420
Dropp 160

Drug(s)
  abuse of 49, 399, 529
  anti-infective 485
  autonomic nervous system **422–441**, 441
  cardiovascular **459–484**
  concentrations of 100
  endocrine **546–555**
  interactions and reactions 20, 21
    analgesics 377
    anesthetics 388
    anti-infectives 505
    antidepressants 505
    autonomic nervous system agents 440
    cardiovascular agents 481
    depressants 415
    endocrine agents 552
    ethanol 203
    therapeutic and diagnostic agents 581
  poisoning treatment 26
Dry cell batteries 292
Dry cleaner
  inflammable *see* Petroleum distillates 228
  noninflammable *see*
    Tetrachloroethylene 182
DTIC-Dome 576
Dual 155
Duco Cement *see* Acetone [90%] 224
Dulcolax 545
Dupont Engine Cleaner *see* Kerosene 228
Dupont Tar Remover *see* Kerosene 228
Duranest 382
Duraset 160
Duricef 492
Dursban *see* Chlorpyrifos 124
Dust(s)
  cloth oil *see* Kerosene 228
  nuisance 338
  organic *see* Sugar cane dust 339
Dybar 154
Dyclone 382
Dyclonine 382
Dye remover 360
Dye(s) 163
  cloth 360
  fish bait 360
  lip 346
  shoe *see* Aniline [1%] 163, 164
  *see also*
    Arsenic 270
    Benzene 231
    Silver nitrate 455
Dyfonate 124
Dylox 125
Dymelor 550

Dymid 153
Dymron 154
DynaCirc 473
Dynex 154
Dyphylline 510
Dyrene 154
Dyrenium 479, 481

Eagle Spirits *see* Methanol 199
Ears, poison diagnosis 45
Eastern coral snake 588
Eastern diamondback rattlesnake 588
Eastern Emulsion Bowl Cleaner *see*
    Hydrochloric acid [22%] 243
Eastern green mamba 589
Eastman 910 *see* Methyl 2-cyanoacrylate 312
Easy-Off *see* Sodium hydroxide [8%] 257
*Ecballium elaterium* 543
Echinacea 570
*Echis carinatus*
  bites 593
  saw-scaled viper 589
Echols Roach Powder *see* Carbaryl [3%] 123,
    126
Echothiophate 415, 431
Econazole 500
Ecstasy 529, 530
Edathamil *see* Edetate 88
Edecrin 479
Edetate 88
Edifenphos 124
Edrophonium 415, 431
EDTA 88
Efavirenz 500
Efosite 124
Ekatin 125
Elapid bites 592, 594
Elase 567
Elaterin 543
Elavil 518
Elco Roach and Ant Powder *see* Sodium
    fluoride [40%] 264
Eldepryl 412
Elderberry 634
Electrolyte and water imbalance 69
Elephant ear 621
Elgetol *see* Dinitrophenol [20%] 135
Ellence 577
Elspar 576
Emadine, see Emedastine 433
Embalming fluid 217
    *see also* Methanol 199
Embark 160
Embutox 117

Emcyt 577
Emedastine 433
Emergency equipment 31
Emergency management **25–34**
Emery 338
Emesis 29
Emetine 495
Eminase 477
Emiron 568
Empire Brush Cleaner *see* Methylene chloride [50%] 184
Empirin *see* Salicylates 367
Enalapril 477
Enamels *see* Lead [1%] 282
Enbrel 567
Endocrine drugs **546–555**
Endocrine system, poison diagnosis 47
Endosulfan 119
Endothall 154
Endrin 119
Enduronyl 480
Energine Charcoal Lighter *see* Kerosene 228
Energine Cleaning Fluid *see* Naphtha 228
Energine Lighter Fluid *see* Petroleum distillates 228
Enflurane 385
    interactions 388
Engine degreaser *see* Kerosene 228
*Enhydrina schistosa*, beaked sea snake 589
Enoxacin 493
Enoxaparin 469
Enstar 159
Entacapone 433
Environmental contamination 16
Enzeon 566
Enzyme induction, interactions 388
Enzymes *see Bacillus subtilis* enzymes 307
Ephedra 570
Ephedrine 425, 426, 441
    and related compounds 426
Epichlorohydrin 197
Epinephrine 88, 425, 426, 494
Epirubicin 577
Epivir 501
EPN 124
Epoetin alfa 553
Epogen 553
Epoprostenol 479, 553
Epoxy catalyst 307
    *see also* Diaminodiphenylmethane 165
Epoxy hardeners 307
Epoxy monomer 307
Epoxy resin 307
Epoxy thinner *see* Xylene 231

Eprosartan 478
Epsom salts *see* Magnesium sulfate 541
Eptam 557
EPTC 557
Eptifibatide 477
*Epyris californicus*, wasp 608
Equanil 391
Erbon 117
Ergamisol 577
Ergocalciferol 571
Ergoloid 437
Ergonovine 437
Ergot 437
Ergotamine 437
Erythrityl tetranitrate *see* Nitrites 467
Erythromycin 491, 506
    interactions 481
Erythromycin estolate 491
Esbiol 159
Esculin *see* Buckeye 631
Eskalith 562
Esmolol 435, 441
Esprocarb 557
Essential oils 536
Estazolam 411, 420
Estradiol 554
Estramustine 577
Estrogens 554
Estropipate 554
Etaconazole 154
Etanercept 567
Ethacrynic acid 479, 480, 483
    interactions 481, 505, 552
Ethalfluralin 157
Ethambutol 501, 506
Ethane 238
Ethanearsonic acid *see* Arsenic 270
Ethanol 89, 202
    interactions 203, 415, 505, 521, 552
    toxicity 205
Ethanolamine 258
Ethchlorvynol 391, 420
Ethephon 160
Ether(s) 225, 385
Ethinyl estradiol 554
Ethiodized oil 575
Ethiofencarb 126
Ethion 124
Ethionamide 501
Ethirimol 154
Ethofumesate 154
Ethoprophos 124
Ethosuximide 393, 420

Ethotoin 393
2-Ethoxy ethanol 213
2-Ethoxy ethyl acetate 213
Ethrane 385
Ethychlozate 110
Ethyl acetate 226
Ethyl acrylate 226
Ethyl alcohol 202
Ethyl aminobenzoate 382
Ethyl amyl ketone 224
Ethyl biscoumacetate 469, 483
Ethyl bromide 197
Ethyl butyl ketone 224
Ethyl chloride 197, 385
Ethyl chlorocarbonate 243
Ethyl ether 385
Ethyl formate 226
Ethyl gasoline *see* Lead 282
Ethyl mercury chloride 295
Ethyl mercury phosphate 295
Ethyl mercury toluene sulfonate 295
Ethyl methacrylate 226
Ethyl methyl ketone *see* Butanone-2 224
Ethyl nitrite 467
Ethyl silicate 226
Ethyl xanthic disulfide 155
Ethyl-4,4′-dichlorobenzilate 110
Ethylamine 258
Ethylbenzene 238
Ethylchloroformate *see* Ethyl
  chlorocarbonate 243
Ethylene 385
Ethylene chlorohydrin 187
Ethylene diamine 166
Ethylene dibromide *see* Dibromoethane 197
Ethylene dichloride 185
Ethylene glycol 109
Ethylene glycol dinitrate 467
Ethylene glycol ethers *see* Ethylene glycol
  209
Ethylene glycol monobutyl ether *see* 2-Butoxy
  ethanol 213
Ethylene glycol monoethyl ether *see* 2-Ethoxy
  ethanol 213
Ethylene glycol monomethyl ether *see*
  2-Methoxy ethanol 213
Ethylene oxide 225
Ethylene tetrachloride *see*
  Tetrachloroethane 178
Ethylenebisdithiocarbamate *see*
  Thiocarbamates 556
1,2-Ethylenediamine 258
Ethylenimine 166
2-Ethylhexanediol-1,3 151

Ethylidene chloride *see* 1,1-Dichloro-
  ethane 197
Ethylidene norbomene 238
Ethylmercaptan 317
Ethylmercuri-*p*-toluenesulfonanilide *see*
  Mercury 294
Ethylmorphine 398
*N*-Ethylmorpholine 166
Ethylpyridine *see* Pyridine 168
Ethynodiol-ethinyl estradiol 553
Ethyol 576
Etidocaine 382, 389
Etidronate 567
Etodolac 377
Etomidate 411
Etoposide 577
Etridazole 154
Etritinate 565
Etrofol 126
Etrofolan 126
Etulos 545
Eucalyptus oil 536
Eugenol *see* Volatile oils 536
Eulexin 577
*Euonymus atropurpureus*, burning bush 632
*Euonymus europaea*, spindle tree 632
Euparen 153
Euparen M 157
*Eupatorium rugosum*, snakeroot 637
*Euphorbia pulcherrima*, poinsettia 636
Eurax 458, 500
European viper 589
  bites 593
Evidence
  legal chain of custody 104
  preservation of 102
Evik 151
Evista 554
Excedrin *see* Aspirin 367
Exemestane 577
Exhaust emissions 236
  *see also* Carbon monoxide 39, 320
ExLax 545
Exosurf 566
Exposure limit, defined 9
Extinguisher, fire
    liquid *see* Carbon tetrachloride 172
    powder *see* Sodium carbonate 258
Eye contamination, treatment 33
Eye wash *see* Boric acid 442
Eyelash dye 345
Eyes, poison diagnosis 44

Face powder 345

Factrel 554
Famciclovir 501
Famfos 124
Famotidine 433
Famphur 124
Famvir 501
Faneron 152
Fansidar 485
Far-go 557
Fareston 579
Fastine 426
Fava bean 619
Favism 619
FD&C yellow No.5 569
Feed insecticides *see* Mercury 294
Felbamate 393
Felbatol 393
Feldene 377
Felodipine 473, 483
Felt Riter *see* Xylene 231
Femara 577
Fenac 117
Fenamiphos 124, 125
Fenarimol 110
Fenbutatin 159
Fenchone *see* Volatile oils 536
Fenfluramine 441
Fenfuram 156
Fenitrothion 124
Fenobucarb 126
Fenofibrate 478
Fenoldopam 479
Fenoprofen 377
    interactions 378
Fenoxaprop 110
Fenoxycarb 126
Fenpropimorph 154
Fentanyl 398, 420
Fenthion 124
Fenuron 154
Fenvalerate 110
Feosol *see* Iron salts 559
Ferbam 556, 557
Fermate *see* Thiocarbamates 556
Ferric dimethyl dithiocarbarnate *see*
    Thiocarbarnates 556
Ferric dimethyl thiocarbamate *see*
    Thiocarbamates 556
Ferric iron 559
Ferric salts 559
Ferrocyanide 312
Ferrosilicon 271
Ferrous salts 559
Ferrous sulfate 559

Ferrovanadium 308
Fertilizer 361
Fertinex 554
Fetal injury 19
Fever, metal fume 304
Feverfew 570
Fexofenidin 402
Fiber glass 399
Fibrinolysin-desoxyribonuclease 567
Ficam 126
Figaron 110
Filefish 611
Filgrastim 578
Film cement *see* Acetone [90%] 224
Film cleaner *see* Trichlorethylene 179
Finasteride 554
Finger cherry 634
Fiolan 479
Fire extinguisher
    liquid *see* Carbon tetrachloride 172
    powder *see* Sodium carbonate 257
Fire starter *see* Kerosene 228
Fire-ant 608
Fireplace colors
    *see*
        Antimony 269
        Arsenic 270
        Copper 533
Fireworks 361
Fish, poisonous 611
Fish berries 516
Fish liver oil *see* Vitamin D 571
Fish toxicants 160
Fixer, photographic 362
Fixer film *see* Boric acid 442
Flagyl 501
Flamprop-isopropyl 110
Flamprop-methyl 110
Flavoxate 422
Flea collar *see* DDVP [9%] 124
Flea powder *see* Naphthalene 234
Flecainide 479, 483
Flex 110
Flexeril 518
Flit Killer *see* Kerosene 228
Flolan 553
Flomax, see Tamsulosin 434
Floor cleaner *see* Kerosene 228
Floor finish *see* Xylene 231
Floraltone 160
Florel 160
Floropryl 431
Flour 338
Floxacillin 506

Floxin 493
Floxuridine 577
Fluazifop-butyl 154
Fluchloralin 154
Fluconazole 492, 501
Flucytosine 501, 506
Fludara 577
Fludarabine 577
Fludrocortisone 547, 552
Flumadine 502
Flumazenil 89
Flunisolide see Corticosteroids 547
Fluoaluminate see Cryolite 263
Fluoboric acid see Hydrogen fluoride 264
Fluocinolone see Corticosteroids 547
Fluocinonide see Corticosteroids 547
Fluometuron 154
Fluoranthrene 238
Fluorescein 577
    diagnostic use 33
Fluorescent lamps 361
Fluoride 263
    salts 263
    toothpaste see Fluoride [0.1%] 264
Fluorine 263
Fluoro-dinitrobenzene see
    Chloronitrobenzenes 165
Fluoroacetamide 137
Fluoroacetanilide 137
Fluoroacetate 137
Fluoroacetic acid 137
Fluoroalkane 191
Fluorocarbons 191, 308
Fluoroform see Chloroform 385
Fluorohydrocortisone see Corticosteroids 547
Fluoromar 385
Fluorometholone see Corticosteroids 547
Fluorophors 275
Fluorosilicate 264
5-Fluorouracil 577, 582
Fluosilicic acid see Fluorosilicate 264
Fluosulfonic acid see Fluorosilicate 264
Fluothane 385
Fluoxetine 523, 530
    interactions 508
Fluoxymesterone 553
Fluphenazine 404, 420
Flurandrenolide see Corticosteroids 547
Flurazepam 411, 420
Flurbiprofen 377
Fluridone 154
Fluroxene 385
Flutamide 577
Fluticasone see Corticosteroids 547

Flutriafol 110
Fluvastatin 478
Fluvoxamine 523
    interactions 481
Fly-Tox see Kerosene 228
Folic acid 89, 567
Folimat 125
Folinic acid 575
Folithion 124
Follitropins 553
Folpet 156
Fomepizole 89
Fomesafen 110
Fomvirsen 501
Fongarid 154
Fonofos 124
Food poisoning **348–355**
Formaldehyde 217, 236
Formalin 217
Formamide 166
Formetanate 126
Formic acid 243
Formothion 124
Fortress 124
Fosamax 565
Fosamine 125
Foscarnet 501
Foscavir 501
Fosetyl 124
Fosfomycin 493
Fosinopril 477
Fosphenytoin 393
Fosthioazate 124
Fowler's solution see Arsenic [0.5%] 270
Foxglove 459
Fragmin 469
Frangula see Cascara 545
Freons 192
Fructose 567
Fthalide 110
Fuberidazol 154
*Fucus* 570
Fuel booster see Diethyl ether 385
Fuel (lighter fluids) see Petroleum
    distillates 228
Fuel oil see Kerosene 228
Fuel tablets 361
Fuji-One 155
Fulvicin 491
Fumaronitrile 312
Fumazone 197
Fume Rite see Nicotine [40%] 138
Fumigants see Carbon tetrachloride 172
Fumigating agents see Cyanide 311

Fungicide(s) 151
  poisoning prevention 6
Funginex 158
Fungizone 491
Funnel-web spider 602, 604
Furadan 126
Furalaxyl 154
2-Furaldehyde 224
Furandantin 502
Furathiocarb 126
Furazolidone, interactions 204, 522
Furfural *see* 2-Furaldehyde 224
Furfuryl alcohol 213
Furniture cleaner *see* Kerosene [50%] 228
Furniture polish 361
Furniture wax *see* Kerosene 228
Furore 110
Furosemide 479, 483
  interactions 378, 482, 505, 552
Fusarex 110
Fusidic acid 506
Fusilade 154

Gabapentin 393
Gabitril 393
Galben 152
*Galerina* sp 624
Gallic acid 449
Gallium arsenide *see* Arsenic 270
Galvanized utensils 533
Galzin 533
*Gambierdiscus toxicus*, seafood poisoning 352
Gamboge 543
Ganciclovir 501
Ganglionic blocking agents 480
Gantanol 485
Gantrisin 485
Garamycin 490
*Garcinia hanburyi* 543
Gardona 125
Gardoprim 157
Garlon 110
Gas
  fumigating *see* Cyanide 311
  illuminating, *see* Carbon monoxide 320
  natural, *see* Methane 238
Gasline Antifreeze *see* Methanol 199
Gasoline 228
  *see also* Lead 282
Gastric lavage, procedure 30
Gatifloxacin 493
GBL 411, 529
*Gelsemium sempervirens*, jessamine 634
Gelusil 542

Gemcitabine 577
Gemfibrozil 478
Gemzar 577
Genitourinary system, poison diagnosis 46
Gentamicin 490, 506
Geraniol *see* Volatile oils 536
Geref 554
Germanium 308
Germanium hydride *see* Arsine 270
Germanium tetrahydride 308
Gesafloc 158
Gesamil 157
GHB 411, 529
Gibberellic acid 160
Gila monster 598
Gildings *see* Benzene [50%] 231
Gingko 570
Gitaligin 459
Gitalin 459
Glass etch *see* Fluoride 263
Glass fiber 339
Glatiramer 567
Glazes *see* Lead [10%] 282
Glazing putty *see* Lead [16%] 282
GLB 570
Glibenclamide 552
Glibomuride 552
Glimepiride 550
Glipizide 550, 552
γ-Globulin 567
*Gloriosa superba*, glory lily 634
Glory lily 634
Glow Fuel Model Airplane Fuel *see*
    Methanol [65%] 199
    Nitromethane [15%] 167
Glucagon 90, 481, 554
Glucophage 550
α-Glucosidase inhibitors 550
Glucotrol 550
Glue sniffing 231
Glutaraldehyde 224
Glutethimide 392, 420
Glyburide 550
Glycerin 213
Glycerol
    *see also* Glycerin 213
    iodinated 445
Glyceryl trinitraie 467
Glycidol 225
Glycobiarsol 272
Glycols **199–215**
Glycopyrrolate 422
Glycosides
    cardiac 459

cyanogenetic 311
Glycyrrhizin 548
Glynase 550
Glyodin 154
Glyphosate 154
Glyset 550
GMB 570
Goal 156
Goatfish 611
Gold sodium thiomalate 377
Gold sodium thiosulfate 377
Gold thioglucose *see* Aurothioglucose 377
Golden chain 635
Golden seal 570
Goltix 155
Gonadorelin 554
Gonal-F 554
*Gonyaulax catenella*, shellfish poisoning 610
Good Boiler Sealer *see* Potassium bichromate
    [5%] 280
Goon *see* Phencyclidine 527
Gopher Corn *see* Strychnine [0.3%] 513
Gopher Go *see* Strychnine [1%] 513
Goserelin 577
Gotu kola 570
Grain alcohol 202
Grain dust 339
Grain fumigant
    *see*
        Carbon tetrachloride [30%] 172
        Ethylene dichloride [70%] 185
Gramoxone *see* Paraquat 145
Granisetron 412
Grapefruit juice, drug interactions 481
Graphite 339
Great Basin rattlesnake 588
Green hellebore *see* Veratrum 630
Greenfield Contact Kill *see* Xylene 231
Greenfield Dandelion Killer *see* Xylene 231
Griseofulvin 491, 506
Grouper 611
Growth hormone 554
Grunerite, fibrous 331
Guaiacol 449
Guaifenesin 567
Guanabenz 433
Guanadrel 433
Guanethidine 433, 441
    interactions 440, 521
Guanfacine 433
Guarana 570
Guazatine 154
Gum, cambogia (gamboge) 543
Gun bluing *see* Selenium [3%] 309

Gusathion-A 124
Guthion 124
*Gymnocladus dioica*, Kentucky coffee
    berry 635
*Gyromitra esculenta* 624
Gyromitrin 625

Hafnium 308
Hair cream 280
Hair dye(s) 345, 346
    vegetable 347
Hair lacquers 346
Hair lighteners 346
Hair lotions *see* Methanol 199
Hair neutralizers *see* Potassium bromate 343
Hair oil 347
Hair straightener 346
Hair tonic 346
Halcinonide *see* Corticosteroids 547
Halcion 412
Haldol 412
Halobenzene derivatives 109, 110
Halobetasol *see* Corticosteroids 547
Halogenated hydrocarbons **172–198**
Halogenated insecticides **109–122**
Haloperidol 412, 420
    interactions 521, 581
Halothane 385
    interactions 388, 482
Halowax 188
Hand cream or lotion 347
Hardener, film *see* Chromate 280
Harmaline 529
Harmine 529
Harvade 160
Hawthorn leaves 570
Headache tablets and powders *see*
    Salicylates 367
Heart failure 59
*Hebeloma* sp 625
Hectorol 571
Hellebore, false 630
*Helleborus niger*, Christmas rose 633
*Heloderma* 598
*Helvella* sp 625
Hemabate 553
Hematopoietic system, poisoning 77
Hemlock 622
Hemodialysis 98
Hemolytic reactions, treatment 80
Henbane 422
Heparin 469, 483
    interactions 482
Heptachlor 119

Heptane 238
Heptanone-2 *see* Ethyl butyl ketone 224
Heptenophos 124
Herbicides 151
   *see also* Arsenic 270
Herbisan 155
Herceptin 569
Heroin 397, 398
Hetacillin *see* Penicillins 489
Hetastarch 478
HETP *see* TEPP 125
Hexabarbital 420
Hexachloroacetone 197
Hexachlorobutadiene 197
Hexachlorocyclohexane 113
Hexachlorocyclopentadiene 197
Hexachloroethane 197
Hexachloronaphthalene 189
Hexachlorophene 449
Hexafluogallate *see* Cryolite 263
Hexafluophosphate *see* Fluoride 263
Hexafluorenium 415
Hexafluoroacetone 192, 197
Hexalen 576
Hexamethyl phosphoramide 166
Hexamethyl phosphoric triamide *see*
   Hexamethyl phosphoramide 166
n-Hexane 238
Hexanes, branched 238
Hexanone-2 224
Hexazinone 155
Hexol *see* Pine oil [50%] 536
Hexone *see* Methylpentanone 225
Hextend 478
Hexyl acetate 226
Hexyl methyl ketone *see* Hexanone-2 224
Hexylene *see* Ethylene 385
Hexylene glycol 214
Hexylresorcinol 449
Hexylthiocarbam 557
Hexythiazox 159
Hibiclens 458
Hinosan 124
*Hippomane mancinella*, manchineel 636
Hismanal 402
Histamine blocking agents 433
Histrelin 554
Hivid 503
Hog *see* Phencyclidine 527
Holly 634
Homatropine 422
Hopcide 126
Horse beans 619
Horse chestnut 632

Hostaquick 124
Hostathion 125
Hourglass spider 601
Household hazards **341–364**
Household poisoning prevention 3
Human chorionic gonadotropin 554
Human growth hormone 554
Humatin 493
Humorsol 431
Hyacinth 634
Hyalgan 567
Hyaluronate 567
Hyaluronidase 567
Hycamtin 579
Hycodan *see* Hydrocodone 398
Hydergine 437
Hydralazine 471, 483
   interactions 482
Hydrangea 634
*Hydrastis* 570
Hydrazine 166
Hydrazinophthalazine *see* Hydralazine 471
Hydrazoic acid 166, 243
Hydrobromic acid 243
Hydrocarbons **228–239**
   aliphatic 228
   aromatic 231
Hydrochloric acid 243
Hydrochlorothiazide 479, 483
Hydrocodone 398, 420
Hydrocortamate *see* Corticosteroids 547
Hydrocortisone 547, 552
   interactions 521
Hydroflumethiazide 479
Hydrofluoric acid 263
Hydrogen bromides *see* Hydrobromic acid 243
Hydrogen chloride *see* Hydrochloric acid 243
Hydrogen cyanide 311, 312, 536
Hydrogen fluoride 263
Hydrogen peroxide 458
Hydrogen selenide 309
Hydrogen sulfide 39, 316
Hydrogen telluride *see* Arsine 270
Hydrol 126
Hydromorphone 398, 420
Hydromox 480
Hydrophilite *see* Calcium chloride 243
Hydroquinone 449
Hydroxocobalamin *see* Cyanocobalamin 86
p-Hydroxybenzoic acid 458
p-Hydroxybenzoic esters 458
γ-Hydroxybutyrate 529
γ-Hydroxybutyric acid 411, 570
Hydroxychloroquine 497

Hydroxyethyl cellulose 347
Hydroxyethylacrylate 226
Hydroxyhexamide, interactions 377
Hydroxylamine 166
Hydroxymercurichlorophenol *see* Mercury 294
Hydroxymercuriphenol 295
Hydroxyprogesterone 554
Hydroxypropylacrylate 226
8-Hydroxyquinoline 153
5-Hydroxytryptamine *see* Selective serotonin
    reuptake inhibitors 523
Hydroxyurea 577
Hydroxyzine 402, 420
Hygroton 479
Hymexazol 155
Hymorphan *see* Dilaudid 398
Hyoscine 441
Hyoscyamine 422
*Hyoscyamus niger* 422
Hypaque 575
Hyperactivity, management 64
*Hypericum* 570
Hyperstat 478
Hypertension remedies *see* Nitrites 467
Hyperthermia, treatment 72
Hypnotics 390
    interactions 203, 415
Hypochlorous acid 356
Hypoglycemia 66
Hypoglycemic agents, interactions 378, 522,
    552
Hyponone *see* Acetophenone 224
Hypothermia, treatment of 73
Hypoxia 52
Hytrin 480

Ibogaine 529
Ibuprofen 377
    interactions 378
Ibutilide 480
Ice camphor *see* Camphor 515
Ice dry *see* Carbon dioxide 307
Idamycin 577
Idarubicin 577
Ifex 577
Ifosfamide 577
Igran 157
*Ilex* sp 634
Illuminating gas *see* Carbon monoxide 320
Ilopan 566
Ilosone 491
Imazalil 110
Imidan 125
Imidazolidinethione 166

Imiglucerase 567
Imipenem 493
Imipramine 518, 519, 530
Imiquimod 567
Imodium 398
Imuran 576
Inapsine 411
Indandione anticoagulants 469
Indane derivatives 119
Indapamide 479
Indelible ink *see* Silver nitrate 455
Indelible pencils 361
Indene 238
Inderal 435
Indian krait 588
Indian tobacco 634
Indinavir 501
Indium 308
Indocin 377
Indomethacin 377
    interactions 377, 378, 481
Industrial chemicals, hazards of 8
Infasurf 565
Infliximab 567, 577
Ingested poisons, management 29
INH 503
Inhaled poisons, treatment 33
Injected poisons, treatment *see* Snakebite 32,
    595
Ink 361
    eradicator 361
    laundry *see* Aniline [1%] 163
    marker *see* Aniline [1%] 163
    writing 361
Inocor 477
*Inocybe* sp 625
Insect spray, household *see* Kerosene 228
Insecticide(s) **109–122**, 158
    poisoning prevention 6
    *see also* Arsenic 270
Insects and arachnids **601–609**
Insulin 550, 552, 554
    interactions 203, 440, 552
Intal 566
Integrilin 477
Interactions
    analgesics, antipyretics, anti-inflammatory
        drugs 377
    anesthetics 388
    anti-infective drugs 505
    antidepressants 521
    autonomic nervous system drugs 440
    cardiovascular drugs 481
    depressants 415

endocrine drugs 552
ethanol 203
therapeutic and diagnostic drugs 581
Interferons 577
Intropin 426
Invirase 502
Iocetamic acid 575
Iodamide 575
Iodate *see* Bromates 343
Iodex *see* Iodine 445
Iodides 445
Iodine 445
Iodipamide 575
Iodobehenate *see* Iodide 445
Iodochlorhydroxyquin 445
Iodoform 445
Iodoquinol 445
Iodostearate *see* Iodide 445
Iopanoic acid 575
Iopidine 426
Iothalamate 575
Ioxynil 110
IPC 157
Ipecac 495
Ipecac syrup 90
Ipodate 575
Ipratropium 422
Iprobenfos 124
Iprodione 159
Iproniazid 508
Irbesartan 478
*Iridaceae* 634
Irinotecan 577
Iris 634
Iron, dicyclopentadienyl 308
Iron dust or fumes 308
Iron oxide 308, 339
Iron pentacarbonyl 308
Iron salts 559
Irritants and rubefacients **532–540**
Isazofos 124
Isazophos 125
Iso-octane *see* Hexane 238
Isoamyl acetate *see* Amyl acetate 226
Isoamyl alcohol *see* Amyl alcohol 213
Isobac *see* Tetrachlorophenol 449
Isobornyl thiocyanoacetate *see* Thanite 142
Isobutyl acetate  *see* Amyl acetate 213
Butyl acetate 226
Isobutyl alcohol, *see* Butyl alcohol 213
Isobutylmethyl ketone *see* 4-Methyl-
pentanone-2 225
Isocarbamid 155
Isocarbamide 126

Isocarboxazid 508
Isoetharine 426
Isofenphos 124
Isoflurane 385
Isoflurphate 431
Isometheptene 426
interactions 508
Isoniazid 503, 506
interactions 415, 505, 522
Isooctyl alcohol *see* Octanol 213
Isophamfos 124
Isophorone 224
Isophorone diisocyanate 166
Isoprocarb 126
Isopropanol 214
Isopropoxyethanol 213
Isopropyl acetate *see* Propyl acetate 226
Isopropyl acetone *see* 4-Methyl-pentanone-
2 225
Isopropyl alcohol 214
*N*-Isopropyl aniline 166
Isopropyl ether 225
Isopropyl glycidyl ether 225
Isopropylamine 258
Isoproterenol 426
Isoprothiolane 155
Isoproturon 155
Isosorbide dinitrate 467, 483
Isotretinoin 565
Isoxathion 124
Isoxsuprine 426, 441
Isradipine 473, 483
Isuprel 426
Itraconazole 492, 501
interactions 481
Ivermectin 147
Ivy
poison 628
extract 568
*Ixodidae* sp, ticks 608

J-O Paste *see* Phosphorus (yellow) [1%] 301
Jack-in-the-pulpit 621
Jalap *see* Aloe 545
Janimine 518
*Jatropha* sp 636
Jelly fire starter *see* Kerosene 228
Jellyfish 614
Jequirity bean 616
Jerusalem cherry 622
Jessamine 634
Jetberry 634
Jetberry bush seeds 311
Jewelry *see* Nickel 308

Jiffy Aluminum Cleaner *see* Hydrofluoric acid [5%] 263
Jiffy Chrome Rust Remover *see* Hydrofluoric acid [5%] 263
Jimsonweed 422
Jute 635

*Kalmia* sp, laurel 635
Kanamycin 490, 506
Kantrex 490
Kaolin 347
Karathane 135
Karaya 545
Karbutilate 126
Karidium *see* Fluoride [2 mg] 263
Karphos 124
Kasugamycin 155
Kasumin 155
Kava kava 570
Kayexalate 461, 568
Keflin 492
Kelthane 110
Kemadrin 422
Kentucky coffee berry 635
Kepone 119
Keppra 393
Kerb 156
Kerlone 435
Kerosene 228
Ketalar 412
Ketamine 412, 415, 420
Ketene 224
Ketoconazole 491, 501
    interactions 481
Ketones 224
Ketoprofen 377
Ketorolac 377
Kidney failure 66
Killer Katz Rat Snax *see* Squill [5%] 459
Kinoprene 159
Kinstex *see* Thallium [3%] 140
*Klebsiella*, seafood poisoning 353
Kloben 156
Klonopin 411
Krait snakes 588
    bites 592
Krenite 125
Krystal *see* Phencyclidine 527
Kutzit *see* Toluene 231
Kwikeeze *see* Toluene 231
Kytril 412

*l*-Arterenol *see* Epinephrine 426
Laam 398

Labetalol 435, 441
Laboratory tests 47
Laburnum 635
*Laburnum anagyroides* 635
*Lachesis mutus*, bushmaster snake 588
Lacquer remover 362
Lacquer thinner *see* Petroleum ether [50%] 228
    Toluene [50%] 231
Lacquer *see* Toluene [75%] 231
*Lactarius* sp 625
Lactic acid 243
Lactofen 110
Lactulose 567
Laetrile 311
Lamarine 500
Lamictal 393
Lamisil 491
Lamivudine 501
Lamotrigine 393
Lanatoside C 459, 483
Lance 126
Lance-headed vipers, bites 590, 591
Lanex 154
Lannate 126
Lanolin 347
Lanray 126
Lantana 635
*Lantana camara*, lantana 635
Lariam 501
Larkspur 538
Lasix 479
Lasso 155
Latanoprost 553
Latex paint 362
*Lathyrus* sp 637
*Latrodectus mactans*, black widow spider 601
Laundry compounds 358
Laurel 635
Lauryl thiocyanate 142
Laxatives
    interactions 416, 482
    *see also* Cathartics 541
LC, defined 35
LD50, defined 35
LD, defined 35
Lead 39, 282
    tetraethyl 282
    tetramethyl 283
Lead arsenate 283
    *see also* Arsenic 270
Lead chromate 280
Lead poisoning, signs and symptoms 286
Leflunomide 567
Legal responsibility in poisonings **102–105**

Lenacil 155
*Lepiota* sp 625
Lepirudin 469
Lescol 478
Lethal concentration, defined 35
Lethal dose, defined 35
Lethane 142
Letrozol 577
Leucovorin 577
Leucovorin calcium 575
Leukeran 576
Leuprolide 577
Leustatin 576
Levamisole 577
Levant berry 516
Levantine viper, bites 593
Levarterenol *see* Norepinephrine 426
Levetiracetam 393
Levo-Dromoran 398
Levobunolol 435
Levocabastine 433
Levocarnitine 567
Levodopa 426, 441
    interactions 440, 521, 552
Levofloxacin 493
Levomethadyl 398
Levonorgestrel 554
Levonorgestrel-ethinyl estradiol 553
Levophed 426
Levorphanol 398, 420
Levothyroxine 552, 555
Levotol 435
Levulan 565
Librium 411
Licorice 548
Lidocaine 382, 389
    interactions 388, 440
Lighter fluid *see* Petroleum distillates 228
Ligroin 228
*Ligustrum vulgare*, privet 636
Lily family 630
Lily of the valley 635
Lima bean 311
Lime
    sulfurated *see* Calcium polysulfide 316
    *see also* Calcium oxide 258
Limonene *see* Turpentine 536
Lincocin 492
Lincomycin 492, 506
Lindane 113
Linezolid 493
Liniment *see* Methyl salicylate 367
Linseed oil, boiled *see* Lead 282
Linuron 155

Lioresal 411
Liothyronine 552, 555
Liotrix 555
Lipitor 478
Liquefied petroleum gas *see* Methane 238
Liquefied phenol 448
Liquid Bright Gold *see* Turpentine 536
Liquid Paper *see* 1,1,1-Trichloroethane 181
Liquid Plumr *see* Potassium hydroxide
    [3%] 257
Liquiprin *see* Acetaminophen [300 mg] 373
Lisinopril 477
Listerine Antiseptic *see* Ethanol [30%] 202
Lithane 562
Lithium 525, 562, 582
    interactions 581
Lithium carbonate 562
Lithium hydride 258
Lithium hydroxide 258
Lithium salts 562
Lithobid 562
Lithonate 562
Lithostat 565
Liver damage 74
Livostin *see* Levocabastine 433
Lixivium *see* Sodium hydroxide 257
Lizard *see* Gila monster 598
*Lobelia inflata*, Indian tobacco 634
Lobeline 138
Local anesthetics 382
Lock Fluid, Graphite *see* Kerosene 228
Locust 635
Lodine 377
Lomefloxacin 493
Lomotil 398
Lomustine 576
Loniten 480
Loperamide 398, 421
*Lophophora williamsii* 529
Lopid 478
Lopressor 435
Loprox 500
Loracarbef 493
Loratidine 402
Lorazepam 62, 412, 421
Lorox 155
Lorsban 124
Losartan 478
Lotensin *see* Benazepryl 477
Lotiprednol *see* Corticosteroids 547
Lotrimin 500
Lovastatin 478
Love beads 616
Lovenox 469

Loxapine 412, 421
*Loxosceles* sp 603, 604
Lozol 479
LPG *see* Methane 238
LSD 529, 530
Lubricating oils 228
Ludiomil 518
Lugol's solution *see* Iodine [5%] 362
Luminal 392
Lupin (lupine) 635
*Lupinus* sp 635
Lupron 577
Lutrepulse 544
Luvox 523
*Lycosa erythrognata*, tarantula spider 604
Lye 257
Lysergic acid diethylamide 529
Lysol Toilet Bowl Cleaner *see* Hydrochloric
   acid [9%] 243

Ma Huang 570
Macbal 126
Mace 193
Machete 152
Mackerel 611
Mafenide 485
Magnesium 308, 421
Magnesium oxide fumes 308, 310
Magnesium salts 541
Magnesium silicate 331
Magnesium sulfate 90, 541
Magnesium trisilicate 567
Magron *see* Chlorates [40%] 453
Maintain 110
Maitotoxin 352
Majic Digester *see* Sulfuric acid 209
Makeup, liquid 347
Malathion 123, 125
Malayan pit viper 588
   bites 590, 591
Maleic anhydride 243
Maleic hydrazide 160
Malmefene 91
Malonaldehyde 224
Malononitrile 312
Mamba 589
   bites 592
Management of poisoning **52–101**
   emergency **25–34**
Manchineel 636
Mandelamine 501
Mandelonitrile 312, 536
Mandole 492
Maneb 557

Manganese 292
Manganese cyclopentadienyl tricarbonyl 292
Manganese tetroxide 292
*Mangifera indica*, mango 636
Mango 636
Mania, management of 64
*Manihot utilissima* 311
Mannitol 480, 483
Mannitol hexanitrate 467
MAOI *see* Monoamine oxidase inhibitors 508
MAPP gas *see* Methylacetylene 238
Maprotiline 518, 519, 530
Marcaine 382
Marezine 402
Marigold, marsh 633
Marihuana 529
Marine animals **610–614**
Marsh marigold 633
Masoprocol 567
Mataven 110
Matches 361
   *see also* Chlorates 453
Matulane 578
Mavik *see* Trandolapril 477
Maxair 426
Maxalt 578
Maxaquin 493
Mayapple 543
Mazindol 441
MBK *see* Hexanone-2 224
MCPA 117
MCPB 117
MCPP 117
MDA 529, 530
MDI 166
MDMA 529, 530
Meadow saffron 579
Mebaral 392
Mebendazole 501
Mecamylamine 480
Mecarbam 125
Mechlorethamine 575, 578
Meclastine 421
Meclizine 402
Meclofenamate 377
Meclomen 377
Mecoprop 117
Medicinal poisons **365–584**
Medroxyprogesterone 554
Medrysone *see* Corticosteroids 547
Mefenamic acid 377
Mefloquine 501
Mefluidide 160
Mefoxin 492

Megace 578
Megestrol 578
Meglitinide analog 550
MEK *see* Butanone-2 224
Melarsoprol 272
*Melia azedarach*, chinaberry 633
Mellaril 404
Melphalan 578
Meltatox 154
Menadiol *see* Vitamin K 581
Menadione *see* Vitamin K 581
*Menispermum canadense*, moonseed 636
Menotropins 554
Mentax 500
Menthol 449
Meobal 126
Mepacrine 497
Mepenzolate 422
Meperidine 398, 421
    interactions 440, 508, 522
Mephentermine, interactions 440
Mephenytoin 393
Mephobarbital 392
Mephosfolan 125
Mephyton, as antidote 471
Mepiquat 145
Mepivacaine 382, 389
Meprobamate 391, 421
Mepron 500
Mepronil 155
Mequinol 569
Meralluride 295
Merbromin 295
Mercaptans 316
2-Mercaptoethanol 317
Mercaptomerin 295
6-Mercaptopurine 578, 592
    interactions 581
Mercocresol 295
Mercresin *see* Phenyl mercuric salts 295
Mercuhydrin *see* Meralluride 295
Mercurial diuretics 295
Mercurials, organic 294
Mercuric chloride 294
Mercurin *see* Mersalyl 295
Mercurochrome *see* Mercury 294
Mercurophylline 295
Mercurous chloride 294
Mercury 39, 294
Mercury oxycyanide *see* Cyanide 311
Mercury protoiodide 295
Merethoxylline 295
Meridia, see Sibutramine 434
Meropenem 493

Merpelan 155
Merphenyl nitrate *see* Mercury 294
Mersalyl 295
Mersolite *see* Phenyl mercuric salts 295
Merthiolate 295
Mertoxol *see* Mercury salts 294
Mesalamine 500
Mesantoin 393
Mescal 529
Mescaline 529
Mesityl oxide 225
Mesitylene *see* Trimethylbenzene 239
Meso-2,3-dimercaptosuccinic acid 97
Mesoridazine 404
Mesothelioma 332
Mestinon 431
Mesurol 126
Metacide 125
Metacrate 126
Metadelphene *see* Deet 151
Metal cleaners and polishes
    *see* miscellaneous acids 242
        Sodium hydroxide 257
Metal fume fever 310
Metal polish *see*
    Cyanide 311
    Oxalic acid [10%] 240
Metal salts 533
Metalaxyl 155
Metaldehyde 219
Metallic poisons **269–310**
Metam 557
Metamitron 155
Metamucil 545
Metandren 553
Metaphen *see* Mercury 294
Metaproterenol 426, 441
Metaraminol 426, 440
    interactions 508
Metasystox-R 125
Metaxolone 412
Metazaclor 155
Metformin 550
Methacholine 430
Methacrifos 125
Methacrylic acid 243
    *see also* Ethyl methacrylate 226
Methacrylonitrile *see* Acrylonitrile 312
Methacycline 490
Methadone 397, 398, 421
Methallyl chloride *see* Allyl chloride 196
Methamidophos 125
Methamphetamine 426, 441
Methandrostenolone, interactions 552

Methane 236, 238
Methane arsonic acid 271
Methanethiol 317
Methanol 39, 199
Methantheline 422
Methapyrilene 403, 421
Methaqualone 421
Methazolamide 478
Methemoglobinemia 77
Methenamine 501, 506
Methicillin 489, 506
Methidathion 125
Methimazole 546, 552
Methiocarb 126
Methocarbamol 412
Methohexital 392
Methomyl 126
Methorphan *see* Dextromethorphan 398
Methotrexate 575, 578, 582
    interactions 378
Methoxamine 426
    interactions 440
Methoxone 117
Methoxsalen 569
2-Methoxy ethanol 213
2-Methoxy ethyl acetate 213
1-Methoxy-2-propanol 213
Methoxychlor 110
Methoxyethylmercury acetate *see* Mercury 294
Methoxyflurane 385
    interactions 505
4-Methoxyphenol 449
Methscopolamine 422
Methsuximide 393, 421
Methyclothiazide 479
Methyl acetate 226
Methyl acrylate 226
Methyl acrylonitrile 312
Methyl alcohol 199
*N*-Methyl aniline 166
Methyl bromide 176
Methyl butyl ketone *see* Hexanone-2 224
Methyl carbitol *see* Ethylene glycol 209
Methyl cellosolve acetate *see* 2-Ethoxy ethyl
    acetate 213
Methyl cellosolve *see* 2-Methoxy ethanol 213
Methyl chloride 176
Methyl 2-cyanoacrylate 312
Methyl demeton 125
Methyl ether *see* Ether 385
Methyl ethyl ketone *see* Butanone-2 224
Methyl formate 227
Methyl hydrazine 166
Methyl iodide 176

Methyl isocyanate 312
Methyl isothiocyamate 167
Methyl manganese cyclopentadienyl
    tricarbonyl 292
Methyl mercury chloride 295
Methyl mercury cyamide 295
Methyl mercury hydroxide 295
Methyl mercury pentachtorophenate 295
Methyl mercury toluene sulfonate 295
Methyl methacrylate monomer 227
Methyl parathion 125
Methyl salicylate 367
Methyl silicate 243
Methyl styrene *see* Styrene 239
Methyl sulfate *see* Dimethyl sulfate 250
Methyl sulfonyl fluoride 264
Methyl trichlorosilane 243
Methyl viologen 145
*N*-Methyl-2-pyrrolidone 167
5-Methyl-3-heptanone *see* Ethyl amyl
    ketone 224
*N*-Methyl-*N'*-nitro-*N*-nitrosoguanidine 167
*N*-Methyl-*N*-nitrosourea 167
Methyl-*p*-aminophenol sulfate *see* *p*-
    Aminophenol 164
4-Methyl-pentanone-2 225
1-Methyl-2-propanol 213
Methylacetylene 238
Methylal 225
Methylamine 258
Methylamyl alcohol *see* Methyl
    isobutylcarbinol 213
Methylamyl ketone 225
Methylated naphthalene *see* Naphthalene 234
Methylbenzethonium chloride 452
Methylcellulose 347, 545
Methylchloroform 181
2-Methyl-4-chlorophenoxy acetic acid 117
Methylchlorothion 125
Methylcyclohexane 239
Methylcyclohexanol 213
Methylcyclohexanone 225
Methyldopa 433, 441
    interactions 440
Methylene aminoacetonitrile 313
Methylene bis(4-cyclohexyl isocyamate) 166
Methylene bisphenyl isocyanate 166
Methylene blue 78, 90, 567
Methylene chloride 39, 184
Methylene dichloride 184
Methylene dioxyamphetamine 529
3,4-Methylene dioxymethamphetamine 529
4,4'-Methylene-bis(2-chloroaniline) 166
Methylergonovine 437

Methylisobutylcarbinol 213
Methylisobutylketone 225
Methylmercaptan 317
Methylmercuric cyanoguanidine *see*
    Mercury 294
Methylmethane sulfonate 225
Methylphenidate 426, 441
    interactions 415
Methylprednisolone 547, 552
4-Methylpyrazole *see* Fomepizole 89
Methyltestosterone 553
Methylvinylketone 225
Methyprylon 421
Methysergide 437
Metipranolol 435
Metiram 557
Metobromuron 155
Metocarb 126
Metoclopramide 431, 441
Metocurine iodide 414
Metol 362
Metolachlor 155
Metolazone 480
Metoprolol 435, 441
Metoxuron 155
Metrazol 516
Metribuzin 155
Metrizamide 575
Metronidazole 204, 501, 506
Metubine 414
Metyrosine 433
Mevacor 478
Mevinphos 125
Mexacarbate 126
Mexican poppy 636
Mexiletine 483
Mexilitene 480
Mexitil 480
Mezlocillin 489
MGK-874 252
MGK-II 151
Mica 339
Micardis 478
Michaelis-Menton kinetics 101
Mickey Finn *see* Chloral hydrate 391
Miconazole 501
Micronase 550
Microsulfon 485
*Micrurus* sp 588
    bites 592
Midamor 477, 479
Midazolam 62, 412, 421
Midodrine 426
Midrin 426

Miglitol 550
Milcurb 153
Milcurb Super 154
Mildew remover *see* Sodium hypochlorite 356
Mildewcide *see* Mercury salts [11%] 294
Mildex *see* Dinitrophenol [20%] 135
Millipedes 608
Milogard 157
Milontin 393
Milrinone 480, 483
Miltown 391
Minamata disease 295
Mineral oil 545
Mineral oil mist 339
Mineral seal oil 228
Mineral spirits 228
Mineral wool fiber *see* Rock fiber 339
Minipress 480
Minocin 489
Minocycline 489
Minoxidil 480
Mintezol 502
Miostat 431
MIPC 126
Miral 125
Mirbane, oil of *see* Nitrobenzene 163
Mirex 119
Mirtazapine 518
Mistletoe 636
Mistral 154
Mithracin 578
Mitomycin 578
Mitoxantrone 578
Mivacron 414
Mivacurium 414
Moban 412
Mocap 124
Moccasin snakes 588
    bites 590, 591
Model airplane cement *see* Ethylene
    dichloride 185
Model fuel *see* Methanol 199
Moderil 480
Modown 117
Moexipril 477
Mojave rattlesnake 588
Mole poison *see* Strychnine [0.5%] 513
Mole-Nots *see* Strychnine [0.4%] 513
Molinate 155
Molindone 412
Mollusk toxicants 160
Mologen *see* Ricin 617
Molybdenum 308
Mometasone *see* Corticosteroids 547

Mond process 299
Monistat 501
Monitor 125
Monkshood 538
Monoacetin 347
Monoamine oxidase inhibitors 508
    interactions 203, 415, 416, 440, 481, 522, 552
Monobenzone 449
Monocid 492
Monocrotophos 124
Monolinuron 155
Monomethylarsonate *see* Arsenic 270
Monomethylhydrazine 625
Monopril *see* Fosinopril 477
Monosodium glutamate 567
Monsel's solution *see* Iron salts 559
Montelukast 567
Monuron 155
Moon fish 611
Moonseed 636
Moray eel 611
Morestan 159
Morfamquat 145
Moricizine 480
Morocide 135
Morphine 397, 398, 421
    interactions 508
Morpholine 167
Moth proofer *see* Fluoride [5%] 263
Moth repellent 234, 362
Motion sickness remedies 401
Motrin 377
Mouth, poison diagnosis 45
Mouth-to-mouth resuscitation 53
Mouthwash *see* Ethanol [50%] 202
Moxifloxacin 493
4MP *see* Fomepizole 89
MPMC 126
MSG 567
MTMC 126
Mucomyst 375
Murfotox 125
Muriatic acid *see* Hydrochloric acid 243
Muromonab-CD3 567
Muscarine 624, 625
Muscle relaxants 413
    interactions 440, 481
Mushrooms 624
Musquash root *see* Cocculus indicus 516
Mussels 610
Mustard gas *see* Bis(2-chloroethyl) sulfide 39, 196
Mustard oil 539
Mustargen 578

Mutamycin 578
Myambutol 501
Mycophenolate 568
Mycostatin 491
Mylabris *see* Cantharidin 532
Myleran 576
Mylone 153
Myochrysine 377
Myoral *see* Gold sodium thiosulfate 377
*Myristica fragrans*, nutmeg 636
Myrrh *see* Volatile oils [5%] 536
Mysoline 393

N-Serve 160
NAA 160
Nabam 557
Nabumetone 377
Nacto Fabric Cleaner *see* Tetrachloroethylene [80%] 198
Nadolol 435, 441
*Naematoloma* sp 625
Nafarelin 554
Nafcillin 489, 506
Naftifine 501
Naftin 501
Nail polish and remover *see* Acetone [100%] 224
*Naja* sp 588
    bites 592
Nalbuphine 398
Naled 124
Nalfon 377
Nalidixic acid 506
Nalmefene 398
Naloxone 91, 397, 398, 421
Naltrexone 398
Nandrolone 553
Naphazoline 425, 426
Naphtha 228
Naphthalene 234
α-Naphthalene acetic acid 160
Naphthol(s) 449
1,4-Naphthoquinone 225
1-Naphthyl-*N*-methylcarbamate 123
Naphthylamine, α or β 167
Naphthylamine mustard 167
α-Naphthylisothiocyanate *see* Methyl isothiocyanate 126
α-Naphthylthiourea 151
Naproanilide 156
Napropamide 153
Naprosyn 377
Naproxen 377
    interactions 378

Naptalam 151
Naqua 479
Narcan 91, 398
*Narcissus pseudonarcissus* 633
Narcotic analgesics 397, 415
Nardil 508
Naropine 382
Nasal sprays *see* Antibiotics 488
Nasco Aluminum Cleaner *see* Hydrofluoric
    acid [1.7%] 263
Natamycin 493
Natrin 117
Natural gas *see* Methane 238
Navane 404
Navelbine 579
Neatsfoot oil 347
Nebcin 490
Nebs *see* Acetaminophen [325 mg] 373
Neburex 156
Neburon 156
Nefazodone 518
    interactions 482, 508
Nelfinavir 502
Nemacur 125
Nemagon *see* Dibromochloropropane 197
Nembutal 392
Neo-Decadron *see* Corticosteroids 547
Neoarsphenamine *see* Arsenic 270
Neocincophen 377
Neohydrin *see* Chlormerodrin 295
Neomycin 491, 506
Neostigmine 415, 430, 431, 440
    interactions 482
Neptazene 478
*Nerium oleander*, oleander 621
Nerve gas *see* Organophosphorus
    derivatives 125
Nesacaine 382
Netilmicin 490
Netromycin 490
Neumega 568
Neuromuscular blocking agents 62, 91, 413
Neuromuscular system, poison diagnosis 47
Neurontin 393
Neutralizer, permanent wave *see* Potassium
    bromate 343
Neutrapen, as antidote 494
Neutrexin 503
Nevirapine 502
Niacinamide 92
Nialamide 508
Nickel 308
Nickel ammonium sulfate 533
Nickel carbonyl 299

Nickel salts 533
Niclosamide 160
Nicorette 138
Nicotinamide 92, 570
Nicotine 138
Nicotinic acid 570
Nicotrol *see* Nicotine [40%] 138
Nicotrox 10-X *see* Nicotine [10%] 138
Nifedipine 92, 483
Nightshade
    deadly 422
    English 422
Nikethamide 516
Nikoban *see* Lobeline [0.5 mg] 138
Nilandrone 578
Nilutamide 578
Nimbex 414
Nimrod 152
Ninhydrin 225
Nipent 578
Niphos *see* TEPP 123
Nipride 480
Nissorun 159
Nitrapyrin 160
Nitrates 467
Nitrazepam 421
Nitric acid 247
Nitric oxide 247
Nitriles *see* Cyanide 311
Nitrilotriacetate 167
Nitrites 467
    sodium and amyl 92
Nitroanilines 163, 167
Nitrobenzene 163, 167
4-Nitrobiphenyl *see* 4-Nitrodiphenyl 167
Nitrochlorobenzene *see*
    Chloronitrobenzenes 165
4-Nitrodiphenyl 167
Nitroethane 167
Nitrofen 156
Nitroferricyanide *see* Nitroprusside 311
Nitrofurantoin 502, 506
Nitrogen compounds **163–171**
Nitrogen dioxide 247
Nitrogen mustard 578
Nitrogen oxides 247
Nitrogen pentoxide 247
Nitrogen tetroxide 247
Nitrogen trifluoride 264
Nitrogen trioxide 247
Nitroglycerin 467, 483
Nitromersol 295
Nitromethane 167
Nitrophenols 167

O-ethyl-O-*p*-Nitrophenyl
   benzenethionophosphonate 124
Nitropropane 167
Nitroprusside 93, 252, 311, 480, 483
Nitrosamines 467
*N*-Nitrosodimethylamine 167
Nitrosyl chloride *see* Nitrogen oxide 247
Nitrosyl fluoride *see* Hydrogen fluoride 263
Nitrotoluene 167
Nitrous oxide 247, 385
Nizatidine 433
Nizoral 491, 501
No-Pest Strip Insecticide *see* DDVP [18%]
   124
Nolvadex 555
Nonane 239
Nonionic detergents 358
Nonsteroidal anti-inflammatory agents **367–378**
Norbormide 151
Norcuron 414
Norepinephrine 426
   interactions 440
Norethindrone 554
Norethindrone-ethinyl estradiol 553
Norethindrone-mestranol 553
Norethynodrel-mestranol 553
Norflex *see* Orphenadrine 402
Norfloxacin 493
Norflurazon 156
Norgestimate-ethinyl estradiol 553
Norgestrel 554
Norgestrel-ethinyl estradiol 553
Norlutate 554
Normeperidine 421
Normiflo 469
Normodyne 435
Nornicotine 138
Noroxin 493
Norpace 478
Norpramin 518
Norpropoxyphene 421
Nortriptyline 419, 518, 530
   interactions 521
Nortron 154, 165
Norvasc 473
Norvir 502
Nose, poison diagnosis 45
*Notechis scutatus*, tiger snake 589
Novantrone 578
Novocaine 382
NTA 167
Nuarimol 110
Nubain 398

Numol *see*
   Camphor [10%] 515
   Methyl salicylate [10%] 367
Numorphan 398
Nuromax 414
Nutmeg 636
Nux vomica *see* Strychnine [0.12%] 513
Nyco Urinakleen *see* Hydrochloric acid
   [21%] 243
Nystatin 491

Obidoxim 130
Octachloronaphthalene 189
Octane 239
Octanol 213
Octreotide 93, 568
Octyl alcohol *see* Amyl alcohol 213
Octyl dimethyl-*p*-aminobenzoic acid 565
2-Octylthioethanol 151
Odor threshold 10
Oflaxacin 493
Oftanol 124
Ofunack 125
Ofurace 156
Ohric 153
Oil spill remover *see* Benzene 231
Oil(s)
   bitter almonds *see* Cyanide 311
   camphorated *see* Camphor 515
   coal *see* Kerosene 228
   mirbane *see* Nitrobenzene 163
   mustard 539
   penetrating *see* Toluene [10%] 231
   pine 536
   turpentine *see* Turpentine 536
   volatile 536
   wintergreen 367
OK Cub Glow Fuel *see*
   Methanol 199
   Nitromethane [15%] 167
Olanzapine 412
Oleander 621
Olopatidine 434
Olsalazine *see* 5-aminosalicylic acid 500
Omethoate 125
Omite 159
Omnopon 398
Oncaspar 578
Oncovin 579
Ondansetron 93, 434
Ontak 577
Ophthaine 382
Ophthalmic medications *see*
   Ephedrine *and related drugs* 426

Silver nitrate 455
Opium 398
   derivatives of 397
Oprelvelkin 568
Opti Kleen *see* Methanol [80%] 199
Optipranolol ophthalmic 435
Oral contraceptives 552, 553
Orap 412
Orbencarb 126
Ordram 155
Organan 469
Organic compounds, atmospheric 236
Organic phosphate pesticides 124, 125
Organophosphorus derivatives 125
Organotins *see* Tributyl tin 309
Orinase 550
Orlistat 568
*Ornithodoros* sp, ticks 608
Orphenadrine 402, 421
Orthene 124
Ortho Crab Grass Killer *see* Mercury 294
Orthoclone OKT3 567
Orudis 377
Oryzalin 156
Osbac 126
Oseltamivir 502
Osmic acid 243
Osmium tetroxide *see* Osmic acid 243
Osmotic diuretics 98
Outflank *see* Permethrin 159
Outfox 153
Oven cleaner *see* Sodium hydroxide [10%] 257
Oxacillin 506
Oxadiazon 156
Oxadixyl 156
Oxalate 240
Oxalic acid 240
Oxamyl 126
Oxandrolone 553
Oxaprozin 377
Oxazepam 412, 421
Oxazolidinones 493
Oxcarbazepine 393
Oxcillin 489
Oxidants 252
Oxitriphylline, see Theophylline 510
Oxybutynin 422
Oxycamphor *see* Camphor 515
Oxycarboxin 156
Oxychloroquine *see* Chloroquine 497
Oxycodone 398, 421
Oxydemeton-methyl 125
Oxydicolchicine 579
Oxyfluorfen 156

Oxygen 93
   poisoning 573, 574
   therapy 572
Oxygen difluoride 264
Oxylone *see* Corticosteroids 547
Oxymetholone 553
Oxymorphone 398
Oxyphenbutazone, interactions 378, 552
Oxyquinoline sulfate 458
*N*-Oxystrychnic acid 513
Oxytetracycline 489
Oxythioquinox 159
Oxytocin 554
*Oxyuranus*, bites 592
Oysters 610
Ozone 252

Paclitaxel 578
Padan 158
PAH 236
Painaway *see* Methyl salicylate [15%] 367
Paint brush cleaner liquid *see* Benzene 231
Paint drier *see* Lead 282
Paint remover 362
Paint thinner 228
Paint(s) 362, 363
   green and blue *see* Lead 282
   marine *see* Xylene [35%] 231
   oil type *see* Petroleum distillates [20%] 228
   spray type
      *see* Acetone [50%] 224
      *see* Toluene [50%] 231
   *see also*, Arsenic 270
   *see also* art *see* Gamboge [1%] 543
   *see also* Benzene 231
Palivizumab 568
Palma christi *see* Castor bean 616
2-PAM *see* Pralidoxime 96, 130
Pamaquine, interactions 505
Pamidronate 565
Pamine 422
PAN 253
*Panaeolus* sp 625
Pancrease 568
Pancrelipase 568
Pancuronium 414
Panoctine 154
Panoram 156
Panretin 565
Pantopon 398
*Papaver somniferum* 398
Papaverine 412
   interactions 440
Papthion 125

Parabens 458
Paracetamol 373
Parachlorobenzene *see* Dichlorobenzene 197
Paradione 393
Paraffin 347
Paraffin wax 239
    fumes 339
Paraflex 411
Paraformaldebyde 217
Paraldehyde 219, 421
Paramethadione 393
Paraplatin 576
Paraquat 145
Parasympathomimetic agents 430
Parathion 123, 125
Paregoric 398
Pargyline 508
    interactions 440, 481
Paricalcetol *see* Vitamin D 571
Paris green *see* Arsenic 270
Parnate 508
Paromomycin 493
Paroxetine 523
Parrot fish 611
Parsley family 622, 623
Particulates, atmospheric **327–340**
PAS 500
Paste
    ant *see* Arsenic 270
    *see also* Starch 347
Patanol *see* Olopatidine 434
Patoran 155
*Paulinia cupana* 570
Pavulon 414
Paxil 523
PBB 188
PCB 189
PCP 527
Pea, sweet 637
Peace pill *see* Phencyclidine 527
Peacemaker 193
Pearl ash *see* Potassium carbonate 257
Pebulate 557
Pectin *see* Algin 347
Pegademase 568
Peganone 393
*Peganum harmala* 529
Pegaspargase 578
Pemirolast 568
Pemoline 426
Penbutolol 435, 441
Penciclovir 502
Pencils
    indelible 361

    yellow or green *see* Lead salts [10%] 282
Penconazole 110
Pendimethalin 156
Penetrating oil *see* Kerosene 228
Penetrex 493
Penicillamine 94
Penicillin G, as antidote 626
Penicillinase, as antidote 494
Penicillin(s) 488, 489, 506
    interactions 481
Pennyroyal 536
Penphos *see* Parathion 123
Pentaborane 442
Pentac 159
Pentachlorobenzene 197
Pentachloroethane 197
Pentachloronaphthalene 189
Pentachloronitrobenzene 167
Pentachlorophenol 448, 449
Pentachlorozincate *see* Zinc salts 533
Pentaerythritol tetranitrate 467
Pentafluorochloropropene 192
Pentamidine isethionate 502
Pentane 239
Pentanone-2 225
Pentasodium tripolyphosphate *see* Sodium
    phosphates 257
Pentazocine 398, 421
Penthrane 385
Pentobarbital 392, 421
Pentosan polysulfate 568
Pentostatin 578
Pentothal 392
    for convulsions 62
Pentoxifylline 510
Pentylenetetrazol 516
Pepcid 433
Pepper 536
Perborate 442
Perch 611
Perchlorethylene 182
Perchloric acid 243
Perchloroethane *see* Hexachloroethane 197
Perchloroethylene *see* Tetrachloroethylene 182
Perchloromethane *see* Carbon tetrachlonde 172
Perchloromethylmercaptan 317
Perchloryl fluoride 264
Percodan 398
Perfl-didone 156
Perfume 346
Pergolide 437
Periactin 402
Peridex 458
Perindopril 477

Periodic acid *see* Perchloric acid 243
Peritoneal dialysis 98
Perlite 339
Permanent wave neutralizer *see*
  Hydrogen peroxide [10%] 458
  Potassium bromate [10%] 343
  Sodium perborate [20%] 442
Permax 437
Permethrin 159
Permitil 404
Peropal 158
Peroxide *see* Hydrogen peroxide 458
Peroxyacetic acid 243
Peroxyacetylnitrate 253
Peroxyvanadate *see* Vanadium 310
Perphenazine 404, 421
  interactions 521
Persantine 477
Perthane 109
Pertofrane 518
Pertussin Actin Cough Medicine *see*
  Dextromethorphan [0.1%] 398
Pesticides 109
  carbamate 126
  cholinesterase inhibitors **123–132**
  miscellaneous **133–160**
Peterman Ant Food *see* Sodium fluoride
  [50%] 264
Peterman Roach Powder and Paste *see* Sodium
  fluoride [50%] 264
Pethidine 398
Petrolatum 228, 545
Petroleum distillates 228
Petroleum ether 228
Petroleum fumes 338
Petroleum gas *see* Methane 238
Petroleum mist 339
Petroleum naphtha 228
Petroleum spirit 228
Peyote 529
Phalloidin 624
Phaltan 156
Pharmacokinetics 100
*Phaseolus lunatus* 311
Phemerol 452
Phenacemide 393
Phenacetin 373
  interactions 378
Phenaphen *see*
  Phenacetin [0.2 g] 373
  Phenobarbital [15 mg] 392
Phenazopyridine 502
Phencyclidine 527, 530
Phendimetrazine 426

Phenelzine 508
Phenergan 404
Phenformin 552
Phenindione 469, 483
Pheniprazine 508
Phenmedipham 156
Phenobarbital 392, 421
  for convulsions 62
Phenol 448, 449
Phenolphthalein 545
Phenothiazine 159
  derivatives 404
  interactions 416, 440
Phenothiol 117
Phenoxybenzamine 434
  interactions 440
2-Phenoxyethanol *see* 2-Ethoxyethanol 213
Phenoxymethylpenicillin 506
Phensuximide 393
Phentermine 426, 441
Phenthoate 125
Phentolamine 94, 434
Phenurone 393
Phenyl ether 225
Phenyl glycidyl ether 225
*o*-Phenyl phenol 449
Phenyl salicylate *see* Salicylates 367
*p*-Phenyl-β-naphthylanune 167
Phenylamine *see* Aniline 163
Phenylbutazone 377
  interactions 378, 415, 481, 552
Phenylcellosolve *see* 2-Ethoxyethanol 213
*p*-Phenylenediamine 167, 362
Phenylephrine 426
  interactions 440, 508
2-Phenylethanol *see* Benzyl alcohol 382
Phenylethyl alcohol *see* Benzyl alcohol 382
Phenylhydrazine 167
Phenylhydroxylamine 167
Phenylmercaptan 316
Phenylmercuric salts 295
Phenylpropanolamine 441
  interactions 508
Phenylsemicarbazide *see* Phenylhydrazine 167
Phenyramidol, interactions 481
Phenytoin 62, 95, 393, 421, 461
  interactions 377, 388, 415, 482, 505, 552
*Philodendron* 621
Phix *see* Mercury salts [22%] 294
*Phoneutria fera*, tarantula spider 604
*Phoradendron flavescens*, mistletoe 636
Phorate 125
Phosalone 125
Phosdrin 125

Phosgene 190
Phosmet 125
Phosphamidon 125
Phosphate(s) 257, 258
   insecticides 123
Phosphides 301
Phosphine 301
Phospholine 431
Phosphoric acid 243
Phosphorous acid *see* Phosphoric acid 243
Phosphorus 301
Phosphorus oxychloride *see* Phosphorus
   pentachloride 243
Phosphorus pentachloride 243
Phosphorus pentasulfide 317
Phosphorus pentoxide *see* Phosphoric acid 243
Phosphorus sesquisulfide 301
Phostex 125
Photofrin 578
Photographic fixative 362
Phoxim 125, 126
Phthalates *see* Dimethylphthalate 151
Phthalide 110
Phthallic anhydride 243
*m*-Phthalodinitrile 312
Phthalthrin 159
Phygon *see* Dichloronaphthoquinone 197
*Physalia* sp 614
Physic nut 636
*Physostigma venenosum*, calabar bean 632
Physostigmine 95, 430, 431
Phytare *see* Cacodylic acid 271
*Phytolacca americana*, pokeweed 621
Phytonadion 95
Phytonadione 571
   as antidote 471
Picloram 156
2-Picoline 167
Picragol 455
Picric acid 167
Picrotoxin 516
Pigment
   black *see* Iron salts 559
   blue *see* Iron salts 559
   brown *see* Lead 282
   green *see* Arsenic 270
   maroon *see* Aniline [1%] 164
   metallic *see* Copper salts 533
   orange *see* Lead 282
   red *see* Mercury 294
   violet *see* Arsenic 270
   white *see* Lead 282
   yellow *see* Lead 282
Pilocarpine 430, 431

Pimozide 412, 421
Pindolol 434, 435, 441
Pindone 469
Pine oil 536
α-Pinene *see* Turpentine 536
Pioglitazone 550
Pipe and drain cleaners *see* Sodium
   hydroxide 257
Pipecuronium 414
*Piper methysticum* 570
Piperacillin 489
Piperalin 156
Piperazine 507
Piperidine 168
Piperine *see* Piperidine 168
Piperonyl butoxide 159
Piperophos 125
Pipron 156
*Piptadenia peregrina* 529
Pirbuterol 426
Pirimicarb 126
Pirimiphos-ethyl 125
Pirimiphos-methyl 125
Pirimor 126
Piroxicam 377
Pit viper 588
   bites 590
Pix 145
Placidyl 391
Plant and animal hazards **585–638**
Plant growth regulators 160
Plant poisoning **615–638**
*Plantago ovata* *see* Psyllium 545
Plantvax 156
Plaquenil 497
Plastic casting resin 362
Plastic menders *see* Ethylene dichloride 185
Plastic resin hardener 363
Plasticizer *see* Triorthocresyl phosphate 216
Plating compounds *see* Cyanide 311
Platinol 576
Platinum 308
Plavix 477
Plegine 426
Plendil 473
Pletal 477
Plicamycin 578
Plictran 158
Pneumoconiosis 329
PNU 143
Poast 157
Podofilox 543
Podophyllum 543
*Podophyllum peltatum* 543

*Poinciana* sp 632
Poinsettia 636
Poison checklist 5
Poison hemlock 622, 623
Poison ivy 628
Poison ivy extract, alum-precipitated 568
Poison ivy wash *see* Iron salts 559
Poison sumac 628
Poisoning
  accidental 105
  diagnosis and evaluation **35–51**
  drug treatment 26
  emergency **25–34**
  homicidal 104
  management **52–101**
  occupational, reporting 105
  prevention **3–24**
  suicidal 17, 104
Pokeweed 621
Polish
  aluminum *see* Benzene [50%] 231
  automobile *see* Kerosene [90%] 228
  car or home *see* Kerosene [50%] 228
  household, aerosol *see* Mineral oil
    [50%] 545
  metal *see* Oxalates [30%] 240
Polyalkylene oxide ethers *see* 2-
  Butoxyethanol 213
Polyamines 168
Polybrominated biphenyls 188
Polychlorinated biphenyls 188
Polychlorinated naphthalene 188
Polycyclic aromatic hydrocarbons 236
Polyethylene glycol *see* Ethylene glycol 209
Polyglycols *see* Ethylene glycol 209
Polymixins, interactions 416
Polymyxin B 491, 507
Polymyxin(s) 491
  interactions 415
Polypropylene glycol 213
Polyram 557
Polysorbate 347
Polysulfides 316
Polytetrafluoroethylene *see* Teflon fumes 308
Polythiazide 479
Polyurethane polymer 309
Polyvinyl acetate 347
Polyvinylchloride polymer 309
Polyvinylpyrrolidone 347
Pompano 611
Ponstel 377
Pontocaine 382
Pool chlorine *see* Sodium hypochlorite
  [15%] 356

Poractant 565
Porcupine fish 611
Porfimer 578
Portland cement 258
Portuguese Man-of-War 614
Potash
  sulfurated *see* Sulfides 316
  *see also* Potassium hydroxide 257
Potassium, imbalance, and drugs 481
Potassium alum 533
Potassium bichromate 280
Potassium bromate 343
Potassium bromide 408
Potassium carbonate 257, 258
Potassium chlorate 453
Potassium chloride 480
Potassium chromate 280
Potassium cyanide 312
Potassium hexametaphosphate 257
Potassium hydroxide 257, 258
Potassium iodide 445
Potassium loss 416
Potassium permanganate 258
Potassium persulfate 256
Potassium polyphosphate 257
Potassium pyrophosphate 257
Potassium tripolyphosphate 257
Potato 621
Povidone-iodine 445
Powder, face or skin *see* Talc 340
Prairie rattlesnake 588
Pralidoxime 96, 130
Pramipexole 412
Pramitol 156
Pramoxine 382
Prandin 544, 550
Pravachol 478
Pravastatin 478
Prazepam 421
Praziquantel 502
Prazosin 480, 483
Precose 550
Prednicarbate *see* Corticosteroids 547
Prednisolone 546, 552
Prednisone 546
Prefar 124
Prefix 153
Pregnancy 19
Preservation of evidence 102
Preservative
  brush *see* Kerosene 228
  concrete *see* Benzene 231
  wood *see* Fluoride 263
Pressor agents, interactions 522

Prevalite 481
Prevention of poisoning **3–24**
Preventive, rust *see* Phosphoric acid 243
Preveon 500
Priftin 502
Prilocaine 382, 389
Primacor 480
Primicid 125
Primidone 393, 421
   interactions 482
Primrose 636
*Primula* sp 636
Princep 157
Prinivil *see* Lisinopril 477
Priscoline 434
Privet 636
Privine 426
Pro-Banthine 422
ProAmatine 426
Proban 124
Probenecid 480, 483
   interactions 378, 481
Procainamide 465, 483
   interactions 388, 416, 440, 482
Procaine 382
   interactions 388, 415
Procarbazine 578
Prochlorperazine 404, 421
Procrit 553
Procyclidine 422
Procymidone 157
Profenal 377
Profenofos 125
Progesterone 544
Progestins 544
Prograf 569
Proleukin 576
Proloprim 503
Promethazine 404, 421
Prometone 156
Prometryne 156
Pronamide 156
Propachlor 156
Propafenone 480, 483
Propamocarb 126
Propane 239
Propane sultone 316
Propanidid, interactions 415
Propanil 157
Propantheline 422, 441
   interactions 440
Propaphos 125
Proparacaine 382
Propargite 159

Propargyl alcohol *see* Propynol 213
Propazine 157
Propecia 554
Propetamphos 125
Propham 126, 157
Propiconazole 157
Propine 426
Propineb 557
β-Propiolactone 225
Propionaldehyde *see* Acetaldehyde 219
Propionic acid 243
Propionitrile 312
Propofol 412
Propoxur 126
Propoxyphene 398, 421
Propranolol 435, 441
   as antidote 626
   interactions 388, 416, 440, 552
Propulside 431
Propyl acetate 227
n-Propyl alcohol 214
Propyl ether *see* Isopropyl ether 225
n-Propyl nitrate 168
n-Propyl nitrite *see* Nitroglycerin 467
Propylene chlorohydrin 197
Propylene dibromide *see* Dicloropropane 197
Propylene dichloride *see* Dichloropropane 197
Propylene *see* Ethylene 385
Propylene glycol 213
Propylene glycol dinitrate 467
Propylene glycol monomethyl ether *see*
   Ethylene glycol 209
Propylene glycol monostearate *see* Ethylene
   glycol 209
Propylene imine 168
Propylene oxide 226
Propylparaben *see* Benzoic acid 458
Propylparasept *see* Benzoic acid 458
Propylthiouracil 546, 552
Propynol 213
Propyzamide 156
Proscar 554
ProSom 411
Prostacyclin 553
Prostigmin 415, 431
Prostin VR 553
Prosulfocarb 557
Protamine 96
Protamine sulfate 568
   as antidote 471
Protective clothing 7
Protective devices, personal 193
Protein hydrolysates 568
*Proteus*, seafood poisoning 353

Prothiophos 125
*Protogonyaulax* sp, shellfish poisoning 354
Protopam 130
Protriptyline 419, 518
Proturf fungicide *see* Phenylmercuric salts [0.7%] 295
Prowl 156
Prozac 523
*Prunus* sp 633
Prussic acid *see* Cyanide 311
Pseudoephedrine 426, 441
Psilocin 529
*Psilocybe* sp 625
   *P. mexicana* 529
Psilocybin 529
Psychotomimetic agents **508–531**
Psyllium hydrophilic mucilloid 545
Puff adder 589, 593
Puffers 611
Pulmonary edema 55
Pulmozyme 566
Purex Bleach 356
Purinethol 578
Putty *see* Lead 282
Pyraclofos 125
Pyramin 153
Pyrazinamide 502
Pyrazolones 377
Pyrazophos 125
Pyrethrin 159
Pyrethrum *see* Pyrethrin 159
Pyributicarb 557
Pyridaphenthion 125
Pyridate 157
Pyridine 168
Pyridine-2-aldoxime methochloride 130
Pyridinethione zinc 458
Pyridium 502
Pyridostigmine 431
Pyridoxine 96
   as antidote 626
   interactions 440
*N*-3-Pyridylmethyl-*N′*-*p*-nitrophenylurea 143
Pyrilamine 403, 421
Pyrimethamine 502, 507
Pyrogallol 449

Quartz 329
Quarzan 422
Quazepam 412, 421
Questran 481, 566
Quetiapine 412
Quicklime *see* Calcium oxide 258
Quinacrine 497, 507

   interactions 204, 505
Quinalbarbital 421
Quinalphos 125
Quinapril 477
Quinethazone 480
Quinidine 462, 483
   interactions 388, 416, 440, 481, 482
Quinine 497, 507
Quinolones 493
Quinone *see* Benzoquinone 168, 224

R-Gen 565
Rabcide 110
Rabon 125
Racumin 469
Raloxifene 554
Ramipril 477
Ramrod 156
Rangado 124
Range oil *see* Kerosene 228
Ranitidine 434
*Ranunculaceae* 633
Rapamune 568
Rat poison *see*
   Arsenic 270
   Cyanide 311
   Fluorides 264
   Phosphorus 301
   Strychnine 513
   Thallium 140
   Warfarin 469
Rattlesnakes 588
   bites 590, 591
Rauwolfia preparations 480
Rayless goldenrod 637
RDX *see* Tetryl 168
Rectal poisoning 33
Red diamond rattlesnake 588
Red oil 347
Red phosphorus 301
Red tides, seafood poisoning 352
Reducing capsules or pills *see*
   Amphetamine 426
   Thyroid 555
Refludan 469
Refrigerants 191
Refrigerator gas *see* Carbon monoxide 320
Regitine, *see also* Phentolamine 94
Reglan 431
Regranex 553
Relafen 377
Relaxants
   muscle 413
      interactions 388, 440, 481

Relenza 503
Remeron 518
Remicade 567, 577
Remifentanil 398
Renacidin 568
Renagel 568
Renal failure 66
Renese 479
Renovue 575
ReoPro 477
Repaglinide 550, 554
Repellents 151
   dog *see*
      Capsicum [15%] 539
      Naphthalene 234
   insect, powdered *see* Naphthalene
      [100%] 234
Reptiles **587–600**
Requip, see Ropinirole 412
Rescinnamine 480
Rescriptor 500
Reserpine 441, 480, 483
   interactions 482
Resins 481
   solvents *see* Polychlorinated
      naphthalene 188
Resmethrin 159
Resorcinol 449
Respiration, depressed 52
Restoril 412
Retavase 477
Reteplase 477
Retin-A 569
Retrovir 503
Revex *see* Nalmefene 91
*Rheum* sp 621
Rhodium 309
Rhodododendron 637
*Rhodomyrtus macrocarpa*, finger cherry 634
*Rhodophyllus* sp 625
*Rhodotypos scandens*, jetberry 634
Rhubarb 240, 621
*Rhus* spp 628
Ribavirine 502
Ricin 617
Ricinoleic ester 545
*Ricinus communis*, castor bean 616
Ridomil 155
Riebeckite, fibrous 331
Rifabutin 493
Rifampin 493, 507
   interactions 482
Rifapentine 502
Rilutek 412

Riluzole 412
Rimactane 493
Rimantidine 502
Rimexolone *see* Corticosteroids 547
Riot control agents 193
Ripcord 158
Risedronate 565
Risperidal 412
Risperidone 412
Ritalin 426
Ritodrine 426
Ritonavir 502
Rituximab 578
Ro-Neet 557
Roach poison *see* Phosphorus 301
Roach powder *see*
   Boric acid 442
   Sodium fluoride 264
Robaxin 412
*Robinia pseudoacacia*, locust 635
Robinul 422
Rock fiber 339
Rocuronium 414
Rodenticide(s) 151
   poisoning prevention 6
   *see also* Arsenic 270
   *see also* Phosphorus 301
Rofecoxib 377
Rogue 157
Romazicon *see* Flumazenil 89
Romilar 398
Ronilan 110
Ronstar 156
Ropinirole 412
Ropivacaine 382
Rosary bean 616
Rosi 347
Rosiglitazone 550
Rotenone 159
Rouge 347
Roundup 154
Rovral 159
Roxatidine 433
Roxin 433
Rubber cement *see* Hexane 238
Rubber patch cement *see* Toluene [60%] 231
Rubbing alcohol *see* Isopropanol 214
Rubefacients **532–540**
Rubigan 110
Rue 536
Rug cleaner *see* Trichloroethylene 179
Russell's viper 588
   bites 593, 594
*Russula* sp 625

Rust remover *see* Phosphoric acid 243
Ryania 159
Rye 437
Rythmol 480

S-bioallethrin 159
Sabril 393
Saccharin 568
Sacrosidase 568
Safety equipment 10
Safrotin 125
St John's wort 570
    interactions 508
Sal soda *see* Sodium carbonate 257
Salagen 431
Salbutamol 426, 441
Salicylamide 367
    interactions 378
Salicylates 367
    interactions 377, 482, 505
Salicylic acid 367
Salmeterol 426
Salsalate, see salicylates 367
Saluron 479
*Sambucus* sp 634
Sandostatin 568
    *see also* Octreotide 93
*Sanguinaria* sp 632
Sani-Chlor 356
Sansert 437
Saponated solution of cresols 449
Saprol 158
Saquinavir 502
Sargramostim 578
Sarin *see* Parathion 123
Sassafras 536
Saturation kinetics 101
Saturn 557
Savin 536
Saw Palmetto 570
Saw-scaled viper 589
    bites 593
Scepter 157
Scheele's green *see* Arsenic 270
Scillaren *see* Digitalis 459
Scilliroside 459
*Scolopendra subspinipes*, centipede 608
Scombroid poisoning 353, 611, 612
Scoparius *see* Digitalis 459
Scopolamine 422
*Scorpaena guttata*, scorpion fish 614
Scorpion fish 614
Scorpion(s) 605
Sea bass 611

Sea snake venom 594
Sea wasp 614
Seafood poisoning 352
Secobarbital 392, 421
Seconal 392
Sectral 435
Sedatives 390
    interactions 203
    *see also* Bromides 408
    *see also* Morphine 398
Seed disinfectant *see* Mercury 238
Seldane 403
Selective serotonin reuptake inhibitors 523
Selective serotonin uptake inhibitors,
    interactions 508
Selegiline 412
Selenate 309
Selenium 309
Selenium hexafluoride 264, 309
Selenium oxide 309
Selenium sulfide 458
Selsun 458
Semeron 153
Semprex-D 433
Sencor 155
Senna 545
Sensorcaine 382
Septra 486
Serax 412
*Serenoa repens* 570
Serentil 404
Serevent 426
Sermorelin 554
Seromycin 491
Seroquel 412
Serotonin *see* Selective serotonin reuptake
    inhibitors 523
Serpasil 480
Serpentine, fibrous 331
Sertraline 523
Serzone 518
Sesame oil 347
Sesone 117
Sethoxydim 157
Sevelamer 568
Sevin 126
Sevoflurane 385
Sheep dip *see* Arsenic 270
    Phenol 448
Shellac *see* Methanol 199
Shellfish poisoning 610
    paralytic 354
Shock 56
Shock-absorber fluid *see* Ethylene glycol 209

Sibutramine 434
Sidewinder rattlesnake 588
Siduron 157
Silane 309
Sildenafil 568
Silica 39, 328
Silica gel 329
Silicofluoride *see* Fluoride 263
Silicon 339
Silicon carbide 339
Silicon tetrahydride 339
    *see also* Silane 309
Silicone 347
Silicosis 329
Silvadene 502
Silver 455
Silver nitrate 455
Silver picrate 455
Silver proteinate 455
Silver salts 455
Silver solder flux *see* Fluoride 263
Silver sulfadiazine 502
Silvex 117
Simazine 157
Simetryn 157
Simulect 565
Simvastatin 478
Sinbar 157
Sinemet 416
Sinequan 518
Singulair 567
Sirolimus 568
Sistan 557
Skelaxin 412
Skelid 565
Skin
    bleach *see* Hydroquinone 449
    contamination 32
    poison diagnosis 42
    protectives 347
Slug insecticide *see* Metaldehyde [20%] 219
Smog 247, 252
Snail insecticide *see* Metaldehyde [20%] 219
Snakeroot 637
Snakes 587
    bites 32, 587
        antisera 596
    venom 588
Snapper 611
Soap 358
Soapstone 339
Sodium acid sulfate 255
Sodium alkyl phosphate 358
Sodium aluminum fluoride 264

Sodium arsenite *see* Arsenic 270
Sodium bicarbonate 97
Sodium bisulfite 256
Sodium borate 442
Sodium bromide 408
Sodium cacodylate *see* Arsenic 270
Sodium carbonate 257, 258
Sodium chlorate 453
Sodium chloride 568
Sodium cyanide 312
Sodium ferro-ferrisilicate 331
Sodium fluoride 264
Sodium fluoroacetate 137
Sodium hexametaphosphate 257
Sodium hydride *see* Sodium hydroxide 257
Sodium hydrosulfite 256
Sodium hydroxide 257, 258
Sodium hypochlorite 356
Sodium iodide 445
Sodium lauryl sulfate 358
Sodium metabisulfite 243, 256
Sodium metal *see* Sodium hydroxide 257
Sodium metasilicate *see* Sodium silicate 258
Sodium morrhuate 481
Sodium nitrite 467
    as cyanide antidote 314
Sodium oleate 358
Sodium perborate 442
Sodium persulfate 256
Sodium phosphate 257, 545
Sodium polyphosphate 257
Sodium polystyrene sulfonate 568
Sodium psylliate 481
Sodium pyrophosphate 258
Sodium restriction and loss, lithium
    toxicity 581
Sodium salicylate 367
Sodium silicate 258
Sodium sulfate 545
    as antidote 134
Sodium sulfite 256
Sodium sulfoxylate 256
Sodium tetradecylsulfate 481
Sodium thiosalicylate 367
Sodium thiosulfate 97, 256, 314, 362, 575
Sodium trichloroacetate 198
Sodium tripolyphosphate 257
Sodium tyropanoate 575
Sodium valproate 393
Softeners, skin 347
Soil fumigant *see* 2,2′-Dichloroethyl ether 197
Solage 569
Solanaceae 621
*Solanum* sp 621, 622

Solatene 566
Solder 309
Soldering flux
    silver *see* Fluoride 263
    *see also* Hydrochloric acid [10%] 243
*Solenopsis saevissima*, fire-ant 608
Solganal 377
Solox 199
Soltalol 441
Soma 391
Somatropin 554, 555
Sonalan 157
Sonar 154
Sorbic acid 347
Soriatane 565
Sotalol 435, 481
Southern Pacific rattlesnake 588
Spanish fly 532
Sparfloxacin 493
Spectazole 500
Spectinomycin 490, 507
Spermaceti 347
Spiders, poisonous 601
Spike 157
Spindle-tree 632
Spirits
    Eagle *see* Methanol 199
    mineral 228
Spironolactone 479, 483
Sporanox 492, 501
Squill 459
SSRIs 523
    interactions 508
Stadol 398
Stamp pad inks 363
Stannic salts *see* Tin salts 533
Stannous chloride 533
Stanozolol 553
*Staphylococcus*, food poisoning 351
Starch 340, 347
Starting fluid *see* Ethyl ether 385
Stavudine 502
Steam iron cleaner 363
Stearates 340
Stearic acid 347
Stelazine 404
*Sterculia* gum 545
Sterno Canned Heat *see*
    Ethanol [80%] 202
    Methanol [4%] 199
Steroids
    adrenal, interactions 552
    anabolic 533

    interactions 481, 552
Stibine 269
Stimulants **508–531**
Sting-ray 614
Stoddard solvent 228
Stonefish 614
Storage batteries *see* Lead 282
Storage of poisons 3, 6
STP 529
Streamer 193
Streptase 477
Streptokinase 477
*Streptomyces avermitilis* 147
Streptomycin 488, 490, 507
Streptozocin 578
Strophanthin *see* Digitalis 459
Strophanthus 459
Strychnine 513
Styrene 239
Sublimate, corrosive *see* Mercury 294
Sublimaze 398
Substance dependency 49
Succimer 97
Succinylcholine 414
    for convulsions 62
    interactions 415, 440, 481, 482
Sucraid 568
Sucralfate 568
Sufenta 398
Sufentanil 398
Suffix BW 110
Sugar cane dust 339
Suicidal poisoning 17, 104
    prevention 18
Sulamyd 485
Sulfabenzamide 485
Sulfacetamide 485
Sulfadiazine 485
Sulfadoxine 485
Sulfafenazole, interactions 552
Sulfamate 157
Sulfamethoxazole 485, 507
Sulfamic acid 243
Sulfamylon 485
Sulfanilamide 485
Sulfanilic acid 168
Sulfasalazine 485, 486, 507
Sulfides 316
Sulfinpyrazone 485
    interactions 378, 481
Sulfisoxazole 485, 507
    interactions 505
Sulfonamides 485
    interactions 481, 505

Sulfonated soaps 358
Sulfone drugs 485
Sulfonylureas 550
  interactions 204, 440, 552
Sulfosalicylic acid 243
Sulfotepp 125
Sulfur 316
  compounds 155, 316
Sulfur dioxide 39, 255
Sulfur hexafluoride 264
Sulfur monochloride 255
Sulfur oxides 255
Sulfur pentafluoride 264
Sulfur tetrafluoride 264
Sulfur trioxide 255
Sulfuric acid 255
Sulfurous acid 255
Sulfuryl fluoride 264
Sulindac 377, 378
Sulprofos 125
Sumac, poison 628
Sumilex 157
Sumithrin 159
Supona 124
Supprelin 554
Supracide 125
Suprane 385
Suprofen 377
Surflan 156
Surgeon fish 611
Surmontil 518
Survanta 565
Sustiva 500
Sutan 557
Sweet pea 637
Swep 126
Symmetrel 500
Sympathetic blocking agents 433
Sympatholytic agents 432
Sympathomimetics, interactions 482
*Symphytum* 570
*Synaceja horrida* 614
Synagis 568
*Synanceja trachynis* 614
Synarel 554
Synthrin 159
Synvisc 567
Systox 125

2,4,5-T 117
t₁/₂, defined 100
T-stuff *see* Hydrogen peroxide [30%] 458
Tabatrex 151
Tabcin *see* Salicylates [360 mg] 367

*Tabernanthe iboga* 529
Tabun *see* Parathion 123
Tachigaren 155
Tacrine 431
Tacrolimus 569
Tagamet 433
Taipan snakes, bites 592
Talc 340
Talcord 159
Talcum powder 328
Talon 469
Talwin 398
Tambocor 479
Tamiflu 502
Tamoxifen 555
Tamsulosin 434
*Tanacetum* 570
Tandex 126
Tannic acid 448, 449
Tanning agents 346
Tansy 536
Tantalum 309
Tapazole 546
Tapioca 311
Tar 449
Tar camphor *see* Naphthalene 234
Tar remover *see* Kerosene 228
Tarantula spider 604
Targretin 576
Tartar emetic 269
Tartaric acid 243
Tartrazine 569
Tavist 402
Taxol 578
Taxoter 577
*Taxus*, yew 622
Tazarotene 569
Tazorac 569
TCDD 109, 117
TCDF 192
TCDFa 192
Tebuthiuron 157
Tecnazene 110
Tedion 110
Teflon fumes 308
Tegison 565
Tegretol 393
Tellurium 309
Tellurium hexafluoride 264
Telmisartan 478
Telone *see* Dichloropropene 197
Temazepam 412, 421
Temik 126
Temodar 578

Temophos 124
Temozolomide 578
Temperature regulation 72
Tenecteplase 477
Teniposide 578
Tenormin 435
Tensilon 431
    use of 415
TEPP 123, 125
Tequin 493
Teratogens 19
Terazol 502
Terazosin 480
Terbacil 157
Terbinafine 491, 502
Terbumeton 157
Terbuphos 125
Terbutaline 426, 441
Terbuthylazine 157
Terbutryn 157
Terconazole 502
Terfenidine 402
Teridox 153
Terphenyls 239
Terpin hydrate 569
Terpineol *see* Turpentine 536
Terpinylthiocyanoacetate *see* Lethane 142
Terramycin 489
Terrazole 154
*p*-Tert-butyltoluene 238
Teslac 578
Tessalon 411
Testolactone 578
Testosterone 553
sym-Tetrabromoethane 198
Tetracaine 382
1,1,1,2-Tetrachloro-2,2-difluoroethane 192
1,1,1,2-Tetrachloro-1,2-difluoroethane 192
Tetrachloro-*p*-dibenzodioxin 117
2,3,7,8-Tetrachlorodibenzodioxin 109, 118
Tetrachlorodifluoroethane 192
Tetrachlorodiphenylsulfone 110
Tetrachloroethane 178
Tetrachloroethylene 182, 198
Tetrachloronaphthalene 189
Tetrachloronitrobenzene 168
Tetrachlorophenol 449
Tetrachlorvinphos 125
Tetracycline(s) 489, 507
    interactions 481, 505
Tetracyn 489
Tetradifon 110
Tetraethyl dithionopyrophosphate 125
Tetraethyl lead 282

Tetraethyl pyrophosphate 123, 125
Tetraethylthiuram disulfide *see* Disulfiram 556
Tetraglycine hydroperiodide 445
Tetrahydro-β-naphthylalmine *see*
    Naphthylamine 167
Tetrahydrofuran 226
Tetrahydrofurfuryl alcohol 213
Tetrahydronaphthalene 239
Tetrahydrozoline 426
Tetralin *see* Tetrahydronaphthalene 239
Tetramethoxysilane *see* Methyl silicate 243
Tetramethrin 159
Tetramethyl lead 283
Tetramethylsuccinonitrile 168
Tetramethylthiuram disulfide *see*
    Disulfiram 556
Tetranitromethane 168
*Tetraodontidae*, puffers 611
Tetraphosphorus trisulfide 301
Tetrasodium edetate 363
Tetrasodium pyrophosphate 258
Tetryl 168
Teveten 478
Thalidomide 569
Thallium 140
THAM 569
Thanite 142
THC 530
Theobromine 510
Theophylline 510, 530
Theophylline ethylenediamine 511
*Thevetia* sp 637
Thevetin *see* Digitalis 459
Thiabendazole 502
Thiamine 571
Thiazide diuretics, interactions 482, 552
Thiazolidinediones 550
Thidiazuron 160
Thiethylperazine 404
Thimerosol 295
Thimet 125
4,4′-Thio-bis(6-tertiary-butyl-*m*-cresol) 448
Thio-TEPP *see* TEPP 125
Thioacetamide 316
Thiobencarb 126, 557
Thiocarbamates 556
    interactions 204
Thiocresol 449
Thiocyanate 312, 483
    insecticides 142
Thiocyclam 159
Thiodan 119
Thiodicarb 126
Thiofanox 126

Thioglycolic acid 243
Thioguanine 578
Thiometon 125
Thionyl chloride 255
Thiopental 392, 421
   for convulsions 62
   interactions 505
Thiophanate 157
Thiophanate-methyl 160
Thioridazine 404, 421
   interactions 415
Thiotepa 578
Thiothixene 404
Thiouracil compounds 546
Thiram 556, 557
Thorazine 404
Thorn apple 422
Threshold limit values 10
Thrombocytopenia 79
Thymol 449
Thyroid 555
Thyroid drugs 555
   interactions 415, 481, 552
Thyroid hormone, interactions 521
Thyroxine 552
   *see also* Thyroid 555
Tiagabine 393
TIBA 160
Ticarcillin 489
Ticks 608
Ticlid 477
Ticlopidine 477
Tigan 402
Tiger snake 589
Tiglium *see* Croton oil 543
Tikosyn 479
Tile cleaner *see* Hydrochloric acid [20%] 243
Tillam 557
Tilt 157
Tiludronate 565
Timber rattlesnake 588
Timolol 435, 441
Tin
   organic compounds *see* Tributyl tin 309
   salts 533
   tetrachloride *see* Stannous chloride 533
Tirofiban 469, 477
TIT *see* Liothyronine 555
Titanium dioxide 340
Titanium oxide 347
Titanium tetrachloride 243
*Tityus* sp 605
Tizanidine 426
TLV 9

TNKase 477
TNT 170
Tobacco 138
   Indian 634
Tobramycin 490, 507
Tocainide 481
α-Tocopherol 571
TOCP 216
Tofranil 518
Toilet bowl cleaner *see* Acids 243
TOK 156
Tokuthion 125
Tolazamide 550, 552
Tolazoline 434
   interactions 204
Tolbutamide 550, 552
   interactions 377, 505, 552
Tolcapone 433
Tolectin 377
*o*-Tolidine 168
Tolinase 550
Tolmetin 377, 378
Tolterodine 422
Toluene 231
Toluene diisocyanate 168
Toluenediamine 168
Toluidine(s) 163, 168
*o*-Tolunitrile 312
Toluol *see* Toluene 231
Tolylfluanid 157
Tomaset 160
Tonic(s) 497
Tonocard 481
Toothpaste fluoridated *see* Fluoride [0.1%] 264
Topamax 393
Topaz 110
Topiramate 393
Topotecan 579
Topsin 157
Toradol 377
Tordon 156
Torecan 404
Toremifene 579
Tornalate 426
Torsemide 479
Toxaphene 115
Toxic screens 48
Toxogonin 130
Toyon 311
Tracrium 414
Tramadol 398
   interactions 508
Trandate 435
Trandolapril 477

Tranquilizers 390
  interactions 203, 415, 481
  *see also* Depressants **390–421**
Tranxene 411
Tranylcypromine 508
Trasuzumab 569
Trasylol 565
Trazodone 518
Trecator 501
Tree fumigant *see* Cyanide 311
Treflan 158
Tremolite-actinolite 331
Tretinoin 569, 579
Trexan 398
Triac *see* Liothyronine 555
Triacetin 347
Triadimefon 157
Triadimenol 158
Triallate 557
Triallyl phosphate 227
Triallylamine 168
Triamcinolone 547, 552
Triamterene 479, 481, 483
Triazolam 412, 421
Triazophos 125
Tribunil 158
Tributyl tin 309
Tributylphosphate 227
S,S,S-Tributylphosphorotrithioate 124
Trichlorfon 125
Trichlormethiazide 479
1,1,2-Trichloro-1,2,2-trifluoroethane 192
Trichloroacetate 198
Trichloroacetonitrile 311
1,2,4-Trichlorobenzene 198
Trichlorobenzoic acid 198
1,1,1-Trichloroethane 181
1,1,2-Trichloroethane 198
Trichloroethylene 179
Trichlorofluoromethane 192
Trichloroisocyanurate 359
Trichloromethyl benzene *see*
  Benzyltrichloride 243
Trichloronaphthalene 189
2,4,5-Trichlorophenoxyacetic acid 117
1,2,3-Trichloropropane 198
Trichlorotrifluoroethane 192
*Tricholoma* sp 625
Triclene *see* Trichloroethylene 179
Triclopyr 110, 158
Tricor 478
Tricresyl phosphate 216
Tricyclazole 158
Tricyclic antidepressants, interactions 440

Tridemorph 158
Tridione 393
Tridymite 329
Trientine 569
Trietazine 158
Triethanolamine 258
Triethyl tin 309
Triethylamine 258
Triethylene glycol *see* Ethylene glycol 209
Triethylenephosphoramide *see*
  Mechlorethamine 575, 578
Triethylenethiophosphoramide 578
Triethylphosphate 227
Triflumizole 110
Triflumuron 110
Trifluoperazine 404
Trifluorobromomethane 192
Trifluoroethylvinyl ether 385
Trifluralin 158
Trifluridine 502
Trifmine 110
Triforine 158
Triggerfish 611
Trihexyphenidyl 422
Trilafon 404
Trilene *see* Trichloroethylene Trilene 179
Trileptal 393
Trimellitic anhydride 226
*Trimeresurus*, bites 590, 591
Trimethacarb 126
Trimethadione 393
Trimethobenzamide 402
Trimethoprim 503, 507
Trimethoprim-sulfamethoxazole 486
Trimethyl phosphate 227
Trimethyl phosphite 227
Trimethylamine 258
Trimethylbenzene 239
Trimethylene trinitramine *see* Tetryl 168
Trimetrexate 503
Trimidal 110
Trimipramine 518, 519
Trinchloroacetic acid 243
Trinitramine *see* Tetryl 168
Trinitrobenzene 170
Trinitrotoluene 170
Triorthocresyl phosphate 216
Triox *see* Arsenic [50%] 270
Trioxsalen 569
Trioxymethylene 217
Tripelennamine 403, 421
Triphenyl tin 309
Triphenylamine 168
Triphenylmethane dyes 361

Triple Sulfa 485
Tripoli 329
Triprolidine 402
Tris(2,3-dibromopropyl)phosphate 227
Tris(hydroxymethyl)-aminomethane 168
Trisodium phosphate *see* Sodium
    phosphates 258
Trisoralen 569
Trobicin 490
Troglitazone 550
Troleandomycin 492
Trolnitrate phosphate 467
Tromethamine 569
Tropex 117
Trovafloxacin 493
Truban 154
Trusopt 478
Tryparsamide 272
*d*-Tubocurarine, interactions 482
Tubocurarine, interactions 416, 440
Tuna 611
Tung nut 637
Tungsten 310
Tupersan 157
*Turnera diffusa* 570
Turpentine 536
Ty *see* Tetryl 168
Tylenol *see* Acetaminophen 373
Type metal *see* Lead 282
Tyramine, interactions 522
Tyropanoate 575
Tyzine 426

Ultane 385
Ultiva 398
Ultracide 125
Ultram 398
Umbelliferone 347
Undecoylium chloride-iodine 445
Undecylenate 458
Univase *see* Moexipril 477
Universal antidote 448
Uracil mustard 579
Uranium salts 310
Urbacid 557
Urecholine 431
Uribest 156
Urine retention 68
Urispas 422
*Urobatis halleri*, sting-ray 614
Urokinase 477
Ursodiol 569
Urushiol 628
Uva ursi 570

Vacor 143
Valacyclovir 503
n-Valeraldehyde 224
Valerian 570
Validacin 158
Validamycin 158
Valium 411
    for convulsions 62
Valproate 421, 525
Valproic acid 393
Valrubicin 579
Valsartan 478
Valstar 579
Valtrex 503
Vamidothion 125
Vanadium 310
Vancocin 490
Vancomycin 490, 507
Vangard 154
Vapam 557
Vapona *see* DDVP 124
Vapotone *see* TEPP 123
Varnish remover 372
Vascor 473
Vasodilan 426
Vasopressors, interactions 416, 482
Vasotec *see* Enalapril 477
Vasoxyl 426
V$_d$, defined 100
Vecuronium 414
Vegetable gums 346
Velban 579
Velpar 155
Velsicol *see* Chlordane 119
Vendex 159
Venlafaxine 518
    interactions 508
Venom
    snake 588
        antisera 596
Venzar 155
Vepesid 577
Verapamil 483, 525
Veratrine *see* Veratrum 630
*Veratrum* sp 630
Vermifuges *see* Worm toxicants 160
Vermox 501
Vernolate 557
Versed 412
Vesanoid 579
Viagra 568
Vibramycin 489
*Vibrio parahaemolyticus* food poisoning 350,
    351

*Vicia faba*, fava bean 619
Vicks Vaporub 515
Vidarabine 503
Vigabatrin 393
Vinblastine 579, 592
Vinclozolin 110
Vincristine 579, 592
Vinorelbine 579
Vinyl acetate 227
Vinyl benzene *see* Styrene 239
Vinyl bromide 198
Vinyl chloride 39, 198
Vinyl cyclohexene 226
Vinyl cyclohexene dioxide 226
Vinyl fluoride 198
Vinylidene chloride *see* 1,1-
    Dichloroethylene 197
Vinylphate 124
Vinyltoluene 239
Vioform 445
Violin spider 603
Vioxx 377
*Vipera* sp 588, 589
    bites 593
Viperid bites 593, 594
Vipers 588, 589
    bites 590, 591, 593
Vira-A 503
Virac 445
Viracept 502
Viramune 502
Virazole 502
Viroptic 502
Visken 434, 435
Vistide 500
Vitamin A 571
Vitamin $B_1$ 571
Vitamin $B_3$ *see* Nicotinamide 92
Vitamin $B_6$ *see* Pyridoxine 96
Vitamin $B_{12}$ 571
    synthetic 86
Vitamin C 571
Vitamin D 571
Vitamin E 571
Vitamin K 571
    interactions 552, 581
Vitamin $K_1$ 571
    *see also* Phytonadione 95
Vitavax 152
Vitravene 501
Vivactil 518
Vleminckx's solution 316
Volatile and gaseous anesthetics 385
Volatile oils 536

Voltaren 377
Volume of distribution, defined 100
Vomiting 69
Vonduron 154
Voronit 154
Vumon 578
Vydate 126

Warfarin 469, 483
    interactions 377, 505
Washing soda *see* Sodium carbonate 257
Wasp 608
Water colors 363
Water and electrolyte imbalance 69
Water hemlock 622, 623
Wave set 346
Welding flux *see* Fluoride 263
Welding fumes 310
    aluminum 338
Wellbutrin 518
Western diamondback rattlesnake 588
Whip 110
White hellebore *see* Veratrum 630
White phosphorus *see* Yellow phosphorus 301
Wild yam 571
Window cleaner 214
Wisteria 637
Wood alcohol 199
Wood bleach *see* Oxalic acid [50%] 240
Wood dust 340
Wood tar 448, 449
Worm toxicants 160
Wormwood 571
Wrasse 611
Wydase 567

Xalatan 553
Xanax 411
Xanthines 510
Xeloda 576
Xenical 568
*p*-Xenylamine *see* 4-Aminodiphenyl 164
XMC 126
Xylene 231
*m*-Xylene-α-α'-diamine 168
Xylidine 168
Xylocaine 382
Xylol *see* Xylene 231
Xylylcarb 126

Yellow jacket 608
Yellow oleander 637
Yellow phosphorus 301
Yew 622

Yocon 555
Yodoxin 445
Yohimbine 555
Yomesan 160
Yttrium salts 310
Yukamate 557
Yutopar 426

Zafirlukast 567
Zagam 493
Zalcitadine 503
Zanaflex 426
Zanamivir 503
Zanosar 578
Zantac 434
Zarontin 393
Zaroxolon 479
Zaroxolyn 480
Zebeta 435
Zectran 126
Zemplar 571
Zemuron 414
Zenapax 566
Zephiran 452
Zerit 502
Zestril *see* Lisinopril 477
Ziagen 500
Zidex 500
Zidovudine 503
Zileuton 569
Zinacef 492

Zinc 310
Zinc acetate 533
Zinc chloride 310
Zinc chromate 280
Zinc fumes 310
Zinc oxide 347, 533
Zinc sulfate 533
Zineb 557
Zinecard 566
Ziram 557
Zirconium oxide and salts 310
Zocor 478
Zofran 434
Zoladex 577
Zoloft 523
Zolone 125
Zolpidem 412, 421
Zonegran 393
Zonisamide 393
Zorial 156
Zotox *see* Zirconium salts 310
Zovirax 500
Zyban 518
Zyflo 569
Zygadenus 630
*Zygadenus venenosus*, death camas 630
Zyloprim 565
Zyprexa 412
Zyrtec 402
Zyvox 493